Discrete Tomography

Foundations, Algorithms, and Applications

Gabor T. Herman
Attila Kuba

Editors

With 155 Figures

Springer Science+Business Media, LLC

Gabor T. Herman
Department of Radiology
University of Pennsylvania
Philadelphia, PA 19104
USA

Attila Kuba
Department of Applied Informatics
József Attila University
Szeged
Hungary, H-6701

Library of Congress Cataloging-in-Publication Data
Discrete tomography : foundations, algorithms, and applications /
  [edited by] Gabor T. Herman, Attila Kuba.
    p.   cm.
  Includes bibliographical references and index.
  ISBN 978-1-4612-7196-3
    1. Geometric tomography.   I. Herman, Gabor T.   II. Kuba, Attila.
  QA639.5.D58   1999
  516.3'62—dc21   99-20171
                                                              CIP

AMS Subject Classifications: 15, 52, 54

Printed on acid-free paper.
© 1999 Springer Science+Business Media New York *Birkhäuser* ®
Originally published by Birkhäuser Boston in 1999
Softcover reprint of the hardcover 1st edition 1999

ISBN 978-1-4612-7196-3   ISBN 978-1-4612-1568-4 (eBook)
DOI 10.1007/978-1-4612-1568-4   SPIN 19901726

Typeset by the editors in LaTeX.

9 8 7 6 5 4 3 2 1

Contents

Preface

Goals of the Book

Over the last thirty years there has been a revolution in diagnostic radiology as a result of the emergence of computerized tomography (CT), which is the process of obtaining the density distribution within the human body from multiple x-ray projections. Since an enormous variety of possible density values may occur in the body, a large number of projections are necessary to ensure the accurate reconstruction of their distribution.

There are other situations in which we desire to reconstruct an object from its projections, but in which we know that the object to be reconstructed has only a small number of possible values. For example, a large fraction of objects scanned in industrial CT (for the purpose of nondestructive testing or reverse engineering) are made of a single material and so the ideal reconstruction should contain only two values: zero for air and the value associated with the material composing the object. Similar assumptions may even be made for some specific medical applications; for example, in angiography of the heart chambers the value is either zero (indicating the absence of dye) or the value associated with the dye in the chamber. Another example arises in the electron microscopy of biological macromolecules, where we may assume that the object to be reconstructed is composed of ice, protein, and RNA. One can also apply electron microscopy to determine the presence or absence of atoms in crystalline structures, which is again a two-valued situation. In many of these applications there are strong technical reasons why only a few projections of the object can be physically collected. This brings us to the central theme of *Discrete Tomography*: How can we make use of the knowledge that the reconstruction should contain only a few values to make up for the lack of availability of the number of projections typically required in CT?

Interestingly, but not surprisingly, mathematicians have been concerned with abstract formulations of this problem before the emergence of the practical applications. For example, although a general function of two variables is not uniquely determined by any finite number of projections even if we know that it is zero-valued outside some bounded convex domain and positive-valued inside it, the situation changes drastically if we also know that the only possible nonzero value of the function is one. (In fact, four projections are then sufficient.) Other much investigated problems are related to combinatorics: for example, under what circumstances can a 0-1 valued matrix be recovered from its row and column sums?

Both X-rays and the mathematical theory of reconstruction from projections was available by 1920, but it took another fifty years before the availability of high-speed computers made CT a medically useful tool. Similarly, for discrete tomography to achieve its potential applicability, it is essential that there should be algorithms that allow us to reconstruct objects with sufficient accuracy and within acceptable times.

This book deals with the three topics described above: the applications, the mathematical foundations, and the algorithms of discrete tomography. The authors of the chapters work in university departments of mathematics and statistics, in the various fields of computing, engineering, and medicine, in biomedical research institutes, and in industrial research laboratories. Accordingly, the potential readership is also very wide: it includes mathematicians, programers, and engineers working in imaging fields and experts in specific areas where discrete tomography can be applied. Anyone wishing to be brought up-to-date in some aspects of the foundations of, algorithms for, and applications of discrete tomography will be able to find in this book useful and timely material written by a leading expert in the field. The results in the book are the latest known at the time of editing; many of them are published here for the first time. Although each chapter is self-contained, much effort has gone into unifying the material so that it can be read as a book rather than as a collection of unrelated chapters. If read from beginning to end, the book provides a journey through the mathematical problems and solutions of discrete tomography (Chapters 1-7), followed by a presentation of many algorithmic techniques that can be used to achieve actual reconstructions from projections (Chapters 8-14), and ending with the description and illustration of a number of application areas (Chapters 15-21). In particular, the first chapter provides a historical overview of the field and, at the same time, points toward some of the noteworthy results in the remaining chapters.

Acknowledgments

First, we wish to thank the National Science Foundation and the Hungarian Academy of Sciences who jointly sponsored the 1988 "US–Hungary Mathematics Workshop on Discrete Tomography." This workshop gave us (and to many of our contributors) the impetus to put together this book.

Second, we wish to thank the International Journal of Imaging Systems and Technology, its publisher (John Wiley and Sons, Inc.), and its editors (Z. H. Cho and L. A. Shepp) for publishing a Special Issue on Discrete Tomography based on some of the presentations given at the workshop.

Finally, we are grateful to a number of people for technical help with putting together this book as a single computer file based on the computer files of the individual chapters; among them we wish to mention Dr. C. L. Tondo, Kálmán Palágyi, László Nyúl, Antal Nagy, Marianna Sebő, Catalina Emese Balogh, and Tibor Csendes.

Gabor T. Herman
Philadelphia, Pennsylvania

Attila Kuba
Szeged, Hungary

December 1998

Contributors

Charles A. Bouman
Purdue University
Department of Electrical and Computer Engineering
West Lafayette, IN 47907-1285, USA
E-mail: bouman@ecn.purdue.edu

Jolyon A. Browne
Advanced Research and Applications Corporation (ARACOR)
425 Lakeside Drive, Sunnyvale, CA 94086, USA
E-mail: browne@aracor.com

José María Carazo
Campus Universidad Autónoma de Madrid
Centro Nacional de Biotecnología
28049 Madrid, Spain
E-mail: carazo@cnb.uam.es

Yair Censor
University of Haifa
Department of Mathematics
Mt. Carmel, Haifa 31905, Israel
E-mail: yair@mathcs2.haifa.ac.il

Michael T. Chan
Rockwell Science Center
1049 Camino Dos Rios, Thousand Oaks, CA 91360, USA
E-mail: mtchan@risc.rockwell.com

Shi-Kuo Chang
University of Pittsburgh
Department of Computer Science
Pittsburgh, PA 15260, USA
E-mail: chang@cs.pitt.edu

Alberto Del Lungo
Universitá di Firenze
Dipartimento di Sistemi e Informatica (DSI)
Via Lombroso 6/17, 50134, Firenze, Italy
E-mail: dellungo@dsi.unifi.it

Raul Figueroa
University of Puerto Rico
Department of Mathematics and Computer Sciences
P.O. Box 23355, Rio Piedras Campus, Puerto Rico 00931
E-mail: rfiguero@goliath.cnnet.clu.edu

Peter C. Fishburn
AT&T Labs-Research
180 Park Avenue, Florham Park, NJ 07932, USA
E-mail: fish@research.att.com

Thomas Frese
Purdue University
Department of Electrical and Computer Engineering
West Lafayette, IN 47907-1285, USA
E-mail: frese@ecn.purdue.edu

Richard J. Gardner
Western Washington University
Department of Mathematics
Bellingham, WA 98225-9063, USA
E-mail: gardner@baker.math.wwu.edu

Peter Gritzmann
Technische Universität München
Zentrum Mathematik
D-80290 München, Germany
E-mail: gritzman@mathematik.tu-muenchen.de

Gabor T. Herman
University of Pennsylvania
Department of Radiology
423 Guardian Drive, Philadelphia, PA 19104-6021, USA
E-mail: gabor@mipg.upenn.edu

Lei Huang
NEC Corp.
C&C Media Research Labs
4-1-1 Miyazaki, Miyamae-ku, Kawasaki, Kanagawa 216-8555, Japan
E-mail: huang@ccm.cl.nec.co.jp

Akira Kaneko
Ochanomizu University
Department of Information Sciences
2-1-1 Otsuka, Bunkyo-ku, Tokyo 112-8610 Japan
E-mail: kanenko@is.ocha.ac.jp

T. Yung Kong
Queens College, CUNY
Department of Computer Science
65-30 Kissena Boulevard, Flushing, NY 11367, USA
E-mail: ykong@turing.cs.qc.edu

Mathew Koshy
Advanced Research and Applications Corporation (ARACOR)
425 Lakeside Drive, Sunnyvale, CA 94086, USA
Email: koshy@aracor.com

Attila Kuba
József Attila University
Department of Applied Informatics
Árpád tér 2., H-6720 Szeged, Hungary
E-mail: kuba@inf.u-szeged.hu

Emanuel Levitan
Technion
Faculty of Medicine
Haifa 31096, Israel
E-mail: rpremnl@technion.ac.il

Roberto Marabini
University of Pennsylvania
Department of Radiology
423 Guardian Drive, Philadelphia, PA 19104-6021, USA
E-mail: roberto@mipg.upenn.edu

Samuel Matej
University of Pennsylvania
Department of Radiology
423 Guardian Drive, Philadelphia, PA 19104-6021, USA
E-mail: matej@mipg.upenn.edu

Ali Mohammad-Djafari
Supelec
Laboratoire des Signaux et Systemes (CNRS-ESE-UPS)
Plateau de Moulon, 91190 Gif-sur-Yvette, France
E-mail: djafari@lss.supelec.fr

Maurice Nivat
Université Denis Diderot
Laboratoire d'Informatique, Algorithmique, Fondements, et Applications
2, place Jussieu 75251 Paris Cedex 05, France
E-mail: Maurice.Nivat@liafa.jussieu.fr

Dietrich G. W. Onnasch
University of Kiel
Department for Pediatric Cardiology and Biomedical Engineering
Schwanenweg 20, D-24105 Kiel, Germany
E-mail: onnasch@pedcard.uni-kiel.de

Sarah K. Patch
General Electric Company Corporate Research and Development
Industrial Electronics Laboratory
KW B405, PO Box 8, Schenectady, NY 12301-0008, USA
E-mail: patch@crd.ge.com

Guido P. M. Prause
University of Bremen
MeVis – Center for Medical Diagnostic Systems and Visualization
Universitatsallee 29, D-28359 Bremen, Germany
E-mail: prause@mevis.de

Eike Rietzel
MPI für med. Forschung
Jahnstr. 29, 69120 Heidelberg, Germany
E-mail: erietzel@mpimf-heidelberg.mpg.de

James Sachs, Jr.
Ford Motor Corporation
Product Development Center, PDC MD-331
20901 Oakwook Blvd, P.O. Box 2053, Dearborn, MI 48121-2053, USA
E-mail: jsachs@ford.com

Pablo M. Salzberg
University of Puerto Rico
Department of Mathematics and Computer Sciences
P.O. Box 23355, Rio Piedras Campus, Puerto Rico 00931
E-mail: psalzber@goliath.cnnet.clu.edu

Ken Sauer
University of Notre Dame
Department of Electrical Engineering
275 Fitzpatrick Hall, Notre Dame, IN 46556-5637, USA
E-mail: sauer@nd.edu

Rasmus Schröder
MPI für med. Forschung
Jahnstr. 29, 69120 Heidelberg, Germany
E-mail: rasmus.schroeder@mpimf-heidelberg.mpg.de

Lawrence A. Shepp
Rutgers University
Department of Statistics
Busch Campus, Piscataway, NJ 08855, USA
E-mail: shepp@stat.rutgers.edu

Carlos O. Sorzano
Campus Universidad Autónoma de Madrid
Centro Nacional de Biotecnología
28049 Madrid, Spain
E-mail: coss@cnb.uam.es

Charles Soussen
Supelec
Laboratoire des Signaux et Systemes (CNRS-ESE-UPS)
Plateau de Moulon, 91190 Gif-sur-Yvette, France
E-mail: soussen@lss.supelec.fr

Avi Vardi
SAS Institute
R4218, Cary, NC 27513, USA
E-mail: avvard@wnt.sas.com

Eilat Vardi
Technion - Technical Institute of Israel
P.O. Box 41, Haifa 32000, Israel
E-mail: seilat@techst02.technion.ac.il

Yehuda Vardi
Rutgers University
Department of Statistics
Piscataway, NJ 08854-8019, USA
E-mail: vardi@stat.rutgers.edu

Andrew E. Yagle
The University of Michigan
Dept. of Electrical Engineering and Computer Science
Ann Arbor, MI 48109-2122, USA
E-mail: aey@eecs.umich.edu

Cun-Hui Zhang
Rutgers University
Department of Statistics
Piscataway, NJ 08854-8019, USA
E-mail: czhang@stat.rutgers.edu

Part I

Foundations

Chapter 1

Discrete Tomography: A Historical Overview

Attila Kuba[1]
Gabor T. Herman[2]

ABSTRACT In this chapter we introduce the topic of discrete tomography and give a brief historical survey of the relevant contributions. After discussing the nature of the basic theoretical problems (those of consistency, uniqueness, and reconstruction) that arise in discrete tomography, we give the details of the classical special case (namely, two-dimensional discrete sets — i.e., binary matrices — and two orthogonal projections) including a polynomial time reconstruction algorithm. We conclude the chapter with a summary of some of the applications of discrete tomography.

1.1 Introduction

We assume that there is a domain, which may itself be discrete (such as a set of ordered pairs of integers) or continuous (such as Euclidean space). We further assume that there is an unknown function f whose range is known to be a given discrete set (usually of real numbers). The problems of *discrete tomography*, as we perceive the field, have to do with determining f (perhaps only partially, perhaps only approximately) from weighted sums over subsets of its domain in the discrete case and from weighted integrals over subspaces of its domain in the continuous case. In many applications these sums or integrals may be known only approximately. From this point of view, the most essential aspect of discrete tomography is that knowing the discrete range of f may allow us to determine its value at points where without this knowledge it could not be determined. Discrete tomography is full of mathematically fascinating questions and it has many interesting applications. The name *discrete tomography* is due to Larry Shepp, who organized the first meeting devoted to the topic (in 1994).

[1] József Attila University, Department of Applied Informatics, Árpád tér 2., H-6720 Szeged, Hungary, E-mail: kuba@inf.u-szeged.hu

[2] University of Pennsylvania, Department of Radiology, Medical Image Processing Group, Blockley Hall, Fourth Floor, 423 Guardian Drive, Philadelphia, PA 19104-6021, USA, E-mail: gabor@mipg.upenn.edu

The reconstruction algorithms used in CT (computerized tomography, see, e.g., [1]) are derived from the not discrete (let us say, general) tomography model in which the range of f is the real numbers. Such reconstruction algorithms are unlikely to be appropriate for discrete tomography. For example, when using such an algorithm we cannot expect to produce a two-valued function, not even in the case when the data are taken from a two-valued f.

Since discrete functions can be considered to be special cases of general functions, discrete tomography (DT) can be thought of as a special kind of CT: it seems natural to apply the results of CT to discrete functions. However, it turns out that DT needs its own theory to answer questions concerning consistency, existence and uniqueness. Another reason for investigating special discrete reconstruction methods is that, since f is discrete, there is hope that it can be determined from less data than what are necessary for general functions. Accordingly, in DT the typical number of projections (a projection is a collection of line sums or line integrals for a set of lines which are either all parallel to each other or diverge from a single point) is two to four, which is much less than what is typically used in CT (a few hundred). General CT reconstruction methods cannot be used effectively if the number of projections is so small.

DT has its own mathematical theory based mostly on discrete mathematics. It has strong connections with combinatorics and geometry. In the rest of this section we give a brief discussion of the connections of DT to other fields of mathematics. The only intent of this discussion is to set DT into its mathematical historical context; for this reason we will use terms here without carefully defining them. The sections that follow are oriented more toward the specific material in this book; in those sections we will be careful to define all terms that form part of the discussion. (Some of these terms will already appear in the current section, but even in such cases we postpone the definitions until the following sections.)

DT has connections to the *analysis of functions*. Lorentz gave in 1949 [2] a necessary and sufficient condition for a function-pair to be the projections of a planar measurable set. This condition can be considered as the first consistency result of DT. He also found a condition on two orthogonal projections of a measurable set by which one can determine if there is no other measurable set with the same projections. He also showed that for any integer n there are always two different bounded sets which have the same n projections. For related results see the works of Rényi [3], Heppes [4] and Kellerer [5–7].

Many problems of DT were first discussed as *combinatorial problems* during the late 1950s and early 1960s. In 1957 Ryser [8] published a necessary and sufficient consistency condition for a pair of integral vectors being the row and column sum vectors of a (0,1)-matrix. (It is interesting that this consistency theorem is the same as Lorentz's result [2] specialized to the case of (0,1)-matrices. The connection between the general and discrete cases is discussed in Chapter 5 by Kaneko and Huang in this book.) By giving a constructive proof of his theorem, Ryser provided the first reconstruction algorithm. He also recognized that the so-called *interchange* is the elementary operation by which any two (0,1)-matrices can be transformed into each other if they have the same row and column sums. In the same year Gale [9] proved the same consistency condition as Ryser, but applying it to flows in networks. In 1960 Ryser introduced the concept of the *structure matrix* [10], which is useful, for example, in leading to a new consistency condition [11, p. 82].

The discussion of the *geometric connections* of DT was started by Hammer (although it was foreshadowed by Jakob Steiner [12] in the 19th century), who in 1961 at the AMS Symposium on Convexity [13] raised the problem: when is a planar convex body uniquely determined from its projections? For projections along parallel lines, an answer is due to Giering [14], who proved that for any planar convex body there exist three projections which uniquely determine it. Gardner and McMullen [15] proved that it is possible to find four projections that will uniquely determine all planar convex bodies. (As a summary of the geometric results connected with tomography we can suggest the excellent book written by Gardner [16].) Although these results of convex geometry or, more exactly, geometric tomography, are about the reconstruction of convex bodies, there are corresponding results for discrete sets. For example, Lorentz [2] gave a method to construct, for any finite number of directions, distinct discrete sets having the same projections along these directions. That is, a finite number of projections are not generally sufficient to reconstruct discrete sets. However, if the number of points in the discrete set to be reconstructed is known, it is possible to find finitely many projections that will guarantee uniqueness [3, 17]. A discrete analogue of Gardner and McMullen's theorem was obtained by Gardner and Gritzmann [18], who showed that convex lattice sets in $\mathbb{Z}^2$ ($\mathbb{Z}^d$ denotes the set of d-dimensional vectors of integers) are determined by certain prescribed sets of four lattice directions.

The interest in DT is well illustrated by the fact that since September 19, 1994, when the first meeting of the topic was held at DIMACS, Rutgers University, a five-day seminar [19] was held in Dagstuhl, Germany in January 1997, a Discrete Tomography Workshop was held in Szeged, Hungary, in August 1997 (some of its lectures were published in a Special Issue of the International Journal of Imaging Systems and Technology [20]), and a workshop of Discrete Tomography and Related Problems has been scheduled for 1999 in Chateau de Volkrange, France.

In the rest of this introductory chapter we roughly follow the structure of the book. In the first section we discuss the theoretical results of discrete tomography related to three basic problems: consistency, uniqueness and reconstruction. After discussing general theoretical results, the special case of reconstructing two-dimensional discrete sets (i.e., binary matrices) from two projections is presented. The problems of consistency, uniqueness and reconstruction are discussed again because the results are much more powerful than in the general case of more than two projections. The applications of DT is the topic of the last section.

Discrete tomography is a relative young and actively studied field. It is therefore inevitable that its terminology has not as yet settled down. This is reflected in our book: the same concepts are given different names by the authors of the various chapters and each chapter introduces its own specific notation. The editors decided that they should not interfere with this aspect of the chapters, not only because they were too lazy to do so, but also because this way the readers are introduced to the full range of terminology and notation in the DT literature. This introductory chapter will have its own definitional and notational quirks, but some (by no means exhaustive) hints will be given to alternatives used below in the book.

1.2   Foundations and algorithms

1.2.1   Definitions, notations, and basic problems

In this subsection we are working in d-dimensional Euclidean space. In such a space a *lattice* is defined as the set of all linear combinations with integer coefficients of a fixed set of d linearly independent vectors. Since any such lattice is isomorphic to the integer lattice $\mathbb{Z}^d$ under a nonsingular linear transformation, in DT it is enough to study the case of the integer lattice $\mathbb{Z}^d$. We will be doing this for the rest of this chapter without further comment.

The finite subsets of $\mathbb{Z}^d$ will be called *lattice sets* or *discrete sets*. The so-called *lattice directions* are represented by any nonzero vectors of $\mathbb{Z}^d$. We are going to use a set of distinct lattice directions, $D = (v^{(1)}, \ldots, v^{(q)})$, $q \geq 2$ (here distinct means that there are no two vectors in D which are parallel to each other). We say that a line ℓ in d-dimensional Euclidean space is a *lattice line* if it is parallel to a vector $v^{(k)} \in D$ and passes through at least one point in $\mathbb{Z}^d$. Let $\mathcal{L}^{(k)}$ denote the set of all lattice lines that are parallel to $v^{(k)} \in D$.

Definition 1.1.   *Let $F \subset \mathbb{Z}^d$ be a lattice set. Its projection in direction $v^{(k)}$ is defined as the function $\mathcal{P}_F^{(k)} : \mathcal{L}^{(k)} \to \mathbb{N}_0$ (the set of nonnegative integers) by*

$$\mathcal{P}_F^{(k)}(\ell) = |F \cap \ell| = \sum_{x \in \ell} f(x) \qquad (1.1)$$

where f denotes the characteristic function of the discrete set F.

Unfortunately, there is no uniform terminology. There are authors using the names X-ray, marginal or line sum for this concept. For example, the notion of lattice directions is closely related to the notion of fundamental direction vectors in Chapter 3 by Kong and Herman in this book, but there is a subtle, but important, difference in the definition of a lattice line above and of a grid line in that chapter.

Let $D = (v^{(1)}, \ldots, v^{(q)})$ be a set of distinct lattice directions. We say that two discrete sets F and F' are *tomographically equivalent* with respect to the directions D if $\mathcal{P}_F^{(k)} = \mathcal{P}_{F'}^{(k)}$ for $k = 1, \ldots, q$. Let $\mathcal{E}$ be a class of finite sets in $\mathbb{Z}^d$. In our terminology the discrete set $F \in \mathcal{E}$ is *determined* by the projections parallel to D in the class $\mathcal{E}$ if there is no tomographically equivalent other set with respect to the directions D in the class $\mathcal{E}$.

Let $\mathcal{E}$ be a class of finite sets in $\mathbb{Z}^d$ and D be a set of directions in $\mathbb{Z}^d$. Let, furthermore, $\mathcal{L} = (\mathcal{L}^{(1)}, \ldots, \mathcal{L}^{(q)})$ $(q \geq 2)$ be the collection of the sets of lattice lines determined by D. We now introduce the problems of consistency, uniqueness and reconstruction for $\mathcal{E}$ and $\mathcal{L}$.

CONSISTENCY$(\mathcal{E}, \mathcal{L})$.

Given: For $k = 1, \ldots, q$, a function $p^{(k)} : \mathcal{L}^{(k)} \to \mathbb{N}_0$ with finite support.

Question: Does there exist an $F \in \mathcal{E}$ such that $\mathcal{P}_F^{(k)} = p^{(k)}$ for $k = 1, \ldots, q$?

For a discussion of this problem see Chapter 4 by Gardner and Gritzmann in this book. A basic result there is that CONSISTENCY$(\mathcal{E}, \mathcal{L})$ is NP-complete for $q \geq 3$. In the case of $q = 2$, which is discussed in detail in Subsection 1.2.2, the problem of CONSISTENCY$(\mathcal{E}, \mathcal{L})$ can be solved in polynomial time.

UNIQUENESS$(\mathcal{E}, \mathcal{L})$.

Given: An $F \in \mathcal{E}$.

Question: Does there exist a different $F' \in \mathcal{E}$ such that F and F' are tomographically equivalent with respect to the directions of D?

Three chapters of this book discuss UNIQUENESS$(\mathcal{E}, \mathcal{L})$. As an introduction to the problem of uniqueness and its connection with computational complexity see Chapter 4 by Gardner and Gritzmann. Special aspects of uniqueness are discussed in Chapter 2 by Fishburn and Shepp. They show that the additivity of the lattice sets, which is necessary and sufficient for the uniqueness in the case of $q = 2$, is sufficient but not necessary if $q \geq 3$ (independently from the dimension of the lattice). Kong and Herman prove in Chapter 3 that in the case of $q \geq 3$ the uniqueness of a discrete set cannot be decided simply by finding certain patterns of 0's and 1's in the discrete space. As it is known from Ryser [8], the situation is just the opposite if $q = 2$, because then the existence of a certain type of 2×2 submatrix is equivalent to nonuniqueness. It is interesting that all of these chapters express clearly that the uniqueness of discrete sets from two projections is basically different from the case when there are more than two projections.

RECONSTRUCTION($\mathcal{E}, \mathcal{L}$).

Given: For $k = 1, \ldots, q$, a function $p^{(k)} : \mathcal{L}^{(k)} \to \mathbb{N}_0$ with finite support.

Task: Construct a finite set $F \in \mathcal{E}$ such that $\mathcal{P}_F^{(k)} = p^{(k)}$ for $k = 1, \ldots, q$.

Suppose that there are given functions $p^{(k)} : \mathcal{L}^{(k)} \to \mathbb{N}_0$ having finite supports with cardinalities m_k for $k = 1, \ldots, q$. Let $M = m_1 + \cdots + m_q$. It is clear that if F is a finite set having projections $p^{(1)}, \ldots, p^{(q)}$ in the directions $v^{(1)}, \ldots, v^{(q)}$, respectively, then $F \subseteq G$, where G consists of lattice points $z \in \mathbb{Z}^d$ for which $p^{(k)}(\ell) > 0$, where ℓ is the lattice line passing through z in direction $v^{(k)}$, for each $k = 1, \ldots, q$. Because the function $p^{(k)}$ has finite support, $k = 1, \ldots, q$, G is also finite, $|G| = N$ (say). Then the discrete reconstruction problem can be reformulated as the following linear feasibility problem:

$$\text{find} \quad P x = b, \quad \text{such that} \quad x \in \{0, 1\}^N, \qquad (1.2)$$

where $P \in \{0, 1\}^{M \times N}$, $b \in \mathbb{N}_0^M$. The matrix P describes the geometric relation between the points of G and the lattice line ℓ; that is, it specifies which points of G are on a line ℓ. Each equation in (1.2) corresponds to a line sum on a lattice line. The vector x represents the set G. The nonnegative integral vector b contains the values of the functions $p^{(k)}$, $k = 1, \ldots, q$ (see Fig. 1.1).

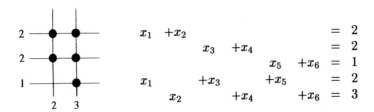

FIGURE 1.1. A lattice set of $\mathbb{Z}^2$, its projections in the directions $(1, 0)$ and $(0, 1)$, and the corresponding linear equation system.

In order to find a solution of the equation system in (1.2) (without the binary constrain $x \in \{0, 1\}^N$) some of the iterative CT reconstruction algorithms (such as ART [21] or its versions [22]) can be used. Of course, they would give a not necessarily binary solution. However, they can be modified in order to get a binary solution. Such a binary ART, called BART, was suggested by Herman [23]. Recently this idea has been developed to a binary steering schema (see Chapter 12 by Censor and Matej in this book) by which an iterative general CT reconstruction algorithm can be steered toward a binary solution. Yagle shows in Chapter 11 of this book how the equation system and also the integrality constraint of (1.2) can be included into a quadratic equation system and solved by algebraic methods.

Alternatively, one can transform (1.2) into the linear programming problem

$$\text{maximize} \quad |\sum_{j=1}^{N} x_j|, \quad \text{subject to} \quad Px = b \quad \text{and} \quad x \in \{0,1\}^N, \quad (1.3)$$

or, by relaxing the integrality constraint in (1.2) to the interval constraint $0 \le x_j \le 1$, for $j = 1, \ldots, N$, into

$$\text{maximize} \quad |\sum_{j=1}^{N} x_j|, \quad \text{subject to} \quad Px = b, \quad \text{and} \quad x \in [0,1]^N. \quad (1.4)$$

These linear programming problems can be solved by the simplex method or by using interior point methods [24].

Another reconstruction method can be deduced by the following approach [25]. After normalizing the equations in (1.2) the EM algorithm can be applied to minimize the nonlinear Kullback-Leibler information divergence criterion. For details, see Chapter 13 by Vardi and Zhang in this book.

If the number of projections is small, the system of linear equations in (1.2) is very undetermined and the number of solutions can be very large. In this case we can try to find only the solution(s) having some a priori property. This property can be given, for example, as a statistical property such as that the image to be reconstructed should have a high probability in a certain distribution. In Chapter 8 by Matej *et al.* in this book, a Metropolis algorithm is described for reconstructing discrete sets on a hexagonal grid from their three projections, when the probability of the occurrence of a discrete set follows some Gibbs distribution. The most probable solution is approached by iterative steps.

In DT we can reconstruct discrete sets of points where the points can have different weights; that is, the function to be reconstructed can have values other than 0 or 1. As it is shown in Chapter 6 by Kuba in this book, if the number of the possible values of these weights is two, then the binary reconstruction methods can be applied even if these two values are not known in advance (see also [26] about two-valued matrices). In the general case of multi-valued discrete images statistical methods, such as Bayesian maximum a posteriory (MAP) estimation, can be applied (see Chapter 10 by Frese, Bouman and Sauer in this book).

Another way of reconstructing discrete images is to use some CT method in the first step and then to postprocess the images using some assumed property. Such a method is described in Chapter 9 by Chan, Herman and Levitan in this book.

It is also possible to reconstruct parametrized objects such as polygons from a few (and noisy) projections. In this case the reconstruction can be considered as a parameter estimation problem, where the discrete set of the vertices of the polygon need to be recovered. The nonlinear problem can be solved by some optimization technique (e.g., maximum likelihood). Such a reconstruction method was suggested by Rossi and Willsky [27]. For the reconstruction of polyhedral shapes another method is presented in Chapter 14 by Muhammad-Djafari and Soussen in this book.

If the projections of the discrete object are defined not only on straight lines but on any path between the source and the detector, then we have the more complicated model of *diffuse tomography* [28]. A recursive algorithm for diffuse planar tomography is described in Chapter 20 by Patch in this book.

1.2.2 Reconstruction of binary matrices from two projections

In this subsection we consider the classical special case of $m \times n$ binary matrices and two projections corresponding to row and column sums. We start with a discussion of the problem of consistency.

Definition 1.2.   Let $R = (r_1, \ldots, r_m)$ and $S = (s_1, \ldots, s_n)$ be nonnegative integral vectors. The class of all binary matrices $A = (a_{ij})$ satisfying the equations

$$\sum_{j=1}^{n} a_{ij} = r_i, \quad i = 1, \ldots, m, \tag{1.5}$$

$$\sum_{i=1}^{m} a_{ij} = s_j, \quad j = 1, \ldots, n, \tag{1.6}$$

is denoted by $\mathfrak{A}(R, S)$. The vectors R and S are called the row and column sum vectors of any matrix $A \in \mathfrak{A}(R, S)$.

Definition 1.3.   A pair (R, S) of vectors is said to be compatible if there exist positive integers m and n such that

(i) $R \in \mathbb{N}_0^m$ and $S \in \mathbb{N}_0^n$;

(ii) $r_i \leq n$, for $1 \leq i \leq m$, and $s_j \leq m$, for $1 \leq j \leq n$;

(iii) $\sum_{i=1}^{m} r_i = \sum_{j=1}^{n} s_j$.

Clearly, if $\mathfrak{A}(R, S)$ is not empty, then (R, S) is compatible. In 1957 Ryser and Gale (independently of each other) gave a necessary and sufficient condition under which the class $\mathfrak{A}(R, S)$ is nonempty [8, 9].

Consider the matrix $\bar{A}$ in which, for $i = 1, \ldots, m$, row i consists of r_i 1's followed by $n - r_i$ 0's. A matrix having this property will be called *maximal*. A maximal matrix $\bar{A}$ is uniquely determined by its row sum vector. Let its column sum vector be denoted by $\bar{S}$. Furthermore, let us denote the nonincreasing permutations of the elements of R and S by R' and S', respectively, that is, $r'_1 \geq r'_2 \geq \cdots \geq r'_m$ and $s'_1 \geq s'_2 \geq \cdots \geq s'_n$.

Theorem 1.1. *Let $R = (r_1, \ldots, r_m)$ and $S = (s_1, \ldots, s_n)$ be a pair of compatible vectors. The class $\mathfrak{A}(R, S)$ is nonempty if and only if*

$$\sum_{j=l}^{n} s'_j \geq \sum_{j=l}^{n} \bar{s}_j, \quad \text{for} \quad 2 \leq l \leq n. \tag{1.7}$$

Proof: Suppose that $\mathfrak{A}(R, S)$ contains a binary matrix A. Then the class $\mathfrak{A}(R, S')$ contains a binary matrix A' constructed from A by a suitable permutations of the columns. $\bar{A}$ can be obtained from A' (if they are different at all) by shifting 1's to the left in the rows of A'. Therefore we have (1.7).

Now let us suppose that (1.7) is true for the vectors R and S. We are going to construct a binary matrix A by the following algorithm, whose output is illustrated in Fig. 1.2.

Algorithm 1.1.

Input: a compatible pair of vectors (R, S) satisfying (1.7);

Step 1. construct S' from S by permutation π;

Step 2. let $B = \bar{A}$ and $k = n$;

Step 3. while $(k > 1)$,
$$\{$$
while $(s'_k > \sum_{i=1}^{m} b_{ik})$,

$$\{$$
let $j_0 = \max_{1 \leq i \leq m} \{j < k \mid b_{ij} = 1, \ b_{i,j+1} = \cdots = b_{ik} = 0\}$;

let row i_0 be where such a j_0 was found;

set $b_{i_0 j_0} = 0$ and $b_{i_0 k} = 1$ (i.e., shift the 1 to the right)
$$\};$$

reduce k by 1
$$\};$$

Step 4. construct the matrix A from B by permutation π^{-1} of the columns;

Output: matrix A.

In order to prove that Algorithm 1.1 produces a matrix A with row sum vector R and column sum vector S, we first prove the following property of Step 3. Suppose that at the beginning of the execution of the code within the outer brackets of Step 3 the matrix B can be written as $(C|D)$, where C is a maximal $m \times k$ matrix and D is an $m \times (n-k)$ matrix (D is an empty matrix when $k = n$), such that

(i) the row sum vector of B is R,

(ii) denoting the column sum vector of B by $T = (t_1, \ldots, t_n)$ we have that

   (a) $s'_j = t_j$, for $k+1 \le j \le n$,

   (b) $\sum_{j=l}^{n} s'_j \ge \sum_{j=l}^{n} t_j$, for $2 \le l \le n$,

   (c) $\sum_{j=1}^{k} s'_j = \sum_{j=1}^{k} t_j$.

Under these circumstances, at the end of the execution of the code within the outer brackets of Step 3 the matrix B will have the same property with k replaced by $k - 1$.

We note that (i) above will certainly be satisfied, since the only type of change that is made to B during Step 3 is the shifting of a 1 to the right (in other words, the interchanging in a row a 1 and a 0).

At the beginning of the execution of the code we have that (observe (a) and (b) above and the fact that $2 \le k \le n$)

$$
\begin{aligned}
s'_k &= \sum_{j=k}^{n} s'_j - \sum_{j=k+1}^{n} s'_j \\
&\ge \sum_{j=k}^{n} t_j - \sum_{j=k+1}^{n} t_j = t_k (= \sum_{i=1}^{m} b_{ik}).
\end{aligned}
\tag{1.8}
$$

If $s'_k = t_k$, we just move the last column of C to become the first column of D and it is clear that (ii) will be satisfied with k replaced by $k - 1$.

Now suppose that $s'_k = t_k + d$, for some $d > 0$. We observe that there has to be at least d values of i ($1 \le i \le m$), such that $b_{ik} = 0$ and $b_{ij} = 1$ for some j, $1 \le j < k$. This is because, by the maximality of C, the definition of S' and (c) above we get

$$
k t_1 \ge \sum_{j=1}^{k} t_j = \sum_{j=1}^{k} s'_j \ge k s'_k = k(t_k + d)
\tag{1.9}
$$

and so $t_1 \geq t_k + d$. This implies that the instructions within the inner while loop can indeed be executed d times; each execution will set to 1 a single $b_{i_0 k}$, which is zero at the beginning of the execution of the while loop. Maximality of the matrix consisting of the first $k-1$ columns of B is retained by the choice of the j_0 and i_0 in Step 3 of the algorithm. When the inner while loop is completed we clearly satisfy $s'_j = t_j$, for $k \leq j \leq n$ (i.e., (ii)(a) with $k-1$ in place of k).

Let j_1 be the maximal value of $j < k$ such that $t_j \geq t_k + d$ at the beginning of the execution of the code. From the way that the j_0 are selected in Step 3, it follows that there are d values of i such that at the beginning of the execution of the code $b_{ik} = 0$ and $b_{ij} = 1$ and at the end of the execution of the code $b_{ik} = 1$ and $b_{ij} = 0$ for some j, $j_1 \leq j < k$, and these are the only $2d$ locations in the matrix that change value. Hence, for $2 \leq l \leq j_1$, the value of $\sum_{j=l}^{n} t_j$ does not change as a result of the execution of the code and the validity of (ii)(b) is preserved. On the other hand, at the end of the execution of the code, $s'_j \geq t_j$, for $j_1 < j \leq n$. For $k \leq j \leq n$, this follows from the already shown fact that (ii)(a) holds at the end of the execution of the code with $k-1$ in place of k. For $j_1 < j < k$, it follows from the definitions of S' and j_1 that at the beginning of the execution of the code $s'_j \geq s'_k = t_k + d > t_j$ and the value of t_j is not increased during the execution of the code. Hence (ii)(b) holds at the end of the execution of the code also for the alternate range $j_1 < l \leq n$.

Trivially, for (ii)(c), the left-hand side is reduced by s'_k (since k is to be replaced by $k-1$) and the right-hand side is reduced by the original t_k (for the same reason) but also by d (corresponding to the d 1's that have been shifted from a column $j < k$ into the kth column during the execution of the code). The preservation of (ii)(c) follows, since $s'_k = t_k + d$ at the beginning of the execution of the code.

Given this behavior of Step 3 it is now easy to complete the proof. First we note that the conditions assumed upon entering the code within the outer brackets of Step 3 are satisfied for the initial entry when $k = n$ with $C = B = \bar{A}$ and D the empty matrix. In this case (ii)(b) is just (1.7) and (ii)(c) follows from the compatibility of R and S. Repeated applications of the code will bring us to the end of execution for the case $k = 2$, at which time will have $s'_j = t_j$ for $1 \leq j \leq n$ (by (ii)(a) and (ii)(c) with $k = 1$), proving that at this time B has row sum vector R (by (i)) and column sum vector S' and, hence, A has row sum vector R and column sum vector S. $\qquad\square$

$$
\begin{array}{cccccc}
2 & 1 & 0 & 1 & 0 & 0 \\
3 & 1 & 1 & 0 & 0 & 1 \\
3 & 1 & 1 & 0 & 1 & 0 \\
1 & 1 & 0 & 0 & 0 & 0 \\
  &   &   &   &   &   \\
  & 4 & 2 & 1 & 1 & 1 \\
\end{array}
$$

FIGURE 1.2. The binary matrix reconstructed from row and column sums $R = (2, 3, 3, 1)$ and $S = (4, 2, 1, 1, 1)$ by Algorithm 1.1.

Remark 1.1.

Note that while the statement of Theorem 1.1 is such that its provides an answer to the consistency problem (for binary matrices from two special projections), the proof of the theorem contains Algorithm 1.1, which provides an answer to the reconstruction problem.

1. The computational complexity of Algorithm 1.1 is $O(nm + n \log n) = O(n \cdot (m + \log n))$. Step 3 can be implemented efficiently if the column indices of the last 1's of each row of C are stored and made use of during the execution.

2. There are several versions of Algorithm 1.1 (see, for example, [8,9,29]) depending on which row i_0 is selected (when there are two or more rows available). Further alternatives can be found in [30–33].

3. The determination of the precise number of matrices in $\mathfrak{A}(R, S)$ is an open problem. Only lower bounds are known, see [34–38].

Definition 1.4.   *For all index sets $I \subseteq \{1, \ldots, m\}$ and $J \subseteq \{1, \ldots, n\}$, let*

$$t(I, J) = |I| \cdot |J| + \sum_{i \notin I} r_i - \sum_{j \in J} s_j. \qquad (1.10)$$

With the help of this function Ford and Fulkerson [11] obtained another necessary and sufficient condition for the nonemptyness of the class $\mathfrak{A}(R, S)$.

Theorem 1.2.   *Let $R = (r_1, \ldots, r_m)$ and $S = (s_1, \ldots, s_n)$ be a pair of compatible vectors. The class $\mathfrak{A}(R, S)$ is nonempty if and only if*

$$t(I, J) \geq 0 \qquad (1.11)$$

for all $I \subseteq \{1, \ldots, m\}$ and $J \subseteq \{1, \ldots, n\}$.

Proof: (Based on [39].) Suppose that there is a binary matrix $A \in \mathfrak{A}(R, S)$. Let $A[I, J]$ denote the submatrix of A obtained from the rows and columns indexed by I and J, respectively. Let, furthermore, $\bar{I} = \{1, \ldots, m\} \setminus I$ and $\bar{J} = \{1, \ldots, n\} \setminus J$. For any binary matrix X, let $\sigma_0(X)$ and $\sigma_1(X)$ denote the number of 0's and 1's in X, respectively. Then it is easy to see that, for any $I \subseteq \{1, \ldots, m\}$ and $J \subseteq \{1, \ldots, n\}$,

$$t(I, J) = \sigma_0(A[I, J]) + \sigma_1(A[\bar{I}, \bar{J}]) \geq 0. \qquad (1.12)$$

Now suppose that (1.11) holds. For $1 \leq k \leq n$, let J be a column index set such that $|J| = k$ and let $I = \{i \mid r_i \geq k\}$. Then

$$\sum_{j \in J} s_j \ \leq \ |I| \cdot |J| + \sum_{i \notin I} r_i = |I| \cdot k + \sum_{i \notin I} r_i$$

$$= \ \sum_{i=1}^{m} \min\{r_i, k\} = \sum_{j=1}^{k} \bar{s}_j \qquad (1.13)$$

and so, specifically,

$$\sum_{j=1}^{k} s_j' \leq \sum_{j=1}^{k} \bar{s}_j. \qquad (1.14)$$

It follows from Theorem 1.1 that $\mathfrak{A}(R, S)$ is not empty. ☐

We now consider binary matrices when not only the row and column sum vectors are given but also certain elements of the matrix are prescribed to be 0 or 1. Fulkerson [40] gave a condition for the existence of a binary matrix having zero trace (i.e., $\sum_{i=1}^{n} a_{ii} = 0$). Anstee published results [41–43] connected with the reconstruction and existence of binary matrices with at most one prescribed 1 or 0 in each row/column. Here we consider the general problem.

Definition 1.5.   *Let Q and P be binary matrices of size $m \times n$. We say that Q covers P if $p_{ij} \leq q_{ij}$ for $i = 1, \ldots, m$, $j = 1, \ldots, n$. We denote this relation as $P \leq Q$. We define*

$$\mathfrak{A}_P^Q(R, S) = \{A \mid P \leq A \leq Q, \ A \in \mathfrak{A}(R, S)\}. \qquad (1.15)$$

Trivially, $\mathfrak{A}_P^Q(R, S) = \mathfrak{A}(R, S)$ if $P = (0)_{m \times n}$ and $Q = (1)_{m \times n}$. Using suitable binary matrices P and Q we can prescribe binary values to any position. The value 0 is prescribed to (i, j) if $q_{ij} = 0$ and 1 is prescribed to (i, j) if $p_{ij} = 1$.

If $A \in \mathfrak{A}_P^Q(R, S)$ then

$$A - P \in \mathfrak{A}_O^{Q-P}(R - R(P), S - S(P)) \qquad (1.16)$$

where $O = (0)_{m \times n}$, and $R(P)$ and $S(P)$ denote the row and column sum vector of P, respectively. It follows that there is no loss of generality if we restrict our studies to the classes $\mathfrak{A}^Q(R, S) = \mathfrak{A}_O^Q(R, S)$, in which the position (i, j) can be classified as *prescribed* (if $q_{ij} = 0$) or *free* (if $q_{ij} = 1$).

Theorem 1.3.   *Let $R = (r_1, \ldots, r_m)$ and $S = (s_1, \ldots, s_n)$ be a pair of compatible vectors. The class $\mathfrak{A}^Q(R, S) \neq \emptyset$ if and only if*

$$\sum_{i \in I} \sum_{j \in J} q_{ij} \geq \max_{I, J}\{\sum_{i \in I} r_i - \sum_{j \notin J} s_j, \ \sum_{j \in J} s_j - \sum_{i \notin I} r_i\} \qquad (1.17)$$

for all $I \subseteq \{1, \ldots, m\}$ and $J \subseteq \{1, \ldots, n\}$.

Theorem 1.3 can be deduced as a special case of two more general theorems by Kellerer ([5] on reconstruction of functions) and Mirsky ([44] on reconstruction of integral matrices).

We now consider the problem of uniqueness for the classical case of binary matrices and two projections.

Definition 1.6. *We say that a binary matrix A is nonunique (with respect to its row and column sums) if there is a binary matrix $B \neq A$ having the same row and column sums as A. Otherwise, A is unique.*

Definition 1.7. *A switching component of a binary matrix A is a 2×2 submatrix of either of the following two forms:*

$$A_1 = \begin{pmatrix} 1 & 0 \\ 0 & 1 \end{pmatrix} \quad or \quad A_2 = \begin{pmatrix} 0 & 1 \\ 1 & 0 \end{pmatrix}. \tag{1.18}$$

A switching (operation) is a transformation of the elements of A that changes a submatrix of type A_1 into type A_2 or vice versa (and leaves all other elements of A unaltered).

Ryser used the name *interchange* [8] for this transformation. In fact, it is called by many different names in the literature; for example, it is referred to as a rectangular 4-switch in Chapter 3 by Kong and Herman in this book. Clearly, switching does not modify the row and column sums. Accordingly, if A has a switching component then it is nonunique. The reverse statement is also true. In fact the material in Section 3.1 provides us not only with the the following necessary and sufficient condition for uniqueness, but also with a proof of Ryser's Theorem [8].

Theorem 1.4. *A binary matrix is nonunique (with respect to its row and column sums) if and only if it has a switching component.*

Theorem 1.5. *(Ryser's Theorem) If A and B are two binary matrices in $\mathfrak{A}(R, S)$ then A is transformable into B by a finite number of switchings (using switching components).*

Now consider the special case of Theorem 1.1, in which (1.7) is replaced by

$$\sum_{j=l}^{n} s'_j = \sum_{j=l}^{n} \bar{s}_j, \quad \text{for} \quad 2 \leq l \leq n. \tag{1.19}$$

In view of the compatibility of (R, S) (1.19) is equivalent to $S' = \bar{S}$. Consequently, no changes are made to the matrix B during the execution of Step

3 in Algorithm 1.1 and so the B of Step 4 is the same as the B of Step 2; namely, $\bar{A}$. Since the 1's of the maximal $\bar{A}$ are in the leftmost positions in their rows, $\bar{A}$ has no switching component. It follows that the A obtained by a permutation of columns of $\bar{A}$ also cannot have a switching component and is consequently (by Theorem 1.4) unique with respect to its row and column sums.

We have just proven that if (R, S) satisfies the conditions of Theorem 1.1 with (1.7) replaced by (1.19), then there is a unique matrix with respect to R and S. Conversely, if the binary matrix A is unique then it has no switching component. Consider two columns of A, say j_1 and j_2. Let us suppose that $s_{j_1} \leq s_{j_2}$. If $a_{ij_1} = 1$ for some i then $a_{ij_2} = 1$. (Otherwise, if $a_{ij_1} = 1$ and $a_{ij_2} = 0$, there is at least one row i' such that $a_{i'j_1} = 0$ and $a_{i'j_2} = 1$, which contradicts to the assumption that A has no switching component.) In other words, the 1's in column j_1 are in the rows in which there is also a 1 in column j_2. This means that if the columns of A are permuted nonincreasingly then we get just the maximal matrix $\bar{A}$. Therefore, $S' = \bar{S}$ and so (1.19) is true.

From the discussion of the previous two paragraphs it follows that if A is a unique binary matrix, then it can be recovered from its row sum R and column sum S using Algorithm 1.1 without Step 3. That is, we can construct the maximal matrix $\bar{A}$ from R and then recover A by a permutation π^{-1} at the columns of $\bar{A}$ (where π is the permutation that produces S' from S). This observation leads us to a remarkable property of unique binary matrices, which is a consequence of the following easily proved result on maximal matrices.

Lemma 1.1.   *If A is a maximal binary matrix, then*

$$a_{ij} = 1 \iff s_j \geq |\{k \mid r_k \geq r_i\}|. \tag{1.20}$$

Now observe that for a unique binary matrix A in $\mathfrak{A}(R, S)$, the maximal matrix $\bar{A}$ is the unique element of $\mathfrak{A}(R, \bar{S}) = \mathfrak{A}(R, S')$. Since A is obtained from $\bar{A}$ by the permutation π^{-1} of the columns, it follows that for a unique binary matrix A in $\mathfrak{A}(R, S)$, (1.20) holds (even if A is not maximal). This leads to yet another characterization of uniqueness.

Definition 1.8.   *An $m \times n$ binary matrix $A = [a_{ij}]$ is additive if there are vectors $X = (x_1, \ldots, x_m) \in \mathbb{R}^m$ and $Y = (y_1, \ldots, y_n) \in \mathbb{R}^n$ such that, for $i = 1, \ldots, m$ and $j = 1, \ldots, n$, $a_{ij} = 1$ if and only if $x_i + y_j \geq 0$.*

Theorem 1.6.   *A binary matrix is unique if and only if it is additive.*

Proof: Let A be an $m \times n$ binary matrix with row and column sum vectors R and S. If A is unique, then it satisfies (1.20). This implies that A is additive with respect to the vectors $x_i = -|\{k \mid r_k \geq r_i\}|$, $i = 1, \ldots, m$, and $y_j = s_j$,

$j = 1, \ldots, n$.

Now let us suppose that A is additive with respect to the vectors $X \in \mathbb{R}^m$ and $Y \in \mathbb{R}^n$. Let $B \in \mathfrak{A}(R, S)$. Consider the function

$$\mathcal{K}(A, B) = \sum_{i=1}^{m} \sum_{j=1}^{n} (x_i + y_j)(a_{ij} - b_{ij}). \qquad (1.21)$$

From Definition 1.8 we see that each term in the sum on the right hand side of (1.21) is nonnegative. Furthermore,

$$
\begin{aligned}
\mathcal{K}(A, B) &= \sum_{i=1}^{m} x_i \sum_{j=1}^{n} (a_{ij} - b_{ij}) + \sum_{j=1}^{n} y_j \sum_{i=1}^{m} (a_{ij} - b_{ij}) \\
&= \sum_{i=1}^{m} x_i (r_i - r_i) + \sum_{j=1}^{n} y_j (s_j - s_j) = 0. \qquad (1.22)
\end{aligned}
$$

This implies that each term in the sum on the right-hand side of (1.21) is in fact zero. Together with Definition 1.8 this implies that if $a_{ij} = 0$ then $b_{ij} = 0$. However, A and B have the same number of 0's, therefore $A = B$. That is, A is unique. $\qquad \square$

As a summary of uniqueness for a nonempty class $\mathfrak{A}(R, S)$, we have the following.

Theorem 1.7.   *Let $R = (r_1, \ldots, r_m)$ and $S = (s_1, \ldots, s_n)$ be vectors of non-negative integers such that there is a binary matrix $A \in \mathfrak{A}(R, S)$. The following conditions are equivalent:*

(1) A is unique with respect to R and S;

(2) A has no switching component;

(3) (1.19) is satisfied;

(4) A is additive.

Condition (2) was found by Ryser [8]. It seems that (1.19) as a necessary and sufficient condition on uniqueness was first published by Wang [33]. The condition given by (1.20) can be considered to be a discrete version of that given in [45]. Additivity was introduced by Fishburn *et al.* [46] in a more general way. Further combinatorial results about the class $\mathfrak{A}(R, S)$ are in [47,48]. The cardinality of the class $\mathfrak{A}_P^Q(R, S)$ is discussed in [35,38].

For the class $\mathfrak{A}(R, S)$ switching components are used to decide the question of uniqueness. For the class $\mathfrak{A}^Q(R, S)$ *switching chains* (a generalization of switching components) can be used for the same purpose.

Definition 1.9.   *Let $A \in \mathfrak{A}^Q(R,S)$. A switching chain is a finite sequence $(i_1, j_1), (i_1, j_2), (i_2, j_2), (i_2, j_3), \ldots, (i_k, j_k), (i_k, j_1)$ of free positions of the matrix A such that*

$$a_{i_1 j_1} = a_{i_2 j_2} = \quad \cdots \quad = a_{i_k j_k} =$$
$$1 - a_{i_1 j_2} = 1 - a_{i_2 j_3} = \quad \cdots \quad = 1 - a_{i_{k-1} j_k} = 1 - a_{i_k j_1} \qquad (1.23)$$

$(k \geq 2)$. The corresponding switching (operation) is defined as changing the 0's and the 1's at all positions in the switching chain.

It is clear that switching in a matrix A does not change the row and column sums of A. As an example, see the following matrices generated from each other by switching (the prescribed elements are denoted by x).

$$\begin{pmatrix} 1 & x & 0 \\ x & 0 & 1 \\ 0 & 1 & x \end{pmatrix} \qquad \begin{pmatrix} 0 & x & 1 \\ x & 1 & 0 \\ 1 & 0 & x \end{pmatrix} \qquad (1.24)$$

The following theorems can be proven in a similar way as for the class $\mathfrak{A}(R,S)$ (see [49]).

Theorem 1.8.   *A binary matrix with prescribed values is nonunique if and only if it has a switching chain.*

Theorem 1.9.   *Let the binary matrices $A, B \in \mathfrak{A}^Q(R,S)$. Then A is transformable into B by a finite number of switchings (using switching chains).*

We now consider the possible values of a matrix element a_{ij} in the class $\mathfrak{A}(R,S)$. The positions can be classified into one of three sets as follows.

Definition 1.10.   *Let $\mathfrak{A} = \mathfrak{A}(R,S)$ be a nonempty class. The position (i,j) is variant if there are matrices $A, B \in \mathfrak{A}$ such that $a_{ij} = 1 - b_{ij}$. A position (i,j) is an invariant 0 or an invariant 1 if $a_{ij} = 0$ or $a_{ij} = 1$ for all $A \in \mathfrak{A}$, respectively. The sets of variant, invariant 0 and invariant 1 positions of the class $\mathfrak{A}$ are denoted by $V(\mathfrak{A})$, $I^{(0)}(\mathfrak{A})$ and $I^{(1)}(\mathfrak{A})$, respectively, and $(V(\mathfrak{A}), I^{(0)}(\mathfrak{A}), I^{(1)}(\mathfrak{A}))$ is called the structure of the class $\mathfrak{A}$.*

For example, the positions of a switching component of a binary matrix $A \in \mathfrak{A}$ are in $V(\mathfrak{A})$. The structure of $\mathfrak{A}(R,S)$ shows which part of the discrete space is ambiguous/unambiguous with respect to the row and column sums. Without loss of generality we present structure results for classes having nonincreasing row and column sum vectors.

Definition 1.11.   *A class $\mathfrak{A}' = \mathfrak{A}'(R',S')$ is called normalized if the elements of the vectors $R' = (r'_1, \ldots, r'_m)$ and $S' = (s'_1, \ldots, s'_n)$ are ordered as $r'_1 \geq r'_2 \geq$*

$\cdots \geq r'_m$ and $s'_1 \geq s'_2 \geq \cdots \geq s'_n$.

In a normalized class $\mathfrak{A}' = \mathfrak{A}'(R', S')$ we define the $(m+1) \times (n+1)$ structure matrix [10] $T = (t_{kl})$ by

$$
\begin{aligned}
t_{kl} &= \min\{t(I, J) \mid |I| = k, \ |J| = l\} \\
&= k \times l + \sum_{i>k} r'_i - \sum_{j\leq l} s'_j
\end{aligned}
\tag{1.25}
$$

for all $k = 0, 1, \ldots, m$ and $l = 0, 1, \ldots, n$.

Rephrasing Theorem 1.2 we can say that a normalized class $\mathfrak{A}'$ is not empty if and only if the structure matrix T of $\mathfrak{A}'$ has no negative elements. If $A \in \mathfrak{A}'$, then from (1.12) we have that

$$
\begin{aligned}
t_{kl} &= \sigma_0(A[\{1, \ldots, k\}, \{1, \ldots, l\}]) + \\
&\quad \sigma_1(A[\{k+1, \ldots, m\}, \{l+1, \ldots, n\}])
\end{aligned}
\tag{1.26}
$$

for any $k = 0, 1, \ldots, m$, $l = 0, 1, \ldots, n$. It follows that if $t_{kl} = 0$ then

$$
\begin{aligned}
\{1, \ldots, k\} \times \{1, \ldots, l\} &\subseteq I^{(1)}(\mathfrak{A}'), \\
\{k+1, \ldots, m\} \times \{l+1, \ldots, n\} &\subseteq I^{(0)}(\mathfrak{A}').
\end{aligned}
\tag{1.27}
$$

We are going to show that the invariant 1 and invariant 0 sets are unions of such discrete rectangles.

Lemma 1.2.   Let $\mathfrak{A}' = \mathfrak{A}(R', S')$ be a normalized class.

(i) If there is a matrix A in the class $\mathfrak{A}'$ such that $a_{ij} = 0$ and $a_{ij'} = 1$ for some $1 \leq i \leq m$ and $1 \leq j < j' \leq n$, then both (i, j) and (i, j') are variant positions of a switching component in A.

(ii) If there is a matrix A in the class $\mathfrak{A}'$ such that $a_{ij} = 0$ and $a_{i'j} = 1$ for some $1 \leq i < i' \leq m$ and $1 \leq j \leq n$, then both (i, j) and (i', j) are variant positions of a switching component in A.

Proof: Statement (i) is true because $s'_j \geq s'_{j'}$ in a normalized class and therefore there is a row i' such that $a_{i'j} = 1$ and $a_{i'j'} = 0$. Part (ii) can be proven analogously.   □

Now let i be any row that contains a variant position and let j and j' be the column indices of the leftmost and rightmost variant positions in row i. It follows that (i, k) is a variant position for $j \leq k \leq j'$. For suppose otherwise. If (i, k) is an invariant 1 position then for some matrix A in the class $a_{ij} = 0$ and $a_{ik} = 1$, which implies that (i, k) is a variant position (by Lemma 1.2 (i)). A similar argument holds if (i, k) is an invariant 0 position. Therefore, the variant positions follow each other in the rows (analogously, also in columns) consecutively.

Furthermore, also on the base of Lemma 1.2 (i), it is easy to show that in the rows of the normalized class the invariant 1, variant and invariant 0 positions (if any) follow in this order from left to right. Similarly, on the base of Lemma 1.2 (ii), it can be proven that in the columns of the normalized class the invariant 1, variant and invariant 0 positions (if any) follow in this order from top to bottom.

In the proof of the following lemma we will make repeated use of the following trivial consequence of Ryser's Theorem (Theorem 1.5). Let $\mathfrak{A} = \mathfrak{A}(R, S)$. If $(i, j) \in V(\mathfrak{A})$, then for any matrix $A \in \mathfrak{A}$, there is a row i' and column j' such that $(i', j) \in V(\mathfrak{A})$, $(i, j') \in V(\mathfrak{A})$ and $a_{ij} = 1 - a_{i'j} = 1 - a_{ij'}$.

Lemma 1.3.   Let $\mathfrak{A}' = \mathfrak{A}(R', S')$ be a normalized class, let i_1 and i_2 be two rows which contain variant positions such that $1 \leq i_1 < i_2 \leq m$ and let $[j_1, j_1']$ and $[j_2, j_2']$ be the corresponding ranges of the (consecutive) variant positions. Then

$$\text{either} \quad j_1 > j_2' \quad \text{or} \quad \text{both} \quad j_1 = j_2 \quad \text{and} \quad j_1' = j_2'. \tag{1.28}$$

Proof: We note that $j_1 < j_2$ is impossible, for then we would have the invariant 1 position (i_2, j_1) below the variant position (i_1, j_1). We complete the proof by showing that the assumption $j_2 < j_1$ implies that $j_1 > j_2'$. (One can prove similarly that $j_1' \neq j_2'$ also implies that $j_1 > j_2'$.)

Since (i_1, j_1) is a variant position, there is an $A \in \mathfrak{A}'$ for which

$$a_{i_1 j_1} = 0. \tag{1.29}$$

Consider the first $j_1 - 1$ columns of A. If $A[\{1, \ldots, m\}, \{1, \ldots, j_1 - 1\}]$ contains only 1's then all positions of $\{1, \ldots, m\} \times \{1, \ldots, j_1 - 1\}$ are invariant 1's (because $t_{m, j_1 - 1} = 0$ and (1.27)), which contradicts the assumption that $j_2 < j_1$. Therefore, there is a 0 somewhere in the first $j_1 - 1$ columns of A. Let i be the index of the uppermost row containing a 0 in the first $j_1 - 1$ columns of A. Then

$$\sigma_0(A[\{1, \ldots, i - 1\}, \{1, \ldots, j_1 - 1\}]) = 0. \tag{1.30}$$

Furthermore, $i > i_1$, because there are only invariant 1's to the left of j_1, and so there can be only invariant 1's above $(i_1, 1), \ldots, (i_1, j_1 - 1)$.

Let j be a column such that

$$a_{ij} = 0. \tag{1.31}$$

Clearly

$$a_{i_1 j} = 1. \tag{1.32}$$

Then $a_{ij_1} = 0$, for otherwise $(i_1, j), (i_1, j_1), (i, j)$, and (i, j_1) would constitute a switching component (see (1.29), (1.31), and (1.32)). Furthermore, if $a_{il} = 1$ for some $l \in (j_1, \ldots, n]$, then on the basis of Lemma 1.2 (i) we can perform a switching on elements $a_{ij_1} = 0$ and $a_{il} = 1$ (and the other two in these columns) getting a new binary matrix $B \in \mathfrak{A}'$ (without altering $a_{i_1 j}$ and $a_{i_1 j_1}$). But in this case $b_{i_1 j} = 1$, $b_{i_1 j_1} = 0$, $b_{ij} = 0$, and $b_{ij_1} = 1$, so these four elements constitute a switching component, which is in contradiction with (i_1, j) being an invariant 1 position. Therefore, $a_{il} = 0$ for $l = j_1, \ldots, n$. Similarly, $a_{kj_1} = 0$ for $k = i, \ldots, m$ (on the basis of Lemma 1.2 (ii)).

Furthermore, for the same reason, all elements of A in the rectangle $\{i, \ldots, m\} \times \{j_1, \ldots, n\}$ are 0, that is

$$\sigma_1(A[\{i, \ldots, m\}, \{j_1, \ldots, n\}]) = 0. \tag{1.33}$$

Summarizing (1.30) and (1.33), we get $t_{i-1, j_1 - 1} = 0$. This implies that the rectangles $\{1, \ldots, i-1\} \times \{1, \ldots, j_1 - 1\}$ and $\{i, \ldots, m\} \times \{j_1, \ldots, n\}$ contain only invariant 1 and invariant 0 positions, respectively. By the assumption that $j_2 < j_1$, this implies that $i_2 \geq i$. That in turn implies that $j_1 > j_2'$, as needed to complete the proof.   □

Theorem 1.10.   *The variant set of a normalized class $\mathfrak{A}' = \mathfrak{A}(R', S') \neq \emptyset$, can always be written as*

$$V(\mathfrak{A}') = \bigcup_{q=1}^{p} I_q \times J_q \tag{1.34}$$

($p = 0$ if there are no variant elements), where

$$I_q = \{i_q, \ldots, i_q'\}, \quad 1 \leq i_1 < i_1' < i_2 < i_2' < \cdots < i_p < i_p' \leq m, \tag{1.35}$$
$$J_q = \{j_q, \ldots, j_q'\}, \quad 1 \leq j_p < j_p' < j_{p-1} < j_{p-1}' < \cdots < j_1 < j_1' \leq n. \tag{1.36}$$

Proof: We define i_q, i_q', j_q, j_q' inductively as follows. We set $i_0' = 0$. Assume that i_q' is already defined. If there is no $i > i_q'$ such that row i contains a variant position, then $p = q$ and we are done. Otherwise, let i_{q+1} be the smallest such i and $[j_{q+1}, j_{q+1}']$ be the associated range of the consecutive variant positions. (Note that $j_{q+1} < j_{q+1}'$ due to the consequence of Ryser's Theorem as stated above in Lemma 1.3.) Let i_{q+1}' be the maximal value of i such that the associated range of consecutive variant positions is still $[j_{q+1}, j_{q+1}']$. (By the same reasoning involving Ryser's Theorem $i_{q+1} < i_{q+1}'$. Also, for all rows i such that $i_{q+1} \leq i \leq i_{q+1}'$, we must have that the range of variant positions is $[j_{q+1}, j_{q+1}']$.) By the properties stated above and in Lemma 1.3, we must also have that $j_{q+1}' < j_q$.   □

Remark 1.2.   *Since the rows/columns of the variant rectangles are between the invariant 1's and 0's, the invariant 1 and invariant 0 sets of the class $\mathfrak{A}'$ are the unions of rectangles of the form (1.27).*

We illustrate the material on the structure of a class in Fig. 1.3 for $R = (4, 4, 10, 13, 11, 7, 10, 9, 1)$ and $S = (1, 7, 4, 7, 9, 8, 5, 7, 7, 6, 1, 3, 4)$. On the left of the figure is an element of $\mathfrak{A}(R', S')$ with the variant positions shaded. It is trivial to check that the shaded positions are indeed variant (all values within either shaded box can be altered by switchings using switching components entirely within that box). The question arises, how do we know that none of the unshaded positions are variant?

R'													
13	1	1	1	1	1	1	1	1	1	1	1	1	1
11	1	1	1	1	1	1	1	1	1	1	1	0	0
10	1	1	1	1	1	1	1	1	1	1	0	0	0
10	1	1	1	1	1	1	1	1	1	1	0	0	0
9	1	1	1	1	1	1	1	1	0	0	1	0	0
7	1	1	1	1	1	1	1	0	0	0	0	0	0
4	1	1	1	1	0	0	0	0	0	0	0	0	0
4	1	1	0	0	1	1	0	0	0	0	0	0	0
1	1	0	0	0	0	0	0	0	0	0	0	0	0
S'	9	8	7	7	7	7	6	5	4	4	3	1	1

R													
4	0	1	0	1	1	1	0	0	0	0	0	0	0
4	0	0	0	0	1	1	0	1	1	0	0	0	0
10	0	1	1	1	1	1	1	1	1	1	0	0	1
13	1	1	1	1	1	1	1	1	1	1	1	1	1
11	0	1	1	1	1	1	1	1	1	1	0	1	1
7	0	1	0	1	1	1	0	1	1	1	0	0	0
10	0	1	1	1	1	1	1	1	1	1	0	0	1
9	0	1	0	1	1	1	1	1	1	1	0	1	0
1	0	0	0	0	1	0	0	0	0	0	0	0	0
S	1	7	4	7	9	8	5	7	7	6	1	3	4

FIGURE 1.3. Illustration of the structure of the class $\mathfrak{A}$. Right: The row and column sum vectors, R and S, and the structure of the class $\mathfrak{A}(R, S)$. The variant positions are shaded. Left: The structure of the normalized class $\mathfrak{A}(R', S')$.

This is, in fact, a consequence of some remarkable general results in [50]. Here we state without proof the applicable special case of Theorem 2.6 (i) of [50]. As it will be easily noted, this result is close in spirit to Theorem 1.6. (In fact, Theorem 1.6 is derived in [50] as a corollary of the results presented there.) Another closely related theorem is stated and proved in Chapter 8 by Matej, Vardi, Herman and Vardi.

Definition 1.12. *Let $A = [a_{ij}]$ be an $m \times n$ binary matrix. A pair of vectors $X = (x_1, \ldots, x_m) \in \mathbb{R}^m$ and $Y = (y_1, \ldots, y_n) \in \mathbb{R}^n$ is said to be compatible with A if, for $i = 1, \ldots, m$ and $j = 1, \ldots, n$,*

$$x_i + y_j = \begin{cases} \geq 0, & \text{if } a_{ij} = 1, \\ \leq 0, & \text{if } a_{ij} = 0. \end{cases} \tag{1.37}$$

Theorem 1.11. *Let $R = (r_1, \ldots, r_m)$ and $S = (s_1, \ldots, s_n)$ be vectors of nonnegative integers such that there is a binary matrix $A \in \mathfrak{A}(R, S)$. Then, for $i = 1, \ldots, m$ and $j = 1, \ldots, n$, (i, j) is not a variant position if and only if there exists a pair of vectors $X = (x_1, \ldots, x_m)$ and $Y = (y_1, \ldots, y_n)$ which is compatible with A such that $x_i + y_j \neq 0$.*

Let $X = (11, 9, 8, 8, 8, 8, 7, 5, 4, 4, 4, 2, 2)$ and $Y = (-1, -3, -4, -4, -4, -6, -8, -8, -10)$. Then it is easy to check that this pair of vectors is compatible with the matrix on the left of Fig 1.3 and that, for all the unshaded positions (i,j), $x_i + y_j \neq 0$. Theorem 1.11 therefore implies that the unshaded positions are in fact not variant positions. Once we have determined the structure of the normalized class $\mathfrak{A}(R', S')$ we can, by performing the reverse permutation of the rows and columns, obtain the structure of the original class $\mathfrak{A}(R, S)$; this is illustrated on the right of Fig 1.3.

The structure of the class of binary matrices was studied first by Ryser [51,52] and Haber [53]. Our summary is based on [54]. We remark that the structure of the class $\mathfrak{A}^Q(R, S)$ is similar to the structure of $\mathfrak{A}(R, S)$ as it was shown in [50]. The same paper describes an algorithm for producing the structure of a nonempty class based on a sample matrix from it; see also [55]. (Such algorithms can be used for finding the vectors X and Y, which we seemed to have pulled out of a hat in the previous paragraph.)

We complete this subsection by considering the problem of reconstruction for the classical case of binary matrices and two projections. As we saw, for a nonempty class $\mathfrak{A}(R, S)$, Algorithm 1.1 constructs a solution in polynomial time.

If we happen to know that there is a unique binary matrix A in $\mathfrak{A}(R, S)$, then we also know that this matrix must satisfy (1.20). This knowledge leads us to the following reconstruction algorithm, which in practice is likely to be much better than Algorithm 1.1. Its output is illustrated in Fig. 1.4. (Algorithms for reconstructing unique binary matrices were described also in [31,56,57].)

Algorithm 1.2.

Input: a compatible pair of vectors, (R, S), satisfying (1.19);

Step 1. $A = O$; (zero matrix)

Step 2. find $i_1, i_2, \ldots, i_m$ such that $r_{i_1} \geq r_{i_2} \geq \cdots \geq r_{i_m}$;

Step 3. for $j = 1$ to n,
*   for $k = 1$ to s_j,*
* $a_{i_k j} = 1$;*

Output: matrix A.

In certain cases the number of binary matrices having given row and column sums can be very high. For example, if $R = S = (1, \ldots, 1)$ $(m = n)$ then $|\mathfrak{A}(R, S)| = n!$. For such reasons it is interesting to study the problem of reconstructing special binary matrices having some special property. Using such a property during the reconstruction, we can hope to reduce the number of possible solutions.

$$
\begin{array}{c|ccccc}
1 & 0 & 0 & 0 & 1 & 0 \\
3 & 0 & 1 & 1 & 1 & 0 \\
5 & 1 & 1 & 1 & 1 & 1 \\
2 & 0 & 1 & 0 & 1 & 0 \\
\\
& 1 & 3 & 2 & 4 & 1
\end{array}
$$

FIGURE 1.4. Reconstruction of a unique binary matrix.

The most frequently used properties are geometrical. For example, let us suppose that the 1's of the binary matrix to be reconstructed follow each other consecutively in the rows and columns.

Definition 1.13.   *A binary matrix is h-convex (respectively, v-convex) if in the rows (respectively, columns) the 1's follow each other consecutively. If a binary matrix is both h- and v-convex then it is hv-convex (see Fig. 1.5). The class of h-convex, v-convex, and hv-convex binary matrices will be denoted by (h), (v), and (hv), respectively.*

$$
\begin{pmatrix}
1 & 1 & 1 & 0 & 0 \\
1 & 1 & 0 & 0 & 0 \\
0 & 1 & 1 & 1 & 1 \\
1 & 0 & 0 & 0 & 0
\end{pmatrix}
\begin{pmatrix}
0 & 1 & 1 & 0 & 0 \\
1 & 1 & 1 & 0 & 1 \\
0 & 1 & 1 & 1 & 0 \\
0 & 0 & 0 & 0 & 0
\end{pmatrix}
\begin{pmatrix}
0 & 1 & 1 & 0 & 0 \\
1 & 1 & 1 & 1 & 1 \\
0 & 1 & 1 & 1 & 0 \\
0 & 0 & 0 & 1 & 0
\end{pmatrix}
$$

FIGURE 1.5. Examples of *h*-convex, *v*-convex, and *hv*-convex binary matrices.

Kuba published an algorithm [58] for reconstructing *hv*-convex binary matrices from their row and column sums.

Definition 1.14.   *The neighbors of the position (i,j) are the positions $(i-1,j)$, $(i,j-1)$, $(i,j+1)$, and $(i+1,j+1)$. We say that two positions of 1's, (i,j) and (k,l) are connected if there is a sequence of positions of 1's*

$$(i,j) = (i_1,j_1),(i_2,j_2),\dots,(i_{t-1},j_{t-1}),(i_t,j_t) = (k,l) \qquad (1.38)$$

$(t \geq 2)$ such that (i_{u+1},j_{u+1}) is one of the neighbors of (i_u,j_u) for all $u = 1,\dots,t-1$. A polyomino is a binary matrix in which every position of 1 is connected to every other position of 1 (see, for example, Fig. 1.6). The class of polyominoes is denoted by (p).

The concept of polyomino is well-known in many other fields but it is usually given a different name. For example, in the picture processing literature [59] a polyomino would be called a digital picture with two levels in which the set of white pixels is 4-connected and in the more general theory

$$\begin{pmatrix} 0 & 1 & 1 & 0 & 0 \\ 1 & 1 & 1 & 0 & 1 \\ 0 & 1 & 1 & 1 & 1 \\ 1 & 1 & 0 & 0 & 0 \end{pmatrix}$$

FIGURE 1.6. A polyomino.

of digital spaces [60] it would be called a finite binary picture over $(\mathbb{Z}^2, \omega_2)$ in which the set of 1-spels is ω_2-connected.

Specifically, the reconstruction theory of the class of hv-convex polyominoes is well developed. There are upper and lower bounds to the maximum number of hv-convex polyominoes having given row and column sum vectors R and S [61]. Reconstruction methods [62–64] have been suggested for this class of binary matrices. A newer method is given in Chapter 7 by Del Lungo and Nivat in this book. An important result for this class of binary matrices is that the computational complexity of the reconstruction problem for hv-convex polyominoes is polynomial [62], but for the classes (p), (h), (v), (p,h) (i.e., h-convex polyominoes), (p,v) (i.e., v-convex polyominoes), and (hv) the problem is NP-complete [65].

1.3   Applications

1.3.1   *Data compression, data coding, and image processing*

Projections can be considered as an encoding of the object. Data coding is interesting from the viewpoints of *data security* and *data compression*. Knowing that the RECONSTRUCTION($\mathcal{E}, \mathcal{L}$) problem is NP-complete if the number of projections is greater than 2, encoding via projections can ensure some security of the data [66].

Let us now consider *data compression*. Let F be a discrete set in $\mathbb{Z}^d$. To store an F of size n^d we need n^d number of bits, while its q projections with size n^{d-1} need $q \cdot \log_2 n \cdot n^{d-1}$ bits for storage. Therefore, the data compression ratio is

$$\frac{n^d}{q \cdot \log_2 n \cdot n^{d-1}} = \frac{n}{q \cdot \log_2 n} \tag{1.39}$$

independently of the dimension d.

From Section 1.2 it is clear that, in general, some information is lost when only the projections are available instead of the discrete set (or, generally, discrete image). However, as Shilferstein and Chien pointed out in [67], several image processing operators have analogous operators on their projections. Further examples are given in [68] for image registration and in [69] for thinning of unique binary images, using only their projections in both cases.

The projections can be used also in image databases. Representing the components (symbols) of the images by their (symbolic) projections, database operations such as spatial reasoning, visualization and browsing can be performed (see Chapter 21 by Chang in this book).

1.3.2 Electron microscopy

Images produced by transmission microscopes can be considered to be projections of the object to be studied. The electron beam transmitted through the specimen can be used to estimate line integrals. If the specimen is composed of a number of homogeneous parts, then DT can be applied for determining the spatial structure. Where only a few noisy projections can be taken from a limited range angles, DT seems to be the only way to reconstruct good quality images.

There are several types of electron microscopy to which the methods of DT had been applied. One of the first experiments was performed by Crew and Crew [70]. They suggested a heuristic discrete algorithm to reconstruct hemoglobin molecules from 3 and 4 projections.

Due to the introduction of a technique [71, 72] called QUANTITEM (QUantitative ANalysis of The Information from Transmission Electron Microscopy), based on high-resolution electron microscopy, it is possible to measure the projections of atomic structures in crystals. The problem of reconstructing discrete sets from their projections for the determination of atomic structures from QUANTITEM data motivated the Mini-Symposium on Discrete Tomography at DIMACS in 1994. Some of the crystalline phantoms designed for testing new reconstruction algorithms are used in a number of chapters of this book as well.

A description of biological problems, which are potentially solvable by electron microscopy and DT, is given in Chapter 18 by Carazo *et al.*

1.3.3 Biplane angiography

For the visualization of a cardiac ventricle it is a standard procedure to inject Roentgen contrast agent into it and to take X-ray images. If we assume that the distribution of the dye is homogeneous and has unit absorption, then we have a binary object consisting of two kinds of points: points of 1's and 0's depending on the presence or absence of the dye. Usually, two orthogonal projections of the ventricle are collected with a conventional biplane X-ray system. The aim is to determine the three-dimensional structure. In practice it is sufficient to reconstruct the two-dimensional cross sections. This problem can be stated as the reconstruction of a binary matrix $A = (a_{ij})_{m \times n}$ from its row and column sum vectors. In general, there is not a unique solution to this problem, as it was shown in Subsection 1.2.2. One way to resolve this ambiguity is to reformulate the reconstruction problem as an optimization problem:

$$\text{minimize} \quad \sum_{i=1}^{m} \sum_{j=1}^{n} c_{ij} a_{ij}, \quad\quad\quad (1.40)$$

under the constraints of (1.5) and (1.6) where the elements of the matrix $C = (c_{ij})_{m \times n}$ represent the costs of assigning the value 1 to the element a_{ij}. With careful selection of C we can hope to get a useful solution [73]. For example, we can use the fact that the successive slices are similar to each other in a ventricular structure. Accordingly, if a section is already reconstructed then we choose C such that the binary matrix of the next section is similar to the previous one. Slump and Gerbrands [74] suggested to use a minimum cost capacitated network flow algorithm to find such an optimal solution. A reconstruction program has been developed to determine the dynamic 3D shape of the left or right heart chamber [75]. A summary of this problem is given in Chapter 17 by Onnasch and Prause in this book.

The first paper discussing the application of binary tomography in cardioangiography seems to be due to Chang and Chow [76]. They reconstructed a clay model of a dog heart from two projections estimated from digitized X-ray films. In order to reduce the ambiguity of the problem they supposed that the cross sections of the heart are convex and symmetric with respect to two orthogonal axes. For a very recent work (which applies the approach of Chapter 8 by Matej, Vardi, Herman, and Vardi in this book to cardioangiography) see [77].

Experiments show that the reconstruction of blood vessels is possible from so-called cone beam projections [78].

1.3.4   Computerized tomography

As it was mentioned in Section 1.1, the methods used in CT are not suitable to reconstruct discrete functions from a few projections. If the number of projections is large enough, then CT is able to generate images that are near to the ideal discrete function. If we know the range of the discrete function to be reconstructed, then by the methods of DT we can hope to get images with better resolution and accuracy; see Chapter 15 by Browne and Koshy in this book, where they write about the technical challenges in DT for CT-assisted engineering and manufacturing.

A possible solution in this direction is given in Chapter 9 by Chan, Herman, and Levitan. Their idea for getting better quality images is a two-step procedure. In the first step a conventional reconstruction technique is used to create PET (positron emission tomography) images. Then these images are used as initial values to an iterative DT method.

1.4   Conclusion

In this chapter we have given a brief historical overview of some of the foundations of, algorithms for, and applications of discrete tomography. To get a more complete coverage of this field, read on!

Acknowledgments

This work was supported by NSF-MTA grants "U.S.-Hungary Mathematics Workshop on Discrete Tomography INT-9602103" and "Aspects of Discrete Tomography Supplement to DMS 9612077" and the Hungarian Ministry of Education Grant FKFP 0908. The second author's work in this area is supported by the U.S. National Institutes of Health under grant no. HL28438 and the U.S. National Science Foundation under grant no. DMS9612077.

References

[1] G. T. Herman, *Image Reconstruction from Projections: The Fundamentals of Computerized Tomography*, (Academic Press, New York), 1980.

[2] G. G. Lorentz, "A problem of plane measure," *Amer. J. Math.* **71**, 417-426 (1949).

[3] A. Rényi, "On projections of probability distributions," *Acta Math. Acad. Sci. Hung.* **3**, 131-142 (1952).

[4] A. Heppes, "On the determination of probability distributions of more dimensions by their projections," *Acta Math. Acad. Sci. Hung.* **7**, 403-410 (1956).

[5] H. Kellerer, "Funktionen auf Produkträumen mit vorgegebenen Marginal-Funktionen," *Math. Ann.* **144**, 323-344 (1961).

[6] H. Kellerer, "Masstheoretische Marginalprobleme," *Math. Ann.* **153**, 168-198 (1964).

[7] H. Kellerer, "Marginalprobleme für Funktionen," *Math. Ann.* **154**, 147-150 (1964).

[8] H. J. Ryser, "Combinatorial properties of matrices of zeros and ones," *Canad. J. Math.* **9**, 371-377 (1957).

[9] D. Gale, "A theorem on flows in networks," *Pacific J. Math.* **7**, 1073-1082 (1957).

[10] H. J, Ryser, "Traces of matrices of zeros and ones," *Canad. J. Math.* **12**, 463-476 (1960).

[11] L. R. Ford, Jr. and D. R. Fulkerson, *Flows in Networks* (Princeton University Press, Princeton, NJ), 1962.

[12] J. Steiner, "Einfache Beweis der isoperimetrischen Hauptsätze," *J. reine angew. Math.* **18**, 289-296 (1838).

[13] P. C. Hammer, "Problem 2," In *Proc. Symp. Pure Math., vol. VII: Convexity* (Amer. Math. Soc., Providence, RI), pp. 498-499, 1963.

[14] O. Giering, "Bestimmung von Eibereichen und Eikörpern durch Steiner-Symmetrisierungen," *Sitzungsberichten Bayer. Akad. Wiss. München, Math.-Nat. Kl.*, pp. 225-253 (1962).

[15] R. J. Gardner and P. McMullen, "On Hammer's X-ray problem," *J. London Math. Soc.* **21**, 171-175 (1980).

[16] R. J. Gardner, *Geometric Tomography* (Cambridge University Press, Cambridge, UK), 1995.

[17] G. Bianchi and M. Longinetti, "Reconstructing plane sets from projections," *Discrete Comp. Geom.* **5**, 223-242 (1990).

[18] R. J. Gardner and P. Gritzmann, "Discrete tomography: Determination of finite sets by X-rays," *Trans. Amer. Math. Soc.* **349**, 2271-2295 (1997).

[19] P. Gritzmann and M. Nivat (Eds.), *Discrete Tomography: Algorithms and Complexity*, (Dagstuhl-Seminar-Report 165, Dagstuhl, Germany), 1997.

[20] G. T. Herman and A. Kuba (Editors), *Discrete Tomography.* Special Issue of Intern. J. of Imaging Systems and Techn., Vol. 9, No. 2/3, 1998.

[21] R. Gordon, R. Bender, and G. T. Herman, "Algebraic reconstruction techniques (ART) for three-dimensional electron microscopy and X-ray photography," *J. Theor. Biol.* **29**, 471-481 (1970).

[22] G. T. Herman, A. Lent, and S. W. Rowland, "ART: Mathematics and applications," *J. Theor. Biol.* **42**, 1-32 (1973).

[23] G. T. Herman, "Reconstruction of binary patterns from a few projections," In A. Günther, B. Levrat and H. Lipps, *Intern, Computing Symposium 1973*, (North-Holland Publ. Co., Amsterdam), pp. 371-378, 1974.

[24] P. Gritzmann, D. Prangenberg, S. de Vries, and M. Wiegelmann, "Success and failure of certain reconstruction and uniqueness algorithms in discrete tomography," *Intern. J. of Imaging Systems and Techn.* **9**, 101-109 (1998).

[25] Y. Vardi and D. Lee, "The discrete Radon transform and its approximate inversion via the EM algorithm," *Intern. J. Imaging Systems and Techn.* **9**, 155-173 (1998).

[26] J. H. B. Kemperman and A. Kuba, "Reconstruction of two-valued matrices from their two projections," *Intern. J. of Imaging Systems and Techn.* **9**, 110-117 (1998).

[27] D. Rossi and A. Willsky, "Reconstruction from projections based on detection and estimation of objects: Performance analysis and robustness analysis," *IEEE Trans. Acoust. Speech Signal Process.* **32**, 886-906 (1984).

[28] J. Singer, F. A. Grünbaum, P. Kohn, and J. Zubelli, "Image reconstruction of the interior of bodies that diffuse radiation," *Science* **248**, 990-993 (1990).

[29] D. R. Fulkerson and H. J. Ryser, "Width sequences for special classes of (0,1)-matrices," *Canad. J. Math.* **15**, 371-396 (1963).

[30] S.-K. Chang and Y. R. Wang, "Three-dimensional reconstruction from orthogonal projections," *Pattern Recognition* **7**, 167-176 (1975).

[31] S.-K. Chang, "The reconstruction of binary patterns from their projections," *Commun. ACM* **14**, 21-25 (1971).

[32] S.-K. Chang, "Algorithm 445. Binary pattern reconstruction from projections," *Commun. ACM* **16**, 185-186 (1973).

[33] Y. R. Wang, "Characterization of binary patterns and their projections," *IEEE Trans. Computers* **C-24**, 1032-1035 (1975).

[34] W. Wandi, "The class $\mathfrak{A}(R,S)$ of (0,1)-matrices," *Discrete Math.* **39**, 301-305 (1982).

[35] W. Honghui, "Structure and cardinality of the class $\mathfrak{A}(R,S)$ of (0,1)-matrices," *J. Math. Research and Exposition* **4**, 87-93 (1984).

[36] S. Jiayu, "On a guess about the cardinality of the class $\mathfrak{A}(R,S)$ of (0,1)-matrices," *J. Tongji Univ.* **14**, 52-55 (1986).

[37] W. Xiaohong, "The cardinality of the class $\mathfrak{A}(R,S)$ of (0,1)-matrices," *J. Sichuan Univ. Nat. Sci. Edition* **4**, 95-99 (1986).

[38] W. Xiaohong, "A necessary and sufficient condition for $|\mathfrak{A}_P^Q(R,S)|$ to equal its lower bound," *J. Sichuan Univ. Nat. Sci. Edition* **24**, 136-143 (1987).

[39] L. Mirsky, *Transversal Theory* (Academic Press, New York), 1971.

[40] D. R. Fulkerson, "Zero-one matrices with zero trace," *Pacific J. Math.* **10**, 831-836 (1960).

[41] R. P. Anstee, "Properties of a class of (0,1)-matrices covering a given matrix," *Canad. J. Math.* **34**, 438-453 (1982).

[42] R. P. Anstee, "Triangular (0,1)-matrices with prescribed row and column sums," *Discrete Math.* **40**, 1-10 (1982).

[43] R. P. Anstee, "The network flows approach for matrices with given row and column sums," *Discrete Math.* **44**, 125-138 (1983).

[44] L. Mirsky, "Combinatorial theorems and integral matrices," *J. Combin. Theor.* **5**, 30-44 (1968).

[45] A. Kuba and A. Volčič, "Characterization of measurable plane sets which are reconstructable from their two projections," *Inverse Problems* **4**, 513-527 (1988).

[46] P. C. Fishburn, J. C. Lagarias, J. A. Reeds, and L. A. Shepp, "Sets uniquely determined by projections on axes II. Discrete case," *Discrete Math.* **91**, 149-159 (1991).

[47] H. J. Ryser, *Combinatorial Mathematics* (The Math. Assoc. Amer., Washington, DC), 1963.

[48] R. A. Brualdi, "Matrices of zeros and ones with fixed row and column sum vectors," *Lin. Algebra and Its Appl.* **33**, 159-231 (1980).

[49] A. Kuba, "Reconstruction of unique binary matrices with prescribed elements," *Acta Cybern.* **12**, 57-70 (1995).

[50] R. Aharoni, G. T. Herman, and A. Kuba, "Binary vectors partially determined by linear equation systems," *Discrete Math.* **171**, 1-16 (1997).

[51] H. J. Ryser, "The term rank of a matrix," *Canad. J. Math* **10**, 57-65 (1958).

[52] H. J. Ryser, "Matrices of zeros and ones," *Bull. Amer. Math. Soc.* **66**, 442-464 (1960).

[53] M. Haber, "Term rank of 0, 1 matrices," *Rend. Sem. Mat. Padova* **30**, 24-51 (1960).

[54] A. Kuba, "Determination of the structure of the class $\mathfrak{A}(R, S)$ of (0,1)-matrices," *Acta Cybernetica* **9**, 121-132 (1989).

[55] W. Y. C. Chen, "Integral matrices with given row and column sums," *J. Combin. Theory, Ser. A* **61**, 153-172 (1992).

[56] S.-K. Chang and G. L. Shelton, "Two algorithms for multiple-view binary pattern reconstruction," *IEEE Trans. Systems, Man, Cybernetics* **SMC-1**, 90-94 (1971).

[57] L. Huang, "The reconstruction of uniquely determined plane sets from two projections in discrete case," *Preprint Series* **UTMS 95-29**, *Univ. of Tokyo* (1995).

[58] A. Kuba, "The reconstruction of two-directionally connected binary patterns from their two orthogonal projections," *Comp. Vision, Graphics, Image Proc.* **27**, 249-265 (1984).

[59] A. Rosenfeld and A. C.Kak, "Digital Picture Processing," (Academic Press, New York) 1976.

[60] G. T. Herman, "Geometry of Digital Spaces," (Birkhäuser, Boston) 1998.

[61] A. Del Lungo, M. Nivat and R. Pinzani, "The number of convex polyominoes reconstructible from their orthogonal projections," *Discrete Math.* **157**, 65-78 (1996).

[62] E. Barcucci, A. Del Lungo, M. Nivat, and R. Pinzani, "Reconstructing convex polyominoes from horizontal and vertical projections," *Theor. Comput. Sci.* **155**, 321-347 (1996).

[63] E. Barcucci, A. Del Lungo, M. Nivat, and R. Pinzani, "Medians of polyominoes: A property for the reconstruction," *Int. J. Imaging Systems and Techn.* **9**, 69-77 (1998).

[64] M. Chrobak and C. Dürr, "Reconstructing hv-convex polyominoes from orthogonal projections," (Preprint, Dept. of Computer Science, Univ. of California, Riverside, CA), 1998.

[65] G. J. Woeginger, "The reconstruction of polyominoes from their orthogonal projections," (Techn. Rep. F003, TU-Graz), 1996.

[66] R. W. Irving and M. R. Jerrum, "Three-dimensional statistical data security problems," *SIAM J. Comput.* **23**, 170-184 (1994).

[67] A. R. Shliferstein and Y. T. Chien, "Some properties of image-processing operations on projection sets obtained from digital pictures," *IEEE Trans. Comput.* **C-26**, 958-970 (1977).

[68] Z. Mao and R. N. Strickland, "Image sequence processing for target estimation in forward-looking infrared imagery," *Optical Engrg.* **27**, 541-549 (1988).

[69] A. Fazekas, G. T. Herman, and A. Matej, "On processing binary pictures via their projections," *Int. J. Imaging Systems and Techn.* **9**, 99-100 (1998).

[70] A. V. Crewe and D. A. Crewe, "Inexact reconstruction: Some improvements," *Ultramicroscopy* **16**, 33-40 (1985).

[71] P. Schwander, C. Kisielowski, M. Seibt, F. H. Baumann, Y. Kim, and A. Ourmazd, "Mapping projected potential, interfacial roughness, and composition in general crystalline solids by quantitative transmission electron microscopy," *Phys. Rev. Letters* **71**, 4150-4153 (1993).

[72] C. Kisielowski, P. Schwander, F. H. Baumann, M. Seibt, Y. Kim, and A. Ourmazd, "An approach to quantitative high-resolution electron microscopy of crystalline materials," *Ultramicroscopy* **58**, 131-155 (1995).

[73] D. G. W. Onnasch, and P. H. Heintzen, "A new approach for the reconstruction of the right or left ventricular form from biplane angiocardiographic recordings," In *Conf. Comp. Card. 1976*, (IEEE Comp. Soc. Press, Washington), pp. 67-73, 1976.

[74] C. H. Slump and J. J. Gerbrands, "A network flow approach to reconstruction of the left ventricle from two projections," *Comp. Graphics and Image Proc.* **18**, 18-36 (1982).

[75] G. P. M. Prause and D. G. W. Onnasch, "Binary reconstruction of the heart chambers from biplane angiographic image sequences," *IEEE Trans. Medical Imaging* **MI-15**, 532-546 (1996).

[76] S.-K. Chang and C. K. Chow, "The reconstruction of three-dimensional objects from two orthogonal projections and its application to cardiac cineangiography," *IEEE Trans. Comput.* **C-22**, 18-28 (1973).

[77] B. M. Carvalho, G. T. Herman, S. Matej, C. Salzberg, and E. Vardi, "Binary tomography for triplane cardiography," In A. Kuba, M. Samal, A. Todd-Pokropek, *Information Processing in Medical Imaging Conference 1999* (Springer-Verlag, Berlin), to be published.

[78] N. Robert, F. Peyrin, and M. J. Yaffe, "Binary vascular reconstruction from a limited number of cone beam projections," *Med. Phys.* **21**, 1839-1851 (1994).

Chapter 2

Sets of Uniqueness and Additivity in Integer Lattices

Peter C. Fishburn[1]
Lawrence A. Shepp[2]

ABSTRACT   A mathematical formulation is provided for inversion problems in which local structures of finite subsets of integer lattices are to be deduced from point counts in prescribed linear manifolds of an n-dimensional space. Notions of uniqueness and additivity for finite lattice sets are defined and characterized by point configurations and by aspects of fractional subsets of the lattice. The latter feature leads to analysis by interior point linear programming, which appears to be a very effective as well as efficient approximation approach to discrete inversion problems.

2.1   Introduction

The central problem of tomography is to reconstruct a faithful image of local relative densities within a physical structure from aggregate density information on linear manifolds that intersect the structure. In practice, the linear manifolds are usually lines, and often are planes for three-dimensional structures or hyperplanes for "structures" of dimensionality greater than three. The usual continuous model for tomography attempts to reconstruct a density function $f(x)$ for x in $\mathbf{R}^2$ or $\mathbf{R}^3$ from knowledge of its line integrals $\int_L f(x)dx$ for lines L through the space. Appropriate quadratures (Shepp and Logan [1]; Shepp and Kruskal [2]) of the Radon inversion formula are used, with Fourier transforms, Jacobians, and other concepts from calculus and continuous mathematics playing the main role. However, when the structure is discrete, say with density 1 on a finite set S of points in the integer lattice $\mathbf{Z}^2$ or $\mathbf{Z}^3$ and density 0 elsewhere, and S is not extremely large, a continuous model is inappropriate and a convolution-backprojection approach [2] seems unlikely to work in practice.

Discrete structures with 0-1 densities have motivated new methods of

---

[1] AT&T Labs-Research, 180 Park Avenue, Florham Park, NJ 07932, USA, E-mail: fish@research.att.com

[2] Department of Statistics, Rutgers University, Busch Campus, Piscataway, NJ 08855, USA, E-mail: shepp@stat.rutgers.edu

analysis, some of which are discussed in ensuing sections. An example of such a structure that is described more fully in Schwander *et al.* [3] and Fishburn, Schwander, Shepp, and Vanderbei [4], concerns atoms' positions in a crystal. It may be possible with refined technology to assess numbers of atoms along certain lines through the crystal. The line counts define the discrete Radon transform of the atomic structure with respect to the family of lines involved. The problem is then to invert the transform, *i.e.*, to deduce the local atomic structure from the line count data. This can be attempted with purely discrete techniques, but these can become unwieldy if S is large. However, there is a way to bring continuous analysis into the picture through interior point linear programming. Although the linear programming approach need not resolve all structural questions, it is computationally efficient and surprisingly effective. We say more about it in Section 2.7 after we develop background on discrete structures.

The next section presents general theory for finite sets in $\mathbb{Z}^n$. We define a discrete Radon base in $\mathbb{R}^n$ as a finite set of linear subspaces of $\mathbb{R}^n$, such as a set of lines through the origin. Translates of the base members give families of "parallel" linear manifolds that are used to define the discrete Radon transform of any finite S in $\mathbb{Z}^n$ by the number of points in S within each manifold. The section then defines notions of uniqueness and additivity for S with respect to the discrete Radon base and proves theorems that characterize these notions in terms of point configurations in $\mathbb{Z}^n$ and fractional subsets of $\mathbb{Z}^n$ that tie in later to interior point linear programming. We note that if S is additive then it is also unique and prove in Section 2.3 that if the discrete Radon base uses only two linear subspaces then additivity and uniqueness are equivalent.

Sections 2.4 through 2.6 supplement the basic theory with results that illustrate special possibilities for finite subsets of $\mathbb{Z}^n$. Section 2.4 shows how the case of two-element bases in Section 2.3 does not extend in a simple way to three-element bases of planes in $\mathbb{Z}^3$. Section 2.5 gives two examples of sets that are additive but not unique. One example uses three lines for a discrete Radon base in $\mathbb{R}^2$; the other uses three planes for the base in $\mathbb{R}^3$. Section 2.6 focuses on line bases in the plane. Its main purpose is to show that when a base uses more than two lines, it may be necessary to consider large subsets of S in an attempt to determine whether S is a set of uniqueness. This contrasts with a two-line base where we need only consider two-element subsets of S to assess uniqueness.

Sections 2.2 through 2.6 provide both theoretical background and practical motivation for the linear programming approach outlined in Section 2.7. We note there that when this approach is applied to an alleged discrete Radon transform with respect to a discrete Radon base, it tells whether any fractional set is consistent with the transform. If the answer is positive, the solution to the linear programming problem gives partial and often complete details about the set or sets in $\mathbb{Z}^n$ that have the given transform.

The final section concludes with a brief summary and a few open problems.

The formulation and results in Sections 2.2 and 2.3 extend [4, 5] to a larger variety of Radon transforms. When [5] was written, we lacked the imagination to consider bases with tilted subspaces, which arose later from the crystal problem raised by Peter Schwander: see [4]. Our work in [4] led to a patent application, but the discrete Radon transform measurements for a real crystal have not been made and their feasibility remains conjectural.

2.2   Uniqueness and additivity

This section presents our basic uniqueness and additivity theorems for nonempty finite subsets S of $\mathbb{Z}^n$, $n \geq 2$. The inputs to each theorem are S and a family $\mathcal{H}$ of linear manifolds in $\mathbb{R}^n$. The two together define the *discrete Radon transform* $v_S : \mathcal{H} \to \{0, 1, 2, \ldots\}$ by

$$v_S(h) = |S \cap h| \quad \text{for all} \quad h \in \mathcal{H} . \tag{2.1}$$

Given S and $\mathcal{H}$, the uniqueness theorem answers the question of whether there is a $T \neq S$ in $\mathbb{Z}^n$ for which $v_T = v_S$, and the additivity theorem answers the question of whether there is a mapping $g : \mathcal{H} \to \mathbb{R}$ such that, for all $x \in \mathbb{Z}^n$,

$$x \in S \Leftrightarrow \sum_{h \in \mathcal{H}} v_x(h)g(h) > 0 . \tag{2.2}$$

Here, and later, v_x is an abbreviation of $v_{\{x\}}$ with

$$v_x(h) = \begin{cases} 1 & \text{if } x \in h \\ 0 & \text{otherwise} . \end{cases} \tag{2.3}$$

As mentioned earlier, there is an intimate one-way relationship between uniqueness and additivity: every additive set is unique, but if $m \geq 3$ in the following definition of a discrete Radon base, then there are sets of uniqueness that are not additive.

The definition we use for $\mathcal{H}$ generalizes previous families of linear manifolds considered for uniqueness and additivity, at no cost of complexity. Each $\mathcal{H}$ will be based on a finite set H of linear manifolds that contain the origin $\mathbf{0}$ of $\mathbb{R}^n$, *i.e.*, of linear subspaces of $\mathbb{R}^n$.

Definition 2.1.   *Let $H = \{h_1, h_2, \ldots, h_m\}$ be a set of linear subspaces of $\mathbb{R}^n$ of dimensions between 1 and $n - 1$ inclusive. Then H is a discrete Radon base if, for all $j, k \in \{1, 2, \ldots, m\}$:*

A1. $\cap_{k=1}^{m} h_k = \{\mathbf{0}\}$;

A2. $j \neq k \Rightarrow h_j \not\subseteq h_k$;

A3. $|h_k \cap \mathbb{Z}^n| \geq 2$.

The predominant type of set H discussed in the literature is a set of lines: see, for example, Crowther, DeRosier, and Klug [6], Gordon and Herman [7], Gardner and McMullen [8], Bianchi and Longinetti [9], Fishburn, Schwander, Shepp, and Vanderbei [4], and Gritzmann and Nivat [10]. At the other dimensional extreme, Fishburn, Lagarias, Reeds, and Shepp [5] consider n hyperplanes that are perpendicular to the axes of $\mathbf{R}^n$.

To describe the effects of **A1–A3**, we first identify $\mathcal{H}$. Given $H = \{h_1, \ldots, h_m\}$, let $\mathcal{H}_k$ be the family of translates of h_k that have nonempty intersections with $\mathbf{Z}^n$, so $h \in \mathcal{H}_k$ if and only if $h = h_k + a$ for some $a \in \mathbf{R}^n$, i.e.,

$$h = \{x + a : x \in h_k\} \quad \text{for some} \quad a \in \mathbf{R}^n , \tag{2.4}$$

and $(h_k + a) \cap \mathbf{Z}^n \neq \emptyset$. We then take

$$\mathcal{H} = \bigcup_{k=1}^m \mathcal{H}_k . \tag{2.5}$$

If $h, h' \in \mathcal{H}_k$ and $h \neq h'$, then $h \cap h' = \emptyset$, so

$$\sum_{h \in \mathcal{H}_k} v_x(h) = 1 \quad \text{for every} \quad x \in \mathbf{Z}^n . \tag{2.6}$$

In other words, if $x \in \mathbf{Z}^n$ then x lies in exactly one member of $\mathcal{H}_k$ for each $k \in \{1, \ldots, m\}$.

It should be apparent from the translates aspect of $\mathcal{H}_k$ that we specify $\mathbf{0} \in h_k$ for each k as a definitional convenience. The roles of **A1–A3** in the definition of a discrete Radon base can be explained as follows.

A1. This implies that every singleton S is a set of uniqueness with respect to H. In particular, if $S = \{x\}$ then x is in exactly one member of $\mathcal{H}_k$ for each k, and the intersection of these m containing linear manifolds equals $\{x\}$. Because every h_k has dimension 1 or more, **A1** requires $m \geq 2$. If $H = \{h_1, h_2\}$, at least one of h_1 and h_2 is a line. If each h_k has dimension $n - 1$, **A1** implies $m \geq n$.

A2. We forbid $h_j \subseteq h_k$ when $j \neq k$ for the sake of parsimony and informational efficiency with respect to Radon transforms. If $h_j \subset h_k$ then h_j is more discerning than h_k because we can always infer v_S on $\mathcal{H}_k$ by aggregation from v_S on $\mathcal{H}_j$. This would render h_k superfluous, so we exclude such inclusions.

A3. Inequality $|h_k \cap \mathbf{Z}^n| \geq 2$ implies that h_k contains a denumerable number of lattice points because any line through two points in $h_k \cap \mathbf{Z}^n$ lies in h_k and intersects $\mathbf{Z}^n$ infinitely often. If $\mathbf{0}$ were the only lattice point in h_k, knowledge of v_S on $\mathcal{H}_k$ would imply knowledge of S and there would be nothing more to say. **A3** also relates to two practical concerns in measuring or assessing v_S when S is not fully known. One is an interest in discerning density differentials for v_S over different members of $\mathcal{H}_k$. The other involves calibrational accuracy within bounded subsets of $\mathbf{Z}^n$, since unrealistically sensitive calibration of a measuring instrument could be implied by $h_k \cap$ (large bounded subset of $\mathbb{Z}^n$ around $\mathbf{0}$) = $\{\mathbf{0}\}$: see [4] for elaboration.

Let H be a discrete Radon base in $\mathbb{R}^n$. We say that finite $S \subseteq \mathbb{Z}^n$ is *a set of uniqueness with respect to H*, or that *S is H-unique*, if $T \subseteq \mathbb{Z}^n$ and $v_T = v_S$ imply $T = S$. Consequently, if $v : \mathcal{H} \to \{0, 1, 2, \ldots\}$ is the (discrete) Radon transform of some set of uniqueness with respect to H, then precisely one S has $v_S = v$. If v is not the Radon transform for some H-unique set, then $\{S \subseteq \mathbb{Z}^n : v_S = v\}$ is empty or has at least two members.

Given H as above, we say that finite $S \subseteq \mathbb{Z}^n$ *is additive with respect to H*, or that *S is H-additive*, if some $g : \mathcal{H} \to \mathbb{R}$ satisfies (2.2) for all $x \in \mathbb{Z}^n$. Because $\sum_\mathcal{H} v_x(h) g(h) > 0$ is preserved when a suitably small positive constant is subtracted from g, we can assume that when S is H-additive and (2.2) holds, we also have

$$\sum_{h \in \mathcal{H}} v_x(h) g(h) < 0 \quad \text{for all} \quad x \in \mathbb{Z}^n \setminus S . \tag{2.7}$$

Additivity is more demanding than uniqueness because every H-additive S is H-unique but, when $m \geq 3$, not all H-unique sets are H-additive. We refer to a unique but nonadditive set as a *nonadditive set of uniqueness*.

Our comparison between uniqueness and additivity will be enriched by considering mappings of $\mathbb{Z}^n$ into $[0, 1]$ as well as into $\{0, 1\}$. We denote the set of mappings into $\{0, 1\}$ by E and into $[0, 1]$ by F subject to

$$f \in E \cup F \Rightarrow \{x \in \mathbb{Z}^n : f(x) > 0\} \text{ is finite} , \tag{2.8}$$

and define $f(\Lambda)$ as $\sum_{x \in A} f(x)$. Given S and H, let

$$E_{S,H} = \{f \in E : f(h \cap \mathbb{Z}^n) = v_S(h) \text{ for all } h \in \mathcal{H}\} , \tag{2.9}$$

$$F_{S,H} = \{f \in F : f(h \cap \mathbb{Z}^n) = v_S(h) \text{ for all } h \in \mathcal{H}\} . \tag{2.10}$$

We refer to members of $F_{S,H}$ as *fractional sets*. Because $f, f' \in F_{S,H}$ and $0 < \lambda < 1$ imply $\lambda f + (1 - \lambda) f' \in F_{S,H}$, $F_{S,H}$ is convex and can be analyzed by continuous methods, including linear programming. Functions in $E_{S,H}$ are extreme members of $F_{S,H}$, each of which is the characteristic function χ_T of some finite $T \subseteq \mathbb{Z}^n$. Our definition of uniqueness says that S is H-unique if and only if $E_{S,H} = \{\chi_S\}$. We prove below that if S is H-additive then $F_{S,H} = E_{S,H}$, and if S is a nonadditive set of uniqueness then $E_{S,H} \subset F_{S,H}$.

The final definitions needed for our basic theorems refer to H-based balances between same-sized lists of sets in S and in $\mathbb{Z}^n \setminus S$. A *K-bad H-configuration* for S, $K \geq 2$, is a pair of lists $x^1, x^2, \ldots, x^K$ of K distinct points in S and $y^1, y^2, \ldots, y^K$ of K distinct points in $\mathbb{Z}^n \setminus S$ such that

$$\sum_{k=1}^{K} v_{x^k}(h) = \sum_{k=1}^{K} v_{y^k}(h) \quad \text{for every} \quad h \in \mathcal{H} . \tag{2.11}$$

A *bad H-configuration* for S is any K-bad H-configuration for S. We refer to a 2-bad H-configuration as a *bad H-rectangle*. Because each point in $\mathbb{Z}^n$ lies in m members of $\mathcal{H}$, bad H-rectangles can exist only when $m = 2$ if all h_k are lines. If $000, 111 \in S$ and $001, 110 \notin S$ for $n = 3$, we have a bad H-rectangle for $m = 3$ when H consists of the three planes through the origin perpendicular to the axes, or when H consists of two such planes and its third member is the line through 000 and 110.

A *weakly K-bad H-configuration* for S is the same as a K-bad H-configuration except that the members of the x and y lists need not be distinct. We sometimes note explicitly the multiplicity of each distinct member in a list. Let $(\gamma_1 z^1, \ldots, \gamma_I z^I)$ denote a list of $\sum \gamma_i$ points in $\mathbb{Z}^n$ in which z^i appears exactly γ_i times, the z^i are distinct, and each γ_i is a positive integer. Then a weakly K-bad H-configuration consists of $(\alpha_1 x^1, \ldots, \alpha_I x^I)$ from S and $(\beta_1 y^1, \ldots, \beta_J y^J)$ from $\mathbb{Z}^n \setminus S$ such that $\sum \alpha_i = \sum \beta_j = K$ and

$$\sum_{i=1}^{I} \alpha_i v_{x^i}(h) = \sum_{j=1}^{J} \beta_j v_{y^j}(h) \quad \text{for every} \quad h \in \mathcal{H} . \tag{2.12}$$

We say that S has a *weakly bad H-configuration* if it has a weakly K-bad H-configuration for some $K \geq 2$.

Our basic theorems characterize uniqueness and additivity, respectively. They apply to all $n \geq 2$, all nonempty finite $S \subseteq \mathbb{Z}^n$, and all discrete Radon bases $H = \{h_1, \ldots, h_m\}$, $m \geq 2$.

Theorem 2.1. *The following are mutually equivalent:*

(1) S is H-unique;

(2) S has no bad H-configuration;

(3) $E_{S,H} = \{\chi_S\}$.

Theorem 2.2. *The following are mutually equivalent:*

(1) S is H-additive;

(2) S has no weakly bad H-configuration;

(3) $F_{S,H} = \{\chi_S\}$.

It follows immediately that S is unique if it is additive, and that S is a nonadditive set of uniqueness if and only if $F_{S,H}$ has an infinity of solutions but only one 0-1 solution, namely χ_S.

We conclude this section with proofs of the theorems, beginning with the proof of Theorem 2.1.

Proof: (1) and (3) are equivalent by the definitions.

(1)⇒(2): If S has a bad H-configuration, uniqueness is contradicted by replacing in S the points in the S list of the bad configuration by those in its $\mathbb{Z}^n \setminus S$ list.

(2)⇒(1): If S is not H-unique because $T \neq S$ and $v_T = v_S$, then $v_{T \setminus (S \cap T)} = v_{S \setminus (S \cap T)}$ and the points in $S \setminus (S \cap T)$ and in $T \setminus (S \cap T)$ form two lists for a bad H-configuration.   □

The following discretized linear separation theorem [11] will be used in the proof of Theorem 2.2. The scalar product of $a, x \in \mathbf{R}^N$, $a_1 x_1 + \cdots + a_N x_N$, is denoted by $\langle a, x \rangle$.

Lemma 2.1.   *Suppose $J \in \{1, 2, \ldots\}$ and $z^1, z^2, \ldots, z^J \in \mathbb{Z}^N$. Then exactly one of [A] and [B] holds:*

[A] *For some $a \in \mathbf{R}^N$, $\langle a, z^j \rangle > 0$ for $j = 1, \ldots, J$;*

[B] *There are $r_1, \ldots, r_J \in \{0, 1, 2, \ldots\}$ with $\sum r_j > 0$ such that*

$$\sum_{j=1}^{J} r_j z_i^j = 0 \quad for \quad i = 1, \ldots, N .$$
(2.13)

Proof: To prove Theorem 2.2, we show that $(2) \Rightarrow (1) \Rightarrow (3) \Rightarrow (2)$.

$(2) \Rightarrow (1)$: We prove that if S is not H-additive then it has a weakly bad H-configuration. Assume that S is not H-additive. Then, for every $g : \mathcal{H} \to \mathbf{R}$,

$$\sum_{h \in \mathcal{H}} v_x(h) g(h) > 0 \text{ for all } x \in S$$

$$\Rightarrow \sum_{h \in \mathcal{H}} v_x(h) g(h) > 0 \text{ for some } x \in \mathbb{Z}^n \setminus S .$$
(2.14)

Define $\mathcal{H}_0 \subset \mathcal{H}$ and $X_0 \subset \mathbb{Z}^n$ by

$$\mathcal{H}_0 = \{h \in \mathcal{H} : v_x(h) = 1 \quad \text{for some} \quad x \in S\}$$
$$= \{h \in \mathcal{H} : x \in h \quad \text{for some} \quad x \in S\} ,$$
(2.15)

$$X_0 = \{x \in \mathbb{Z}^n : v_x(h) = 0 \quad \text{for all} \quad h \in \mathcal{H} \setminus \mathcal{H}_0\}$$
$$= \{x \in \mathbb{Z}^n : v_x(h) = 1 \quad \text{for } m \quad h \in \mathcal{H}_0\} .$$
(2.16)

Clearly, $S \subseteq X_0$. Let

$$N = |\mathcal{H}_0| \leq m|S| ,$$
(2.17)

$$J = |X_0| \leq \binom{N}{m} .$$
(2.18)

By making g highly negative on $\mathcal{H} \setminus \mathcal{H}_0$, we can get $\sum v_x(h)g(h) < 0$ for all $x \in \mathbf{Z}^n \setminus X_0$ without affecting the sums for X_0. Therefore, failure of additivity implies that, for all $g : \mathcal{H}_0 \to \mathbf{R}$,

$$\sum_{\mathcal{H}_0} v_x(h)g(h) > 0 \quad \text{for all} \quad x \in S \Rightarrow \sum_{\mathcal{H}_0} v_x(h)g(h) > 0 \quad \text{for some} \quad x \in X_0 \setminus S .$$

Let b map $\mathcal{H}_0$ onto $\{1, 2, \ldots, N\}$ and c map X_0 onto $\{1, 2, \ldots, J\}$. Then define $z^{c(x)} \in \mathbf{R}^N$ for $x \in X_0$ by

$$x \in S : \qquad z^{c(x)}_{b(h)} = \begin{cases} 1 & \text{if } x \in h \\ 0 & \text{otherwise} , \end{cases}$$

$$x \in X_0 \setminus S : \quad z^{c(x)}_{b(h)} = \begin{cases} -1 & \text{if } x \in h \\ 0 & \text{otherwise} , \end{cases}$$

and define $a \in \mathbf{R}^N$ by $a_{b(h)} = g(h)$. Our presumed failure of additivity says that there is no $a \in \mathbf{R}^N$ such that $\langle a, z^j \rangle > 0$ for $j = 1, \ldots, J$, in view of (2.7). Hence [A] of Lemma 2.1 is false. Therefore, by [B], there are nonnegative integers $r_1, \ldots, r_J$ with $\sum r_j > 0$ such that

$$\sum_{j=1}^{J} r_j z^j_{b(h)} = 0 \quad \text{for every} \quad h \in \mathcal{H}_0 , \tag{2.19}$$

or, equivalently,

$$\sum_{x \in S} r_{c(x)} v_x(h) = \sum_{x \in X_0 \setminus S} r_{c(x)} v_x(h) \quad \text{for every} \quad h \in \mathcal{H}_0 . \tag{2.20}$$

This holds also on $\mathcal{H} \setminus \mathcal{H}_0$ because $v_x(h) = 0$ for all $x \in X_0$ when $h \in \mathcal{H} \setminus \mathcal{H}_0$. It therefore defines a weakly K-bad H-configuration with $K = \sum_S r_{c(x)} = \sum_{X_0 \setminus S} r_{c(x)}$. The α_i for (2.12) are the $r_{c(x)} > 0$ for $x \in S$, and the β_j are the $r_{c(x)} > 0$ for $x \in X_0 \setminus S$.

(1) $\Rightarrow$ (3): Suppose S is H-additive and f is a fractional set in $F_{S,H}$. We show that $f = \chi_S$. Let $g : \mathcal{H} \to \mathbf{R}$ satisfy (2.2) and (2.7). By definition, $f : \mathbf{Z}^n \to [0, 1]$ satisfies $f(\mathbf{Z}^n \cap h) = v_S(h)$ for all $h \in \mathcal{H}$. Therefore

$$\begin{aligned} 0 &= \sum_{h \in \mathcal{H}} g(h)[v_S(h) - f(\mathbf{Z}^n \cap h)] \\ &= \sum_{h \in \mathcal{H}} g(h) \sum_{x \in \mathbf{Z}^n \cap h} [\chi_S(x) - f(x)] \\ &= \sum_{x \in \mathbf{Z}^n} [\chi_S(x) - f(x)] \sum_{h \in \mathcal{H} : x \in h} g(h) . \end{aligned} \tag{2.21}$$

If we sum first on $\mathcal{H}$, holding $x \in \mathbf{Z}^n$ fixed, then for $x \in S$ we have $\sum_{h \in \mathcal{H} : x \in h} g(h) > 0$ by (2.2), along with $\chi_S(x) - f(x) \geq 0$ because $\chi_S(x) = 1$ when $x \in S$ and $0 \leq f(x) \leq 1$, so the term for x in (2.21) is nonnegative. On the other hand, if $x \in \mathbb{Z}^n \setminus S$, then $\sum_{h \in \mathcal{H}: x \in h} g(h) < 0$ by (2.7), along with $\chi_S(x) - f(x) \leq 0$ because $\chi_S(x) = 0$, so the term for x in (2.21) is again nonnegative. Since the outside sum over $\mathbb{Z}^n$ in (2.21) equals 0, it follows that $\chi_S(x) - f(x) = 0$ for all $x \in \mathbb{Z}^n$, i.e., that $f = \chi_S$.

(3) $\Rightarrow$ (2): We show that if S has a weakly bad H-configuration then $f \neq \chi_S$ for some $f \in F_{S,H}$. Assume that S has a weakly bad H-configuration as characterized by (2.12). For small $\lambda > 0$ let

$$b_j = \lambda \beta_j \quad \text{and} \quad a_i = 1 - \lambda \alpha_i \quad \text{for} \quad i = 1, \ldots, I \quad \text{and} \quad j = 1, \ldots, J .$$

Then $0 < b_j < 1$ and $0 < a_i < 1$ for all i and j. Also, by (2.12), for all $h \in \mathcal{H}$

$$\sum_{i=1}^{I} a_i v_{x^i}(h) + \sum_{j=1}^{J} b_j v_{y^j}(h) = \sum_{i=1}^{I} v_{x^i}(h) . \tag{2.22}$$

Define $f : \mathbb{Z}^n \to [0,1]$ by

$$\begin{aligned}
f(x^i) &= a_i & i &= 1, \ldots, I , \\
f(y^j) &= b_j & j &= 1, \ldots, J , \\
f(z) &= \chi_S(z) & \text{for all } & z \in \mathbb{Z}^n \setminus \{x^1, \ldots, x^I, y^1, \ldots, y^J\}.
\end{aligned} \tag{2.23}$$

Then, for all $h \in \mathcal{H}$,

$$\sum_{x \in \mathbf{Z}^n \cap h} f(x) = v_S(h) = \sum_{x \in \mathbf{Z}^n \cap h} \chi_S(x) , \tag{2.24}$$

so $f \in F_{S,H}$. By definition, $f \neq \chi_S$. $\square$

2.3 Bad rectangles

In contrast to our claim that there can be nonadditive sets of uniqueness when $m \geq 3$ for a discrete Radon base, we prove in this section that additivity and uniqueness are equivalent when $m = 2$. We recall that when $H = \{h_1, h_2\}$ is a discrete Radon base, at least one of h_1 and h_2 must be a line. If h_1 is a line and $h_1 \not\subseteq h_2$, as in **A2**, then for every $x \in \mathbb{Z}^n$, $x \in h \cap h'$ for $h \in \mathcal{H}_1$ and $h' \in \mathcal{H}_2$ implies that $h \cap h' = \{x\}$.

Theorem 2.3. *Suppose $H = \{h_1, h_2\}$ is a discrete Radon base and S is a nonempty finite subset of $\mathbb{Z}^n$. Then the following are mutually equivalent:*

(1) S is H-unique;

(2) S is H-additive;

(3) $F_{S,H} = \{\chi_S\}$;

(4) S has no weakly bad H-configuration;

(5) S has no bad H-configuration;

(6) S has no bad H-rectangle.

Proof: We know by the definitions and Theorems 2.1 and 2.2 that (4) $\Rightarrow$ (3) $\Rightarrow$ (2) $\Rightarrow$ (1) $\Rightarrow$ (5) $\Rightarrow$ (6). We complete the proof of Theorem 2.3 by showing that (6) $\Rightarrow$ (5) and (5) $\Rightarrow$ (4).

(5) $\Rightarrow$ (4): We prove that if S has a weakly bad H-configuration then it has a bad H-configuration. Here and later we write

$$x =_j y \Leftrightarrow (x, y \in \mathbb{Z}^n, \ x \text{ and } y \text{ are in same } h \in \mathcal{H}_j) \ . \tag{2.25}$$

Suppose S has a weakly bad H-configuration as in (2.11), multiplicities allowed. Let $a^1 = x^1$ and form an alternating sequence

$$a^1 =_1 b^1 =_2 a^2 =_1 b^2 =_2 a^3 =_1 b^3 =_2 \cdots \ , \tag{2.26}$$

where each a^i is an $x^k \in S$ and each b^i is a $y^k \in \mathbb{Z}^n \setminus S$. The construction is validated by (2.11). Because K is finite, we encounter a term used previously. When this first occurs, we obtain an alternating cycle by trimming the sequence just before the previous twin and can assume with no loss of generality that

$$a^1 =_1 b^1 =_2 a^2 =_1 b^2 =_2 \cdots =_2 a^r =_1 b^r =_2 a^1 \tag{2.27}$$

with all a^i and b^i distinct. We have, say

$$\begin{aligned} a^i, b^i \in h_1^i \in \mathcal{H}_1 \quad &\text{for} \quad i = 1, 2, \ldots, r \ , \\ b^i, a^{i+1} \in h_2^i \in \mathcal{H}_2 \quad &\text{for} \quad i = 1, 2, \ldots, r \ (a^{r+1} = a^1). \end{aligned} \tag{2.28}$$

It follows that $\sum_i v_{a^i}(h) = \sum_i v_{b^i}(h)$ for all $h \in \mathcal{H}$, so we have an r-bad H-configuration.

(6) $\Rightarrow$ (5). Suppose S has the r-bad H-configuration of the preceding paragraph. We show that S has a bad H-rectangle. We are done if $r = 2$, so suppose $r \geq 3$:

$$a^1 =_1 b^1 =_2 a^2 =_1 b^2 =_2 a^3 =_1 b^3 =_2 \cdots \ . \tag{2.29}$$

Assume without loss of generality that $h_1 \in H$ is a line. Because $a^2 \neq b^2$ and $a^2 =_1 b^2$, a^2 and b^2 are on the same $\mathcal{H}_1$ line but in different members of $\mathcal{H}_2$, and the one of these which contains b^2 also contains a^3 since $b^2 =_2 a^3$. Let t be the point on the $\mathcal{H}_1$ line through a^3 where this line intersects the member of $\mathcal{H}_2$ that contains a^2, so

$$a^2 =_2 t =_1 a^3 \ . \tag{2.30}$$

The point t is distinct from a^2, b^2 and a^3, and lies in $\mathbb{Z}^n$ by the lattice structure. We also have

$$b^1 =_2 t =_1 b^3 \tag{2.31}$$

by transitivity: $\{t =_2 a^2, a^2 =_2 b^1\} \Rightarrow t =_2 b^1$; $\{t =_1 a^3, a^3 =_1 b^3\} \Rightarrow t =_1 b^3$. If $t \notin S$, we have a bad H-rectangle with S list a^2, a^3 and $\mathbb{Z}^n \setminus S$ list b^2, t. If $t \in S$, we replace $(a^2 =_1 b^2 =_2 a^3)$ in the initial display of this paragraph by t to obtain a shorter sequence

$$a^1 =_1 b^1 =_2 t =_1 b^3 =_2 \cdots , \tag{2.32}$$

and continue, as needed, until a bad H-rectangle appears.   □

2.4 No bad rectangles

This section is the first of three that illustrates facets of uniqueness and additivity going beyond Theorems 2.1, 2.2, and 2.3. We focus here on bad rectangles.

When $n = 3$, $m = 3$, and H consists of three planes through $\mathbf{0}$ that are perpendicular to the axes, many $S \subseteq \mathbf{Z}^3$ that are not H-unique have bad H-rectangles. This is true, for example, of $S = \{000, 111\}$ and, more generally of any S that contains ijk and $\alpha\beta\gamma$ but not $i\beta\gamma$ or αjk. On the other hand, and in distinction to $m = 2$ in Theorem 2.3, there are S for this context that have no bad H-rectangle and are not sets of uniqueness. The following example from Fishburn et al. [5] shows this for a 14-point S within $\{1, 2, 3\}^3$. Let

$$S_1 = \{111, 222, 333, 113, 121, 122, 123, 131, 133, 221, 223, 231, 233, 323\} .$$

Theorem 2.4. *Suppose $n = 3$ and $H = \{h_1, h_2, h_3\}$ with each h_j a plane perpendicular to an axis of R^3. Then S_1 has no bad H-rectangle and it is not a set of uniqueness with respect to H.*

Proof: S_1 is not H-unique because the S_1 list $111, 222, 333$ and the $\mathbf{Z}^3 \setminus S_1$ list $132, 213, 321$ define a 3-bad H-configuration: see Theorem 2.1.

To show that S_1 has no bad H-rectangle, suppose to the contrary that it has a bad H-rectangle whose four points form a set $C \subseteq \{1, 2, 3\}^3$. Suppose that some point in $S_1 \cap C$ ends in 2. Then, since only 122 and 222 from S_1 end in 2, one of the two points in $(\{1, 2, 3\}^3 \setminus S_1) \cap C$ has 2 in its second position. Since the only such points are 321 and 322, some point in $S_1 \cap C$ has 3 in its first position and must be either 323 or 333. Therefore, some point in $(\{1, 2, 3\}^3 \setminus S_1) \cap C$ has 3 in its third position and can be only 213 or 313. Hence

$S_1 \cap C$ contains either 122 or 222, and either 323 or 333;
$(\{1, 2, 3\}^3 \setminus S_1) \cap C$ contains 321 or 322, and 213 or 313.

However, no choices here produce a bad H-rectangle.

It follows that neither point in $S_1 \cap C$ ends in 2. Similarly, neither point in $(\{1, 2, 3\}^3 \setminus S_1) \cap C$ ends in 3. When all points that end in 2 or 3 are deleted from $\{1, 2, 3\}^3$, we are left with

S_1 points 111, 121, 131, 221 and 231;
$\{1, 2, 3\}^3 \setminus S_1$ points 211, 311, 321 and 331.

Since nothing left in $\{1, 2, 3\}^3 \setminus S_1$ begins with 1, and nothing left in S_1 begins with 3, further reductions leave only 221 and 231 from S_1 and 211 from $\{1, 2, 3\}^3 \setminus S_1$, and it follows that S_1 has no bad H-rectangle. $\qquad\square$

2.5 Nonadditive sets of uniqueness

This section presents two examples of nonadditive sets of uniqueness. The first, from [4], uses three lines for H in the plane and an 11-point S. The second, from [5], uses three hyperplanes for H in R^3 and a 60-point S in $\{1, 2, 3, 4, 5\}^3$.

   Although we have found it hard to construct small-S examples of nonadditive sets of uniqueness, it seems likely for large S that such sets are abundant. It might be true for some fixed H with $m \geq 3$ that the proportion of nonsimilar sets of uniqueness that are also additive goes to 0 as $|S| \to \infty$, but we do not presently have a good way of attacking the problem.

   Our first example of nonadditive uniqueness takes $S \in \mathbf{Z}^2$ with $H = \{l_1, l_2, l_3\}$, where each l_k is a line through the origin. We denote a nonorigin point on l_1, l_2, and l_3 by (α_1, α_2), (β_1, β_2), and (γ_1, γ_2), respectively. By A3, α_1 through γ_2 can be assumed to be integers. We refer to (α_1, α_2) as the *direction* of l_1, and do likewise for other lines through the origin.

Theorem 2.5.   *Suppose $n = 2$ and $H = \{l_1, l_2, l_3\}$ is a discrete Radon base. Every such H has an 11-point nonadditive set of uniqueness.*

Proof: Suppose that $S \subseteq \mathbf{Z}^2$ is a nonadditive set of uniqueness with respect to directions $(\alpha_1, \alpha_2) = (1, 0)$, $(\beta_1, \beta_2) = (0, 1)$, and $(\gamma_1, \gamma_2) = (1, 1)$. Given any other (α_1, α_2), (β_1, β_2) and (γ_1, γ_2), A2 implies that $\alpha_1\beta_2 \neq \alpha_2\beta_1$, $\alpha_1\gamma_2 \neq \alpha_2\gamma_1$ and $\beta_1\gamma_2 \neq \beta_2\gamma_1$, and the 2×2 matrix

$$T = \begin{bmatrix} \alpha_1 c_1 & \gamma_1 c_2 \\ \alpha_2 c_1 & \gamma_2 c_2 \end{bmatrix} \qquad c_1 = \beta_1\gamma_2 - \beta_2\gamma_1, \;\; c_2 = \alpha_1\beta_2 - \alpha_2\beta_1 \qquad (2.33)$$

is nonsingular. We use T to define a transform on $\mathbf{Z}^2$, which maps (i, j) into

$$T(i, j)' = (i\alpha_1 c_1 + j\gamma_1 c_2, i\alpha_2 c_1 + j\gamma_2 c_2)' , \qquad (2.34)$$

where the prime denotes transposition. The transform maps $\mathbf{Z}^2$ into $\mathbf{Z}^2$ and preserves the parallel aspect of the lines in each $\mathcal{H}_k$. It then follows that $\{Ts' : s \in S\}$ is a nonadditive set of uniqueness with respect to (α_1, α_2), (β_1, β_2), and (γ_1, γ_2).

It remains to show that there is an 11-point nonadditive set of uniqueness with respect to directions $(1,0)$, $(0,1)$, and $(1,1)$. Our 11 points for this are

a	$=$	$(10,11)$	d	$=$	$(11,0)$	g	$=$	$(0,32)$	j	$=$	$(38,24)$
b	$=$	$(7,9)$	e	$=$	$(24,19)$	h	$=$	$(48,70)$	k	$=$	$(49,8)$.
c	$=$	$(9,7)$	f	$=$	$(16,35)$	i	$=$	$(35,25)$

Let rst denote a point in $\mathbb{Z}^2$ and not in $S = \{a, \ldots, k\}$ that lies in the horizontal line through $r \in S$, the vertical line through $s \in S$, and the 45° line through $t \in S$. There are 13 rst points. One is $kac = (10,8)$. The other 12 are

$$acb, gah, bdc, chk, afe, kba, egf, fkj, dai, iea, jid, hjg .$$

These 12 give the $\mathbb{Z}^2 \setminus S$ list of a weakly 12-bad H-configuration whose S list is $a, a, b, c, d, e, f, g, h, i, j, k$. By Theorem 2.2, S is not H-additive.

We now show that S has no bad H-configuration, so by Theorem 2.1 it is a set of uniqueness. If rst is in the $\mathbb{Z}^2 \setminus S$ list of a bad configuration then this list must have triples with r second, r third, s first, s third, t first, and t second. We use this fact to prove by contradiction that there is no bad configuration.

Suppose S has a bad H-configuration with S list A and $\mathbb{Z}^2 \setminus S$ list B. Suppose kac is in B. Then c is in A, so acb is in B; then b is A, so bdc is in B. But then c appears twice in the third position of B members, $i.e.$, in kac and bdc, so c would have multiplicity two or more in the A list, a contradiction to distinct terms in each list for a bad H-configuration. We conclude that kac is not in B.

Suppose h appears in some triple of the B list. Then all letters in $\{a, b, \ldots, k\}$ appear in B. In particular, since the only rst triples with h are hjg, chk, and gah, each of j, g, c, k and a is involved in B's triples; since the only triples with j in first or third position are jid and fkj, each of i, d and f appears in B; then i's presence requires e (by iea) and d's presence requires b (by bdc). We remark also that if any letter other than h appears in B, then h also is involved in B by similar reasoning. It follows that all 12 of the rst triples other than kac are in B. This is a contradiction because A can have at most $|S| = 11$ terms. $\square$

Our second example of nonadditive uniqueness takes $S \subseteq \{1, 2, 3, 4, 5\}^3$ with $H = \{h_1, h_2, h_3\}$ in which the h_k are the planes through the origin of $\mathbf{R}^3$ that are perpendicular to the axes. We denote by S_2 the 60 points in Fig. 2.1 identified by a 1 or a z. Point (x_1, x_2, x_3) in $\{1, \ldots, 5\}^3$ is located in the figure by row x_1 (bottom up), column x_2 (left-to-right), and level x_3 (left array to right array). The points identified by a 0 or a w are in $\mathbb{Z}^3 \setminus S_2$.

Theorem 2.6. S_2 is a nonadditive set of uniqueness.

Proof: S_2 has the weakly 6-bad H-configuration with S_2 list z^1, z^1, z^3, z^4, z^5, z^6 and $\mathbb{Z}^3 \setminus S_2$ list w^1, w^2, w^3, w^4, w^5, w^6. This is easily seen from the fact that, counting z^1 twice, there are equal numbers of z's and w's in each array and

	$x_3 = 1$	$x_3 = 2$	$x_3 = 3$	$x_3 = 4$	$x_3 = 5$
5	$1\ 1\ w^1\ 0\ 0$	$z^3\ 0\ \ 0\ 0\ 0$	$0\ \ 0\ \ 0\ 0\ 0$	$0\ 0\ 0\ 0\ \ 0$	$0\ 0\ 0\ \ 0\ \ 0$
4	$1\ 1\ 1\ \ z^1\ 0$	$1\ \ w^3\ 0\ 0\ 0$	$w^4\ 0\ \ 0\ 0\ 0$	$0\ 0\ 0\ 0\ \ 0$	$0\ 0\ 0\ \ 0\ \ 0$
x_1 \quad 3	$1\ 1\ 1\ \ 1\ \ w^2$	$1\ \ 1\ \ \ 0\ 0\ 0$	$1\ \ z^4\ 0\ 0\ 0$	$0\ 0\ 0\ 0\ \ 0$	$0\ 0\ 0\ \ 0\ \ 0$
2	$1\ 1\ 1\ \ 1\ \ 1$	$1\ \ 1\ \ \ 1\ 1\ 1$	$1\ \ 1\ \ 1\ 1\ 1$	$1\ 1\ 1\ w^5\ 0$	$1\ 1\ z^6\ 0\ \ 0$
1	$1\ 1\ 1\ \ 1\ \ 1$	$1\ \ 1\ \ \ 1\ 1\ 1$	$1\ \ 1\ \ 1\ 1\ 1$	$1\ 1\ 1\ 1\ \ z^5$	$1\ 1\ 1\ \ w^6\ 0$
	$\overline{1\ 2\ 3\ \ 4\ \ 5}$				

x_2

FIGURE 2.1. Nonadditive uniqueness.

in each row and column of the arrays take together. By Theorem 2.2, S_2 is not H-additive.

But S_2 is H-unique. This is verified by three steps:

Step 1. If a z point is removed from S_2, what remains is H-additive and therefore H-unique;

Step 2. Given v_{S_2}, if $T \subseteq \{1, \ldots, 5\}^3$ and $v_T = v_{S_2}$, and if T contains any z point, then $T = S_2$;

Step 3. If no z point is in T, then $v_T \neq v_{S_2}$.

Some details follow.

Step 1. For notational ease, the plane in $\mathbf{R}^3$ that is perpendicular to the x-axis (respectively, y-axis, z-axis) and cuts the axis at x_1 (respectively, x_2, x_3) will be denoted by x_1 (respectively, x_2, x_3). Then $\mathcal{H}_k = \mathbf{Z}$ for each k. We index the $\mathcal{H}_k$ so that $(x_1, x_2, x_3) \in \mathbf{Z}^3$ lies in $x_1 \in \mathcal{H}_1$, $x_2 \in \mathcal{H}_2$ and $x_3 \in \mathcal{H}_3$. For additivity considerations let

$$g(h) = f_k(h) \quad \text{when} \quad h = x_k \in \mathcal{H}_k . \tag{2.35}$$

Then, by (2.2), S is H-additive if and only if, for all $x \in \mathbf{Z}^3$,

$$(x_1, x_2, x_3) \in S \Leftrightarrow f_1(x_1) + f_2(x_2) + f_3(x_3) > 0 . \tag{2.36}$$

In what follows, let $f_k(t) = -10^{10}$ except when $t \in \{1, \ldots, 5\}$, so that $\sum f_i(x_i) < 0$ whenever $x \in \mathbf{Z}^3 \setminus \{1, \ldots, 5\}^3$.

We claim that $S_2 \setminus \{z^j\}$ is H-additive for $j \in \{1, 3, 4, 5, 6\}$. The following f_k values are used for z^1:

	t				
	1	2	3	4	5
f_1	1450	1400	-1948	-2000	-2048
f_2	1300	1250	-1948	-2000	-2048
f_3	3995	749	699	599	549

Thus, $\sum f_k(x_k)$ is $1450 + 1300 + 3995$ for $(x_1, x_2, x_3) = (1, 1, 1)$, $\sum f_k(z_k^1) = f_1(4) + f_2(4) + f_3(1) = -2000 - 2000 + 3995 = -5$, and $\sum f_k(x_k) = -2048 +$

$1300 + 749 = 1$ for $(x_1, x_2, x_3) = (5, 1, 2)$. It is routine to check that (2.36) holds when $S = S_2 \setminus \{z^1\}$, so $S_2 \setminus \{z^1\}$ is H-additive.

The same procedure is used for the other z^j. The values used for z^j are identical to those for z^1 except for the following new values:

$$z^3 : \quad f_1(4) = -1994, \quad f_2(1) = 1294, \quad f_3(2) = 743$$
$$z^4 : \quad f_1(4) = -1994, \quad f_2(2) = 1244, \quad f_3(3) = 693$$
$$z^5 : \quad f_1(1) = 1444, \quad f_2(4) = -1994, \quad f_3(4) = 593$$
$$z^6 : \quad f_1(2) = 1394, \quad f_2(4) = -1994, \quad f_3(5) = 543 .$$

It follows from (2.36) that $S_2 \setminus \{z^j\}$ is H-additive for $3 \leq j \leq 6$.

Step 2. Let the row (x_1), column (x_2) and level (x_3) marginal counts (which are obtained from Fig. 2.1 when $z^j \to 1$ and $w^j \to 0$) for S_2 be denoted respectively by

$$(\alpha_1, \ldots, \alpha_5) \quad = \quad (23, 21, 8, 5, 3) \tag{2.37}$$
$$(\beta_1, \ldots, \beta_5) \quad = \quad (17, 15, 12, 9, 7) \tag{2.38}$$
$$(\gamma_1, \ldots, \gamma_5) \quad = \quad (20, 14, 12, 8, 6) . \tag{2.39}$$

For example, $\alpha_1 = 23$ because the only points in row 1 not in S_2 are w^6 and its right-hand neighbor in level 5; $\gamma_3 = 12$ because S_2 has 12 points in level 3. Each point in S_2 is counted in one row, one column and one level, so $\sum \alpha_i = \sum \beta_i = \sum \gamma_i = 60$. Each α_i, β_i and γ_i is a Radon value $v_{S_2}(h)$ for $h \in \mathcal{H}$. For example, $v_{S_2}(x_2 = 2) = 15$ since 15 points in S_2 lie in the $\mathcal{H}_2$ plane characterized by $x_2 = 2$.

Suppose z^1 is removed from S_2 and the marginals are reduced accordingly: α_4 from 5 to 4, β_4 from 9 to 8, γ_1 from 20 to 19. By Step 1, the modified marginals identify an H-unique set, namely $S_2 \setminus \{z^1\}$. That is, without making any assumptions whatever about which of the 124 points in $\{1, \ldots, 5\}^3 \setminus \{z^1\}$ are in the set of uniqueness S_2', we must get $S_2' = S_2 \setminus \{z^1\}$ from the modified marginals. Consequently, *if we assume at the outset that z^1 is in S_2, then the original marginals imply that S_2 itself is a set of uniqueness.*

The same logic applies to the other z^j. Hence, if any one of the five z^j is presumed to be in S_2, then S_2 is a set of uniqueness. It follows that the only possible way for S_2 *not* to be a set of uniqueness is for some T that contains no z^j to have the same marginals as S_2.

Step 3. To prove that no such T exists, we suppose to the contrary and obtain a contradiction. Since the supposed T excludes all z^j, we place 0's in their cells but leave all others empty in a $5 \times 5 \times 5$ array like that in Fig. 2.1. With the understanding that 0 indicates *not in T*, and 1 indicates *in T*, the proof now proceeds through a sequence of steps that attempt to construct T with the marginals of S_2. We eventually conclude that this is impossible. We omit most of the details of this process, which are fully described in [5], but will illustrate its logic in the next paragraph.

At the beginning we have $\alpha_1 = 23$, so there must be 23 1's and two 0's in the 25 cells of row 1. Because $z^5 = (1, 5, 4)$, we already know the location of one 0 and attempt to discern the position of the other 0 in row 1. Suppose the last level ($x_3 = 5$) has five 1's in its first row. Because $\gamma_5 = 6$, there is then only one 1 above row 1 in level 5. Because $\alpha_2 = 21$ for row 2, this 1 must be in the second row of level 5, with solid 1's in row 2 at all previous levels. Moreover, since $\alpha_1 = 23$ and $\gamma_4 = 8$, the other 0 for row 1 must be in level 4, so there are solid 1's in row 1 at levels 1, 2 and 3. We then have eight 1's in column 5, two each in the first three levels and one each in the last two levels. However, $\beta_5 = 7$, so we arrive at a contradiction and conclude that the second 0 for row 1 must be in level 5.

The next two steps show that row 2 of level 4 has exactly four 1's, and that row 2 of level 5 has exactly two 1's. The process continues until we obtain a final contradiction to the supposed existence of T. $\square$

2.6   Planar sets and lines

Theorem 2.3 says that if $m = 2$ then uniqueness and additivity can be assessed by looking only at two-point subsets of S regardless of the cardinality of S. Our next theorem shows that there is no upper bound on K, apart from $|S|$, in deciding whether S has a K-bad H-configuration for $m = 3$ when $n = 2$ and each $h \in H$ is a line. Theorem 2.8 gives related results for four-line discrete Radon bases in the plane. Both theorems apply to uniqueness. We do not have similar results for additivity but note that Fishburn [12], [13] addresses the additivity question in a slightly different context. (See also Chapter 3 written by Kong and Herman.)

Theorem 2.7.   *Suppose $n = 2$ and $H = \{l_1, l_2, l_3\}$ in a three-line discrete Radon base. Then for every $K \geq 3$ there is an $S \subseteq \mathbb{Z}^2$ with $|S| = K$ such that S is not H-unique but every nonempty proper subset of S is H-unique.*

Proof: We prove the theorem for directions $(1, 0)$, $(0, 1)$, and $(1, 1)$. Transformation T in the proof of Theorem 2.5 then shows that the result holds for every triple of directions for which $\{l_1, l_2, l_3\}$ is a discrete Radon base.

Define x^k and y^k for $k = 1, \ldots, K$, $K \geq 3$, by

$$
\begin{aligned}
x^1 &= (1, K-1) & y^1 &= (2, K), \\
x^k &= (k+1, K-k+2) & y^k &= (k-1, K-k) & &\text{for even } k < K, \\
x^k &= (k-1, K-k) & y^k &= (k+1, K-k+2) & &\text{for odd } k, 3 \leq k < K
\end{aligned}
$$

and

$$
\begin{aligned}
x^K &= (K, 2) & y^K &= (K-1, 1) & &\text{if } K \text{ is even}, \\
x^K &= (K-1, 1) & y^K &= (K, 2) & &\text{if } K \text{ is odd}.
\end{aligned}
$$

Figure 2.2 illustrates this for $K = 6, 7$.

Take $S = \{x^1, \ldots, x^K\}$ and let an alleged bad configuration have S list A and $\mathbb{Z}^2 \setminus S$ list B. All points in B must be in $\{1, \ldots, K\}^2$.

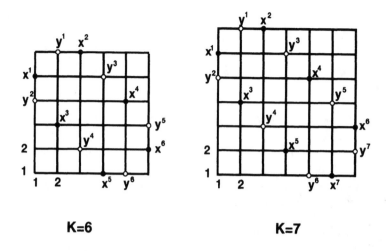

K=6   K=7

FIGURE 2.2. Planar arrays for three directions.

Suppose x^1 is in A. Then y^1 is in B because y^1 is the only non-S point in $\{1, \ldots, K\}^2$ on the 45° line through x^1. Also, x^2 is in A because it is the only S point on the horizontal line through y^1. The possible positions for a B match for x^2 on its 45° line are $(2, K-1)$ and $(1, K-2) = y^2$, but the first of these is infeasible because y^1 is on the same vertical line and there is only one S point on that line, namely x^3, which must be in A. The only feasible point for B on the 45° line through x^3 is $y^3 = (4, K-1)$ because rows one and three (top down on Fig. 2.2) and column one already have points (y^1 and y^2) in B. Next, x^4 is in A because it is the only S point in the row of y^2, and y^4 is in B because it is the only non-S point in $\{1, \ldots, K\}^2$ on the 45° line through x^4 that does not already have a B point in the same row or column. Continuation implies that the bad configuration has every x^k in A and every y^k in B. It is evident that these lists form a K-bad configuration.

Suppose x^1 is not in A. Then there is no B point in the row, column, or 45° line through x^1, and it follows that x^2 is not in A. Then there is no B point in the row, column, or 45° line through x^2, and it follows (consider the 45° line through x^3) that x^3 is not in A. Continuation implies that $A = \emptyset$, a contradiction, and we conclude that S has no J-bad configuration for $J < K$.   □

In the language of logic (Scott and Suppes [14]), Theorem 2.7 says that the planar theory of uniqueness for three directions is not axiomatizable by a universal sentence. The next theorem shows that this is true also for four direction, at least when they are the most natural ones, i.e., horizontal, vertical, 45°, and −45°.

Theorem 2.8. *Suppose $n = 2$ and $H = \{l_1, l_2, l_3, l_4\}$ with directions $(1, 0)$, $(0, 1)$, $(1, 1)$ and $(-1, 1)$. For every even $K \geq 4$ there is an $S \subseteq \mathbb{Z}^2$ with $|S| = K$ such that S is not H-unique but every nonempty proper subset of S is H-unique. For every odd $K \geq 7$ there is an $S \subseteq \mathbb{Z}^2$ with $|S| = K$ that has a K-bad H-configuration.*

Proof: Given the hypotheses, the construction of the proof of Theorem 2.7 shows that every even $K \geq 4$ has a K-point S with a K-bad H-configuration but no J-bad H-configuration for $J < K$. This is not true for odd K because the construction is not balanced in the $-45°$ direction.

The conclusion of Theorem 2.8 for odd $K \geq 7$ is obtained by splicing a mirror image of our preceding $|S| = 4$ array onto an $|S| = K - 3$ array by placing the left-most y of the $|S| = 4$ array on top of the right-most x of the $|S| = K - 3$ array and deleting those two from the joined lists. This corrects the $-45°$ defect in our preceding odd-K array and yields a K-bad H-configuration. However, S in these cases also has a 4-bad H-configuration, so at least one proper subset of S is not H-unique.   □

Theorem 2.8 leaves two questions for its four-directional H. The first is whether any odd $K \geq 7$ has an S with $|S| = K$ that is not H-unique while every nonempty proper subset is H-unique. We leave this open.

The second concerns $K = 5$. An example in Bianchi and Longinetti [9] shows that, when $|S| = 5$, most families of four directions admit an S with a 5-bad configuration. Because their analysis is not confined to $\mathbb{Z}^2$, we generalize and allow lines that contain only the origin in $\mathbb{Z}^2$.

Theorem 2.9. *Suppose $n = 2$ and lines l_1 through l_4 through the origin have directions $(1, 0)$, $(0, 1)$, $(1, r)$ and $(-1, s)$ with r and s any positive numbers. Then there exist disjoint $A, B \subseteq \mathbb{R}^2$ with $|A| = |B| = 5$ such that every line parallel to one of l_1 through l_4 contains the same number of A points as B points if, and only if, $r \neq s$.*

The conclusion for $r = s = 1$ says that, in sharp contrast to Theorem 2.8 for odd $K \geq 7$, there is no five-point S with a 5-bad H-configuration. Theorem 2.9 corrects an oversight in the preceding paper which alleged a 5-bad configuration for every set of four directions. We conclude this section with its proof.

Proof: Let $n = 2$ with directions $(1, 0)$, $(0, 1)$, $(1, r)$ and $(-1, s)$, $r, s > 0$. Suppose $r \neq s$. Fig. 5 in [4], which is similar to Fig. 2 in [9], displays a 10-point set in which five points for a set A and the other five for a set B satisfy the line-balance conclusion of Theorem 2.9. However, if $r = s$ then two points in the figures coincide, and their deletion (one from A, the other from B) leaves a 4-bad configuration.

We now prove that a 5-bad configuration for the line-balance conclusion of the theorem is impossible when $r = s$. Assume that $r = s$ and let

$$d^1 = (1,0), \quad d^2 = (0,1), \quad d^3 = (1,r), \quad d^4 = (-1,r) . \qquad (2.40)$$

Also let $xd^j y$ mean that x and y lie on a line parallel to the line through $(0,0)$ and d^j. We will say that geometric conclusions implied by $r = s$ follow "by the geometry." For example, if x and y lie on a rectangle's top horizontal edge, u and v lie on the rectangle's right edge, z and w lie on its bottom edge, and $xd^4 v d^3 z$, $yd^4 u d^3 w$, and $xd^2 w$ (same vertical line), then $yd^2 z$ by the geometry.

Suppose, contrary to Theorem 2.9, that disjoint

$$A = \{a_1, a_2, a_3, a_4, x\} \quad \text{and} \quad B = \{b_1, b_2, b_3, b_4, y\} \qquad (2.41)$$

have equal numbers of points on every line parallel to some l_k. Let R be the smallest rectangle that includes $A \cup B$. We assume the following with no loss of generality:

(i) $\{a_1, b_1\}$, $\{a_2, b_2\}$, $\{a_3, b_3\}$, and $\{a_4, b_4\}$ lie in the left, top, right, and bottom edge of R, respectively.

(ii) The bad-configuration matches in B for x in directions d^3 and d^4 lie below x. Then for balance, the bad-configuration matches in A for y in directions d^3 and d^4 lie above y. Horizontal balance then implies that x and y lie in the interior of R.

(iii) a_2 is to the left of b_2 on the top edge of R.

Three exclusive possibilities for x versus y are

(I) $xd^3 y$: x above y on a line sloping upward to the right;
(II) $xd^4 y$: x above y on a line sloping upward to the left;
(III) neither $xd^3 y$ nor $xd^4 y$.

We consider them in turn and show that they yield contradictions.

(I) $xd^3 y$ implies $xd^2 b_4$ or $xd^2 b_2$.

Suppose $xd^2 b_4$. Then $xd^4 b_3$, $b_2 d^2 a_4$ and $a_2 d^2 y$. Because three B points are below x (i.e., b_4, b_3 and y), we need a_1 and a_3 below x for d^1 matches with b_3 and y, respectively. Then $xd^1 b_1$. We then require $b_1 d^3 a_2$, $a_1 d^3 b_2$, $a_4 d^4 b_1$ and $yd^4 a_1$. See Fig. 2.3(Ia) for a slightly warped picture. The last four d^j relationships in conjunction with $a_2 d^2 y$ and $b_2 d^2 a_4$ imply $yd^1 a_4$ by the geometry. But then y is on the lower edge of R, a contradiction.

Suppose $xd^2 b_2$. Then $b_4 d^2 a_2$, $yd^2 a_4$, $xd^4 b_3$, $a_2 d^4 y$ and, because three B points lie below x, $a_1 d^1 b_3$, $yd^1 a_3$ and $b_1 d^1 x$. Balance also requires $b_1 d^3 a_2$, $a_1 d^3 b_2$, $a_1 d^4 b_4$ and $b_1 d^4 a_4$. An inaccurate picture appears in Fig. 2.3(Ib). The last four d^j along with $a_2 d^2 b_4$ imply $b_2 d^2 a_4$ by the geometry. This forces $yd^2 x$, a contradiction.

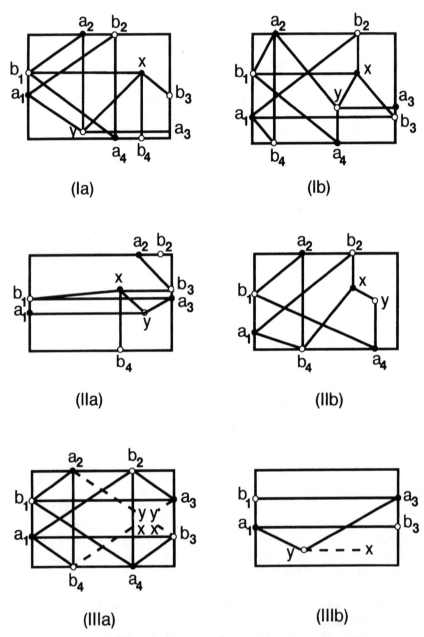

FIGURE 2.3. Case analysis for four directions.

(II) xd^4y implies xd^2b_4 or xd^2b_2.

Suppose xd^2b_4. Then xd^3b_1 and xd^1b_3. Because b_1, y and b_4 are below x, we have a_3 and a_1 below x. Then $b_3d^4a_2$. But this forces a_3 below b_3 and, since b_2 is to the right of a_2, there is no d^4 match for b_2: see Fig. 2.3(IIa).

Suppose xd^2b_2. Then $a_2d^2b_4$, $a_2d^3b_1$, $a_1d^3b_2$, xd^3b_4, yd^2a_4, $a_1d^4b_4$, and $b_1d^4a_4$: se Fig. 2.3(IIb). By the geometry, $b_2d^2a_4$. This forces yd^2x, a contradiction.

(III) Neither xd^3y nor xd^4y implies $a_2d^4yd^3a_3$ or $a_1d^4yd^3a_3$. ($a_1d^4yd^3a_2$ forces $a_1d^3b_2$, placing b_2 left of a_2.)

Suppose $a_2d^4yd^3a_3$. Then $a_2d^2b_4$, $a_3d^1b_1$, $b_1d^3a_2$ (x is to the right of a_2 for its vertical match), and a_1 is below b_1 for a_1's d^3 match. Also, $b_2d^4a_3$, $b_4d^3xd^4b_3$, $a_1d^4b_4$, $a_1d^3b_2$, $b_1d^4a_4$ and, by the geometry, $a_4d^2b_2$. In addition, $a_4d^3b_3$ and, by the geometry, $a_1d^1b_3$: see Fig. 2.3(IIIa). This requires both xd^1y and xd^2y, a contradiction.

Suppose $a_1d^4yd^3a_3$. Then $a_1d^1b_3$ and $a_3d^1b_1$. These require xd^1y: see Fig. 2.3(IIIb). Then b_4 is the only B point below x, and this contradicts (ii).

Because (I)–(III) yield contradictions, there do not exist five-point disjoint A and B with equal numbers of points on every line parallel to some l_k. $\square$

2.7   Linear programming

The preceding section suggests that if $m \geq 3$ and if finite $S \subseteq \mathbb{Z}^n$ is large, it may be quite difficult to determine whether S is H-unique. See, for example, Gritzmann, Prangenberg, de Vries, and Wiegelmann [15]. Moreover, if $m \geq 3$ and we know a discrete Radon transform of some S but do not know S, it may be hard to reconstruct S or another set with the same transform when S is not H-unique. Irwing and Jerrum [16] proves that the problem of reconstructing S from v_S is generally NP-hard, so we expect on the basis of NP-completeness theory that no algorithm that runs in polynomial time in $|S|$ can be found.

A route around intractability was suggested to us a few years ago by Ron Aharoni and Gabor Herman (see Aharoni, Herman, and Kuba [17]) by way of linear programming. Pursuit of that route resulted in Fishburn, Schwander, Shepp, and Vanderbei [4]. We summarize here the aspects of that paper which bear on analysis by linear programming.

As indicated in Section 2.2, we formulated the problem in terms of fractional sets to take advantage of continuous methods. Given a discrete Radon transform $v : \mathcal{H} \to \{0, 1, \ldots\}$ for a specified discrete Radon base, the problem is to

$$\text{minimize } 0$$
$$\text{subject to } \sum_{x \in h \cap \mathbb{Z}^n} f(x) = v(h) \text{ for all } h \in \mathcal{H}_I \qquad (2.42)$$
$$\text{and } 0 \leq f(x) \leq 1 \text{ for all } x \in I,$$

where "minimize 0" initiates a feasibility check, I is a finite subset of $\mathbb{Z}^n$

that is sure to contain S, and $\mathcal{H}_I$ is the set of members of $\mathcal{H}$ that intersect I. It is well-known that there are interior point methods for this problem that run in polynomial time, and we favor these not only because of efficiency but because they produce solutions that lie in the center of the face of optimality (Adler and Monteiro [18]).

The main features of this approach in terms of the three possible outputs of the linear program are as follows.

1. If the output indicates infeasibility then no f, and in particular no S, satisfies its constraints and v is not the discrete Radon transform of any S.

2. If there is a solution and it has $f(x) \in \{0, 1\}$ for all x, it follows from the interior point method, convexity, and Theorems 2.2 and 2.1 that the corresponding S is H-additive and is a set of uniqueness.

3. If there is a solution and it has $0 < f(x) < 1$ for some x, then the situation for pure sets is ambiguous. If there is exactly one extreme solution to the problem, its corresponding S is H-unique but not H-additive (Theorem 2.2). If there are no extreme solutions or more than one extreme solution, then there is no set of uniqueness. Because of the interior point method, if there are extreme solutions $S_1, S_2, \ldots$, then every x with $f(x) = 0$ is excluded from every S_i, and every x with $f(x) = 1$ is included in every S_i. Hence in the ambiguous-output case, the interior-point solution f can provide a great deal of information about S sets, if any, that satisfy the constraints.

Section 7 in [4] reports on experience with an interior point method described in Vanderbei [19]. Several S sets with about 600 points were chosen in a two-dimensional grid according to arrays that were believed to have some semblance of reality to problems of discrete tomography. We then computed v_S for each set using a discrete Radon base of three lines with directions $(1, 0)$, $(0, 1)$ and $(1, 1)$. Because each case was feasible by construction, the outputs were of types 2 and 3 above. A few reconstructions by the interior point method were of type 2, meaning that the S used to compute v_S was a set of uniqueness. Other f solutions were of type 3. The simplest of these had six fractional $f(x)$ values strictly between 0 and 1 that corresponded to two S sets, the one used to compute v_S and another with an identical discrete Radon transform.

2.8   Discussion

Our main purpose has been to explicate structures of finite subsets of integer lattices in terms relevant to discrete tomography as well as other areas in which one is interested in deducing local structure from aggregate data. Basic theory toward this end was presented in Sections 2.2 and 2.3 through the notions of discrete Radon bases, discrete Radon transforms, sets of uniqueness, and additivity. Sections 2.4 through 2.6 then explored special possibilities for subsets of integer lattices that supplement our basic results, and Section 2.7 described how an interior point linear programming approach can be exploited to provide full or partial details of sets that might generate a given discrete Radon transform. We note also that Vardi and Lee [20] proposes a nonlinear programming technique that promises better performance than linear programming in the presence of additive noise. However, until we see actual measurements, we will not know the nature of the noise.

Several open questions were mentioned. One asks whether it is true for certain discrete Radon bases that the proportion of sets S of uniqueness that are not also additive approaches 1 as S gets large (Section 2.5). Another concerns the maximum size of subsets of S that may need examination to determine if S is additive (Section 2.6). For the four-directions base of Theorem 2.8, it is true for each odd $K \geq 7$ that there is an S with K points that has a K-bad configuration but no J-bad configuration for $J < K$? Similar questions can be raised for bases in $\mathbb{Z}^2$ that use more than four lines.

References

[1] L. A. Shepp and B. F. Logan, "The Fourier reconstruction of a head," *IEEE Trans. Nucl. Sci.* **NS-21**, 21–43 (1974).

[2] L. A. Shepp and J. B. Kruskal, "Computerized tomography: the new medical X-ray technology," *Amer. Math. Monthly* **85**, 420–439 (1978).

[3] P. Schwander, C. Kisielowski, M. Seibt, F. H. Baumann, Y. Kim, and A. Ourmazd, "Mapping projected potential, interfacial roughness, and composition in general crystalline solids by quantitative transmission electron microscopy," *Phys. Rev. Lett.* **71**, 4150–4153 (1993).

[4] P. Fishburn, P. Schwander, L. Shepp, and R. J. Vanderbei, "The discrete Radon transform and its approximate inversion via linear programming," *Discrete Appl Math.* **75**, 39–61 (1997).

[5] P. C. Fishburn, J. C. Lagarias, J. A. Reeds, and L. A. Shepp, "Sets uniquely determined by projections on axes II: Discrete case," *Discrete Math.* **91**, 149–159 (1991).

[6] R. A. Crowther, D. J. DeRosier and A. Klug, "The reconstruction of a three-dimensional structure from projections and its application to electron microscopy," *Proc. Royal Soc. London Ser. A* **317**, 319–340 (1970).

[7] R. Gordon and G. T. Herman, "Reconstruction of pictures from their projections," *Commun. ACM* **14**, 759–768 (1971).

[8] R. J. Gardner and P. McMullen, "On Hammer's X-ray problem," *J. London Math. Soc.* **21**, 171–175 (1980).

[9] G. Bianchi and M. Longinetti, "Reconstructing plane sets from projections," *Discrete Comput. Geom.* **5**, 223–242 (1990).

[10] P. Gritzmann and M. Nivat, Eds., "Discrete Tomography: Algorithms and Complexity," Dagstuhl Seminar Report 165, *Internat. Beg. Forsch. Infor.*, Schloss Dagstuhl, Germany, 1997.

[11] P. C. Fishburn, *Mathematics of Decision Theory* (Mouton, Paris), 1972.

[12] P. C. Fishburn, "Finite linear qualitative probability," *J. Math. Psychol.* **40**, 64–77 (1996).

[13] P. C. Fishburn, "Failure of cancellation conditions for additive linear orders," *J. Combin. Designs* **5**, 353–365 (1997).

[14] D. Scott and P. Suppes, "Foundational aspects of theories of measurement," *J. Symbolic Logic* **23**, 113–128 (1958).

[15] P. Gritzmann, D. Prangenberg, S. de Vries, and M. Wiegelmann, "Success and failure of certain reconstruction and uniqueness algorithms in discrete tomography," *Int. J. Imaging Sci. Tech.* **9**, 101–109 (1998).

[16] R. W. Irwing and M. R. Jerrum, "Three-dimensional statistical data security problems," *SIAM J. Comput.* **23**, 170–184 (1994).

[17] R. Aharoni, G. T. Herman, and A. Kuba, "Binary vectors partially determined by linear equation systems," *Discrete Math.* **171**, 1–16 (1997).

[18] I. Adler and R. D. C. Monteiro, "Limiting behavior of the affine scaling continuous trajectories for linear programming," *Math. Programming* **50**, 29–51 (1991).

[19] R. J. Vanderbei, *An interior point code for quadratic programming*, SOR 94-15, Princeton University, Princeton, NJ, 1994.

[20] Y. Vardi and D. Lee, "Discrete Radon transform and its approximate inversion via the EM algorithm," *Int. J. Imaging Sci. Tech.* **9**, 155–173 (1998).

Chapter 3

Tomographic Equivalence and Switching Operations

T. Yung Kong[1]
Gabor T. Herman[2]

ABSTRACT A binary picture on an arbitrary grid is a mapping f from the set of all grid points to $\{0,1\}$ such that $f(x) = 1$ for only finitely many grid points x. If two binary pictures f_1 and f_2 on the same grid have the property that for every grid line ℓ the sets $\{p \in \ell \mid f_1(p) = 1\}$ and $\{p \in \ell \mid f_2(p) = 1\}$ contain exactly the same number of grid points, then we say that f_1 and f_2 are tomographically equivalent. Given a binary picture f on the usual 2-dimensional square grid, there may exist an upright rectangle R (of any size) whose sides are grid lines, such that $f = 1$ at two diagonally opposite corner points of R and $f = 0$ at the other two corner points. If so, then we call the process of changing the value of the picture f from 1 to 0 and 0 to 1 at the four corner points of R (without changing the value of f at any other grid point) a rectangular 4-switch. Ryser showed in the 1950s that two binary pictures on the square grid are tomographically equivalent if and only if one picture can be transformed to the other by a finite sequence of rectangular 4-switches. We present a few different versions of this theorem, describe an application, and also give a proof of the result. We then show that the result has no analog on grids that have grid lines in three or more directions (such as the 3-dimensional cubic grid), because on such grids one can find for every integer L two tomographically equivalent binary pictures that differ at more than L grid points and are not tomographically equivalent to any other binary picture.

3.1 Ryser's theorem for binary pictures on the square grid

Ryser showed in the 1950s [1] that if one matrix of 0's and 1's has the same row and column sums as another such matrix then the first matrix

---

[1]Queens College, CUNY, Department of Computer Science, 65-30 Kissena Boulevard, Flushing, NY 11367, U.S.A., E-mail: ykong@turing.cs.qc.edu

[2]University of Pennsylvania, Medical Image Processing Group, Department of Radiology, Blockley Hall, 4th Floor, 423 Guardian Drive, Philadelphia, PA 19104, U.S.A., E-mail: gabor@mipg.upenn.edu

can be transformed into the second by a finite sequence of simple switching operations each of which changes two 1's to 0's and two 0's to 1's. This can be regarded as a result of discrete tomography, since matrices of 0's and 1's can be viewed as binary pictures on the 2-dimensional square grid; two matrices that have the same row and column sums correspond to two binary pictures that are tomographically equivalent (with respect to projections in the directions of the grid lines). Ryser's theorem then raises the question of whether there are analogous results for binary pictures on grids other than the square grid.

In this chapter we state Ryser's theorem (in terms of binary pictures on the square grid) in a number of different ways, describe an application of the theorem, and prove the result. Then we prove the possibly surprising fact that there is no analogous result on any grid that has grid lines in three or more directions. (It follows, for example, that there is no analog of Ryser's theorem on the 2-dimensional hexagonal grid shown in Fig. 3.1, nor on the 3-dimensional cubic grid.)

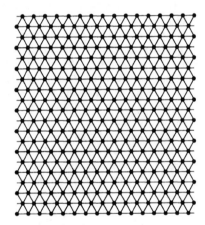

FIGURE 3.1. A part of the isometric hexagonal grid (which is so-called because the grid points are the centers of the hexagons in a tiling of the plane by regular hexagons). When the straight lines shown here are extended to infinity (in both directions), the set of grid points on each line constitutes a grid line.

3.1.1   Binary and ternary pictures on the square grid

A *binary picture* (or *binary image*) on the (2-dimensional) square grid is a mapping $f : \mathbf{Z}^2 \to \{0, 1\}$ that is nonzero at only finitely many points of $\mathbf{Z}^2$; here $\mathbf{Z}$ denotes the set of all integers, so that $\mathbf{Z}^2$ is the infinite rectangular lattice consisting of all points in the Euclidean plane with integer coordinates. A point $p \in \mathbf{Z}^2$ is called a 1 or a 0 of a binary picture f according to whether $f(p) = 1$ or $f(p) = 0$. A *ternary picture* on the square grid is a mapping $f : \mathbf{Z}^2 \to \{-1, 0, 1\}$ that is nonzero at only finitely many points. In particular, every binary picture is a ternary picture.

In this chapter we are mainly interested in binary pictures. However, if f_1 and f_2 are binary pictures then $f_1 - f_2$ need not be a binary picture, but is always a ternary picture. For brevity we will sometimes use the unqualified term *picture* to mean a binary picture.

For all $i, j \in \mathbf{Z}$, each of the sets $\{(i, y) \mid y \in \mathbf{Z}\}$ and $\{(x, j) \mid x \in \mathbf{Z}\}$ is called a *grid line* of the square grid. For each point $p \in \mathbf{Z}^2$, we write ℓ_p^x and ℓ_p^y for the grid lines through p that are parallel to the x-axis and the y-axis, respectively. (Thus $\ell_p^y = \{(i, y) \mid y \in \mathbf{Z}\}$, where i is the x-coordinate of p, and $\ell_p^x = \{(x, j) \mid x \in \mathbf{Z}\}$ where j is the y-coordinate of p.) For any grid line ℓ and any ternary picture f on the square grid, the *line sum* of f along ℓ is the sum $\sum_{p \in \ell} f(p)$. (This is essentially a finite sum, since f is nonzero at only finitely many points.) If f is a binary picture, then this sum is just the number of points on the grid line ℓ at which f has value 1.

3.1.2   Four statements of Ryser's theorem

Two binary pictures on the square grid, f and f', are said to be *tomographically equivalent* if f has the same line sum as f' along every grid line. Our first version of Ryser's theorem is:

Theorem 3.1.   *Let f and f' be tomographically equivalent binary pictures on the square grid. Then there is a finite sequence of tomographically equivalent binary pictures $f = f_0, f_1, \ldots, f_n = f'$ on the square grid such that, for $0 \le i < n$, f_{i+1} differs from f_i at exactly four points of $\mathbf{Z}^2$.*

Before giving other formulations of the theorem, it is convenient to introduce some notation and a lemma.

The l_1-*norm* of a ternary picture f, denoted by $\|f\|_1$, is the number of points p for which $f(p) \ne 0$. The l_1-*distance* (also called the *Hamming distance*) between two binary pictures f_1 and f_2 is $\|f_1 - f_2\|_1$ — i.e., the number of grid points at which the f_1 differs from f_2.

For any rectangle R whose sides are parallel to the x- and y-axes and whose corner points are in $\mathbf{Z}^2$, and any binary picture f that has value 1 at two diagonally opposite corner points of R and value 0 at the other two corner points of R, we refer to the process of simultaneously changing the value of f from 1 to 0 and 0 to 1 at the four corner points of R — without changing the value of f elsewhere — as a *rectangular 4-switching operation* or, more briefly, a *rectangular 4-switch* (*on* f).

The term *switching component* is used by some authors to denote the set of two 1's and two 0's that are changed in value by a rectangular 4-switch.

Such sets are the simplest nonempty sets of 1's and 0's having the property that the picture's line sums are all unchanged when each 1 is changed to a 0 and each 0 to a 1; some authors refer to a set of 1's and 0's with this property as a *switching set*. When S is the set of all 1's of the picture and H is the set consisting of the x- and the y-axes in the Euclidean plane, these concepts of switching component and switching set are closely related to the concepts of a *bad H-rectangle for S* and a *bad H-configuration for S* that are used in the previous chapter (by Fishburn and Shepp).

Lemma 3.1.   *Let f and f' be distinct tomographically equivalent binary pictures. Then the following three conditions are equivalent.*

(i) $\|f - f'\|_1 = 4$.

(ii) $\|f - f'\|_1 \leq 4$.

(iii) f can be transformed into f' by a single rectangular 4-switching operation.

Proof: Clearly (i) implies (ii), and (iii) implies (i). To show that (ii) implies (iii) we proceed as follows. Suppose (ii) holds, so that f differs from f' at no more than four points. Let a be a point at which f differs from f'. Then f must also differ from f' at another point b on ℓ_a^x, and at another point c on ℓ_a^y (for otherwise f would not have the same line sum as f' along ℓ_a^x and ℓ_a^y). As f differs from f' at b and at c, f must also differ from f' at another point d on ℓ_b^y and at another point e on ℓ_c^x (for otherwise f would not have the same line sum as f' along ℓ_b^y and ℓ_c^x). Note that $e \notin \{a, b\}$ since ℓ_c^x passes through neither a nor b (which lie on the parallel grid line ℓ_a^x), and similarly $d \notin \{a, c\}$ since ℓ_b^y passes through neither a nor c. Thus the four points a, b, c and d are distinct, as are the four points a, b, c and e. So since f differs from f' at no more than four points, $d = e$. Thus a, b, c and $d = e$ are the four corner points of some rectangle R whose sides are parallel to the x- and the y-axes, and a is diagonally opposite to d. Now f cannot have the same value at a and b for otherwise f' would have the opposite value at those points and f would not have the same line sum as f' along ℓ_a^x. Similarly, f cannot have the same value at a and c, and cannot have the same value at c and d. So f must have value 1 at a and d and value 0 at b and c, or vice versa, and the replacement of f by f' is a rectangular 4-switch. $\square$

A sequence of binary pictures $f_0, f_1, \ldots, f_n$ will be called a *k-switching chain* (that *links f_0 to f_n*) if $\|f_i - f_{i+1}\|_1 \leq k$ for $0 \leq i < n$; if in addition each f_i belongs to a set of binary pictures $\mathcal{F}$, then we will say that the k-switching chain is *in $\mathcal{F}$*. In view of the equivalence of (i) and (ii) in Lemma 3.1, Theorem 3.1 is equivalent to the following:

Theorem 3.2.   *Let $\mathcal{F}$ be any tomographic equivalence class of binary pictures on the square grid, and let $f, f' \in \mathcal{F}$. Then there is a 4-switching chain in $\mathcal{F}$ that links f to f'.*

Our next version of Ryser's theorem says that every tomographic equivalence class of binary pictures on the square grid is connected in a sense that we now define. The l_1-distance between two sets of binary pictures $\mathcal{F}_1$ and $\mathcal{F}_2$ is defined to be $\min\{\|f_1 - f_2\|_1 \mid f_1 \in \mathcal{F}_1, f_2 \in \mathcal{F}_2\}$. For any integer $k > 0$, a set $\mathcal{F}$ of binary pictures is $(l_1 \leq k)$-*disconnected* if $\mathcal{F}$ can be partitioned into two nonempty subsets $\mathcal{F}_A$ and $\mathcal{F}_B$ such that the l_1-distance between $\mathcal{F}_A$ and $\mathcal{F}_B$ exceeds k; otherwise, $\mathcal{F}$ is $(l_1 \leq k)$-*connected*.

Let $\mathcal{F}$ be an arbitrary set of binary pictures and let $f \in \mathcal{F}$. We now claim that $\mathcal{F}$ is $(l_1 \leq k)$-connected if and only if for each f' in $\mathcal{F}$ there exists a k-switching chain in $\mathcal{F}$ that links f to f'. To see this, write $\mathcal{F}_f^k$ for the set $\{f' \in \mathcal{F} \mid$ there is a k-switching chain in $\mathcal{F}$ that links f to $f'\}$. Our claim is that $\mathcal{F}$ is $(l_1 \leq k)$-connected if and only if $\mathcal{F}_f^k = \mathcal{F}$. Since it is evident that $\mathcal{F}_f^k$ is $(l_1 \leq k)$-connected, the "if" part of our claim is true. Conversely, if $\mathcal{F}_f^k \neq \mathcal{F}$ then the l_1-distance between the sets $\mathcal{F}_f^k$ and $\mathcal{F}\backslash\mathcal{F}_f^k$ evidently exceeds k, so $\mathcal{F}$ is $(l_1 \leq k)$-disconnected.

Theorem 3.2 can now be restated as follows:

Theorem 3.3.   *Every tomographic equivalence class of binary pictures on the square grid is $(l_1 \leq 4)$-connected.*

It follows from the equivalence of (i) and (iii) in Lemma 3.1 that Ryser's theorem can also be stated as follows. (Of the four statements of Ryser's theorem in this subsection, the following is closest to Ryser's own statements of the result [1,2].)

Theorem 3.4.   *If two binary pictures on the square grid are tomographically equivalent, then one picture can be transformed to the other by a finite sequence of rectangular 4-switches.*

3.1.3   Metropolis algorithms based on Ryser graphs

Let $\mathcal{C}$ be any tomographic equivalence class of binary pictures on the square grid. Consider the graph whose vertices are in $1 - 1$ correspondence with the binary pictures in $\mathcal{C}$, in which two vertices are adjacent if and only if the picture corresponding to one vertex can be obtained from the picture corresponding to the other by a single rectangular 4-switch. We will call this the *Ryser graph* of the tomographic equivalence class $\mathcal{C}$.

The Ryser graph is a finite graph since each tomographic equivalence class is finite. (Indeed, if M is an integer such that both coordinates of every 1 of a binary picture f lie in the interval $[-M, M]$, then both coordinates of every 1 of any binary picture that is tomographically equivalent to f must also lie in $[-M, M]$.) In view of Theorem 3.4, the Ryser graph is connected.

We now give an application of the Ryser graph. Let $\mathcal{P}$ be the set of all binary pictures on the square grid. Suppose we have defined a "goodness" function $\gamma : \mathcal{P} \to (0, \infty)$ that we regard as a measure of the quality of a binary picture — the higher the value of γ, the more we like the picture. Consider the following problem: Given a binary picture $f \in \mathcal{P}$, find a picture in f's tomographic equivalence class for which γ has a relatively high value. (Ideally, we would like to find a picture that maximizes γ, but we do not expect to always achieve this.)

We will describe (two versions of) an iterative stochastic algorithm that, given any finite connected graph with vertex set V and any function $\gamma : V \to (0, \infty)$, aims to find a vertex $v \in V$ for which $\gamma(v)$ has a relatively high value. The algorithm is a typical instance of a class of algorithms known in the literature as Metropolis algorithms [3]. Since the Ryser graph of a tomographic equivalence class on a square grid is finite and connected, the algorithm is applicable to our problem.

Our first version of the algorithm uses a positive integer constant N with the property that no vertex of the graph has more than N neighbors. It uses a vertex variable $current\_v$ that may be initialized to any vertex of the graph, and a second vertex variable v'. At each iteration, v' is randomly set equal either to $current\_v$ or to one of the neighbors of $current\_v$ with the following probabilities: For each neighbor of $current\_v$, the probability that v' is set to that neighbor is $1/N$; the probability that v' is set to $current\_v$ is therefore $1 - d/N$, where d is the number of neighbors of the vertex $current\_v$. This is called the *proposal step* of the iteration. Now there are three cases:

1. If $v' = current\_v$ then the algorithm leaves $current\_v$ unchanged.

2. If v' is a neighbor of $current\_v$ such that $\gamma(v') \geq \gamma(current\_v)$ then $current\_v$ is changed to v'.

3. If v' is a neighbor of $current\_v$ such that $\gamma(v') < \gamma(current\_v)$ then $current\_v$ is changed to v' with a probability of $\gamma(v')/\gamma(current\_v)$ (and is left unchanged with a probability of $1 - \gamma(v')/\gamma(current\_v)$).

A real variable max_gamma and a vertex variable $best\_vertex$ are also used; max_gamma is initialized to 0 prior to the first iteration. In case 2 above, if $\gamma(v') > max\_gamma$ then the value $\gamma(v')$ is stored in max_gamma and the vertex v' is stored in $best\_vertex$. (Thus max_gamma stores the greatest value attained by $\gamma(current\_v)$ in the current and previous iterations, and $best\_vertex$ stores the vertex at which this value of γ was first attained.)

Some stopping condition must be specified; a simple stopping condition would be that the number of iterations has reached a certain bound. When the stopping condition is satisfied the algorithm outputs the values of $best\_vertex$ and max_gamma, and then stops.

Our second version of the algorithm uses the same variables, but the proposal step of each iteration is different: At each iteration v' is randomly set to one of the neighbors of $current\_v$, in such a way that it has the same probability of being set to any neighbor of *current_v*. Unlike the first version of the algorithm, this version never sets v' to *current_v* in its proposal step (and does not use N). The rest of the algorithm is the same as for the first version, except that case 1 above cannot occur.

Note that in the first version of the algorithm, when v' is set to a neighbor of *current_v* it is no more likely to be set to one neighbor than to another. Thus if we redefine our concept of iteration so that iterations where v' is set to *current_v* are not counted, then the first version of the algorithm becomes an instance of the second version. Thus the second version is, in a sense, an "accelerated" version of the first.

For any positive integer n, let $p_n(v_0, v)$ denote the probability, for the first version of the algorithm, that if *current_v* is initially the vertex v_0 then after n iterations *current_v* is the vertex v. As n tends to infinity, it can be shown [3, Theorem 8.2.2(a)] that, for all initial vertices v_0, $p_n(v_0, v)$ converges to a probability distribution on the set V of all vertices that is proportional to $\gamma(v)$: So *current_v* is likely to spend more iterations in a subset of the vertices on which γ has high values than in a subset of the same size on which γ has low values.

For the algorithm to be practical it is important that (1) the proposal step can be efficiently implemented, and (2) it is computationally easy to evaluate $\gamma(v')/\gamma(current\_v)$.

We first consider (2). It is common to use a function $\gamma(v)$ of the form $e^{-\beta H(v)}$, where β is a positive constant and H is a function such that $H(current\_v) - H(v')$ is easy to compute. Then since $\gamma(v')/\gamma(current\_v) = e^{\beta(H(current\_v) - H(v'))}$, condition 2 is satisfied. In the case where the algorithm is applied to a Ryser graph, using f_v to denote the binary picture corresponding to the vertex v, H might (for example) be such that when v' is a neighbor of *current_v* the value of $H(current\_v) - H(v')$ depends only on the values of $f_{current\_v}$ and $f_{v'}$ at grid points close to the four points where $f_{current\_v}$ differs from $f_{v'}$.

Now we turn our attention to (1) in the case where the algorithm is applied to a Ryser graph, and describe one possible implementation of the proposal step for the first version of the algorithm.

An *invariant element* of a binary picture f is a grid point p such that $f'(p) = f(p)$ for all binary pictures f' that are tomographically equivalent to f. Any grid point that does not have this property is a *variant element* of f. Our implementation of the proposal step will depend on our being able to find the variant elements of an arbitrary binary picture f. We now state a result that enables us to do this efficiently.

Let L_x and L_y be the grid lines in the x- and the y-directions, respectively, that contain at least one 1 of the picture f. We first number the grid lines in each of the sets L_x and L_y in decreasing order of f's line sums along those lines. For $1 \le i \le |L_x|$ and $1 \le j \le |L_y|$, let r_i and s_j denote f's line sums along the grid line numbered i in L_x and the grid line numbered j in L_y, respectively. (Thus $r_1 \ge r_2 \ge \cdots \ge r_{|L_x|}$ and

$s_1 \geq s_2 \geq \cdots \geq s_{|L_y|}$.) Let $r'_j = |\{i \mid r_i \geq j\}|$ and $s'_i = |\{j \mid s_j \geq i\}|$. Thus r'_j (respectively, s'_i) is the number of grid lines in the x-direction (respectively, y-direction) for which f's line sum is greater than or equal to j (respectively, i). Let $1 \leq i'_1 < i''_1 < i'_2 < i''_2 < \cdots < i'_m < i''_m \leq |L_x|$ and $1 \leq j'_n < j''_n < j'_{n-1} < j''_{n-1} < \cdots < j'_1 < j''_1 \leq |L_y|$ (where $m, n \geq 0$; note that the order of indexing is different for the i's and the j's) be the integers for which the following equations hold:

$$\bigcup_{1 \leq t \leq m} \{k \mid i'_t \leq k < i''_t\} = \{k \leq |L_x| \mid \sum_{i=1}^{k} s'_i > \sum_{i=1}^{k} r_i\} \qquad (3.1)$$

$$\bigcup_{1 \leq t \leq n} \{k \mid j'_t \leq k < j''_t\} = \{k \leq |L_y| \mid \sum_{j=1}^{k} r'_j > \sum_{j=1}^{k} s_j\}. \qquad (3.2)$$

It can be shown that $m = n$.

Before stating the result that enables us to find the variant elements of f, we note that it is a straightforward matter to compute the i's, i''s, j's and j''s. In fact, once L_x, L_y and the line sums of f along those grid lines have been determined, the i's, i''s, j's, and j''s can be computed in $O(|L_x| + |L_y|)$ time. One way to do this is as follows. We first use counting sort [4, p. 176] to create two sorted lists, one containing a record for each grid line in L_x, the other containing a record for each grid line in L_y. The record for each grid line in L_x (respectively, L_y) contains the y-coordinate (respectively, x-coordinate) of the grid line and f's line sum along that line. Both lists of records are sorted with respect to the latter field. The value of each r_i and s_j can be obtained from these sorted lists. It is also easy to compute the value of each r'_j and s'_i from the two lists. But this is in fact unnecessary because arrays that contain the values of $|L_y| - r'_j$ for $1 \leq j \leq |L_y|$ and of $|L_x| - s'_i$ for $1 \leq i \leq |L_x|$ are generated as a part of the process of creating the sorted lists using counting sort. Now for k from 1 to $|L_x|$ we can easily compute $\sum_{i=1}^{k} s'_i$ and $\sum_{i=1}^{k} r_i$ from $\sum_{i=1}^{k-1} s'_i$ and $\sum_{i=1}^{k-1} r_i$, and hence determine whether that value of k is an i', an i'' or neither. The j's and j''s can be computed in a similar way.

For $1 \leq t \leq m = n$, let I_t be the union of the grid lines in L_x whose line numbers lie between i'_t and i''_t (inclusive) and let J_t be the union of the grid lines in L_y whose line numbers lie between j'_t and j''_t (inclusive). Then, by a result due to Kuba [5, Theorem 4.1], the set of variant elements of the picture f is $\bigcup_{1 \leq t \leq m} T_t$, where T_t denotes the set $I_t \cap J_t$. Thus $\{T_t \mid 1 \leq t \leq m\}$ is a partition of the set of variant elements of f. (Generalizations of this result are given by Aharoni, Herman, and Kuba in [6].)

For any rectangular 4-switch on the picture f the four points whose values are changed must all lie in the same one of the m sets T_t [5, Consequence 4.2]. It follows from this, and Theorem 3.4, that for $1 \leq t \leq m$ the number of pairs of 1's in T_t such that no grid line passes through both 1's is the same for any binary picture that is tomographically equivalent to f. Let

$\nu_1(t)$ denote this number, and let $\nu_0(t)$ denote the analogous number for 0's in T_t. Let $\nu(t) = \min(\nu_0(t), \nu_1(t))$; $\nu(t)$ is readily computed.

For $1 \leq t \leq m$ we maintain an array A_t. If $\nu(t) = \nu_0(t)$ then A_t contains the coordinates of the points in T_t that are 0's of the picture corresponding to *current_v*; but if $\nu(t) = \nu_1(t) < \nu_0(t)$ then A_t contains the coordinates of the points in T_t that are 1's of that picture.

At each iteration we first pick a value of t in the range $1 \leq t \leq m$, in such a way that the probability of picking a value t^* is $\nu(t^*)/\sum_{t=1}^{m} \nu(t)$. Then we pick two elements of the array A_t (for the selected value of t) at random in such a way that all pairs of elements have the same probability of being picked. If the corresponding pair of points in T_t are equal or lie on the same grid line in either direction, then we reject the elements we picked and randomly pick two other elements of A_t. This is repeated if necessary until we pick two elements of A_t that correspond to distinct points of T_t which do not lie on the same grid line in either direction.

Then there is a unique grid rectangle that has those two points of T_t as diagonally opposite corner points. If f has the opposite value at both of the other two corner points of that rectangle, then we apply the rectangular 4-switch that changes the picture at those four points and set v' to the vertex that corresponds to the resulting picture; otherwise we set v' to *current_v*. In the former case we also update the array A_t by replacing the coordinates of the two points corresponding to the elements we picked with the coordinates of the other two points that are affected by the rectangular 4-switch. It is readily confirmed that this process implements the proposal step of the first version of the algorithm with $N = \sum_{t=1}^{m} \nu(t)$.

When $\gamma(v)$ is defined as $e^{-\beta H(v)}$, the "goodness ordering" on the vertices depends only on H and is independent of the value of the positive constant β. Indeed, $e^{-\beta H(v_1)} \leq e^{-\beta H(v_2)}$ if and only if $H(v_1) \geq H(v_2)$. Regardless of the value of β, maximization of γ is equivalent to minimization of H. However, the value of β affects the number of iterations that are likely to be needed to find a vertex at which H's value is close to its minimum.

If β is very large then the algorithm will have a tendency to be trapped in the vicinity of local minima of H: When *current_v* enters the vicinity of a vertex v where H's value attains a local minimum, it is likely to take very many iterations to escape from that vicinity, regardless of the difference between the local minimum value $H(v)$ and the global minimum of H. On the other hand, if β is very small then the influence of H on the random movements of *current_v* from vertex to vertex will be very weak, so that it may take very many iterations to find a vertex at which H is small. For any given function H, one needs to use a value of β for which the algorithm has acceptable performance. But in some cases no such value of β exists.

In a variant of this algorithm β is slowly increased as the algorithm progresses. More precisely, if $\gamma(v') < \gamma(current\_v)$ at the ith iteration then *current_v* is changed to v' with a probability of $e^{\beta_i(H(current\_v) - H(v'))}$, where $\beta_1, \beta_2, \beta_3, \ldots$ is a slowly increasing unbounded infinite sequence. This is called *Metropolis annealing* [3].

We will show later that there is no analog of Ryser's theorem, and hence no analog of the Ryser graph of a tomographic equivalence class, for grids with grid lines in three or more directions. Even for such grids, Metropolis algorithms may be applicable to the problem of finding a binary picture in a given tomographic equivalence class that is good according to a numerical measure. However, a different kind of graph must be used. Chapter 8 by Matej, Vardi, Herman, and Vardi describes an experimental study that illustrates this for the isometric hexagonal grid.

3.1.4   A proof of Ryser's theorem

We now give a proof of Ryser's theorem. (For other proofs see [1, 2, 7].) Since Theorems 3.1–3.4 are equivalent, it is enough to prove Theorem 3.2.

Suppose Theorem 3.2 is false. Then there exists a tomographic equivalence class $\mathcal{F}$ of binary pictures on the square grid and binary pictures g_A, g_B in $\mathcal{F}$ such that g_A and g_B are not linked by any 4-switching chain in $\mathcal{F}$. For $\alpha = A$ and B, let $\mathcal{F}_\alpha$ denote the set of all binary pictures f in $\mathcal{F}$ such that there is a 4-switching chain in $\mathcal{F}$ that links g_α to f. Then $\mathcal{F}_A$ and $\mathcal{F}_B$ are disjoint. Moreover, for $\alpha = A$ or B and all binary pictures f and f', if $f \in \mathcal{F}_\alpha$ and $\|f - f'\|_1 \leq 4$ then $f' \in \mathcal{F}_\alpha$.

Let f_A and f_B be binary pictures in $\mathcal{F}_A$ and $\mathcal{F}_B$, respectively, such that $\|f_A - f_B\|_1$ is as small as possible — i.e., $\|f_A - f_B\|_1 \leq \|f'_A - f'_B\|_1$ for all f'_A in $\mathcal{F}_A$ and f'_B in $\mathcal{F}_B$. Since f_A and f_B both lie in the same tomographic equivalence class, f_A has the same line sum as f_B along every grid line.

In the rest of this subsection we will use the term *interchange cycle* to denote a sequence of points $p_0, p_1, \ldots, p_n$ (where $n \geq 0$) in $\mathbf{Z}^2$ that have the following three properties:

1. For $0 \leq i < n$, p_{i+1} has the same y-coordinate as p_i if i is even and has the same x-coordinate as p_i if i is odd.

2. $p_n = p_0$, but the points $p_0, p_1, \ldots, p_{n-1}$ are distinct.

3. $f_A(p_0) - f_B(p_0) = 1$ or -1 and, for $1 \leq i \leq n$, $f_A(p_i) - f_B(p_i) = -(f_A(p_{i-1}) - f_B(p_{i-1}))$.

Property 3 implies that there is no i for which $p_{i-1} = p_i$: Consecutive points in the sequence cannot be equal. The integer n will be referred to as the *length* of the interchange cycle. Properties 2 and 3 imply that n is even. In view of property 1, it is easily verified that $n \neq 2$.

Although we do not need this fact, we note that if $p_0, p_1, \ldots, p_n$ is any interchange cycle then the pair of subsequences $(p_{2i} \mid 0 \leq i < n/2)$ and $(p_{2i+1} \mid 0 \leq i < n/2)$ constitute a *bad H-configuration* in the sense of the previous chapter either for the 1's of f_A or for the 1's of f_B, in the case where H consists of the x- and y-axes in the Euclidean plane.

We now show that an interchange cycle of length > 0 must exist. Consider the set of all nonnegative integers n for which there exists a sequence of *distinct* points $p_0, p_1, \ldots, p_n$ that have properties 1 and 3 above. This set is nonempty (and contains 0), since $f_A \neq f_B$ implies there is some point q such that $f_A(q) \neq f_B(q)$, and the one-point sequence consisting just of that point q has properties 1, 2 and 3 with $n = 0$. Moreover, the set is finite (and has at most $\|f_A - f_B\|_1$ elements) since property 3 implies $f_A(p_i) \neq f_B(p_i)$ for $1 \leq i \leq n$. Let k be the largest number in this set.

Let $p_0^*, p_1^*, \ldots, p_k^*$ be a sequence of distinct points that have properties 1 and 3 with $n = k$. There must be points p^x and p^y on the grid lines $\ell_{p_k^*}^x$ and $\ell_{p_k^*}^y$, respectively, such that $f_A(p^x) - f_B(p^x) = f_A(p^y) - f_B(p^y) = -(f_A(p_k^*) - f_B(p_k^*))$, for otherwise f_A would not have the same line sum as f_B along $\ell_{p_k^*}^y$ and $\ell_{p_k^*}^x$. Let p_{k+1}^* be p^x or p^y according to whether k is even or odd. Then $p_{k+1}^* = p_r^*$ for some r in the range $0 \leq r < k$, for otherwise $p_0^*, p_1^*, \ldots, p_{k+1}^*$ would be distinct points that have properties 1 and 3 above for $n = k + 1$, contrary to the definition of k. The sequence $p_r^*, p_{r+1}^*, \ldots, p_{k+1}^*$ has all three properties above for $n = k + 1 - r$ and is therefore an interchange cycle of length > 0, as required.

Let $p_0, p_1, \ldots, p_n$ be a shortest interchange cycle of length > 0. We already know n is even and $n > 2$. Let p^* be the point where the grid lines $\ell_{p_0}^y$ and $\ell_{p_2}^x$ intersect. If $f_A(p^*) - f_B(p^*) = f_A(p_0) - f_B(p_0)$, then $p^*, p_3, p_4, \ldots, p_{n-1}, p^*$ is an interchange cycle of length $n - 2$, which contradicts the fact that the shortest interchange cycle is of length n.

Thus we may assume $f_A(p^*) - f_B(p^*) \neq f_A(p_0) - f_B(p_0)$. Consider the ternary picture $g : \mathbf{Z}^2 \to \{-1, 0, 1\}$ such that $g(p) = f_A(p) - f_B(p)$ for $p \in \{p_0, p_1, p_2\}$, $g(p^*) = -(f_A(p_0) - f_B(p_0))$, and $g(p) = 0$ for all points $p \in \mathbf{Z}^2 \setminus \{p_0, p_1, p_2, p^*\}$. It follows from property 3 that g has a line sum of 0 along every grid line.

We now show that at all points $p \in \mathbf{Z}^2 \setminus \{p^*\}$, both $f_A(p) - g(p)$ and $f_B(p) + g(p)$ lie in $\{0, 1\}$. This is clearly so if $p \in \mathbf{Z}^2 \setminus \{p_0, p_1, p_2, p^*\}$ since $g(p) = 0$ at such points. But it is also true if $p \in \{p_0, p_1, p_2\}$, because $f_A - g = f_B$ and $f_B + g = f_A$ at those three points. As $f_A(p^*) - f_B(p^*) \neq f_A(p_0) - f_B(p_0)$, either $f_A(p^*) - f_B(p^*) = 0$ or $f_A(p^*) - f_B(p^*) = -(f_A(p_0) - f_B(p_0))$. In the latter case $g(p^*) = f_A(p^*) - f_B(p^*)$, and both $f_A - g = f_B$ and $f_B + g = f_A$ are binary pictures. In the former case, $f_A(p^*) = f_B(p^*)$ implies that one of $f_A - g$ and $f_B + g$ must have a value of 0 or 1 at p^*, so that it is a binary picture.

In either case let f be one of $f_A - g$ and $f_B + g$ that is a binary picture. Then f is tomographically equivalent to f_A and f_B, because g has a line sum of 0 along every grid line. If $f = f_A - g$ then $\|f - f_A\|_1 = \|g\|_1 \leq 4$, so $f \in \mathcal{F}_A$. But in this case $\|f - f_B\|_1 < \|f_A - f_B\|_1$: At p_0, p_1 and p_2, $f = f_B$ but (by property 3) $f_A \neq f_B$; at all points in $\mathbf{Z}^2 \setminus \{p_0, p_1, p_2, p^*\}$, $f = f_A$. This contradicts the fact that f_A and f_B were defined to be such that $\|f_A - f_B\|_1 \leq \|f_A' - f_B'\|_1$ for all f_A' in $\mathcal{F}_A$ and f_B' in $\mathcal{F}_B$.

Similarly, if $f = f_B + g$ then $\|f - f_B\|_1 = \|g\|_1 \leq 4$ so that $f \in \mathcal{F}_B$, but $\|f - f_A\|_1 < \|f_A - f_B\|_1$ contrary to the definition of f_A and f_B. This completes the proof of Theorem 3.2.

3.2   Nonexistence of analogs on m-grids with $m > 2$

The definition of tomographic equivalence can also be applied to binary pictures on non-square grids such as the isometric hexagonal grid shown in Fig. 3.1. One might guess that Ryser's theorem has analogs for binary pictures on such grids: Specifically, one might well expect that for any such grid $\mathcal{G}$ there would be an integer $n_{\mathcal{G}}$ and switching operations (analogous to rectangular 4-switching operations) that change the value of a picture at no more than $n_{\mathcal{G}}$ points, such that any binary picture can be transformed to any other tomographically equivalent picture by a finite sequence of such operations.

However, we will show that no such integer $n_{\mathcal{G}}$ exists unless $\mathcal{G}$ is iso-morphic to the 2-dimensional square grid. In order to be able to state this result precisely and prove it, we now generalize the definitions given in Subsections 3.1.1 and 3.1.2 to admit non-square grids.

3.2.1   m-grids

Let m be any integer such that $m \geq 2$. In the rest of this chapter an *m-grid* is a pair (Γ, P) where:

1. P is a set $\{v_1, \ldots, v_m\}$ of m nonzero vectors in a Euclidean space (of any dimensionality), no two of which are parallel.

2. Γ is the (infinite) set of all linear combinations with integer coeffi-cients of the vectors in P: Thus $\Gamma = \{\sum_{i=1}^{m} k_i v_i \mid k_1, \ldots, k_m \in \mathbf{Z}\}$.

We use the term *grid* to mean an m-grid for some $m \geq 2$. The elements of P are called the *fundamental direction vectors* of the grid (Γ, P): These vectors define the "projection directions" that are used with the grid. The elements of Γ are the *grid points* of the grid (Γ, P); note that Γ is actually determined by P. Here are three examples of grids:

1. The 2-grid (Γ, P) where $P = \{(1, 0), (0, 1)\}$ (so that $\Gamma = \mathbf{Z}^2$) is the square grid considered in Section 3.1 above.

2. The 3-grid (Γ, P) where $P = \{(1, 0, 0), (0, 1, 0), (0, 0, 1)\}$ (so that $\Gamma = \mathbf{Z}^3$) is the *cubic grid*.

3. The 3-grid (Γ, P) where $P = \{(1, 0), (-1/2, \sqrt{3}/2), (-1/2, -\sqrt{3}/2)\}$ is referred to in this chapter as the *isometric hexagonal grid*. This is shown in Fig. 3.1.

If p is any grid point and v any fundamental direction vector of a grid then the set of grid points $\{p + kv \mid k \in \mathbf{Z}\}$ is called a *grid line* and, more precisely, the *grid line through p in the direction of v*. A grid line ℓ of a grid (Γ, P) is said to *pass through* a grid point $p \in \Gamma$ if $p \in \ell$. For example, in the grid $(\mathbf{Z}^2, \{(3,0), (0,1), (2,2)\})$ the grid line through the grid point $(0,0)$ in the direction of $(2,2)$ passes through the grid point $(4,4)$ but does not pass through the grid point $(5,5)$.

A *binary picture* on a grid (Γ, P) is a map $f : \Gamma \to \{0,1\}$ such that f is nonzero at only finitely many grid points. A grid point q is called a 1 (of f) if $f(q) = 1$; q is called a 0 (of f) if $f(q) = 0$. A *ternary picture* on a grid (Γ, P) is a map $f : \Gamma \to \{-1, 0, 1\}$ such that f is nonzero at only finitely many grid points.

The definitions of the line sum along a grid line and of tomographic equivalence are the same for arbitrary grids as for the special case of the square grid. Thus the line sum of a ternary picture f along a grid line ℓ of an arbitrary grid (Γ, P) is $\sum_{p \in \ell} f(p)$, and two binary pictures on (Γ, P), f and f', are said to be tomographically equivalent if f has the same line sum as f' along every grid line of (Γ, P).

The definitions of a k-switching chain, the l_1-norm of a ternary picture, the l_1-distance between two binary pictures, the l_1-distance between two sets of binary pictures, and $(l_1 \leq k)$-connectedness of a set of binary pictures are also the same for arbitrary grids as for the square grid.

Two grids $\mathcal{G}_1 = (\Gamma_1, P_1)$ and $\mathcal{G}_2 = (\Gamma_2, P_2)$ are said to be *isomorphic* if there is a bijection of Γ_1 to Γ_2 that induces a bijection of the grid lines of $\mathcal{G}_1$ to the grid lines of $\mathcal{G}_2$; the bijection of Γ_1 to Γ_2 is called a *grid isomorphism*. Evidently, any grid isomorphism of one grid to another induces a bijection of the binary pictures on the first grid to the binary pictures on the second grid, and the induced bijection preserves tomographic equivalence.

3.2.2 Validity of Ryser's theorem for arbitrary 2-grids

A grid $\mathcal{G}$ is isomorphic to the square grid if and only if $\mathcal{G}$ is a 2-grid. Indeed, if $\mathcal{G}$ is an m-grid then each grid point of $\mathcal{G}$ lies on m grid lines of $\mathcal{G}$, so if $\mathcal{G}$ is isomorphic to the square grid then $m = 2$. Conversely, it is easily verified that the map $\theta : \Gamma \to \mathbf{Z}^2$ such that $\theta(\lambda_1 v_1 + \lambda_2 v_2) = (\lambda_1, \lambda_2)$ for all integers λ_1 and λ_2 is a grid isomorphism of the 2-grid $(\Gamma, \{v_1, v_2\})$ to the square grid.

It follows that Theorems 3.1–3.3 remain valid if we substitute any 2-grid for the square grid. The same is true of Theorem 3.4 if we generalize the concept of a rectangular 4-switching operation in the obvious way to arbitrary 2-grids.

3.2.3   The main result

The situation is quite different for m-grids where $m \geq 3$. In fact we will prove the following, which is the main result of this chapter:

Theorem 3.5.   *Let $\mathcal{G}$ be an m-grid for some $m \geq 3$. Then there is no integer L for which every tomographic equivalence class of binary pictures on $\mathcal{G}$ is ($l_1 \leq L$)-connected.*

This theorem is a corollary of the following proposition, which will be established below.

Proposition 3.1.   *Let $\mathcal{G}$ be an m-grid, where $m \geq 3$, and let L be any positive integer. Then there exist binary pictures f_A and f_B on $\mathcal{G}$ such that:*

(i) *f_A and f_B differ at more than L points.*

(ii) *f_A and f_B are tomographically equivalent.*

(iii) *f_A and f_B are not tomographically equivalent to any other binary picture on $\mathcal{G}$.*

Note that properties (ii) and (iii) in this proposition imply that $\{f_A, f_B\}$ is a tomographic equivalence class, and (i) implies that this tomographic equivalence class is not ($l_1 \leq L$)-connected.

3.3   A proof of the main result

Let m be any integer such that $m \geq 3$. Let $v_1, v_2, \ldots, v_m$ be vectors and Γ a set of points such that $(\Gamma, \{v_1, v_2, \ldots, v_m\})$ is an m-grid. Let L be an arbitrary positive integer.

We write $\mathcal{G}$ for the grid $(\Gamma, \{v_1, v_2, \ldots, v_m\})$ and say that each of two points in Γ is a *$\mathcal{G}$-mate* of the other if the points are distinct and there is a grid line of $\mathcal{G}$ that passes through both points.

Recall that a graph is said to be *bipartite* if its vertices can be partitioned into two subsets in such a way that none of the edges joins two vertices in the same subset. Equivalently, a graph is bipartite if and only if it is possible to color each of its vertices in one of two colors in such a way that no two adjacent vertices are given the same color.

Main Claim.   There is a finite set $D \subset \Gamma$ such that:

D1. $|D| > L$.

D2.   For every grid point $q \in \Gamma \setminus D$, there is a grid line of $\mathcal{G}$ that passes through q but does not pass through any point of D.

D3. Each grid line of $\mathcal{G}$ that passes through a point in D passes through one and only one other point in D. (This implies that each point in D has exactly m $\mathcal{G}$-mates in D.)

D4. The graph with vertex set D in which each vertex is adjacent to (and only to) its m $\mathcal{G}$-mates in D is a connected bipartite graph.

In the next subsection we will prove that Proposition 3.1 follows from the Main Claim. Then, in Subsection 3.3.2, we will justify the Main Claim by constructing a set D that satisfies conditions D1–D4. But first we state and prove a simple general lemma about connected bipartite graphs; this lemma will be used in Subsection 3.3.2 to show that the set D constructed there satisfies condition D4.

Lemma 3.2.   *Let G_1 and G_2 be isomorphic connected bipartite graphs with disjoint vertex sets V_1 and V_2, respectively, and let $\theta : V_1 \rightarrow V_2$ be a graph isomorphism of G_1 to G_2. Let G_3 be the graph with vertex set $V_1 \cup V_2$ whose edge set consists of (i) all edges of G_1, (ii) all edges of G_2, and (iii) $\{(x, \theta(x)) \mid x \in V_1\}$. Then G_3 is connected and bipartite.*

Proof: We may assume V_1 and V_2 are nonempty — otherwise the result is trivially valid. To see that G_3 is connected, let v and w be any two vertices of G_3. Since G_1 and G_2 are connected, if v and w are both in V_1 or both in V_2 then there is a path from one to the other along edges of G_1 or edges of G_2. If one of them, say v, is in V_1 and the other is in V_2, then a path of G_3 from v to w is obtainable by concatenating the edge from v to $\theta(v)$ with a path along edges of G_2 from $\theta(v)$ to w. This shows that G_3 is connected.

Since G_1 and G_2 are bipartite, there is a partition $\{V_1^A, V_1^B\}$ of V_1 such that if v and w are both in V_1^A or both in V_1^B then v and w are not adjacent in G_1 (and hence also not adjacent in G_3). As $\theta : V_1 \rightarrow V_2$ is an isomorphism of G_1 to G_2, $\{\theta[V_1^A], \theta[V_1^B]\}$ is a partition of V_2, and if v and w are both in $\theta[V_1^A]$ or both in $\theta[V_1^B]$ then v and w are not adjacent in G_2 (and hence also not adjacent in G_3). Moreover, if $v \in V_1^A$ and $w \in \theta[V_1^B]$ or if $v \in V_1^B$ and $w \in \theta[V_1^A]$, then v is not adjacent to w in G_3. Thus $\{V_1^A \cup \theta[V_1^B], V_1^B \cup \theta[V_1^A]\}$ is a partition of the vertex set of G_3, and if v and w are both in $V_1^A \cup \theta[V_1^B]$ or both in $V_1^B \cup \theta[V_1^A]$ then v is not adjacent to w in G_3. Hence G_3 is bipartite.   □

3.3.1   Derivation of the main result from the Main Claim

Assuming that the Main Claim is valid, let D be a subset of Γ that satisfies conditions D1–D4. We now define two binary pictures f_A and f_B on $\mathcal{G}$ that have the properties (i), (ii), and (iii) stated in Proposition 3.1.

Condition D4 implies that there is a partition $\{A, B\}$ of the set D such that the $\mathcal{G}$-mates in D of each point of A all lie in B, and the $\mathcal{G}$-mates in D of each point of B all lie in A. For each grid line ℓ, condition D3 implies that *either* (a) ℓ does not pass through any point in D *or* (b) ℓ passes through just one point in A and just one point in B. We will say that ℓ is a grid line of type (a) or type (b) accordingly.

Let f_A and f_B be the binary pictures on $\mathcal{G}$ such that $f_A(p) = 1$ if and only if $p \in A$, and $f_B(p) = 1$ if and only if $p \in B$. f_A and f_B differ at all points in $A \cup B = D$. Condition D1 says $|D| > L$, so f_A and f_B have property (i).

Each grid line of type (a) passes through no 1's of f_A and no 1's of f_B. Each grid line of type (b) passes through just one 1 of f_A and just one 1 of f_B. So f_A and f_B are tomographically equivalent: They have property (ii).

It remains to show that f_A and f_B also have property (iii). Suppose f is a binary picture on $\mathcal{G}$ that is tomographically equivalent to f_A and f_B: We need to show that either $f = f_A$ or $f = f_B$. This will follow from the next two lemmas.

Lemma 3.3.   *Let q be any point in $\Gamma \setminus D$. Then q is a 0 of f as well as of f_A and f_B.*

Proof: By condition D2, there is a grid line ℓ_q through q that does not pass through any 1 of f_A or f_B. As f is tomographically equivalent to f_A and f_B, the grid line ℓ_q also does not pass through any 1 of f, and so q must be a 0 of f.   □

Lemma 3.4.   *Let d and d' be points in D that are $\mathcal{G}$-mates of each other, and suppose $f = f_A$ at d. Then $f = f_A$ at d'.*

Proof: Let $\ell_{d,d'}$ be the grid line of $\mathcal{G}$ that passes through d and d'. By condition D3, d and d' are the only points on $\ell_{d,d'}$ that are in D: So all points on $\ell_{d,d'}$ other than d and d' are 0's of f_A, and (by Lemma 3.3) 0's of f.

By the definition of the set A, just one of the $\mathcal{G}$-mates d and d' is in A. So just one of d and d' is a 1 of f_A. It follows that just one point on $\ell_{d,d'}$ is a 1 of f_A, which implies that just one point on $\ell_{d,d'}$ is a 1 of f, since f is tomographically equivalent to f_A. So just one of d and d' is a 1 of f (for, as we saw in the first paragraph, d and d' are the only points on $\ell_{d,d'}$ at which f can have value 1).

As just one of d and d' is a 1 of f_A, and just one of d and d' is a 1 of f, if $f = f_A = 1$ at d then $f = f_A = 0$ at d', and if $f = f_A = 0$ at d then $f = f_A = 1$ at d'. In both cases $f = f_A$ at d', so the lemma is true.   □

Lemma 3.4 and condition D4 imply that if $f = f_A$ at any one point in D, then $f = f_A$ at all points in D, which in turn implies that $f = f_A$ (as Lemma 3.3 says that $f = f_A = f_B = 0$ at all points outside D). Symmetrically, if $f = f_B$ at any one point in D, then $f = f_B$.

Now let d_0 be an arbitrary point in D. Then f_A and f_B have opposite values at d_0 (as d_0 lies in just one of A and B) so either $f = f_A$ at d_0 or $f = f_B$ at d_0. Hence either $f = f_A$ or $f = f_B$. This shows that no other binary picture on $\mathcal{G}$ is tomographically equivalent to f_A and f_B. Thus f_A and f_B have property (iii).

This proves Proposition 3.1, but only under the assumption that the Main Claim is valid.

3.3.2 Justification of the Main Claim

To complete our proof of Proposition 3.1 (and hence of our main result, Theorem 3.5), we now construct a set D that satisfies the conditions of the Main Claim. Our construction of D will be based on a family of "staircase-like" sets, which we now define.

For every $a \in \Gamma$ and all integers $h \geq 1$ and $k \geq 2$, let $X_{a,h,k}$ denote the set $\{x_i \mid 1 \leq i \leq 2k\}$, where the x's are the grid points in Γ that are given by the following rules:

1. $x_1 = a$.

2. For $1 \leq i \leq k - 1$, $x_{2i} = x_{2i-1} + v_1$ and $x_{2i+1} = x_{2i} + hv_2$.

3. $x_{2k} = x_{2k-1} - (k-1)v_1 = a + (k-1)hv_2$.

Figure 3.2 shows what $X_{a,3,5}$ may look like. Note that v_1 and v_2 are the only two fundamental direction vectors of the grid $\mathcal{G}$ that appear in the definition of $X_{a,h,k}$. However, an analogous set could be defined for any other pair of vectors in $\{v_1, v_2, \ldots, v_m\}$, and any such set could be used in essentially the same way to construct a set D that satisfies D1 – D4.

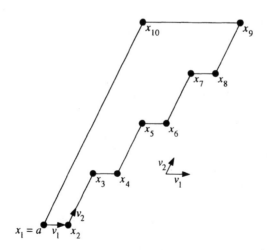

FIGURE 3.2. An example of a set $X_{a,3,5}$.

It is readily confirmed that $X_{a,h,k}$ has the following two properties for all $a \in \Gamma$, $h \geq 1$ and $k \geq 2$:

X1. $|X_{a,h,k}| = 2k$ (i.e., no two of the x's in the above definition of $X_{a,h,k}$ are equal).

X2. If a grid line of $\mathcal{G}$ in the direction of v_1 or v_2 passes through a point of $X_{a,h,k}$, then it passes through just one other point of $X_{a,h,k}$.

We claim that conditions D1–D4 are satisfied when $D = C_m$, where the $m - 1$ sets $C_2, \ldots, C_m$ are defined as follows. (We will not define any set C_1.) Let a be an arbitrary grid point in Γ, and let k be any integer such that $2^{m-1}k > L$. We define $C_2 = X_{a,h_2,k}$, where h_2 is some integer for which both of the following conditions hold:

X3. No grid line of $\mathcal{G}$ in any of the $m - 2$ directions $v_3, \ldots, v_m$ passes through more than one point of $X_{a,h_2,k}$.

X4. For each point $q \in \Gamma \setminus X_{a,h_2,k}$, at least one of the three grid lines through q in the directions v_1, v_2, and v_3 does not pass through any point in $X_{a,h_2,k}$.

That such an integer h_2 exists will follow from Lemma 3.5 below.

For $2 \le i < m$, we inductively define $C_{i+1} = C_i \cup (C_i + h_{i+1}v_{i+1})$, where h_{i+1} is an integer such that the following conditions C1, C2 and C3 all hold. (Note that condition C2 actually implies condition C1.)

C1. C_i and $C_i + h_{i+1}v_{i+1}$ are disjoint.

C2. No grid line of $\mathcal{G}$ in a direction other than v_{i+1}'s direction passes through both a point in C_i and a point in $C_i + h_{i+1}v_{i+1}$.

C3. For each point q in $\Gamma \setminus (C_i \cup (C_i + h_{i+1}v_{i+1}))$, at least one of the three grid lines through q in the directions v_1, v_2 and v_3 does not pass through any point in $C_i \cup (C_i + h_{i+1}v_{i+1})$.

That such an integer h_{i+1} exists will follow from Lemma 3.7 below.

Figure 3.3 shows an example of the set C_3 when C_2 is the set $X_{a,3,5}$ shown in Fig. 3.2. In this case one can confirm by inspection of the broken lines in Fig. 3.3 that conditions C2 and C3 are satisfied for $i = 2$ (and that the set $X_{a,3,5}$ satisfies conditions X3 and X4).

Lemma 3.5.   *Conditions X3 and X4 hold provided h_2 is sufficiently large.*

Proof: We first prove that X3 holds if h_2 is sufficiently large; in fact we prove more generally that the following is true if h is sufficiently large:

Assertion. No grid line of $\mathcal{G}$ in any of the $m - 2$ directions $v_3, \ldots, v_m$ passes through two distinct points p and q of Γ for which $q - p \in \{\alpha_1 v_1 + \alpha_2 h v_2 \mid \alpha_1, \alpha_2 \in \mathbf{Z}$ and $|\alpha_1| \le k - 1\}$.

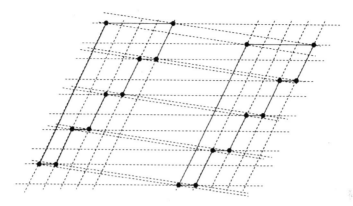

FIGURE 3.3. An example of the set C_3.

Indeed, suppose that for some integer i in the range $3 \leq i \leq m$ two distinct points p and q of Γ lie on a grid line of $\mathcal{G}$ in the direction of v_i, and suppose $q - p = \alpha_1 v_1 + \alpha_2 h v_2$, where α_1 and α_2 are integers and $|\alpha_1| \leq k - 1$. Since p and q lie on a grid line in the direction of v_i, there is a nonzero integer λ such that $\lambda v_i = q - p = \alpha_1 v_1 + \alpha_2 h v_2$; equivalently,

$$\alpha_1 v_1 = \lambda v_i - \alpha_2 h v_2. \tag{3.3}$$

The α's are nonzero, since v_1 and v_2 are not parallel to v_i (as $\mathcal{G}$ is a grid).

As v_i is not parallel to v_2, they are linearly independent and so for each value of α_1 there is at most one value of λ and of $\alpha_2 h$ for which (3.3) holds. It follows that there are at most $2k - 1$ values of λ and $\alpha_2 h$ for which (3.3) holds with $|\alpha_1| \leq k - 1$. So since $|\alpha_2 h| \geq h$, there is an integer H_i such that (3.3) cannot hold with $|\alpha_1| \leq k - 1$ when $h > H_i$. This implies that the Assertion is true for all $h > \max_{3 \leq i \leq m} H_i$.

Let h_2 be any integer such that $h_2 > \max_{3 \leq i \leq m} H_i$. Then X3 holds, since the Assertion holds for $h = h_2$. We will now show that X4 also holds.

Let $q \in \Gamma \setminus X_{a,h_2,k}$. If the grid line through q in the direction of v_1 does not pass through any point in $X_{a,h_2,k}$, then X4 holds.

Now suppose that the grid line does pass through some point q' in $X_{a,h_2,k}$. Then $q - q' = \lambda v_1$ for some integer λ. Moreover, since $q' \in X_{a,h_2,k}$, $q' = a + \alpha_1' v_1 + \alpha_2' h_2 v_2$ for some integers α_1' and α_2' such that $0 \leq \alpha_1' \leq k - 1$. It follows that $q = a + (\alpha_1' + \lambda) v_1 + \alpha_2' h_2 v_2$. If $\alpha_1' + \lambda$ does not lie between 0 and $k-1$ (inclusive) then the grid line through q in the direction of v_2 does not pass through any point in $X_{a,h_2,k}$ and again X4 holds. In the case where $0 \leq \alpha_1' + \lambda \leq k - 1$, if p is any point in $X_{a,h_2,k}$ then $q - p \in \{\alpha_1 v_1 + \alpha_2 h_2 v_2 \mid \alpha_1, \alpha_2 \in \mathbf{Z} \text{ and } |\alpha_1| \leq k - 1\}$, and the Assertion implies that the grid line of $\mathcal{G}$ in the direction of v_3 which passes through q cannot pass through p. Thus X4 also holds in this case. $\qquad\square$

This lemma shows that the integer h_2 used in the definition of C_2 exists.

Now we show that the integers h_{i+1} used in our definition of C_{i+1} for $2 \leq i < m$ also exist. But first we state a very easy lemma:

Lemma 3.6.   *Let ℓ be any grid line of $\mathcal{G}$, and let v be any vector in Γ. Then:*

(1) *The set $\ell + v$ is a grid line of $\mathcal{G}$ in the same direction as ℓ.*

(2) *If S_1 and S_2 are subsets of Γ such that ℓ passes through a point q_1 in S_1 and a different point q_2 in S_2, then $\ell + v$ passes through the point $q_1 + v$ in $S_1 + v$ and the point $q_2 + v$ in $S_2 + v$, and these two points are different.*

Proof: We confidently leave this to the reader. $\square$

Lemma 3.7.   *Let C^* be any finite subset of Γ and let j be an integer in the range $1 \leq j \leq m$. Then the following are true for all sufficiently large integers h:*

(1) *No grid line of $\mathcal{G}$ in a direction other than v_j's direction passes through both a point in C^* and a point in $C^* + hv_j$.*

(2) *If each point $q \in \Gamma \setminus C^*$ has the property that at least one of the three grid lines through q in the directions v_1, v_2 and v_3 does not pass through any point in C^*, then each point q in $\Gamma \setminus (C^* \cup (C^* + hv_j))$ has the property that at least one of the three grid lines through q in the directions v_1, v_2 and v_3 does not pass through any point in $C^* \cup (C^* + hv_j)$.*

Proof: We first consider (1). Suppose that C^* fails to satisfy (1) for some value of h, say $h = h^*$. Then there exist an integer $i \neq j$ in the range $1 \leq i \leq m$, points $p \in C^*$, $p' \in C^* + h^* v_j$, and an integer λ such that $p' - p = \lambda v_i$. Here it is possible that p and p' are the same point.

Since $p' \in C^* + h^* v_j$ there is a point $p'' \in C^*$ such that $p' = p'' + h^* v_j$. Thus $(p'' + h^* v_j) - p = \lambda v_i$, or, equivalently, $p'' - p = \lambda v_i - h^* v_j$. As $i \neq j$, v_i and v_j are nonparallel and hence linearly independent. It follows that h^* is uniquely determined by v_i and the pair of points p'' and p in C^*. Since there are just $|C^*|^2$ different ordered pairs of points in C^*, and just $m - 1$ different values of $i \neq j$ in the range $1 \leq i \leq m$, there are at most $(m - 1)|C^*|^2$ different possible values of h^*. Thus (1) can fail for at most $(m - 1)|C^*|^2$ different values of h. So we have proved that (1) holds for all sufficiently large integers h.

Now we consider (2). Suppose that for each point $q \in \Gamma \setminus C^*$ at least one of the three grid lines through q in the directions v_1, v_2 and v_3 does not pass through any point in C^*. Suppose further that there is a positive integer h^{**} for which condition (2) fails when $h = h^{**}$.

Then there exists a point $q \in \Gamma \setminus (C^* \cup (C^* + h^{**} v_j))$ such that each of the three grid lines through q in the directions v_1, v_2 and v_3 passes through a point in $C^* \cup (C^* + h^{**} v_j)$. Let ℓ_1, ℓ_2 and ℓ_3 be these three grid lines, where ℓ_i is in the direction of v_i for $i = 1, 2, 3$. By hypothesis at least one of ℓ_1, ℓ_2 and ℓ_3 does not pass through any point in C^*. Similarly, at least one of the three does not pass through any point in $C^* + h^{**}v_j$ (for otherwise $\ell_1 - h^{**}v_j$, $\ell_2 - h^{**}v_j$ and $\ell_3 - h^{**}v_j$ would be the three grid lines of $\mathcal{G}$ in the directions of v_1, v_2 and v_3 that pass through $q - h^{**}v_j \in \Gamma \setminus C^*$, and they would each pass through a point in C^*, by Lemma 3.6 with $S_1 = \{q\}$, $S_2 = C^* + h^{**}v_j$ and $v = -h^{**}v_j$).

Let (C, C') be a permutation of $\{C^*, C^* + h^{**}v_j\}$, and (a, b, c) a permutation of $\{1, 2, 3\}$, such that ℓ_c passes through a point $q_c \in C$ while ℓ_a passes through a point $q'_a \in C'$ and ℓ_b passes through a point $q'_b \in C'$. (Such permutations exist, by the remarks in the previous paragraph.) Note that ℓ_c does not pass through any point in C', for if it did then all three of ℓ_a, ℓ_b and ℓ_c would pass through a point in C'. In view of the definitions of q'_a, q'_b and q_c, the following three equations hold for some integers λ'_a, λ'_b and λ_c:

$$q - q'_a = \lambda'_a v_a \tag{3.4}$$

$$q - q'_b = \lambda'_b v_b \tag{3.5}$$

$$q - q_c = \lambda_c v_c \tag{3.6}$$

Let κ be the element of $\{h^{**}, -h^{**}\}$ such that $C' = C + \kappa v_j$, and let q'_c be the point $q_c + \kappa v_j$ in C'. By equation (3.6)

$$q - q'_c = \lambda_c v_c - \kappa v_j \tag{3.7}$$

Hence $c \neq j$, for if $v_c = v_j$ then (3.7) would imply that ℓ_c passes through a point in C' (namely q'_c), which is not so. Hence v_c and v_j are linearly independent. Thus for any given pair of points q and q'_c there cannot be more than one pair of integers (λ_c, κ) for which (3.7) holds.

Equations (3.4) and (3.5) imply

$$q'_a - q'_b = \lambda'_b v_b - \lambda'_a v_a \tag{3.8}$$

For any given pair of points q'_a and q'_b there cannot be more than one pair of integers λ'_a and λ'_b for which (3.8) holds (since v_a and v_b are linearly independent), and so there cannot be more than one point q for which (3.4) and (3.5) hold.

It follows from the two preceding paragraphs that for any given triple of points q'_a, q'_b and q'_c in C' there cannot be more than one point q and one quadruple of integers $(\lambda'_a, \lambda'_b, \lambda_c, \kappa)$ for which equations (3.4), (3.5), and (3.7) all hold. So since there are just $|C'|^3$ different triples (q'_a, q'_b, q'_c), there are at most $|C'|^3 = |C^*|^3$ different values of κ for which these three equations can be satisfied.

But whenever (2) fails for $h = h^{**} > 0$, these equations hold with $\kappa = h^{**}$ or $\kappa = -h^{**}$ for one of the two permutations (C, C') of $\{C^*, C^* + h^{**}v_j\}$ and one of the 3! permutations (a, b, c) of $\{1, 2, 3\}$. As there are just $2 \times 3! = 12$ possible pairs of permutations, and at most $|C^*|^3$ possible values of κ for each pair, there are at most $12|C^*|^3$ positive integer values of h^{**} for which condition (2) fails when $h = h^{**}$. Hence (2) holds for all sufficiently large integers h. $\square$

We now use this lemma to show that for $2 \leq i < m$ there always exists an integer h_{i+1} for which conditions C1, C2 and C3 in the definition of

C_{i+1} are satisfied. When $C^* = C_i$ and $j = i + 1$, statement (1) of the lemma implies that C2 holds if $h_{i+1} = h$. Hence C2 holds provided h_{i+1} is sufficiently large, and (since C2 implies C1) so does C1. The hypothesis of statement (2) of the lemma holds when $C^* = C_2 = X_{a,h_2,k}$ (since X4 holds), so C3 holds when $i = 2$ provided h_3 is sufficiently large. Moreover, if the value of h_n is such that C3 holds for $i = n - 1$ (where $3 \leq n < m$), then when we define $C_n = C_{n-1} \cup (C_{n-1} + h_n v_n)$ the hypothesis of (2) holds for $C^* = C_n$, and so C3 holds for $i = n$ provided h_{n+1} is sufficiently large. It follows (by induction) that, for all i in the range $2 \leq i < m$, C3 holds provided h_{i+1} is sufficiently large.

Note that C1 implies $|C_{i+1}| = 2|C_i|$. As $2^{m-1}k > L$ and (by X1) $|C_2| = 2k$, it follows that condition D1 holds for $D = C_m$. The case $i = m - 1$ of C3 implies that condition D2 holds for $D = C_m$, since $C_m = C_{m-1} \cup (C_{m-1} + h_m v_m)$. That condition D3 holds for $D = C_m$ will follow from the next three lemmas.

Lemma 3.8.   *For $2 \leq i < m$, if a grid line of $\mathcal{G}$ in any of the $m - i$ directions $v_{i+1}, \ldots, v_m$ passes through a point of C_i, then it passes through no other point of C_i; if a grid line in any of these directions passes through a point of $C_i + h_{i+1} v_{i+1}$, then it passes through no other point of $C_i + h_{i+1} v_{i+1}$.*

Proof: The second assertion is an immediate consequence of the first assertion and Lemma 3.6 (with $S_1 = S_2 = C_i + h_{i+1} v_{i+1}$ and $v = -h_{i+1} v_{i+1}$). We now prove the first assertion by induction on i. The assertion holds for $i = 2$, by X3. Assume as an induction hypothesis that the first assertion holds when $i = n - 1$ (where $3 \leq n < m$). Let p and q be two points in $C_n = C_{n-1} \cup (C_{n-1} + h_n v_n)$. If one of p and q is in C_{n-1} and the other is in $C_{n-1} + h_n v_n$, then p and q cannot lie on a grid line in any of the $m - n$ directions $v_{n+1}, \ldots, v_m$, by the case $i = n-1$ of C2. But the same is true if p and q are both in C_{n-1}, by the induction hypothesis, or if they are both in $C_{n-1} + h_n v_n$, by the induction hypothesis and Lemma 3.6. Hence the first assertion holds for $i = n$, and we are done. $\square$

Lemma 3.9.   *For $2 \leq i \leq m$, no three points of C_i lie on the same grid line of $\mathcal{G}$.*

Proof: The lemma holds for $i = 2$, by conditions X2 and X3. Assume as an induction hypothesis that it holds for $i = n - 1$, where $3 \leq n \leq m$.

Suppose three points in $C_n = C_{n-1} \cup (C_{n-1} + h_n v_n)$ lie on the same grid line ℓ of $\mathcal{G}$. By the induction hypothesis, the three points cannot all lie in the same one of the sets C_{n-1} and $C_{n-1} + h_n v_n$, so at least one of the points lies in C_{n-1} and at least one lies in $C_{n-1} + h_n v_n$. The case $i = n - 1$ of C2 now implies that the grid line ℓ must be in the direction of v_n. But two of the three points must lie in the same one of C_{n-1} and $C_{n-1} + h_n v_n$, so the fact that ℓ is in the direction of v_n contradicts Lemma 3.8 (with $i = n - 1$). $\square$

Lemma 3.10.   *For $2 \leq i \leq m$, if a grid line of $\mathcal{G}$ in any of the i directions $v_1, \ldots, v_i$ passes through a point of C_i, then it passes through another point of C_i.*

Proof: Suppose $1 \leq j \leq m$, $i \geq \max\{j, 2\}$ and ℓ is a grid line of $\mathcal{G}$ in the direction of v_j that passes through a grid point p in C_i. We assert that ℓ passes through another grid point in C_i; if we can prove this assertion, then we will have proved the lemma.

If $j = 1$ or $j = 2$ then the assertion is true in the case $i = 2$, by X2. Now suppose $j \geq 3$ and $i = j$. Then $p \in C_j = C_{j-1} \cup (C_{j-1} + h_j v_j)$. If $p \in C_{j-1}$ then $p + h_j v_j$ lies in $C_{j-1} + h_j v_j \subset C_j = C_i$ and lies on ℓ. If $p \in C_{j-1} + h_j v_j$ then $p - h_j v_j$ lies in $C_{j-1} \subset C_j = C_i$ and lies on ℓ. So if $j \geq 3$ then the assertion is true when $i = j$. Thus, for $1 \leq j \leq m$, the assertion is true when $i = \max\{j, 2\}$.

For any j in the range $1 \leq j \leq m$, assume as an induction hypothesis that the assertion is true when $i = j + n$, where n is some integer such that $n \geq 0$ and $j + n < m$. Note that this hypothesis is satisfied when $n = \max\{j, 2\} - j$ (so that $i = j + n = \max\{j, 2\}$). Suppose $i = j + n + 1$.

Since $p \in C_i = C_{j+n} \cup (C_{j+n} + h_{j+n+1} v_{j+n+1})$, either p or $p - h_{j+n+1} v_{j+n+1}$ lies in C_{j+n}. In the first case it follows from the induction hypothesis that ℓ passes through another point in $C_{j+n} = C_{i-1} \subset C_i$. Thus the assertion is true in this case. In the second case $\ell - h_{j+n+1} v_{j+n+1}$ is a grid line that passes through $p - h_{j+n+1} v_{j+n+1} \in C_{j+n}$ (by Lemma 3.6), so it follows from the induction hypothesis that the grid line $\ell - h_{j+n+1} v_{j+n+1}$ passes through another point besides $p - h_{j+n+1} v_{j+n+1}$ in C_{j+n}. Hence ℓ passes through another point besides p in $C_{j+n} + h_{j+n+1} v_{j+n+1} \subset C_i$, and so the assertion is true in this case too.

Thus the assertion is true by induction, and we have proved the lemma.   □

On putting $i = m$ in Lemmas 3.9 and 3.10, we deduce that condition D3 holds for $D = C_m$. It remains only to establish that condition D4 holds for $D = C_m$. We will deduce this from Lemma 3.2. For $2 \leq i \leq m$, write $G^{(i)}$ for the graph with vertex set C_i in which each vertex is adjacent to and only to its $\mathcal{G}$-mates in C_i. Then when $D = C_m$ condition D4 is the assertion that $G^{(m)}$ is connected and bipartite. We now prove, by induction on i, the more general fact that $G^{(i)}$ is connected and bipartite for $2 \leq i \leq m$.

Since $C_2 = X_{a, h_2, k}$, it follows from the definition of $X_{a, h, k}$ and conditions X1 – X3, that $G^{(2)}$ is a cycle of length $2k$ and is therefore connected and bipartite. Now suppose that for some i in the range $2 \leq i < m$ the graph $G^{(i)}$ is connected and bipartite. Let $V_1 = C_i$ and $V_2 = C_i + h_{i+1} v_{i+1}$. By C1, the sets V_1 and V_2 are disjoint. Let $G_1 = G^{(i)}$ and let G_2 be the graph with vertex set V_2 in which each vertex is adjacent to, and only to, its $\mathcal{G}$-mates in V_2. Let $\theta : V_1 \to V_2$ be the bijection defined by $\theta(x) = x + h_{i+1} v_{i+1}$. Both θ and θ^{-1} map $\mathcal{G}$-mates to $\mathcal{G}$-mates, so θ is a graph isomorphism of $G_1 = G^{(i)}$ to G_2.

For each vertex v in $V_1 = C_i$, $\theta(v) = v + h_{i+1} v_{i+1}$ is a vertex in $V_2 = C_i + h_{i+1} v_{i+1}$ that is a $\mathcal{G}$-mate of v. Moreover, C2 and Lemma 3.9 imply that $\theta(v)$ is the only $\mathcal{G}$-mate of v in V_2.

Let $G_3 = G^{(i+1)}$. G_3's vertex set is $C_{i+1} = C_i \cup (C_i + h_{i+1} v_{i+1}) = V_1 \cup V_2$. In G_1, G_2 and G_3 two vertices are adjacent if and only if they are $\mathcal{G}$-mates of each other. So (in view of the observations in the previous paragraph) two vertices v and w of G_3 are adjacent in G_3 in just the following three cases: (i) v and w both lie in V_1 and are adjacent in G_1; (ii) v and w both lie in V_2 and are adjacent in G_2; (iii) $v \in V_1$, $w \in V_2$ and $w = \theta(v)$, or $v \in V_2$, $w \in V_1$ and $v = \theta(w)$. As G_1 and G_2 are connected and bipartite with disjoint vertex sets, it follows from Lemma 3.2 that $G_3 = G^{(i+1)}$ is also connected and bipartite. This completes the inductive proof that $G^{(i)}$ is connected and bipartite for $2 \leq i \leq m$.

We have now shown that all four conditions of the Main Claim hold when $D = C_m$. This completes the proof of Proposition 3.1 and hence of our main result, Theorem 3.5.

3.4   Concluding remarks

We have shown that on any grid $\mathcal{G}$ with more than two fundamental direction vectors there is no integer L for which every tomographic equivalence class of binary pictures is ($l_1 \leq L$)-connected. In other words, there does not exist any integer L such that an arbitrary binary picture on $\mathcal{G}$ can be transformed to any other tomographically equivalent binary picture on $\mathcal{G}$ by a sequence of steps each of which preserves tomographic equivalence and changes the picture at no more than L points. This is in sharp contrast to Ryser's theorem for the 2-dimensional square grid, which says that every tomographic equivalence class of binary pictures on the square grid is ($l_1 \leq 4$)-connected.

In [8] the same result is stated and proved for a more general concept of "grid" than has been used in this chapter. In that paper a grid is defined as a pair (Γ, P), where Γ is an infinite Abelian group and:

1. P is a finite set of two or more elements that generates the group Γ.

2. If v and w are any two distinct elements of P and $m, n \in \mathbf{Z}$, then $mv = nw$ only if $m = n = 0$.

Evidently, every grid (Γ, P) in the sense of the present chapter satisfies these conditions. However, these conditions allow the group Γ to contain elements of finite order; they admit certain "grids" in three- and higher-dimensional analogs of cylindrical and toroidal surfaces. With minor changes our proof of the main result in Section 3.3 above is valid even for this more general definition of a grid.

A polynomial-time algorithm for determining whether a binary picture on the square grid is tomographically nonunique (i.e., is tomographically equivalent to at least one other binary picture or, equivalently, has at least one variant element) can be derived from Ryser's theorem. That theorem implies that a binary picture f on the square grid is tomographically nonunique if and only if a rectangular 4-switch can be performed on f. If the x- and y-coordinates of the 1's of f are known to lie in the range $[a, a + h]$ for some integers a and $h \geq 0$, then the existence or nonexistence of such a rectangular 4-switch can obviously be determined in $O(h^4)$ time by testing all pairs of 1's to see if they are diagonally opposite corner points of a grid rectangle whose other corner points are 0's. (It can be done more efficiently, using the observation that no rectangular 4-switch can be performed on f if and only if, for every pair of grid lines ℓ and ℓ' parallel to the x-axis, the set of x-coordinates of the 1's on ℓ is a subset or superset of the set of x-coordinates of the 1's on ℓ'. This condition can be checked in $O(h^2)$ time if we first sort the y-coordinates of the grid lines parallel to the x-axis with respect to the line sums of f along those grid lines.)

It follows from our main result that on grids with grid lines in three or more directions there is no analogous way to determine whether a binary picture is tomographically nonunique. In fact this problem has recently been shown by Gardner, Gritzmann, and Prangenberg [9] to be NP-complete. We refer the reader to Chapter 4 (by Gardner and Gritzmann) for further details. As Gritzmann et al. observe in [10, Sect. 4], this NP-completeness result actually implies that our main result is true unless $P = NP$.

Acknowledgments

The second author's work in this area is supported by the U.S. National Institutes of Health under grant no. HL28438 and the U.S. National Science Foundation under grant no. DMS9612077.

References

[1] H. J. Ryser, "Combinatorial properties of matrices of zeros and ones," *Can. J. Mathematics* **9**, 371–377 (1957).

[2] H. J. Ryser, *Combinatorial Mathematics* (Mathematical Association of America, Washington, DC), 1963, Chapter 6.

[3] G. Winkler, *Image Analysis, Random Fields and Dynamic Monte Carlo Methods* (Springer-Verlag, Berlin), 1995.

[4] T. H. Cormen, C. E. Leiserson, and R. L. Rivest, *Introduction to Algorithms* (MIT Press, Cambridge, Massachusetts), 1990.

[5] A. Kuba, "Determination of the structure of the class $\mathcal{A}(R,S)$ of (0,1)-matrices," *Acta Cybernetica* **9**, 121–132 (1989).

[6] R. Aharoni, G. T. Herman, and A. Kuba, "Binary vectors partially determined by linear equation systems," *Discrete Mathematics* **171**, 1–16 (1997).

[7] R. P. Anstee, "The network flows approach for matrices with given row and column sums," *Discrete Mathematics* **44**, 125–138 (1983).

[8] T. Y. Kong and G. T. Herman, "On which grids can tomographic equivalence of binary pictures be characterized in terms of elementary switching operations?" *Int. J. Imaging Syst. Technol.* **9**, 118–125 (1998).

[9] R. J. Gardner, P. Gritzmann, and D. Prangenberg, "On the computational complexity of reconstructing lattice sets from their X-rays," to appear in *Discrete Mathematics*.

[10] P. Gritzmann, D. Prangenberg, S. De Vries, and M. Wiegelmann, Success and failure of certain reconstruction and uniqueness algorithms in discrete tomography, *Int. J. Imaging Syst. Technol.* **9**, 101–109 (1998).

Chapter 4

Uniqueness and Complexity in Discrete Tomography

Richard J. Gardner[1]
Peter Gritzmann[2]

ABSTRACT We study the discrete inverse problem of reconstructing finite subsets of the n-dimensional integer lattice $\mathbb{Z}^n$ that are only accessible via their line sums (discrete X-rays) in a finite set of lattice directions. Special emphasis is placed on the question of when such sets are uniquely determined by the data and on the difficulty of the related algorithmic problems. Such questions are motivated by demands from the material sciences for the reconstruction of crystalline structures from images produced by quantitative high-resolution transmission electron microscopy.

4.1   Introduction

Let $\mathcal{E}$ be a class of *lattice sets*, finite subsets of the integer lattice $\mathbb{Z}^n$, and let $\mathcal{L}$ be a finite set of lines containing the origin and at least one other point in $\mathbb{Z}^n$. We consider the following questions, mainly focusing on the case $n = 2$.

Question 4.1.1 *Can a set $E \in \mathcal{E}$ be distinguished from any other set in $\mathcal{E}$ by its X-rays parallel to the lines in $\mathcal{L}$?*

This is the basic uniqueness problem in discrete tomography. The answer depends on $\mathcal{E}$ and $\mathcal{L}$. The present state of our knowledge is summarized in Section 4.3.

Question 4.1.2 *What is the complexity of the associated algorithmic problems?*

At the same time it is natural to consider the complexity of the associated algorithmic problems of data consistency and of reconstruction of a set from the data. What is known is set out in Section 4.4.

---

[1] Western Washington University, Department of Mathematics, Bellingham, WA 98225-9063, USA, E-mail: gardner@baker.math.wwu.edu
[2] Technische Universität München, Zentrum Mathematik, D-80290 München, Germany, E-mail: gritzman@mathematik.tu-muenchen.de

The problem of reconstructing lattice sets from their X-rays has various interesting applications and connections to image processing, graph theory, scheduling, statistical data security, game theory, material sciences, and so on. Some of these topics are discussed in the final chapters. The principal motivation is in the attempt to reconstruct crystalline structures from their images obtained by high-resolution transmission electron microscopy, and the setting for the two questions above is suggested by this application. In fact, [1] and [2] show how a quantitative analysis of images from high-resolution transmission electron microscopy can be used to determine the number of atoms in atomic columns in certain directions. The goal is to use this technique for quality control in VLSI (Very Large Scale Integration) technology. In particular, the interfacial topography of a material is vital in the manufacture of silicon chips.

Other questions can be asked, of course. In remarks scattered in Sections 4.3 and 4.4 we shall mention extensions and variations, and Section 4.5 is also devoted to such matters. The reader searching for research topics will find plenty of unsolved problems; see in particular Remarks 4.3.4(iv), 4.3.11(iv), (v), and (vi), 4.4.7(iii), and Sections 4.5.1 and 4.5.3.

Among the topics *not* treated in depth here are the connections between uniqueness, additivity, and the existence of switching components or bad configurations (see Chapter 2 by Fishburn and Shepp in this book), and recent developments concerning reconstruction algorithms, though we will touch on these issues.

We provide full proofs where space allows. Where some details are omitted, references to sources where the missing details can be found are given in the various remarks.

4.2   Definitions and preliminaries

If A is a set, we denote by $|A|$ and conv A the *cardinality* and *convex hull* of A, respectively. The *symmetric difference* of two sets A and B is $A \triangle B = (A \setminus B) \cup (B \setminus A)$. The *vector sum* of A and B is

$$A + B = \{x + y : x \in A, \, y \in B\}. \tag{4.1}$$

If $x \in \mathbb{R}$, then $\lfloor x \rfloor$ and $\lceil x \rceil$ signify the greatest integer less than or equal to x, and the smallest integer greater than or equal to x, respectively.

Let F be a finite subset of Euclidean n-space $\mathbb{E}^n$, and L a line through the origin. The *(discrete) X-ray of F parallel to L* is the function $X_L F$ defined by

$$X_L F(T) = |F \cap T|, \tag{4.2}$$

for each line T parallel to L. The function $X_L F$ is in effect the projection, counted with multiplicity, of F on $L^\perp$. Some authors refer to $X_L F$ as a projection. In this chapter we shall omit the word "discrete" and simply write

X-ray, but we note that this term has often been used for the continuous X-ray; see [3].

Let $\mathcal{E}$ be a class of finite sets in $\mathbb{E}^n$ and $\mathcal{L}$ a finite set of lines through the origin. We say that $E \in \mathcal{E}$ is *determined* by the X-rays parallel to the lines in $\mathcal{L}$ if whenever $E' \in \mathcal{E}$ and $X_L E' = X_L E$ for all $L \in \mathcal{L}$, we have $E' = E$.

One might consider the scenario in which X-rays parallel to $L \in \mathcal{L}$ of sets in $\mathcal{E}$ are only known up to a translation (depending on L). However, assuming $|\mathcal{L}| \geq 2$, sets in $\mathcal{E}$ are then determined up to a translation if and only if they are determined by X-rays parallel to the lines in $\mathcal{L}$ in the sense of the definition above. The proof given for continuous X-rays in [3, Theorem 1.2.4] is easily modified to apply to the discrete case.

A *lattice* is a finite subset of $\mathbb{Z}^n$. The class of lattice sets in $\mathbb{Z}^n$ is denoted by $\mathcal{F}^n$. A *convex lattice set* is a finite set F such that $F = \mathbb{Z}^n \cap \operatorname{conv} F$, and the class of such sets is denoted by $\mathcal{C}^n$. A *lattice line* is a line containing two or more points of $\mathbb{Z}^n$. The class of lattice lines *containing the origin* in $\mathbb{E}^n$ is denoted by $\mathcal{L}^n$.

If L is a line through the origin that is not a lattice line, then lattice sets are determined by the single X-ray parallel to L. Unfortunately, this is completely useless in the electron microscopy application. In this chapter our main interest is therefore in the *lattice situation*, in which we consider only X-rays parallel to lattice lines of lattice sets. Occasionally we shall refer to the *non-lattice situation*, in which X-rays parallel to arbitrary lines through the origin are taken of arbitrary finite subsets of $\mathbb{E}^n$.

A *convex polygon* is the convex hull of a finite set of points in $\mathbb{E}^2$. A *convex lattice polygon* is a convex polygon with its vertices in $\mathbb{Z}^2$. (More generally, a *convex lattice polytope* is a convex polytope with its vertices in $\mathbb{Z}^n$.) By a *regular polygon* we shall always mean a nondegenerate convex regular polygon.

Let $\mathcal{L}$ be a finite set of lines through the origin in $\mathbb{E}^2$. We call a nondegenerate convex polygon P an *$\mathcal{L}$-polygon* if it has the following property: If v is a vertex of P, and T is a line containing v and parallel to some $L \in \mathcal{L}$, then T also contains a different vertex v' of P. Clearly $\mathcal{L}$-polygons have an even number of vertices. Note that an affinely regular polygon with an even number of vertices is an $\mathcal{L}$-polygon if and only if each line in $\mathcal{L}$ is parallel to one of its edges.

Let $\mathcal{L}$ be a finite set of lines through the origin in $\mathbb{E}^n$. An *$\mathcal{L}$-switching component* is a finite set $A \cup B$ such that A and B are disjoint and nonempty, and

$$|A \cap (x + L)| = |B \cap (x + L)| \tag{4.3}$$

for all $x \in \mathbb{E}^n$ and $L \in \mathcal{L}$. Note that if A and B are two sets of alternate vertices of an $\mathcal{L}$-polygon, then $A \cup B$ is an $\mathcal{L}$-switching component.

4.3   Uniqueness results

In this section we summarize what we know about Question 4.1.1.

Theorem 4.3.1 *Let $\mathcal{L}$ be a finite subset of $\mathcal{L}^2$. There are sets in $\mathcal{F}^2$ that cannot be determined by X-rays parallel to the lines in $\mathcal{L}$.*

Proof: Suppose $\mathcal{L}$ contains only one line L. If $F_i = \{x_i\}$, $i = 1, 2$, where x_1 and x_2 are different points on L, then F_1 and F_2 have the same X-ray parallel to L. Suppose the theorem has been proved when $|\mathcal{L}| = k$, and suppose that $|\mathcal{L}| = k + 1$. Let G_1 and G_2 be different lattice sets with the same X-rays parallel to some k of the lines in $\mathcal{L}$, and let L be the remaining line in $\mathcal{L}$. Choose a nonzero vector $v \in L \cap \mathbb{Z}^2$ of large enough magnitude that $(G_1 \cup G_2) + v$ is disjoint from $G_1 \cup G_2$. (The disjointness is not essential, but aids visualization.) Let $F_1 = G_1 \cup (G_2 + v)$ and $F_2 = G_2 \cup (G_1 + v)$. Then F_1 and F_2 are different lattice sets with the same X-rays parallel to the lines in $\mathcal{L}$.   □

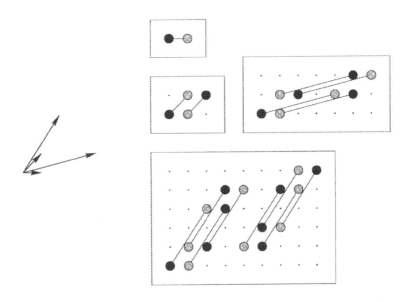

FIGURE 4.1. Construction of different lattice sets with equal X-rays in four directions.

Remark 4.3.2 (i) Theorem 4.3.1 extends without difficulty to higher dimensions and to the general non-lattice situation in $\mathbb{E}^n$; see, for example, [3, Lemma 2.3.2]. In $\mathbb{E}^2$, it was noted by Lorentz [4]. It has been rediscovered several times, for example by Ron Graham, who at the DIMACS mini-conference in 1994 referred to it as "the dark side of the force"! It is indeed a fundamental source of difficulties in discrete tomography.

(ii) The proof is equivalent to noting that there is a lattice parallelepiped P of dimension $|\mathcal{L}|$ whose vertices can be projected into $\mathbb{Z}^2$ so that the projections of the two sets of $2^{|\mathcal{L}|-1}$ alternate vertices of P have the same X-rays parallel to the lines in $\mathcal{L}$. See Fig. 4.1 for an illustration of the case $|\mathcal{L}| = 4$.

(iii) Consider any rectangular array F of consecutive points in $\mathbb{Z}^2$ large enough to contain the sets F_1 and F_2 constructed in the proof of Theorem 4.3.1. Then $F_1' = F \setminus F_1$ and $F_2' = F \setminus F_2$ also have the same X-rays parallel to the lines in $\mathcal{L}$. Whereas the points in F_1 and F_2 are widely dispersed over a region, those in F_1' and F_2' are contiguous in a way similar to atoms in a crystal; see Fig. 4.2.

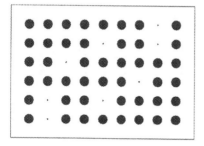 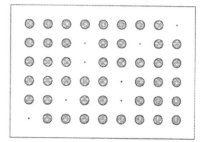

FIGURE 4.2. Contiguous lattice sets with equal X-rays parallel to four lattice lines.

Theorem 4.3.3 *Let $m \in \mathbb{N}$, and let $\mathcal{F}^2(m)$ be the class of sets in $\mathcal{F}^2$ of cardinality less than or equal to m. Let $\mathcal{L} \subset \mathcal{L}^2$ with $|\mathcal{L}| \geq m + 1$. Then the sets in $\mathcal{F}^2(m)$ are determined by X-rays parallel to the lines in $\mathcal{L}$.*

Proof: (First version.) Let F be a set in $\mathcal{F}^2(m)$. If $F' \in \mathcal{F}^2(m)$ has the same X-rays as F parallel to the lines in $\mathcal{L}$, then $|F'| = |F|$ and

$$F' \subset G = \cap\{(L + F) : L \in \mathcal{L}\}. \tag{4.4}$$

However, $G = F$, since the existence of a point in $G \setminus F$ implies the existence of at least $|\mathcal{L}| \geq m + 1$ points in F. Therefore $F = F'$. □

Proof: (Second version.) Let F be a set in $\mathcal{F}^2(m)$. From the X-rays of F parallel to the lines in $\mathcal{L}$, we can construct the set $\mathcal{S}$ of all supporting lines to conv F that are parallel to a line in $\mathcal{L}$. Then $|\mathcal{S}| \geq 2m + 1$ (and $|\mathcal{S}| = 2m + 1$ only in the case that all the points in F lie on a line). The lines in $\mathcal{S}$ also support a convex polygon P containing the points in F.

If a point $x \in \mathbb{Z}^2$ lies on at least three lines in $\mathcal{S}$, it must belong to F, since each of these lines contains a point of F, and at least one of the lines contains no point of P other than x. Moreover, there must be at least one $x \in \mathbb{Z}^2$ lying on three or more lines in S, since there are only m points in F and at least $2m + 1$ lines in S. Now we know $x \in F$. For each $L \in \mathcal{L}$, we replace $X_L F(T)$ by $X_L F(T) - 1$, where T is the line parallel to L containing x. The modified X-rays are those of the set $F \setminus \{x\}$ of $m - 1$ points. Repeating this procedure, we can find F in at most m steps. $\square$

Remark 4.3.4 (i) Theorem 4.3.3 is due to Rényi [5], who attributes the second proof above to Hajós. Both proofs work equally well in the non-lattice situation, the second even when the points are given different weights. Rényi was interested in this since his paper concerned the determination of probability distributions from marginals, the result here corresponding to a finite distribution. Heppes [6] extended the general result to higher dimensions.

(ii) The second proof yields a procedure by which a set in $\mathcal{F}^2(m)$ can actually be reconstructed from $m + 1$ X-rays.

(iii) Consider a regular $2m$-gon P in the plane, and let F_1 and F_2 be two sets of m alternate vertices of P. Clearly F_1 and F_2 have equal X-rays parallel to any of the m lines through the origin parallel to the edges of P. Therefore the number $m + 1$ in Theorem 4.3.3 is the best possible in the non-lattice situation, without further restriction on the set $\mathcal{L}$ of lines. The sets of six black and six gray points in Fig. 4.5 show that this is also true for the lattice situation when $m \leq 6$.

(iv) In the non-lattice situation, Theorems 4.3.1 and 4.3.3 and their proofs show that sets in the class of planar sets of at most m points can be determined by $m + 1$ X-rays but not by $\lfloor \log_2 m \rfloor$ X-rays, no matter how the lines in $\mathcal{L}$ are chosen. A deep result of Bianchi and Longinetti [7] states, roughly speaking, that apart from examples of the type mentioned in (iii) above, sets of m points in $\mathbb{E}^2$ are determined by X-rays parallel to any set $\mathcal{L}$ of lines through the origin, provided

$$|\mathcal{L}| \geq m + \frac{3 - \sqrt{m + 9}}{2}. \tag{4.5}$$

(It would be interesting to see whether a better bound could be achieved in the lattice situation.) They also show that given any set of four such lines (or lattice lines), there are two different sets of no more than five points in $\mathbb{E}^2$ (or $\mathbb{Z}^2$, respectively) with equal X-rays parallel to these lines. (See also Chapter 2 by Fishburn and Shepp, Theorem 2.9.)

In order to reduce the number of X-rays required to guarantee uniqueness, we now consider the class of convex lattice sets. The first step is to reduce the problem to understanding certain kinds of convex lattice polygons.

Lemma 4.3.5 Let $\mathcal{L} \subset \mathcal{L}^2$. The following statements are equivalent.

(i) Sets in $\mathcal{C}^2$ are determined by X-rays parallel to the lines in $\mathcal{L}$.

(ii) There does not exist a lattice $\mathcal{L}$-polygon.

Proof: (Sketch.) The relevance of lattice $\mathcal{L}$-polygons will be clear when we suppose that one, P, say, exists. Let V_1 and V_2 be disjoint sets of alternate vertices of P, let I be the set of lattice points in the interior of P, and let $F_i = I \cup V_i$, $i = 1, 2$. Then F_1 and F_2 are different convex lattice sets with equal X-rays parallel to the lines in $\mathcal{L}$. See Fig. 4.3, which illustrates this construction for a special set of four lines in $\mathcal{L}^2$ parallel to the vectors shown.

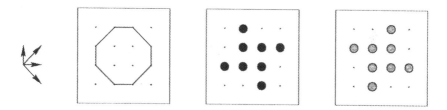

FIGURE 4.3. An $\mathcal{L}$-polygon and different convex lattice sets with equal X-rays.

For the converse, we first note that if $|\mathcal{L}| \leq 3$, it is quite easy to construct a lattice $\mathcal{L}$-hexagon. Therefore, we may suppose that $|\mathcal{L}| \geq 4$. Assume that there exist two different convex lattice sets, F_1 and F_2, with equal X-rays parallel to the lines in $\mathcal{L}$, and let $K_i = \operatorname{conv} F_i$, $i = 1, 2$. One proves readily that K_1 and K_2 are either both 1-dimensional or both 2-dimensional convex polygons. In the former case it is clear that K_1 and K_2, and hence F_1 and F_2, must be equal. If K_1 and K_2 are both 2-dimensional, then since they are different, there is a nonempty component C_0 of $K_1 \triangle K_2$. Given any $L \in \mathcal{L}$, it is reasonable to conclude that there should be another component C_1 of $K_1 \triangle K_2$, such that $C_0 \cap \mathbb{Z}^2$ and $C_1 \cap \mathbb{Z}^2$ are disjoint and have equal X-rays parallel to L. (In fact this is not quite true, and one has to work with finite unions of components, but this is a minor adjustment that need not concern us here.) In particular, $|C_1 \cap \mathbb{Z}^2| = |C_0 \cap \mathbb{Z}^2|$, and one can check that $C_0 \cap \mathbb{Z}^2$ and $C_1 \cap \mathbb{Z}^2$ have their centroids lying on the same line parallel to L.

From C_0, a sequence $\{C_m\}$ of components of $K_1 \triangle K_2$ can be generated inductively, by applying the above procedure to any previously constructed component and with respect to any $L \in \mathcal{L}$. Since each new lattice set $C_m \cap \mathbb{Z}^2$ must either coincide with a previous one, or be disjoint with $|C_m \cap \mathbb{Z}^2| = |C_0 \cap \mathbb{Z}^2|$, the sequence $\{C_m\}$ is actually finite. It follows that the set of centroids of the sets $C_m \cap \mathbb{Z}^2$ form the vertices of an $\mathcal{L}$-polygon P. The vertices of P need not be lattice points, of course, but since each is a centroid of a finite subset of $F_1 \cup F_2$, each can be given rational coordinates with the same denominator s. Then the dilate sP of P is the required lattice $\mathcal{L}$-polygon. ☐

Lemma 4.3.6 *Suppose that there exists an $\mathcal{L}$-polygon. Then there is a* *nonsingular linear transformation ϕ such that the set $\{\phi L : L \in \mathcal{L}\}$ is a subset of a set of equiangular lines through the origin, that is, the angle between each adjacent pair is the same.*

Proof: (Sketch.) Let P be an $\mathcal{L}$-polygon, and suppose, by translating P if necessary, that its centroid is at the origin. The midpoint polygon $M(P)$ of P, formed by taking the convex hull of the midpoints of the edges of P, is also an $\mathcal{L}$-polygon, as is its second midpoint polygon $M^2(P) = M(M(P))$. A very beautiful old result of Darboux states that the sequence $\{M^{2m}P\}$ of successive second midpoint polygons, when these are dilated so that their areas are all the same, converges to the image ψQ of a regular polygon Q under a nonsingular linear transformation ψ. Since ψQ must also be an $\mathcal{L}$-polygon, the lines in $\mathcal{L}$ are parallel to the edges of ψQ. Let $\phi = \psi^{-1}$. Then the lines in the set $\{\phi L : L \in \mathcal{L}\}$ are parallel to the edges of Q and so form a subset of a set of equiangular lines. □

Lemma 4.3.7 *Let $\mathcal{L} \subset \mathcal{L}^2$ with $|\mathcal{L}| \geq 4$, and suppose that there exists a lattice $\mathcal{L}$-polygon. Then the cross ratio of the slopes of any four lines in $\mathcal{L}$, arranged in order of increasing angle with the positive x-axis, is $4/3$, $3/2$, 2, 3, or 4.*

Proof: (Sketch.) Let $\mathcal{L}$ be as in the statement of the theorem. Each line in $\mathcal{L}$ has a rational slope, so if we select any four such lines L_j, $j = 1,\ldots,4$, then the cross ratio of their slopes is a rational number q.

By Lemma 4.3.6, there is a nonsingular linear transformation ϕ such that the set $\{\phi L_j : j = 1,\ldots,4\}$ is a subset of a set of equiangular lines through the origin. Since linear transformations preserve cross ratio, the cross ratio of the slopes of these lines also equals q. To derive an expression for this cross ratio, note that there is an $m \in \mathbb{N}$ such that each line ϕL_j is parallel to a direction that can be represented by a complex number of the form $e^{h_j \pi i / m}$, where $h_j \in \mathbb{N}$, $0 \leq h_j \leq m - 1$ and we can assume that the h_j's increase with j. Then the cross ratio is

$$\frac{(\tan\frac{h_3\pi}{m} - \tan\frac{h_1\pi}{m})(\tan\frac{h_4\pi}{m} - \tan\frac{h_2\pi}{m})}{(\tan\frac{h_3\pi}{m} - \tan\frac{h_2\pi}{m})(\tan\frac{h_4\pi}{m} - \tan\frac{h_1\pi}{m})} = \frac{\sin\frac{(h_3-h_1)\pi}{m} \sin\frac{(h_4-h_2)\pi}{m}}{\sin\frac{(h_3-h_2)\pi}{m} \sin\frac{(h_4-h_1)\pi}{m}} = q. \quad (4.6)$$

The fact that a ratio of products of sines of rational multiples of π must be a rational number would seem to be a rather restrictive condition. The equation certainly has some solutions; for example, one can take $m = 4$, $h_1 = 1$, $h_2 = 2$, $h_3 = 3$, $h_4 = 4$, and $q = 2$. But we need to find *all* solutions of such an equation.

The first step is to switch to complex numbers. Let $k_1 = h_3 - h_1$, $k_2 = h_4 - h_2$, $k_3 = h_3 - h_2$, and $k_4 = h_4 - h_1$. Then $1 \leq k_3 < k_1, k_2 < k_4 \leq m - 1$ and $k_1 + k_2 = k_3 + k_4$. Using $\sin\theta = -e^{-i\theta}(1 - e^{2i\theta})/2i$, we obtain the crucial cyclotomic equation

$$\frac{(1 - \omega_m^{k_1})(1 - \omega_m^{k_2})}{(1 - \omega_m^{k_3})(1 - \omega_m^{k_4})} = q \in \mathbb{Q}, \quad\quad (4.7)$$

where $\omega_m = e^{2\pi i/m}$ is the primitive mth root of unity.

The very form of (4.7) suggests trying to apply Galois theory. Recall that the Galois group $G(\mathbb{Q}(\omega_m)/\mathbb{Q})$ is the group of all automorphisms of the field $\mathbb{Q}(\omega_m)$ (containing the polynomials in ω_m with coefficients in $\mathbb{Z}$) leaving $\mathbb{Q}$ fixed. This Galois group consists of the automorphisms mapping ω_m to some ω_m^s where s and m are coprime. One can apply such an automorphism to (4.7), knowing that the right-hand side, q, will remain unchanged, while the exponents on the left-hand side will change according to the rule $\omega_m \to \omega_m^s$. Every such application yields a relation between factors like those on the left-hand side of (4.7), and one can try to use these to find solutions or eliminate possible solutions. However, there are situations that cannot be dealt with this way, so a more powerful tool is needed: p-adic valuations.

At their most basic level, p-adic valuations appear to have little to do with Galois theory. If p is a prime number, the p-adic valuation is first defined on $\mathbb{Z}$ to be the function v_p such that $v_p(n)$ is the highest power of p that divides n (and $v_p(0) = \infty$). Naturally, this is essentially a log function that can be extended to $\mathbb{Q}$ by the rule

$$v_p\left(\frac{a}{b}\right) = v_p(a) - v_p(b), \tag{4.8}$$

for nonzero integers a and b. Note that v_p is integer-valued on $\mathbb{Q}\backslash\{0\}$. Now comes the big extension, requiring most of the machinery of Galois theory. The function v_p can be extended to the algebraic closure $\bar{\mathbb{Q}}_p$ of a field $\mathbb{Q}_p$, whose elements are called p-adic numbers, containing $\mathbb{Q}$. Note that $\bar{\mathbb{Q}}_p$ contains the algebraic closure of $\mathbb{Q}$ and hence all the algebraic numbers. On $\bar{\mathbb{Q}}_p \backslash \{0\}$, v_p takes values in $\mathbb{Q}$, and satisfies

$$v_p(xy) = v_p(x) + v_p(y) \tag{4.9}$$

and

$$v_p\left(\frac{x}{y}\right) = v_p(x) - v_p(y). \tag{4.10}$$

Armed with this new weapon, we can return to the cyclotomic equation (4.7) and see what happens when we apply v_p to both sides. The p-adic valuation $v_p(q)$ of the right-hand side is an integer. To find the p-adic valuation of the left-hand side, it suffices, by (4.9) and (4.10), to find the p-adic valuation of the four individual factors. Then one can apply the following facts (long familiar to experts in the field). Suppose that r, $s \in \mathbb{N}$ and that r and s are coprime. If r is not a power of p, then

$$v_p(1 - \omega_r^s) = 0. \tag{4.11}$$

If r is a power of p, say $r = p^t$, then

$$v_p(1 - \omega_r^s) = \frac{1}{p^{t-1}(p-1)}. \tag{4.12}$$

To see how helpful p-adic valuations are in dealing with cyclotomic equations, consider the problem of finding the solutions of the simpler equation

$$(1 - \omega_m^{l_1})(1 - \omega_m^{l_2}) = q' \in \mathbb{Q}, \tag{4.13}$$

where l_1, $l_2 \in \mathbb{N}$, $l_1 \le l_2 < m$ and the greatest common divisor of l_1, l_2, and m is 1. Suppose that $q' \ne 1$. Then $v_p(q') \ne 0$ for some prime p, so by (4.11) and (4.12), $l_j/m = s_j/p^{t_j}$, where p and s_j are coprime, for at least one value of j, $j = 1, 2$. Let t be the minimum value of t_j, $j = 1, 2$. Since q' is a nonzero rational, $v_p(q') \in \mathbb{N}$. Taking the p-adic valuation of both sides of (4.13) and using (4.9), (4.11), and (4.12), we see that

$$1 \le v_p(q) = v_p((1 - \omega_m^{l_1})(1 - \omega_m^{l_2})) = v_p(1 - \omega_m^{l_1}) + v_p(1 - \omega_m^{l_2}) \le \frac{2}{p^{t-1}(p-1)}, \tag{4.14}$$

which implies that $p^t \le 4$. If $p = 2$ and $t = 1$, we must have $l_1 = l_2 = 1$ and $m = 2$, so $(1 - \omega_2)(1 - \omega_2) = 4$ is a solution. If $p = 3$ and $t = 1$, we similarly get only $(1 - \omega_3)(1 - \omega_3^2) = 3$, and if $p = 2$ and $t = 2$, we obtain only $(1 - \omega_4)(1 - \omega_4^3) = 2$. The case $q' = 1$ in (4.13) can be dealt with by trigonometry, and gives only the new solution $(1 - \omega_6)(1 - \omega_6^5) = 1$.

To summarize, the power of p-adic valuations lies in their ability to reduce the problem of finding all solutions of an equation such as (4.13) to the consideration of a few special cases. With the same combination of p-adic valuations and trigonometry, all solutions of (4.7) can be found. It turns out that there is an infinite family of solutions of the following type:

$$\frac{(1 - \omega_m^{2k})(1 - \omega_m^s)}{(1 - \omega_m^k)(1 - \omega_m^{k+s})} = 2, \tag{4.15}$$

where $m = 2s$ and $1 \le k \le s/2$ (or $s/2 \le k < s$ if the two factors in the numerator are interchanged). Apart from this, there are precisely 12 "sporadic" solutions, all of which can be written as a solution when $m = 12$. For example, we have

$$\frac{(1 - \omega_2)(1 - \omega_2)}{(1 - \omega_3)(1 - \omega_3^2)} = \frac{(1 - \omega_{12}^6)(1 - \omega_{12}^6)}{(1 - \omega_{12}^4)(1 - \omega_{12}^8)} = \frac{4}{3}, \tag{4.16}$$

corresponding to taking the ratio of two of the solutions of (4.13) found above. The only values of q in any of these solutions are those listed in the statement of the theorem. $\square$

Theorem 4.3.8 *There is a set $\mathcal{L} \subset \mathcal{L}^2$ with $|\mathcal{L}| = 4$ such that sets in $\mathcal{C}^2$ are determined by X-rays parallel to the lines in $\mathcal{L}$.*

Proof: By Lemmas 4.3.5 and 4.3.7, we can take $\mathcal{L}$ to be any set of four lines in $\mathcal{L}^2$ whose cross ratio of slopes, arranged in order of increasing angle with the positive x-axis, is not 4/3, 3/2, 2, 3, or 4. For example, let $\mathcal{L}$ be the set of lines in $\mathcal{L}^2$ parallel to $(2, 1)$, $(3, 2)$, $(1, 1)$, and $(2, 3)$, for which the cross ratio is 5/4 (see Fig. 4.4). $\square$

Lemma 4.3.9 *Let $\mathcal{L} \subset \mathcal{L}^2$ and suppose that there exists a lattice $\mathcal{L}$-polygon. Then $|\mathcal{L}| \le 6$.*

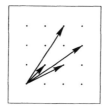

FIGURE 4.4. Directions for determining convex lattice sets by four X-rays.

Proof: Let $|\mathcal{L}| \geq 7$ and suppose there is an $\mathcal{L}$-polygon. Either some four of these lines meet the first quadrant or some four meet the second. Suppose, without loss of generality, that some four meet the first quadrant. We can apply the argument of Lemma 4.3.7 to these four lines. The corresponding solution of (4.7) cannot be of the form (4.15), since it is clear from the exponents in (4.15) that at least one line would meet the interior of the second quadrant.

Therefore the solution must correspond to one of the 12 "sporadic" solutions when $m = 12$ mentioned in the proof of Lemma 4.3.7. Each line $L_j \in \mathcal{L}$ corresponds to an integer h_j in the set $\{0, 1, \ldots, 11\}$, so we already know that $|\mathcal{L}| \leq 12$. To do better, one has to use the above argument for all sets of four lines from $\mathcal{L}$. Each such set yields one of the 12 solutions of (4.7) with $m = 12$ and an associated subset $\{k_1, k_2, k_3, k_4\}$ of $\{0, 1, \ldots, 11\}$. The task now is to examine which subsets A of $\{0, 1, \ldots, 11\}$ are such that *every* 4-integer subset of A corresponds to a solution of (4.7). It turns out that $A = \{0, 2, 4, 6, 8, 10\}$ has this property, but that there is no such A with more than six elements.   □

Theorem 4.3.10 *Let $\mathcal{L} \subset \mathcal{L}^2$ with $|\mathcal{L}| \geq 7$. Then the sets in $\mathcal{C}^2$ are determined by X-rays parallel to the lines in $\mathcal{L}$.*

Proof: This is a direct consequence of Lemmas 4.3.5 and 4.3.9.   □

Remark 4.3.11 (i) Theorems 4.3.8 and 4.3.10 were proved in [8]. The main part of Lemma 4.3.5 is a discrete form of an argument employed in [9] for solving the corresponding continuous problem. For an excellent introduction to p-adic valuations, see the book of Gouvêa [10].

(ii) Theorem 4.3.8 is in a sense the best possible. As we noted in the proof of Lemma 4.3.6, for each set $\mathcal{L}$ of three lines in $\mathcal{L}^2$, there is an $\mathcal{L}$-hexagon (see [8, Lemma 4.4], or, for an even stronger statement, Chapter 2 by Fishburn and Shepp, Theorem 2.7). This shows that less than four X-rays will not work. Also, it is observed in [11] that if $\mathcal{L}$ is a set of four lines in $\mathcal{L}^2$ whose slopes, arranged in order of increasing angle with the positive x-axis, have cross ratio $4/3$, $3/2$, 2, 3, or 4, then there is an $\mathcal{L}$-polygon.

(iii) Theorem 4.3.10 is also in a sense the best possible. Figure 4.5 displays an $\mathcal{L}$-polygon for a special set $\mathcal{L}$ of six lines in $\mathcal{L}^2$ parallel to the vectors

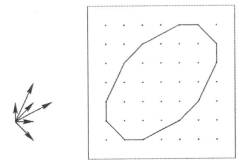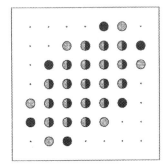

FIGURE 4.5. The lattice $\mathcal{L}$-polygon and convex lattice sets of Remark 4.3.11(iii).

shown. On the right of this figure are different convex lattice sets (one in black and halftone, the other in gray and halftone) with equal X-rays parallel to the lines in $\mathcal{L}$.

(iv) The papers [11] and [12] deal with X-rays of polyominoes; see also Chapter 7 by Del Lungo and Nivat. (For our purposes, a *polyomino* is a set in $\mathcal{F}^2$ that is connected in the graph on $\mathbb{Z}^2$ whose edges are the pairs $\{(a_1, a_2), (b_1, b_2)\}$ with $|a_1 - b_1| + |a_2 - b_2| = 1$.) In particular, the question is discussed in [11] to which extent Theorems 4.3.8 and 4.3.10 extend to polyominoes whose intersections with lines parallel to the coordinate axes are all convex. We shall refer to the latter as *hv-convex polyominoes*; they are called convex polyominoes in the articles just mentioned, but this conflicts with normal usage of the word "convex."

The two hv-convex polyominoes (black and halftone, gray and halftone) depicted on the left in Fig. 4.6 have equal X-rays parallel to the set $\mathcal{L}$ of lines in $\mathcal{L}^2$ parallel to $(1, 0)$, $(1, 1)$, $(0, 1)$, and $(-1, 1)$. Moreover, no other hv-convex polyomino has the same X-rays parallel to these lines. The symmetric difference of the two hv-convex polyominoes in Fig. 4.6 is the $\mathcal{L}$-switching component shown on the right.

This $\mathcal{L}$-switching component is not an $\mathcal{L}$-polygon and neither is its convex hull. This shows that the techniques of Lemma 4.3.5 do not apply to HV-polyominoes. It is not known whether there exists a set of four lines in $\mathcal{L}^2$ (including the two coordinate axes) such that hv-convex polyominoes are determined by the corresponding X-rays. A specific candidate is the set of lines in $\mathcal{L}^2$ parallel to $(1, 0)$, $(2, 1)$, $(0, 1)$, and $(-1, 2)$.

(v) Theorems 4.3.8 and 4.3.10 raise the question of how to reconstruct a convex lattice set from its X-rays parallel to a set of lines in $\mathcal{L}^2$ that guarantees a unique solution. This problem is unsolved, even for the class of convex lattice sets that are also polyominoes. (Note that there are convex lattice sets of arbitrary size that are not polyominoes.)

(vi) Theorems 4.3.8 and 4.3.10 continue to hold in higher dimensions, provided the lines in $\mathcal{L}$ all lie in the same 2-dimensional subspace; in par-

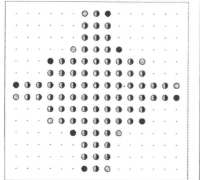 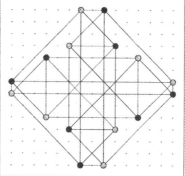

FIGURE 4.6. *hv*-convex polyominoes and associated switching component.

ticular, there are sets of four lines in $\mathcal{L}^n$ such that the corresponding X-rays determine sets in $\mathcal{C}^n$. However, it is unknown, even when $n = 3$, which finite subsets of $\mathcal{L}^n$ in general position will guarantee uniqueness. It seems possible that for each n there is a $k \in \mathbb{N}$ such that any subset $\mathcal{L}$ of $\mathcal{L}^n$ with $|\mathcal{L}| \geq k$ has this property. For remarks on the corresponding problem for continuous X-rays, see [3, Section 2.2] and [13, Problem 1]. In [3, Theorem 2.2.2] it is shown that for continuous X-rays such a number — if it exists — must be at least 7. In the lattice situation, however, we only know of an example that shows $k \geq 6$ is the smallest possible value. This is supplied by two sets of alternate vertices of a lattice truncated octahedron (see Scott [14] for a proof that the truncated octahedron can be realized as a convex lattice polyhedron).

4.4 Complexity results

In this section we consider Question 4.1.2.

In most practical applications we have some a priori information about the sets that are to be reconstructed. Mathematically, this information is modeled in terms of a subclass $\mathcal{E}$ of $\mathcal{F}^n$ to which the solution must belong. For algorithmic purposes, an *efficient membership test* for $\mathcal{E}$ must be available, that is, a polynomial-time algorithm that accepts as input a set $E \in \mathcal{F}^n$ and decides whether $E \in \mathcal{E}$. This section will mainly focus on the full class $\mathcal{F}^n$ in the case $n = 2$. However, most of the results hold for a great variety of other subclasses $\mathcal{E}$ as well, without any significant change in their statement or their proofs. With this understanding, we can state the basic decision problems of data consistency and uniqueness for a given subclass $\mathcal{E}$ of $\mathcal{F}^n$ and a given finite set $\mathcal{L}$ of lines in $\mathcal{L}^n$.

CONSISTENCY($\mathcal{E}, \mathcal{L}$).

    Instance: For each $L \in \mathcal{L}$, a function $f_L : \mathcal{D}(L) \to \mathbb{N}_0$, where $\mathcal{D}(L)$ is a finite set of lattice lines parallel to L.

    Question: Does there exist an $E \in \mathcal{E}$ such that $X_L E = f_L$ for all $L \in \mathcal{L}$?

UNIQUENESS($\mathcal{E}, \mathcal{L}$).

    Instance: An $E \in \mathcal{E}$.

    Question: Does there exist an $E' \in \mathcal{E} \setminus \{E\}$ such that $X_L E' = X_L E$ for all $L \in \mathcal{L}$?

We say there is a solution for a given instance of a decision problem if the corresponding question has an affirmative answer.

We can also define the reconstruction problem RECONSTRUCTION($\mathcal{E}, \mathcal{L}$) in a way similar to CONSISTENCY($\mathcal{E}, \mathcal{L}$), the input being the same but the question replaced by the task of constructing a solution if one exists.

We are using informal definitions in this paper, since they are easier to understand and to use in obtaining the complexity results. They can be made precise to allow a formal treatment in the usual binary Turing machine model.

A necessary condition that there is a solution $E \in \mathcal{E}$ for an instance $\mathcal{I}$ of CONSISTENCY($\mathcal{E}, \mathcal{L}$) is that the sums

$$\sum \{f_L(T) : T \in \mathcal{D}(L)\}, \tag{4.17}$$

$L \in \mathcal{L}$, are all equal to some $N \in \mathbb{N}$, the cardinality of any solution. This condition can be checked efficiently. We assume that the condition is satisfied and denote by $N = N(\mathcal{I}) \in \mathbb{N}$ this cardinality.

The input to CONSISTENCY($\mathcal{E}, \mathcal{L}$) — that is, an instance $\mathcal{I}$ of the problem — allows us to compute a lattice set $G = G(\mathcal{I})$ called the *grid* for $\mathcal{I}$, defined by

$$G = \mathbb{Z}^2 \cap \bigcap \{\mathcal{D}(L) : L \in \mathcal{L}\}. \tag{4.18}$$

Note that if there is a solution $E \in \mathcal{E}$ for $\mathcal{I}$, then $E \subset G$, so the grid is a lattice set containing all possible solutions for $\mathcal{I}$.

It is easy to see that G can be computed in polynomial time. It follows that CONSISTENCY($\mathcal{E}, \mathcal{L}$) belongs to NP. In fact, since G contains at most N^2 points we may simply guess a set E of N points of G. Then we check whether $E \in \mathcal{E}$ (using the efficient membership test) and, by counting, whether E has X-rays consistent with the input. This can be done in polynomial time.

Theorem 4.4.1 *Let $\mathcal{L} \subset \mathcal{L}^2$ with $|\mathcal{L}| = 2$. Then* CONSISTENCY($\mathcal{F}^2, \mathcal{L}$), UNIQUENESS($\mathcal{F}^2, \mathcal{L}$), *and* RECONSTRUCTION($\mathcal{F}^2, \mathcal{L}$) *can be solved in polynomial time.*

See Chapter 1 by Kuba and Herman for an efficient algorithm of this type. Theorem 4.4.1 also follows from the fact that the natural formulation of CONSISTENCY$(\mathcal{F}^2, \mathcal{L})$ as an integer linear program involves coefficient matrices that are totally unimodular; see [15, Chapters 19–21]. Of course, Theorem 4.4.1 holds for any subclass $\mathcal{E}$ of $\mathcal{F}^2$ that can be defined by a property that does not destroy total unimodularity. This includes subclasses that are obtained by excluding or prescribing certain lattice points. Hence the positive result of Theorem 4.4.1 extends to the problem of checking whether a given subset of a solution is *invariant*, i.e., whether it belongs to *all* solutions. Note, however, that a convexity condition does not seem to fall into this category. Chapter 7 by Del Lungo and Nivat discusses the situation where $\mathcal{F}^2$ in Theorem 4.4.1 is replaced by various subclasses of $\mathcal{F}^2$ consisting of sets with a polyomino and/or weak convexity property; see, in particular, Table 7.1 of that chapter. However, the complexities of CONSISTENCY$(\mathcal{C}^2, \mathcal{L})$, UNIQUENESS$(\mathcal{C}^2, \mathcal{L})$, and RECONSTRUCTION$(\mathcal{C}^2, \mathcal{L})$ remain open even for $|\mathcal{L}| = 2$.

Lemma 4.4.2 *Let $\mathcal{L}$ be a finite subset of $\mathcal{L}^2$, and suppose $M \in \mathcal{L}^2 \setminus \mathcal{L}$ and $\mathcal{M} = \mathcal{L} \cup M$. There is a polynomial-time transformation from* CONSISTENCY$(\mathcal{F}^2, \mathcal{L})$ *to* CONSISTENCY$(\mathcal{F}^2, \mathcal{M})$. *If the former problem is NP-complete, then so is the latter.*

Proof: (Sketch.) Suppose that $\mathcal{I} = \{f_L : L \in \mathcal{L}\}$ is a given instance of CONSISTENCY$(\mathcal{F}^2, \mathcal{L})$, and let G be the grid for $\mathcal{I}$. We have to define an instance $\mathcal{J} = \{f_L : L \in \mathcal{M}\}$ of CONSISTENCY$(\mathcal{F}^2, \mathcal{M})$ in such a way that there is a solution for $\mathcal{J}$ if and only if there is a solution for $\mathcal{I}$.

The idea is to define $\mathcal{J}$ so that its grid is the union of G and a suitable translate $v + G$ of G, where $v \in \mathbb{Z}^2$ is parallel to M. The translate is sufficiently far away from G that no line parallel to any $L \in \mathcal{L}$ meets both G and its translate. Moreover, we want that $F \subset G$ is a solution for $\mathcal{I}$ if and only if $F' = F \cup (v + (G \setminus F))$ is a solution for $\mathcal{J}$.

To achieve this, we simply define the functions f_L for $L \in \mathcal{M}$ so that they will agree with the X-rays of F' when it arises from a solution F for $\mathcal{I}$ as above. That is, for each $L \in \mathcal{L}$ we add to $\mathcal{D}(L)$ those lines T parallel to L that meet $v + G$, and for such T define $f_L(T) = |G \cap (T - v)| - f_L(T - v)$. Then we define $\mathcal{D}(M)$ to be the set of lines T parallel to M that meet G, and for such T define $f_M(T) = |G \cap T|$. □

The previous lemma shows that any polynomial-time algorithm for the consistency problem with $|\mathcal{L}| = m+1$ can be used to construct a polynomial-time algorithm for the consistency problem with $|\mathcal{L}| = m$. We already know that the case $|\mathcal{L}| = 2$ can be solved in polynomial time, so it will suffice to prove that the case $|\mathcal{L}| = 3$ is NP-complete. By applying a suitable linear transformation, if necessary, we need only consider the special set $\mathcal{L}^* = \{L_1^*, L_2^*, L_3^*\}$, where for $i = 1, 2, 3$, L_i^* is the line in $\mathcal{L}^2$ parallel to v_i, with $v_1 = (1, 0)$, $v_2 = (0, 1)$, and $v_3 = (1, 1)$.

Theorem 4.4.3 CONSISTENCY$(\mathcal{F}^2, \mathcal{L}^*)$ *is NP-complete.*

Proof: (Sketch.) The proof uses a transformation from the following NP-complete problem.

1-IN-3-SAT.

    Instance: *Positive integers r, s, a set V of r variables, a set C of s clauses over V, where each clause consists of three literals.*

    Question: *Is there a satisfying truth assignment for C that sets exactly one literal true in each clause?*

Let $\mathcal{I} = (r, s; V, C)$ be an instance of 1-IN-3-SAT. We need to construct an instance $\mathcal{I}^*$ of CONSISTENCY$(\mathcal{F}^2, \mathcal{L}^*)$ such that there is a solution for $\mathcal{I}^*$ if and only if there is one for $\mathcal{I}$.

The instance of $\mathcal{I}^*$ consists of functions $f_i = f_{L_i^*}$, $i = 1, 2, 3$ defined on horizontal, vertical, and diagonal (parallel to $v_3 = (1, 1)$) lattice lines, respectively. (From now on, "diagonal" will always mean parallel to L_3^*.) A solution for $\mathcal{I}^*$ is a lattice set F contained in the grid G for $\mathcal{I}^*$ (the set of points that for each $i = 1, 2, 3$ are contained in a lattice line on which f_i has a nonzero value) such that the X-ray of F parallel to L_i^* is precisely f_i, $i = 1, 2, 3$. The grid G is determined by the functions f_i and the supports of the functions f_i are determined by G. The construction proceeds in stages, and it is convenient to toggle between defining the functions f_i and defining G.

The grid G will be a subset of the lattice points in the rectangle

$$B = [0, 11p + 5q + 5] \times [-4p - 2q - 2, 0], \tag{4.19}$$

where p and q are natural numbers to be specified later, with $q \geq 3p + 2$. See Fig. 4.7; the size parameters are $\alpha_1 = -p$, $\alpha_2 = -3p - 1$, $\alpha_3 = -4p - q - 2$, $\alpha_4 = -4p - 2q - 2$, $\beta_1 = p + q$, $\beta_2 = 4p + q + 1$, $\beta_3 = 6p + 3q + 3$, and $\beta_4 = 11p + 5q + 5$. We call B the *circuit board*, by analogy with an electronic circuit. In fact, G (and hence any solution for $\mathcal{I}^*$) will be confined to a small part of B, namely, the union of the six small squares and one larger square indicated in Fig. 4.7.

All the action takes place within these seven subsquares of the circuit board. In fact, we define $f_i(T) = 0$ for $i = 1, 2, 3$ and any line T parallel to L_i^* not meeting one of the seven squares. Every lattice point outside the seven squares belongs to at least one such line T, and so cannot belong to any solution for $\mathcal{I}^*$. No diagonal line meets more than one of the seven squares, so in checking the values of f_3 for a possible solution F for $\mathcal{I}^*$, one can check the part of F lying in each square separately. Also, no horizontal or vertical line meets more than two of the squares, and we will have

$$f_i(T) = 1 \quad \text{if and only if} \quad G \cap T \neq \emptyset, \tag{4.20}$$

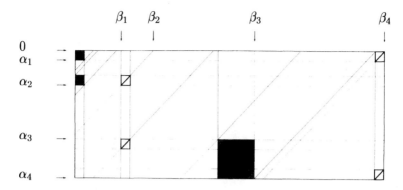

FIGURE 4.7. The circuit board.

for any line T parallel to L_i^*, $i = 1, 2$. A consequence of (4.20), crucial for the whole construction, is that if $x \in F$ lies in one of the seven squares, there can be no point in F on the horizontal or vertical lines through x in any other square.

All seven subsquares of the circuit board have an internal structure designed to guarantee a one-to-one correspondence between satisfying truth assignments for $\mathcal{I}$ and lattice sets that are solutions for $\mathcal{I}^*$. To continue the analogy with an electronic circuit, we refer to these seven squares with their internal structure as chips. The two black squares of side length p contain copies of an *initializing chip* that encodes a truth assignment for the instance $\mathcal{I}$ of 1-IN-3-SAT. The larger square of side length q contains a *clause chip* that encodes the clauses in $\mathcal{I}$. Finally, the four white squares of side length p contain *connector chips* that transfer a truth assignment from the initializing chips to the clause chip and back to close the circuit.

A satisfying truth assignment for $\mathcal{I}$ assigns to each of the r variables in V the value true or false, and the opposite value to its negation. There are $2r$ literals in r pairs, each pair containing a variable and its negation. The idea is to define the grid G so that it intersects the upper initializing chip (with upper left corner at the origin) in exactly $2r$ points x_j, x_j', $j = 1, \ldots, r$, where x_j represents the literal of the jth variable in V, and x_j' represents the literal of its negation. Their position is important. Each pair $\{x_j, x_j'\}$ lies on a diagonal line, and no horizontal or vertical line contains more than one of the $2r$ points. Examples of initializing chips for $r = 1, 2, 3$ are illustrated in Fig. 4.8, where the large black dots show the positions of the points representing literals. An order is established; in J_1, for example, we have $x_1 = (1, 0)$, $x_1' = (0, -1)$, $x_2 = (3, -2)$, and $x_2' = (2, -3)$, where the upper left lattice point is the origin. Generally, the order from top to bottom is $x_1, x_1', x_2, x_2', \ldots, x_r, x_r'$. The functions f_i must be defined appropriately, of course. We use (4.20), as always, for the values of f_1 and f_2, so that for J_2 in Fig. 4.8, we would have $f_1 = 1$ on the upper and lower four horizontal lines, and $f_1 = 0$ on the middle two. Then we define $f_3(T) = 1$ if T is one of the r diagonal lines containing one of the r pairs of points, and $f_3(T) = 0$ for other diagonal lines that meet the initializing chip. This forces any solution F for $\mathcal{I}^*$ to contain exactly one point in each of the r pairs and is equivalent to assigning a value, true or false, to the corresponding variable in V.

J_0 J_1 J_2

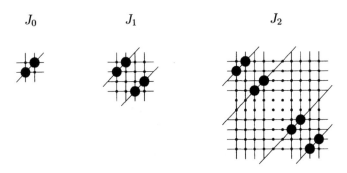

FIGURE 4.8. Examples of initializing chips.

It is useful at this point to study again J_2 in Fig. 4.8. No point other than the eight large black dots can belong to G, since every other lattice point belongs to a horizontal, vertical, or diagonal line on which the corresponding function f_i has zero value. To achieve this, the large black dots must be spaced out somewhat. For example, it is not possible to fit them into a square of side length eight. An initializing chip for eight variables would be contained in a square of side length 27; its upper left and lower right subsquares of side length nine would have exactly the same structure as J_2. If r is not a power of two, the initializing chip square is constructed for the smallest power of two larger than r, and then cut down, to obtain the smallest square containing the first $2r$ points representing literals. The side length p of the initializing chip square is trebled when the number r of variables is doubled, so its size is polynomially bounded in r.

The structure of the lower initializing chip (with its upper left corner at $(0, -2p - 1)$) is exactly the same as the first. That is, its intersection with G is just a translate of the set $\{x_j, x_j' : j = 1, \ldots, r\}$ by the vector $(0, -2p - 1)$, with values of the functions f_i on lines meeting its containing square defined, in a way similar to that above, to ensure this. Each point $x_j + (0, -2p - 1)$ or $x_j' + (0, -2p - 1)$ represents the corresponding literal, just as x_j or x_j' did in the upper initializing chip.

We can already begin to see how a truth assignment for the instance $\mathcal{I}$ of 1-IN-3-SAT will provide a solution F for $\mathcal{I}^*$. Suppose, for example, that $r = 2$ (whence $p = 3$) and that the first variable is assigned the value true and the second the value false. Consider a lattice set F whose intersection with the upper initializing chip consists of the two of the $2r = 4$ points that represent the *false* literals, namely $x_1' = (0, -1)$ and $x_2 = (3, -2)$ in J_1 in Fig. 4.8. Note that the X-rays of this part of F match the values of the functions f_i on the lines meeting the upper initializing chip square. (Conversely, if F is a solution for $\mathcal{I}^*$, the values of the functions f_i force F to contain exactly one of each pair $\{x_j, x_j'\}$, $j = 1, \ldots, r$, and these will correspond to false literals in a truth assignment for $\mathcal{I}$.) Moreover, the truth assignment is transmitted to the lower initializing chip, because by (4.20) (specifically, the values of f_2), the part of F in the lower initializing chip must consist of the two points that represent the *true* literals, namely $x_1 + (0, -7)$ and $x'_2 + (0, -7)$.

The connector chips have a very simple structure. We define $f_3(T) = 0$ for any diagonal line T meeting one of the four white subsquares of B in Fig. 4.7 and not containing their diagonal. We also define $f_3(T) = r$ for the four diagonal lines T containing these diagonals. This means that the intersection of G with any of the connector chip squares is contained within its diagonal.

Figure 4.9 shows, schematically, the lower initializing chip when $r = 4$ on the left and the connector chip on the same horizontal level on the right. The important thing to note is that the values of f_1 already fixed for these 10 horizontal lattice lines mean that G intersects the connector chip square in eight points, indicated by the large black dots, on its diagonal. These again represent the literals, in the order inherited from that in the lower initializing chip. By (4.20) again, any solution F for $\mathcal{I}^*$ will contain the point in each pair $\{x_j, x'_j\}$ corresponding to the *false* literal in a truth assignment for $\mathcal{I}$.

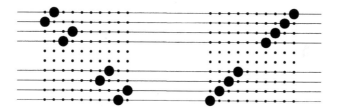

FIGURE 4.9. An initializing chip (left) and the corresponding connector chip (right).

Looking again at the circuit board in Fig. 4.7, we can see how a truth assignment will be transmitted around the circuit. By (4.20) (applied alternately to the function f_1 and f_2), any solution F for $\mathcal{I}^*$ intersects each initializing or connector chip square in r points that represent the false literals in the upper initializing chip, the true literals in the lower one, the false literals in the connector chip to the right, the true literals in the next connector chip below, and so on. The structure of the clause chip has yet to be described, but at its top left is an *input* and at its bottom right an *output*, each with the same structure as a connector chip. The construction will ensure that any solution F for $\mathcal{I}^*$ intersects the input and output in sets of r points that represent the false literals and the true literals, respectively. Then F intersects the lower and upper connector chip squares on the right of Fig. 4.7 in sets of r points that represent the false literals and the true literals, respectively, completing the circuit.

So far no account has been taken of the clauses in $\mathcal{I}$. This job is done by the clause chip. We begin by showing how a single clause is encoded. Consider the clause $C = (w_{i_1} \vee w_{i_2} \vee w_{i_3}) \in \mathcal{C}$, where $w_{i_j} \in \{v_{i_j}, \neg v_{i_j}\}$. The corresponding clause chip square has side length $q = 4p + 3$, illustrated in Fig. 4.10 for the case $r = 4$ and $C = (v_1 \lor v_2 \lor \neg v_4)$. The grid G intersects this square in the points indicated by large black dots, all of which are contained in the diagonals of six subsquares of side length p. We denote these subsquares by M_j, $j = 1, \ldots, 6$, with the first three on the left and the last three on the right, ordered top to bottom.

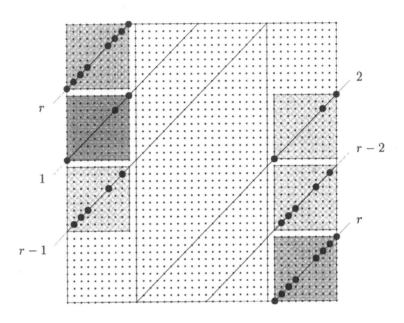

FIGURE 4.10. The clause chip for the single clause $(v_1 \lor v_2 \lor \neg v_4)$.

The squares M_1 and M_6 contain the input and output referred to above. These are essentially connector chips with $2r$ grid points, representing literals, in their diagonals. The squares M_2 and M_4 actually encode the clause $(w_{i_1} \lor w_{i_2} \lor w_{i_3})$. The three points in $M_2 \cap G$ are vertical translates of the points in M_1 that represent the literals $w_{i_1}, w_{i_2}, w_{i_3}$, while the $(2r - 3)$ points in $M_3 \cap G$ are vertical translates of the points in $M_1 \cap G$ representing the remaining literals. The sets $M_4 \cap G$ and $M_5 \cap G$ are the appropriate horizontal translates of $M_2 \cap G$ and $M_3 \cap G$, respectively. The functions f_1 and f_2 have their values dictated, as always, by (4.20) on the horizontal and vertical lines meeting the clause chip, while f_3 is zero on each diagonal line meeting the clause chip except for those containing a diagonal of one of the squares M_j. The values of f_3 for these six lines is indicated in Fig. 4.10.

This is how the clause chip works. Suppose there is a solution for $\mathcal{I}$. Then the corresponding truth assignment selects for each j either x_j or x'_j in the upper initializing chip, whichever represents a false literal. This assignment is transferred in negated form, as described above, via the lower initializing chip and two connector chips to the input M_1, where the original truth assignment is preserved, in the same order. We can use all $5r$ corresponding representative points to begin building a solution F for $\mathcal{I}^*$. In particular, F will contain the r points on the diagonal of M_1 representing the false literals in the truth assignment. The truth assignment sets exactly one literal true in C, and we add to F the corresponding point on the diagonal of M_2. On the diagonal of M_3, we add to F the $(r - 1)$ points representing the remaining true literals. On the diagonal of M_4, we add to F the two literals in C that are false, and on the diagonal of M_5, we add to F the $(r - 2)$ points representing the remaining false literals. On the diagonal of M_6, we add to F the r points representing the true literals in the truth assignment. The part of F defined in this way is consistent with F being a solution for $\mathcal{I}^*$. Conversely, the specified values of f_3 force any solution for $\mathcal{I}^*$ to contain exactly one point on the diagonal of M_2, and the corresponding literal can then be regarded as the one in the clause C that is true.

If there is only one clause, the truth assignment is directly transferred again via the other two connector chips on the right of Fig. 4.7, back to the upper initializing chip. When we add the corresponding $2r$ representative points to F, we have completed the construction of a solution F for $\mathcal{I}^*$.

When there is more than one clause, the clause chip is built recursively, following a doubling procedure very similar to that employed for the upper initializing chip. The general structure is shown in Fig. 4.11. Thus, if there are two clauses, the square shown in Fig. 4.10 for the first clause would be the black square at the top left of Fig. 4.11, and the black square at the bottom right would have a similar structure to encode the second clause. Two additional connector chips have to be included at each stage to transmit the truth assignment from top left to bottom right.

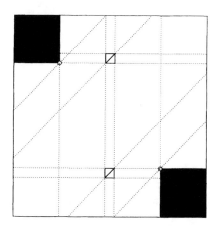

FIGURE 4.11. The doubling procedure for the clause chip.

The side length q of the clause chip increases by a factor of about four when the number of clauses is doubled. In fact, one can show that $q < 12s^2(5r^2 + 1)$, so q is polynomially bounded in s and r.

This completes the definition of the instance $\mathcal{I}^*$ of CONSISTENCY($\mathcal{F}^2, \mathcal{L}^*$). The construction guarantees that G is precisely the grid for $\mathcal{I}^*$. If F is a solution for $\mathcal{I}^*$, then $F \subset G$, and the intersection of F with the lower initializing chip yields a truth assignment for $\mathcal{I}$. In the chip for each clause in $\mathcal{C}$, there is a diagonal line T such that $G \cap T$ consists of three points representing the literals in that clause. The single point $F \cap T$ indicates which of these three literals is true, so we obtain a solution for $\mathcal{I}$. Conversely, a solution for $\mathcal{I}$ provides a satisfying truth assignment that yields a solution $F \subset G$ for $\mathcal{I}^*$ via the correspondence explained above. Finally, we note that the transformation runs in polynomial time. $\square$

We can now state the main result of this section.

Theorem 4.4.4 *Let $\mathcal{L} \subset \mathcal{L}^2$ with $|\mathcal{L}| \geq 3$. Then* CONSISTENCY($\mathcal{F}^2, \mathcal{L}$) *is NP-complete.*

Corollary 4.4.5 *Let $\mathcal{L} \subset \mathcal{L}^2$ with $|\mathcal{L}| \geq 3$. Then* RECONSTRUCTION($\mathcal{F}^2, \mathcal{L}$) *is NP-hard.*

Theorem 4.4.6 *Let $\mathcal{L} \subset \mathcal{L}^2$ with $|\mathcal{L}| \geq 3$. Then* UNIQUENESS($\mathcal{F}^2, \mathcal{L}$) *is NP-complete.*

Proof: (Sketch.) Clearly UNIQUENESS($\mathcal{F}^2, \mathcal{L}$) is in the class NP. The basic idea is to use a polynomial-time parsimonious transformation from the following problem.

UNIQUE-1-IN-3-SAT.

Instance: *Positive integers r, s, a set V of r variables, a set $\mathcal{C}$ of s clauses over V, where each clause consists of three literals, and a truth assignment for which exactly one literal in each clause is true.*

Question: *Is there a truth assignment different from the given one for which exactly one literal in each clause is true?*

It can be shown that UNIQUE-1-IN-3-SAT is NP-complete. Assuming this, let $\mathcal{J}$ be an instance of UNIQUE-1-IN-3-SAT. Then $\mathcal{J}$ contains a solution for the corresponding instance $\mathcal{I}$ of 1-IN-3-SAT. By following the proof of Theorem 4.4.4, we obtain from $\mathcal{I}$ an instance $\mathcal{I}'$ of CONSISTENCY($\mathcal{F}^2, \mathcal{L}$) for which we know one solution, and therefore a corresponding instance $\mathcal{J}'$ of UNIQUENESS($\mathcal{F}^2, \mathcal{L}$). Now there is a solution for $\mathcal{J}'$ if and only if there is one for $\mathcal{J}$, because all the transformations used preserve uniqueness. $\square$

Remark 4.4.7 (i) Detailed proofs of all the NP-completeness results in this section can be found in [16].

(ii) Some variations of the above problems are also considered in [16] and [17]. For example, the associated problem #(CONSISTENCY($\mathcal{F}^2, \mathcal{L}$)) that asks for the number of solutions is shown to be #P-complete when $|\mathcal{L}| \geq 3$. Also, the corresponding problems in which, for an arbitrary positive

ε, the position of $N - N^\varepsilon$ points in a solution is prescribed are proved to be NP-complete when $|\mathcal{L}| \geq 3$.

(iii) Among problems of the type considered so far, only the complexity of $\#(\text{CONSISTENCY}(\mathcal{F}^2, \mathcal{L}))$ when $|\mathcal{L}| = 2$ remains open. We conjecture that it is #P-complete. Note that the problem of counting the solutions that contain a given set of prescribed points includes the well-known #P-complete problem of computing the permanent of a binary matrix.

(iv) All the above results hold in higher dimensions, that is, when $\mathcal{F}^2$ and $\mathcal{L}^2$ are replaced by $\mathcal{F}^n$ and $\mathcal{L}^n$, $n \geq 2$; see [16] and [18]. In particular, [16] contains an alternative proof of the result in [19, Corollary 4.2] that $\text{CONSISTENCY}(\mathcal{F}^3, \mathcal{L})$ is NP-complete when $\mathcal{L}$ consists of the three coordinate axes in $\mathbb{E}^3$.

(v) When a real object is X-rayed and the data is exact, consistency is guaranteed. Under the additional *promise* that the instance is consistent, a polynomial-time algorithm for reconstruction might seem possible even when $|\mathcal{L}| \geq 3$. However, this is not true unless P = NP; see [16].

(vi) The constructions leading to Theorems 4.4.4, 4.4.5, and 4.4.6 may seem somewhat irrelevant for the application to electron microscopy, since crystals do not have their atoms distributed extremely sparsely over a huge region. However, as in Remark 4.3.2(iii) and Fig. 4.2 we can replace the entire construction by its complement in a rectangular array of lattice points that contains it.

(vii) In [20] and [21, Theorem 4], it is shown that when $\mathcal{L} \subset \mathcal{L}^n$ and $|\mathcal{L}| = 2$, a set in $\mathcal{F}^n$ is determined by its X-rays parallel to the lines in $\mathcal{L}$ if and only if it is *additive*; see Chapter 2 by Fishburn and Shepp, Theorem 2.3. Theorem 4.4.6 reflects the difficulty in extending this characterization of uniqueness from $|\mathcal{L}| = 2$ to $|\mathcal{L}| \geq 3$. The additivity of a lattice set can be detected in polynomial time, and it follows that $\text{UNIQUENESS}(\mathcal{F}^n, \mathcal{L})$ can be solved in polynomial time when $|\mathcal{L}| = 2$. Since $\text{UNIQUENESS}(\mathcal{F}^n, \mathcal{L})$ is NP-hard for $|\mathcal{L}| \geq 3$, this shows that unless P = NP, there exists a non-additive set in $\mathcal{F}^3$ that is determined by its X-rays parallel to the three coordinate axes. This conditional answer to a problem posed by A. Kuba was confirmed definitively by specific examples in [22].

If there is a solution E' for an instance E of $\text{UNIQUENESS}(\mathcal{E}, \mathcal{L})$, then $E \triangle E' = (E \setminus E') \cup (E' \setminus E)$ is an $\mathcal{L}$-switching component that transforms E to E' (or vice versa). When $|\mathcal{L}| = 2$, it has long been known (see [23]) that there is a finite sequence of such transformations that takes E to E' via simple $\mathcal{L}$-switching components each consisting of four points. A consequence of Theorem 4.4.6 is that when $|\mathcal{L}| \geq 3$, there is no constant $c \in \mathbb{N}$ such that E can always be transformed to E' via a sequence of $\mathcal{L}$-switching components each consisting of no more than c points; see [17]. A stronger result is proved in [24]: Instances E_k, $k \in \mathbb{N}$ are constructed for which there is exactly one solution E_k' and $|E_k \triangle E_k'| \to \infty$ as $k \to \infty$.

(viii) Given an instance of $\text{RECONSTRUCTION}(\mathcal{F}^n, \mathcal{L})$ with $|\mathcal{L}| \geq 3$, a natural reconstruction scheme is to begin by finding an *invariant pair* of sets

(F_1, Z_1), where F_1 is a subset of *all* solutions while Z_1 is disjoint from *any* solution. A modified instance could then be obtained by subtracting the X-ray of F_1 parallel to L from the function f_L, for all $L \in \mathcal{L}$ and replacing $\mathbb{Z}^2$ by $\mathbb{Z}^2 \setminus Z_1$. One could then either attempt to solve the modified reconstruction problem by any algorithm or find a new invariant pair (F_2, Z_2) and repeat the procedure. However, it is shown in [17] that the complexity results of this section imply that all steps of such an approach are in general bound to fail or to require exponential time. In fact, unless P = NP there is no polynomial-time algorithm to determine whether a set of points is contained in any solution for a given instance of CONSISTENCY$(\mathcal{F}^n, \mathcal{L})$ when $|\mathcal{L}| \geq 3$. The same is true for the problem of determining whether a set is excluded from all solutions. The NP-hardness also applies to the task of extending a "kernel" of invariant points to a complete solution of a given problem. See [17] for a discussion of other algorithmic paradigms.

4.5   Further extensions and variations

In this section we briefly examine some extensions and variations of the problems considered above, without even sketching proofs.

4.5.1   Higher-dimensional X-rays

The following is a natural generalization of the notion of an X-ray. Let F be a finite subset of $\mathbb{E}^n$, let $k \in \mathbb{N}$, $1 \leq k \leq n-1$, and let L be a k-dimensional subspace. The *k-dimensional X-ray of F parallel to L* is the function $X_L F$ defined by

$$X_L F(T) = |F \cap T|, \tag{4.21}$$

for each k-dimensional plane T parallel to L. Of course, the X-ray considered in earlier sections of this paper is the special case when $k = 1$.

Very much less is known about k-dimensional X-rays when $k > 1$. For a summary of work on continuous k-dimensional X-rays, see [3, Chapter 2]. In the lattice situation, we restrict attention to k-dimensional X-rays of sets in $\mathcal{F}^n$ parallel to *lattice subspaces*, that is, subspaces that are spanned by vectors in $\mathbb{Z}^n$. We denote the class of k-dimensional lattice subspaces of $\mathbb{E}^n$ by $\mathcal{L}_k^n$.

We are not aware of any uniqueness results, analogous to those in Section 4.3, for k-dimensional X-rays of lattice sets when $k > 1$ that do not follow more or less trivially from the definition or from the case $k = 1$. To give just one example of our ignorance, it is unknown whether there is a finite subset $\mathcal{L}$ of $\mathcal{L}_2^3$ such that convex lattice sets are determined by their 2-dimensional X-rays parallel to the subspaces in $\mathcal{L}$.

A few complexity results are known. (In defining the decision problems for $k > 1$, one has to be a little more careful since $\cap\{L : L \in \mathcal{L}\}$ can have dimension greater than 0.) The following generalization of Theorem 4.4.1 can be found in [18].

Theorem 4.5.1 *Let $1 \leq k \leq n - 1$, and suppose that $\mathcal{L} \subset \mathcal{L}_k^n$ with $|\mathcal{L}| = 2$. Then the problems* CONSISTENCY($\mathcal{F}^n, \mathcal{L}$), UNIQUENESS($\mathcal{F}^n, \mathcal{L}$), *and* RECONSTRUCTION($\mathcal{F}^n, \mathcal{L}$) *can be solved in polynomial time.*

The preliminary study [25] contains some partial results on the problem when $|\mathcal{L}| \geq 3$. A couple of these are stated in the next theorem.

Theorem 4.5.2 *If $k \geq 2$ and $\mathcal{L} \subset \mathcal{L}_k^n$, then* CONSISTENCY($\mathcal{F}^n, \mathcal{L}$) *is NP-complete under either of the following additional assumptions.*

(i) $|\mathcal{L}| \geq 3$ and the dimension of $\cap\{L : L \in \mathcal{L}\}$ is $k - 1$.

(ii) $|\mathcal{L}| \geq 4$ and $k = 2$.

The simplest unresolved case, one possibly requiring new methods, is when $k = 2$, $n = 3$, and $\mathcal{L}$ consists of the three coordinate planes. The apparent difficulty disappears if we allow sets of points weighted by non-negative integers, in which case the problem can be solved in polynomial time.

4.5.2 Successive determination

The following interactive notion of determining sets by X-rays was introduced by Edelsbrunner and Skiena [26] for continuous X-rays. We refer the reader to [3, Chapters 1 and 2] for background.

Let $\mathcal{E}$ be a class of finite sets in $\mathbb{E}^n$. We say that $E \in \mathcal{E}$ can be *successively determined* by m X-rays if we can inductively choose lines L_i, $i = 1, \ldots, m$ containing the origin, the choice of L_j depending on $X_{L_i} E$, $i = 1, \ldots, j - 1$, such that if $E' \in \mathcal{E}$ and $X_{L_i} E' = X_{L_i} E$ for $i = 1, \ldots, m$, then $E' = E$.

Successive determination by m X-rays parallel to k-dimensional subspaces is defined analogously. The next result was proved in [8].

Theorem 4.5.3 *Let $1 \leq k \leq n - 1$. Sets in $\mathcal{F}^n$ can be successively determined by $\lceil n/(n - k) \rceil$ k-dimensional X-rays parallel to lattice subspaces.*

The number $\lceil n/(n - k) \rceil$ is the best possible. Note that a k-dimensional X-ray parallel to a k-dimensional subspace L is effectively the (orthogonal) projection, with multiplicity, on the $(n - k)$-dimensional subspace $L^\perp$. It is slightly surprising that the values of the X-rays in the previous theorem are not needed, but only their supports. In other words, sets in $\mathcal{F}^n$ can be successively determined by $\lceil n/(n-k) \rceil$ (orthogonal) projections on $(n-k)$-dimensional lattice subspaces.

When $k = 1$, Theorem 4.5.3 implies that sets in $\mathcal{F}^n$ can be successively determined by just two X-rays parallel to lines in $\mathcal{L}^n$ (or even by two projections on $(n-1)$-dimensional lattice subspaces). Unfortunately, there seems to be little hope of applying this result in electron microscopy at present. The two X-rays must generally be taken at a small angle apart, resulting in at least one image of poor resolution.

Remarkably, Theorem 4.5.3 holds for the non-lattice situation in $\mathbb{E}^n$ when $\lceil n/(n-k) \rceil$ is replaced by $(\lfloor n/(n-k) \rfloor + 1)$, and again, this is the best possible. The difference shows when $n = 2$, in which case the successive determination of finite subsets of the plane generally require three X-rays, not two.

For another uniqueness result in the spirit of successive determination, see [27].

4.5.3   The polyatomic case

If Questions 4.1.1 and 4.1.2 are mathematical models of problems associated with the location of atoms in a crystal by means of X-rays, then one must also consider the variants in which there are $c \geq 2$ types of atom present and each X-ray gives the number of atoms of each type lying on each line in a family of parallel lattice lines. We refer to this as the *polyatomic* case.

The consistency problem for the polyatomic case is as follows.

$\text{POLY}_c\text{CONSISTENCY}(\mathcal{E}, \mathcal{L})$.

Instance: For each $i = 1, \ldots, c$ and $L \in \mathcal{L}$, a function $f_{i,L} : \mathcal{D}_i(L) \to \mathbb{N}_0$, where $\mathcal{D}_i(L)$ is a finite set of lattice lines parallel to L.

Question: Do there exist disjoint sets $E_i \in \mathcal{E}$ such that $X_L E_i = f_{i,L}$ for all $i = 1, \ldots, c$ and $L \in \mathcal{L}$?

The corresponding uniqueness and reconstruction problems are defined analogously. In view of the results of Section 4.4, it suffices to consider the case when $|\mathcal{L}| = 2$, so by applying an affine transformation one can restrict attention to X-rays parallel to the two coordinate axes.

The paper [28] considered the case $c = 2$, but the only published complexity results, as far as we know, are those of [29] and Chrobak and Dürr [30]. The following theorem was proved in [30]. (The paper [29] gave the result for $c \geq 6$ and the conjecture that it holds for $c \geq 3$.)

Theorem 4.5.4 *Let $c \geq 3$ and let $\mathcal{L} \subset \mathcal{L}^2$ with $|\mathcal{L}| \geq 2$. Then the problems $\text{POLY}_c\text{CONSISTENCY}(\mathcal{F}^2, \mathcal{L})$ and $\text{POLY}_c\text{UNIQUENESS}(\mathcal{F}^2, \mathcal{L})$ are NP-complete, and the problem $\text{POLY}_c\text{RECONSTRUCTION}(\mathcal{F}^2, \mathcal{L})$ is NP-hard.*

It is an open question whether the previous theorem holds for $c = 2$.

Acknowledgments

First author supported in part by the Alexander von Humboldt Foundation and by U.S. National Science Foundation Grants DMS-9501289 and DMS-9802388; second author supported in part by a Max Planck Research Award and by the German Federal Ministry of Education, Science, Research, and Technology Grant 03-GR7TM1.

References

[1] C. Kisielowski, P. Schwander, F.H. Baumann, M. Seibt, Y. Kim, and A. Ourmazd, "An approach to quantitative high-resolution transmission electron microscopy of crystalline materials," *Ultramicroscopy* **58**, 131–155 (1995).

[2] P. Schwander, C. Kisielowski, M. Seibt, F.H. Baumann, Y. Kim, and A. Ourmazd, "Mapping projected potential, interfacial roughness, and composition in general crystalline solids by quantitative transmission electron microscopy," *Physical Review Letters* **71**, 4150–4153 (1993).

[3] R. J. Gardner, *Geometric Tomography* (Cambridge University Press, New York) 1995.

[4] G. G. Lorentz, "A problem of plane measure," *Amer. J. Math.* **71**, 417–426 (1949).

[5] A. Rényi, "On projections of probability distributions," *Acta Math. Acad. Sci. Hung.* **3**, 131–142 (1952).

[6] A. Heppes, "On the determination of probability distributions of more dimensions by their projections," *Acta Math. Acad. Sci. Hung.* **7**, 403–410 (1956).

[7] G. Bianchi and M. Longinetti, "Reconstructing plane sets from projections," *Discrete Comp. Geom.* **5**, 223–242 (1990).

[8] R. J. Gardner and P. Gritzmann, "Discrete tomography: Determination of finite sets by X-rays," *Trans. Amer. Math. Soc.* **349**, 2271–2295 (1997).

[9] R. J. Gardner and P. McMullen, "On Hammer's X-ray problem," *J. London Math. Soc. (2)* **21**, 171–175 (1980).

[10] F. Q. Gouvêa, *p-adic Numbers* (Springer, New York), 1993.

[11] E. Barcucci, A. Del Lungo, M. Nivat, and R. Pinzani, "X-rays characterizing some classes of digital pictures," (Technical Report RT 4/96, Dipartimento di Sistemi e Informatica, Universita di Firenze, Firenze), 1996.

[12] E. Barcucci, A. Del Lungo, M. Nivat, and R. Pinzani, "Reconstructing convex polyominoes from their horizontal and vertical projections," *Theor. Comput. Sci.* **155**, 321–347 (1996).

[13] R. J. Gardner, "Geometric tomography," *Notices Amer. Math. Soc.* **42**, 422–429 (1995).

[14] P. R. Scott, "Equiangular lattice polygons and semiregular lattice polyhedra," *College Math. J.* **18**, 300-306 (1987).

[15] A. Schrijver, *Theory of Linear and Integer Programming* (Wiley, New York), 1987.

[16] R. J. Gardner, P. Gritzmann, and D. Prangenberg, "On the computational complexity of reconstructing lattice sets from their X-rays," *Discrete Math.* **202**, 45–71 (1999).

[17] P. Gritzmann, D. Prangenberg, S. de Vries, and M. Wiegelmann, "Success and failure of certain reconstruction and uniqueness algorithms in discrete tomography," *Intern. J. Imaging Syst. Techn.* **9**, 101–109 (1998).

[18] R. J. Gardner, P. Gritzmann, and D. Prangenberg, "On the reconstruction of binary images from their discrete Radon transforms," *Proc. Intern. Symp. Optical Science, Engineering, and Instrumentation, SPIE*, pp. 121–132 (1996).

[19] R. W. Irving and M. R. Jerrum, "Three-dimensional statistical data security problems," *SIAM J. Comput.* **23**, 170–184 (1994).

[20] P. C. Fishburn, J. C. Lagarias, J. A. Reeds, and L. A. Shepp, "Sets uniquely determined by projections on axes. II. Discrete case," *Discrete Math.* **91**, 149–159 (1991).

[21] P. C. Fishburn, P. Schwander, L. A. Shepp, and J. Vanderbei, "The discrete Radon transform and its approximate inversion via linear programming," *Discrete Appl. Math.* **75**, 39–62 (1997).

[22] P. Gritzmann and M. Wiegelmann, "On combinatorial patterns given by cross-characteristics: Uniqueness versus additivity," in preparation.

[23] H. J. Ryser, "Combinatorial properties of matrices of zeros and ones," *Canad. J. Math.* **9**, 371–377 (1957).

[24] T. Y. Kong and G. T. Herman, "On which grids can tomographic equivalence of binary pictures be characterized in terms of elementary switching operations," *Intern. J. Imaging Syst. Techn.* **9**, 118–125 (1998).

[25] R. J. Gardner, P. Gritzmann, and D. Prangenberg, "On the computational complexity of inverting higher-dimensional discrete X-ray transforms," in preparation.

[26] H. Edelsbrunner and S. S. Skiena, "Probing convex polygons with X-rays," *SIAM. J. Comp.* **17**, 870–882 (1988).

[27] S. Patch, "Iterative algorithm for discrete tomography," *Intern. J. Imaging Syst. Techn.* **9**, 132–134 (1998).

[28] Y.-C. Chen and A. Shastri, "On joint realization of (0,1) matrices," *Linear Algebra Appl.* **112**, 75–85 (1989).

[29] R. J. Gardner, P. Gritzmann, and D. Prangenberg, "On the computational complexity of determining polyatomic structures by X-rays," *Theor. Comput. Sci.*, to appear.

[30] M. Chrobak and C. Dürr, "Reconstructing polyatomic structures from discrete X-rays: NP-completeness proof for three atoms," preprint.

Chapter 5

Reconstruction of Plane Figures from Two Projections

Akira Kaneko[1]
Lei Huang[2]

ABSTRACT In this chapter, reconstruction of plane figures from their two-projection data is discussed together with its stability, based on the discrete approximation. For this purpose, we introduce the notion of type 1 modification against nonuniquely reconstructed figures, and a kind of weight function to classify them. Many interesting open problems remain concerning theoretical justification of proposed algorithms for nonunique cases.

5.1 Review of the problem and known results

In this chapter, we shall explain how to obtain a reconstruction of plane figures from their two projection data in a general setting. The argument is based on the limit process from the reconstruction for the discrete approximation by small squares. Our actual computational results are all for the approximative discrete data. In this first section, however, we introduce the original work on the reconstruction of continuous figures by G. Lorentz [1], who first discussed this problem in 1949. The discrete version of this problem falls in the category of combinatorial theory, known as reconstruction of binary matrices, that is, the problem of finding a matrix with only two kinds of entries 0,1, given the number of elements 1 in each row and each column. This latter was studied by Ryser with several years delay independently of Lorentz's work (see Ryser [2]). In this chapter, however, keeping the plane figures in mind, we understand by a discrete object the union of squares in ε-mesh, instead of binary matrices.

Lorentz's original theory is of measure theoretic nature. Here for the sake of avoiding sophisticated arguments on measurability, we assume that the figures we are treating are not mere measurable sets but usual nice geometric figures. (What "nice" means will be made precise in Section

[1]Department of Information Sciences, Ochanomizu University, 2-1-1 Otsuka, Bunkyo-ku, Tokyo 112-8610 Japan, E-mail: kanenko@is.ocha.ac.jp
[2]C&C Media Research Labs., NEC Corp., 4-1-1 Miyazaki, Miyamae-ku, Kawasaki, Kanagawa 216-8555, Japan, E-mail: huang@ccm.cl.nec.co.jp

5.3.) For more historical details thereafter, see the introductory chapter by Kuba and Herman.

Let F be a plane figure. (In most situations it may simply be a measurable set, bounded or not. But you may simply imagine rather good geometric figures as remarked above.) We consider its two axial projections, or the length functions of the cut: $f_y(t) = \lambda_1(F \cap \{x = t\})$ and $f_x(t) = \lambda_1(F \cap \{y = t\})$, where in general $\lambda_n(\cdot)$ denotes the n-dimensional Lebesgue measure (this time the "length"). In the discrete case, the projection functions $f_y(x)$ etc. become step functions with step width ε. The problem is to reconstruct the original plane figure F (or more precisely, one of the possible figures) from these two data, hopefully by a fixed deterministic algorithm.

As mentioned above, this problem was first introduced by G. Lorentz, who gave a necessary and sufficient condition for the projection functions f_y, f_x in order that there exists a plane figure F, and also a necessary and sufficient condition in order that such F is uniquely determined from the data. To state these results Lorentz employed the important idea of rearrangement, which had been introduced by F. Riesz and found to be very efficient in proving various inequalities of analysis. (Lorentz continues to use this idea for his lifework on Lorentz spaces in functional analysis.) Here we are adopting the notation of Kuba-Volčič [3] rather than the original one of Lorentz. We shall employ, however, part of his notation in the proof of his theorem below; For example, by the x-projection we mean in the sequel not only the function $f_y(x)$ but also its below-graph set $P = \{(x, y); 0 \leq y \leq f_y(x)\}$, and likewise $Q = \{(x, y); 0 \leq x \leq f_x(y)\}$.

We denote by $f_{xy}(x)$ the re-projection of $f_x(y)$ or Q to the x-axis, which is defined by

$$f_{xy}(x) = \lambda_1(\{y; x \leq f_x(y)\}). \tag{5.1}$$

The corresponding below-graph set will be denoted by P_1. This apparently complex notation will become familiar if it is noticed that the last suffix always indicates the axis along which the last projection was made. We define $f_{yx}(y)$ in a similar way, replacing the role of x, y, together with its below-graph set Q_1. We further denote by $f_{yxy}(x)$ the re-projection of $f_{yx}(y)$. Since f_{yx} is already non-increasing, the below-graph set of f_{yxy} is the same as Q_1 of f_{yx} as a plane figure. But as functions they are categorically distinguished, because f_{yx} is a function of y, while f_{yxy} is of x, hence can be compared directly rather with $f_{xy}(x)$. See Fig. 5.1 for the illustration of these.

The function $f_{yxy}(x)$ is called the (non-increasing) *rearrangement* of the function $f_y(x)$. By abuse we shall call Q_1 the rearrangement of P. The rearrangement has the following properties which explain its name:

Lemma 5.1.   (1) *For each $y \geq 0$, we have*

$$\lambda_1(\{x; f_{yxy}(x) \geq y\}) = \lambda_1(\{x; f_y(x) \geq y\}). \tag{5.2}$$

(2) *There exists a decomposition of the supports of f_{yxy} and f_y into uncountably many subsets of measure 0:*

$$\text{supp} f_{yxy} = \bigcup_{\alpha \in A} K_\alpha, \qquad \text{supp} f_y = \bigcup_{\alpha \in A} K'_\alpha, \tag{5.3}$$

such that for each α f_{yxy} resp. f_y takes a common constant value c_α on K_α resp. K'_α, and that for any index set $\Gamma \subset A$, $\bigcup_{\alpha \in \Gamma} K_\alpha$ is measurable if and only if $\bigcup_{\alpha \in \Gamma} K'_\alpha$ is, and in that case their measures agree.

(3) *For each $c \geq 0$ we can find a measurable set $B \subset \mathbf{R}$ such that $\lambda_1(B) = c$ and that*

$$\int_0^c f_{yxy}(x)dx = \int_B f_y(x)dx. \tag{5.4}$$

Proof: (1) is obvious from the definition of rearrangement. The decomposition in (2) is provided as follows: For those c for which the sets

$$\{x; f_{yxy} = c\}, \qquad \{x; f_y(x) = c\} \tag{5.5}$$

have measure 0, we adopt c as the index and define K_c, K'_c by the above. In the opposite case, the above sets still have equal measure from the definition of rearrangement. Thus we can augment the index by means of

$$\phi_1(t) = \lambda_1(\{x \leq t; f_{yxy} = c\}), \qquad \phi_2(t) = \lambda_1(\{x \leq t; f_y(x) = c\} \tag{5.6}$$

in such a way that $K_{c,c'}$, resp. $K'_{c,c'}$ is defined as the set of t resp. t' for which $\phi_1(t)$ and $\phi_2(t')$ takes the same value c'. The measurability follows naturally. Finally, to show (3), let $\Gamma = \{\alpha \in A; K_\alpha \subset [0, c]\}$. Then it suffices to set

$$B = \bigcup_{\alpha \in \Gamma} K'_\alpha. \tag{5.7}$$

$\square$

Notice that if the rearrangement f_{yxy} is strictly decreasing, K_α reduces to a single point. Even in the general non-decreasing case, almost every K_α is a single point. On the contrary, we cannot in general reduce K'_α to a single point and define thereby a univalent measurable point correspondence from the support of f_{yxy} to that of f_y. To see this, imagine a typical mountain-like smooth figure with axially symmetric f_y, for which K'_α consists of two points in symmetry, except for the summit. When we are dealing with *pixels*, the rearrangement is not strictly decreasing, and for the last example, two vertical segments of equal height are produced except for the summit. Thus in the discrete case, we can define such point correspondence.

Now we present the main results of Lorentz.

Theorem 5.1.   (G. Lorentz) (1) *There exists a plane figure with the given x-resp. y-projection f_y and f_x if and only if for any $c \geq 0$ we have*

$$\int_0^c f_{xy}(x)dx \geq \int_0^c f_{yxy}(x)dx, \tag{5.8}$$

and equality holds for $c = \infty$.

(2) *There exists a unique plane figure with the given x- resp. y-projection f_y and f_x if and only if $f_{xy}(x) = f_{yxy}(x)$ a.e. or equivalently $P_1 = Q_1$.*

Proof: We shall present the proof of Lorentz, omitting the measure theoretical details. It is worth reading because it contains germinal ideas of several fundamental notions now widely employed.

(1) *Necessity.* We first show that for any measurable set $B \subset \mathbf{R}$ satisfying $\lambda_1(B) \leq c$ we have

$$\int_B f_y(x)dx \leq \int_0^c f_{xy}(x)dx. \tag{5.9}$$

Set

$$C = \{(x,y) \in F; \, x \in B\}, \qquad C_1 = \{(x,y) \in Q; \, 0 \leq x \leq c\}. \tag{5.10}$$

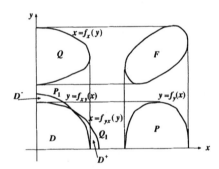

FIGURE 5.1. Illustration of the projections.

Then the projection function $f_x^C(y)$ of the set C satisfies

$$f_x^C(y) \leq \min\{f_x(y), c\}. \tag{5.11}$$

Integrating over $-\infty < y < \infty$ we obtain $\lambda_2(C) \leq \lambda_2(C_1)$, hence

$$\int_B f_y(x)dx = \lambda_2(C) \leq \lambda_2(C_1) = \int_0^c f_{xy}(x)dx, \tag{5.12}$$

as desired.

From this inequality and Lemma 5.1 (3), we can find B such that $\lambda_1(B) = c$ and that

$$\int_0^c f_{yxy}(x)dx = \int_B f_y(x)dx \leq \int_0^c f_{yx}(y)dy. \tag{5.13}$$

Sufficiency. Set

$$D = P_1 \cap Q_1, \qquad D^+ = Q_1 \setminus D, \qquad D^- = P_1 \setminus D. \qquad (5.14)$$

$D^{\pm}$ represent the excessive parts. We have obviously $\lambda_2(D^+) = \lambda_2(D^-)$. Because of the monotone property of the boundary curves of P_1, Q_1, not only D^+ and D^- are disjoint from each other, but so are also their projections onto both directions. (By "disjoint" we mean "of measure 0 intersection.") We apply the "multiresolution analysis" to these sets: Introducing the decomposition of the plane of mesh size 2^{-n}, $n = 0, 1, 2, \ldots$ with the lattice points at $x = 2^{-n}k$, $y = 2^{-n}\ell$, $k, \ell \in \mathbb{Z}$, we decompose $D^{\pm}$ into the unions of disjoint squares

$$D^+ = \bigcup_{i=1}^{\infty} D_i^+, \qquad D^- = \bigcup_{i=1}^{\infty} D_i^- \qquad (5.15)$$

in such a way that the mesh size of D_i^+ and D_i^- is the same for each i, and is non-increasing with i. In fact, starting from $n = 1$ we number the squares of size 2^{-n} contained in $D^{\pm}$ in an arbitrary order. If some squares of this size remain in either of $D^{\pm}$, we halve these and pass to the next mesh $n + 1$, and repeat the numbering for these finer squares, and so on.

Now we explain the reconstruction algorithm. First we assume that the projection functions $f_y(x)$, $x \geq 0$, $f_x(y)$, $y \geq 0$ are non-increasing. In this case, modulo coordinate translation we can assume that $P = Q_1$, $Q = P_1$ agree with their rearrangements. We start from P and deform it little by little to a desired figure F by moving a square of the same size and height as D_i^+ to a vacant place at the height of D_i^- for $i = 1, 2, \ldots$ Let $F_0 = P$, and assume that we have made up to a figure F_{k-1}, processing $D_1^{\pm}, \ldots, D_{k-1}^{\pm}$ already. Let D_k^+ lie in the strip $y_1 \leq y \leq y_2$, and D_k^- in $y_3 \leq y \leq y_4$, with $y_2 - y_1 = y_4 - y_3 = \delta$ and $y_3 \geq y_2$. We have

$$\lambda_1(F_{k-1} \cap \{y = y_2\}) \geq f_x(y_2) + \delta \geq f_x(y_3) + \delta, \qquad (5.16)$$

since f_x is non-increasing and D_k^+ is not yet processed. By the same reason, we have

$$\lambda_1(F_{k-1} \cap \{y = y_3\}) \leq f_x(y_3) - \delta, \qquad (5.17)$$

since the strip of D_k^- still lacks a square of mesh δ. Because the original strip $P \cap \{y_1 \leq y \leq y_2\}$ was connected and the squares were removed from it with size of $2^k\delta$, $k \geq 0$, the region $F_{k-1} \cap \{y_1 \leq y \leq y_2\}$ still contains squares of size δ not less than

$$\left[\frac{f_x(y_3) + \delta}{\delta} \right] = \left[\frac{f_x(y_3)}{\delta} \right] + 1. \qquad (5.18)$$

On the other hand, $F_{k-1} \cap \{y_3 \leq y \leq y_4\}$ can be covered by squares of size δ no more than

$$\left[\frac{f_x(y_3) - \delta}{\delta} \right] + 1 = \left[\frac{f_x(y_3)}{\delta} \right]. \qquad (5.19)$$

Thus for at least one square in F_{k-1} of the same mesh and at the same height as D_k^+, the place above it is vacant in the strip of D_k^-. Thus shifting this square to the above, we can make F_k. Thus the induction proceeds to obtain the final figure F.

To obtain a reconstruction for general projections we modify the figure G reconstructed from the rearrangements by the above procedure. Recall the decomposition (5.3). With exception of measure 0 we can assume that $(K_\alpha \times \mathbf{R}) \cap G = K_\alpha \times G_\alpha$ for some measurable set G_α. Then we obtain a figure above P by $\mathcal{P}_x[G] := \bigcup_{\alpha \in A} K'_\alpha \times G_\alpha$. Let us denote by $\mathcal{P}_y$ a similar operation for the y-coordinates. Then the desired figure will be obtained by $F = \mathcal{P}_y[\mathcal{P}_x[G]]$.

(2) Assume that the condition of the theorem holds. This implies that the figure G reconstructed from the rearranged projections agree with the rearrangements P_1, Q_1 themselves. Thus for a.e. y_1, y_2, $f_{xyx}(y_1) \le f_{xyx}(y_2)$ trivially implies $G \cap \{y = y_1\} \subset G \cap \{y = y_2\}$. Since the operations $\mathcal{P}_x$, $\mathcal{P}_y$ obviously preserve this relation, our special reconstruction given in (1) also satisfies

$$\text{for a.e. } y_1, y_2, \quad f_x(y_1) \le f_x(y_2) \quad \Rightarrow \quad F \cap \{y = y_1\} \subset F \cap \{y = y_2\}. \quad (5.20)$$

Next we show that property (5.20) implies the uniqueness. Assume that there exists another figure F', which has the same projections as F and differs from F by a positive measure. This means that there exists $\varepsilon > 0$ and a set of positive measure $B \subset \mathbf{R}$ such that

$$y \in B \quad \Rightarrow \quad \lambda_1(F_y \setminus F'_y) \ge \varepsilon. \quad (5.21)$$

By shrinking B if necessary, we can assume without loss of generality that $f_x(y)$ is continuous on B. Then we can find $y_0 \in B$ such that for some $\delta > 0$ we have $\lambda_1(\{|y - y_0| < \delta\} \cap B) > 0$ and

$$y \in B, \ |y - y_0| < \delta \quad \Rightarrow \quad \lambda_1(F_y \ominus F_{y_0}) < \frac{\varepsilon}{2}, \quad (5.22)$$

where $F_y \ominus F_{y_0} = (F_y \setminus F_{y_0}) \cup (F_{y_0} \setminus F_y)$ denotes the *symmetric difference*. Then, for such y

$$\lambda_1(F_{y_0} \cap F_y) > \lambda_1(F_{y_0}) - \frac{\varepsilon}{2}. \quad (5.23)$$

On the other hand, we have

$$\lambda_1(F_{y_0} \cap F'_y) = \lambda_1(F_{y_0}) - \lambda_1(F_{y_0} \setminus F'_y) \le \lambda_1(F_{y_0}) - \lambda_1(F_y \setminus F'_y) + \lambda_1(F_y \ominus F_{y_0}). \quad (5.24)$$

Hence from (5.21) – (5.23) we conclude that for such y we have

$$\lambda_1(F_{y_0} \cap F'_y) < \lambda_1(F_{y_0} \cap F_y). \quad (5.25)$$

Employing (5.20), however, we can show below that for a.e. y these two agree. The obtained contradiction will prove the uniqueness.

From the equality of x-projections we have

$$\lambda_2((F_{y_0} \times \mathbf{R}) \cap F) = \int_{F_{y_0}} f_y(x)dx = \lambda_2((F_{y_0} \times \mathbf{R}) \cap F'). \quad (5.26)$$

Viewing this "horizontally," we find that

$$\int_{-\infty}^{\infty} \lambda_1(F_{y_0} \cap F_y)dy = \int_{-\infty}^{\infty} \lambda_1(F_{y_0} \cap F_y')dy. \tag{5.27}$$

If $\lambda_1(F_y) \le \lambda_1(F_{y_0})$, then from the assumption (5.20) we have $F_y \subset F_{y_0}$, hence

$$\lambda_1(F_{y_0} \cap F_y) = \lambda_1(F_y) = \lambda_1(F_y') \ge \lambda_1(F_{y_0} \cap F_y'). \tag{5.28}$$

If $\lambda_1(F_y) \ge \lambda_1(F_{y_0})$, we have similarly $F_y \supset F_{y_0}$, hence

$$\lambda_1(F_{y_0} \cap F_y) = \lambda_1(F_{y_0}) \ge \lambda_1(F_{y_0} \cap F_y'). \tag{5.29}$$

Thus we have always $\lambda_1(F_{y_0} \cap F_y) \ge \lambda_1(F_{y_0} \cap F_y')$. In view of (5.27) they must agree a.e.

We show finally that the uniqueness implies $P_1 = Q_1$. If $P_1 \ne Q_1$, the reconstruction algorithm of (1) shows that there are two solutions for these rearranged projection data as follows: In the first step, in processing D_1^+ we have at least two choices: either we move D_1^+ up to the height of D_1^-, or move the square just below D_1^- at the height of D_1^+ up to D_1^-. In the successive processes, the fact that the place of D_1^+ is voided or the place of D_1^- is filled remains unchanged, whereas the fact that D_1^+ kept its place may be destroyed in the later processes. We can make the same argument, however, with respect to y-coordinates, changing the role of $D_1^{\pm}$ and assure the existence of a solution in which the place of D_1^+ is filled in the first step, hence forever. Thus we knew the existence of at least two different solutions. On the operation of $\mathcal{P}_x$ or $\mathcal{P}_y$ these two solutions obviously remain distinguished.   □

Since the existence proof for F by Lorentz was not fully algorithmic, further work has been done toward producing a reconstruction algorithm. Actually, Lorentz's algorithm is implementable in the discrete case assuming that all $D_j^{\pm}$ are of the same size. Nevertheless, it is less efficient than Ryser's algorithm, which we shall introduce now in a slightly modified manner. Let $f_y(x)$ and $f_x(y)$ be two projection functions satisfying the compatibility condition (5.8) as well. But since we need to view it from the x-axis, we rather consider the below-graph set of $f_x(y)$ as made of y-rows parallel to the y-axis. In the discrete case, the re-projection f_{xy} simply corresponds to the procedure of translating these rows along the y-axis in such a way as they stand as columns on the x-axis. The rearrangement f_{yxy} is the permutation of columns of f_y in the decreasing order. We identify these functions with the corresponding set of x-columns resp. y-rows made of squares of a fixed side length ε as before. The permutation achieving the rearrangement can be fixed to define its inverse procedure $\mathcal{P}_x$: The first column of $f_{yxy}(x)$ comes from the tallest column of $f_y(x)$. If there are many such for the latter, we make the convention that we choose the leftmost one from the columns of $f_y(x)$ of the same height, and so on. Now, by the condition (1) of Theorem 5.1, the base row of the y-projection $f_x(y)$ in general has width bigger than the height of the first x-column. Thus we pick up the same number of squares from this base y-row as contained in the x-column, choosing their places from the highest y-columns of the graph of $f_x(y)$. If there are y-columns of the same height, we make the convention that we first choose the lowest one, that is, the one closest to the x-axis. Using these as the x- resp. y-projection, we draw a patch of squares in the plane as the first part of our F.

In the next step we replace the x-projection by the one $f_y'(x)$ obtained from the original $f_y(x)$ by deleting the above chosen column, and the y-projection by the one $f_x'(y)$ obtained from $f_x(y)$ by deleting the above chosen base squares and then crashing the vacuum thus made toward the y-axis (or equivalently, diminishing the height of the corresponding y-columns by one unit). Then we newly obtain a pair of projections which, as we can see easily, satisfies the compatibility condition again. Since this new pair never requires any square on the strip along the first chosen column from the x-projection, we can repeat this process to construct the remaining part of a requested figure without the fear of overlapping. Thus we obtain

Theorem 5.2.   *The above procedure gives a plane figure F with the given x- and y-projections, in as many number of steps as the number of columns in the original x-projection $f_y(x)$.*

In Ryser [2], reconstruction is made from the smaller parts first. When treating only binary problems, this would be simpler as algorithms. But we preferred to attack from the largest part here, because in the discrete problems coming from continuous ones, the smaller parts are very flexible and should eventually be ignored as errors.

In the special case where uniqueness holds, the above algorithm reduces to the following easier one. The first part of the theorem was, as we saw above, contained in the proof of Lorentz. But it was perceived by A. Kuba [4] and L. Huang [5] to be useful of reconstruction for unique figures.

Theorem 5.3.   (1) *A plane figure F is uniquely reconstructed from its two projections if and only if for any two columns F_{x_1}, F_{x_2} of F, $\lambda_1(F_{x_1}) \leq \lambda_1(F_{x_2})$ implies $F_{x_1} \subset F_{x_2}$.*

(2) *(L. Huang [5]) F can be reconstructed from the two projections $f_y(x)$, $f_x(y)$ by the following deterministic algorithm: From the columns of the x-projection $f_y(x)$, we pick up the tallest one (say, the leftmost one if there are many such). This corresponds to the base row (that is, the one touching the y-axis) of the y-projection. Hence we place a patch of squares with these as x- resp. y-projection. Then we repeat this procedure picking up the second tallest column from the x-projection and the corresponding second wide row from the y-projection, and so on.*

5.2 Choice of good reconstruction for the discrete case

In order to pass to the continuous limit, we have to know what kind of reconstruction solutions we have. It seems that giving an efficient description of the whole solutions is still an open problem. Thus in this section we shall try to choose a standard model among the reconstructions which are stable enough to pass to the continuous limit. Here we do not pose a priori additional constraints such as existence of connected solutions as is discussed in [6] or in Chapter 3 by Kong and Herman.

For this purpose we first recall the notion of a switching component, which presents the essential obstruction to the uniqueness (cf. Section 3.1.2 in Chapter 3). This notion was introduced by Ryser [2] in the discrete case, and later adapted by Kuba-Volčič [3] to continuous case. It is now generalized by Gardner to the case of more than two projections (see [7]).

For the convenience of description, we label a component square S of our "discrete" figure by its center coordinates as $S(x_j, y_j)$. In the combinatorial case, $S(x_j, y_j)$ may be identified with a square of side-length 1 centered at the integral lattice point (x_j, y_j). Either of the two pairs of squares, $S(x_1, y_1)$, $S(x_2, y_2)$, or its reflection $S(x_1, y_2)$, $S(x_2, y_1)$ is called a *switching pair* (see Fig. 5.2). For later use, we shall call as type 1 a pair such that the line from the lower square to the upper one forms a positive inclination, and as type 2 the other pair. We shall call these pairs *associated to each other*. A switching pair in itself gives a typical example of nonunique plane figures. More generally, we say that a figure contains a *switching component* if it contains one such pair and does not contain the associated pair. A theorem of Kuba-Volčič [3] and of Ryser in the discrete case says that the reconstruction is nonunique if and only if a reconstructed figure contains a switching component. We shall use the word "type 1 or 2" for the corresponding switching components, too.

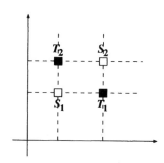

FIGURE 5.2. Switching pair (S_j:type 1, T_j: type 2).

Thus in the nonunique case we can obtain new figures with the same x- and y-projections, by replacing the switching pairs by their associated pairs.

The following result says that this exhausts the variety of reconstruction:

Theorem 5.4.   (Ryser [2]) *Any discrete plane figure with the given x- and y-projections is obtained from a special solution by repeating the procedure of replacing a switching component contained in it by its associated switching component.*

For a proof see Chapter 3 by Kong and Herman.

In order to numerically measure the effect of changing the type of a switching component, we shall introduce a kind of *weight function*. Its general form is as follows:

$$\mu(F) = \sum_{S(x,y)\subset F} \alpha(x)\beta(y). \tag{5.30}$$

We require that

(1) The replacement of a switching component of type 2 by the associated component of type 1 increases the value of μ.

Here the word "increase" may be replaced by "decrease," since μ has the same effect as $-\mu$ in our discussion. The functions α, β may be arbitrary if only they are strictly increasing. In fact, if $S(x_i, y_j)$, $i, j = 1, 2$, $x_1 < x_2$, $y_1 < y_2$ constitute a set of switching pairs, we have

$$\alpha(x_1)\beta(y_1) + \alpha(x_2)\beta(y_2) - \{\alpha(x_1)\beta(y_2) + \alpha(x_2)\beta(y_1)\}$$
$$= \{\alpha(x_2) - \alpha(x_1)\}\{\beta(y_2) - \beta(y_1)\} \geq \delta^2 > 0, \tag{5.31}$$

where δ is the minimal increment of the functions α, β for the mesh step in the considered region. Notice that the sum of the form

$$\sum_{S(x,y)\subset F} \alpha(x) \qquad \text{or} \qquad \sum_{S(x,y)\subset F} \beta(y) \tag{5.32}$$

does not change its value by interchange of switching pairs, because it is determined from the projection data. Thus maximizing μ is equivalent with minimizing the sum

$$\sum_{S(x,y)\subset F} (\alpha(x) - \beta(y))^2. \tag{5.33}$$

This suggests that the figures maximizing μ are those most concentrated around the curve $\alpha(x) = \beta(y)$.

If we wish to make distinction of all the reconstructions by this function, we also have to require the following:

(2) The function μ has different values for the different reconstructions from the same projection data.

We still do not know what is the best choice, or if there exists a weight function satisfying all these requirements in continuous case. (In the case of integral lattice, the function $\sum_{S(x,y)\subset F}\alpha^x\beta^y$, where α,β are two algebraically independent numbers, fulfills all. For continuous figures, however, the level curves of $\alpha^x\beta^y$ are straight lines, and counter-example for nonuniqueness against 3 projections by Gardner ([7], Theorem 2.3.4) shows that this does not satisfy (2). We may eventually use several such weight functions simultaneously, composing them with an increasing function of several variables (e.g., product of several positive weight functions).

Here we shall employ the simplest function

$$\mu_1(F) = \sum_{S(x,y)\subset F} xy. \tag{5.34}$$

An elementary calculation shows that the maximization of this is equivalent with minimization of the moment of inertia of F around the line $x = y$. A similar calculation also shows that this function is essentially invariant under the translation of coordinates:

$$\sum_{S(x,y)\subset F} (x - a)(y - b) \tag{5.35}$$

$$= \sum_{S(x,y)\subset F} xy - b \sum_{S(x,y)\subset F} x f_y(x) - a \sum_{S(x,y)\subset F} y f_x(y) + ab.$$

In particular, the shape of the maximizer of μ_1 does not change by coordinate translation. This function is favorable also on the point that if F consists of squares of side length ε centered at (x,y), then the integral can replace the sum:

$$\iint_F xy\,dx\,dy = \varepsilon^2 \sum_{S(x,y)\subset F} xy. \tag{5.36}$$

Notice that for continuous figures the barycentre (x_G, y_G) of F or the moment of inertia around it are all determined from the projection data:

$$x_G = \frac{1}{\lambda_2(F)} \iint_F x\,dx\,dy = \frac{1}{\lambda_2(F)} \int x f_y(x)\,dx, \quad \text{etc.} \tag{5.37}$$

Our basic assertion is the following

Theorem 5.5.   ([8]) *After a finite number of replacements of type 2 switching components by their associated type 1 switching components, we obtain a figure with no type 2 switching component.*

In fact we can perform the replacement in a fixed order. For example,

Algorithm 5.1.   *(1) We take a square from a column of F in the order from the leftmost column rightward, and from the top square downward in the chosen column.*

(2) We search another square in the order from the rightmost column leftward, and from the bottom square upward in the chosen column, in such a way that this together with the square in (1) makes a type 2 switching component.

(3) We replace this pair by its associated type 1 switching pair.

This procedure obviously does not produce new squares to the left and to the upper side of the first chosen square. Thus we can continue this procedure until we sweep over the figure. Unfortunately, this process gives rise to new type 2 switching components in which squares in already swept region take part in, because the procedure may produce new available holes for them. Thus we have to repeat the process several times. The termination of this several round processes is assured by the measuring function μ: It cannot increase forever, since all the reconstructed figures are contained in some fixed bounded region determined from the projection data, hence μ is bounded from above by some constant. We still do not know how many rounds are necessary in general, hence how is the complexity of the whole process. Computer experiments show that usually 4 or 5 rounds are enough.

We shall call a reconstruction containing only switching components of type 1 a *type 1 reconstruction*. We might call it a standard reconstruction. But unfortunately, they are not unique. Figure 5.3 will show the reason.

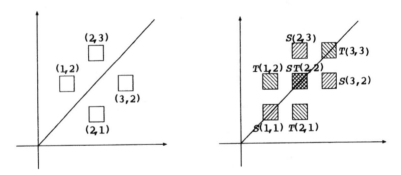

FIGURE 5.3. *S* and *T* **denote two type 1 modifications.**

One may think that such an example is rare. But the fact is that this phenomenon is rather common in the nonunique case. Figure 5.4 shows such an example. The indicated figures are placed in the range of 300×300 pixels. The attached values are those of μ_1 in (5.34). These values show that, unfortunately, the algorithm 5.2 of Theorem 5.2 does not necessarily give the one which attains the maximum of μ_1. According to computer experiments, the maximum of μ_1 is attained by the original slant ellipse in this case.

Also our computer experiment shows that we can recover the original ellipse through very many repetitions of perturbation by type 2 regression and type 1 modification which in pair increase the value of μ_1. Even if the

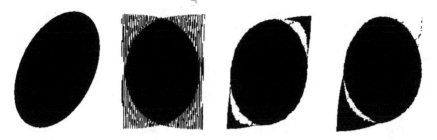

FIGURE 5.4. (1) Original figure (μ_1 = 697567002). **(2) Reconstruction by Ryser** (μ_1 = 667087303). **(3) Type 1 modification by Theorem 5.2** (μ_1 = 687592243). **(4) Another example of type 1 reconstruction** (μ_1 = 686960379).

original figure is convex, however, our type 1 reconstruction maximizing μ_1 may in general give an interesting figure different from the original one; cf. Fig. 5.5. Other fascinating examples in the non-convex case are shown in Figs. 5.6 and 5.7. The pixel numbers are all the same as before. We do not know analytically the exact final form of the maximizer in these examples. But two narrow lunar holes in Fig. 5.6, e.g., should survive in its final shape in order to compensate the circular holes in the original pattern which are individually unique figures. In spite of the example in Fig. 5.3, we conjecture that for projection data coming from natural continuous figures, the maximizer is unique under a rather mild condition.

It will be an interesting problem to study the effect of the choice of weight function against the type 1 reconstruction which maximizes it, including the uniqueness of the maximizer. An easy choice gives figures less beautiful than those supplied by μ_1.

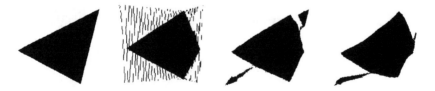

FIGURE 5.5. (1) Original figure (μ_1 = 359614103). **(2) Reconstruction by Ryser** (μ_1 = 353048774). **(3) Type 1 modification by Theorem 5.2** (μ_1 = 360271755). **(4) Near-final form of the maximizer of** μ_1 (μ_1 = 363080237).

The above examples suggest that an algorithm giving the reconstruction with maximum value of μ_1 might be useful. (Notice that a figure maximizing μ_1 is automatically of type 1.) But we still do not know a good algorithm giving such, or any other kind of standard reconstruction, for general case. In the next section we take this for granted to pass to the

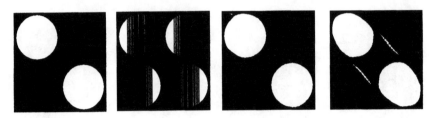

FIGURE 5.6. **(1) Original figure** ($\mu_1 = 1534540950$). **(2) Reconstruction by Ryser** ($\mu_1 = 1414901418$). **(3) Type 1 modification by Theorem 5.2** ($\mu_1 = 1534879614$). **(4) Near-final form of the maximizer of μ_1** ($\mu_1 = 1538741836$).

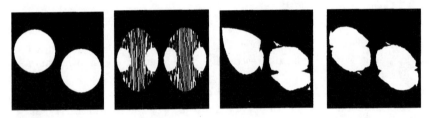

FIGURE 5.7. **(1) Original figure** ($\mu_1 = 1439169120$). **(2) Reconstruction by Ryser** ($\mu_1 = 1376304470$). **(3) Type 1 modification by Theorem 5.2** ($\mu_1 = 1442458405$). **(4) Near-final form of the maximizer of μ_1** ($\mu_1 = 1444388833$).

continuous limit.

5.3   Passage to continuous limit

Now we discuss the stability of the (standardized) reconstruction and examine the convergence to the continuous case as $\varepsilon \to 0$.

In the unique case, A. Kuba and A.Volčič [3] have given the following beautiful reconstruction formula:

$$F = \{(x, y); f_y(x) \geq f_{xy}(f_x(y))\}. \tag{5.38}$$

Since in this case also, we have to discretize the matter for the practical calculation of reconstruction, it will be meaningful to employ the discrete approximation and discuss the passage to the continuous limit.

The general recipe including nonunique case is as follows:

Algorithm 5.2.   *(1) Given $\varepsilon > 0$, we draw lattice of mesh ε, and take the outer approximation $f_x^\varepsilon(y)$ of $f_x(y)$, and the inner approximation $f_y^\varepsilon(x)$ of $f_y(x)$. These two approximations satisfy the inequality (5.8) because they are separated by $f_x(y)$ and $f_y(x)$, which satisfy (5.8).*

(2) Since the areas of these two approximated projections are not equal, we add ε-squares to $f_y^\varepsilon(x)$ of height ε to the right of the rightmost column of $f_y^\varepsilon(x)$, as many number as to equate the total area. Obviously, this does not destroy the inequality (5.8).

(3) Now we can apply the algorithm of Section 5.2 to these modified approximated projections to obtain an ε-discretized reconstruction F^ε.

(4) We modify this F^ε to a type 1 reconstruction $\widetilde{F}^\varepsilon$ by exchange of switching pairs of type 2 to the associated ones of type 1 in a canonical way as explained in Theorem 5.2 of the preceding section.

(5) If the figure thus obtained seems not good enough, we modify it by random application of sets of type 2 regression and type 1 modification to maximize the weight function μ_1 (or any other).

(6) We let $\varepsilon \to 0$, and expect that $\widetilde{F}^\varepsilon$, or the one further modified by step (5), converges to a continuous figure $\widetilde{F}$ by some metric, and gives a figure with the original projection functions f_y, f_x.

In practical calculation, we do not need to take care of thin tails produced by the adjusting process of (2), because they are outside the original region and should finally disappear. Computer experiments show that this process works well in practice and seems to give a stable reconstruction image. Notice, however, that in nonunique case standardization in some sense of the discrete approximate reconstructions is indispensable to have a reasonable limit. This complicates the matter much for theoretical justifications in contrast with the unique case. We shall show this by an example.

Example. Let the two projections be the rectangle with base $[3,5]$ and height 1. These are obtained as the projections of a figure F consisting of the two squares $Q_1 = \{3 \le x, y \le 4\}$, $Q_2 = \{4 \le x, y \le 5\}$. If we apply either Ryser's algorithm or our modified one in Section 5.1 to the ε-discretization (which we assume for the sake of simplicity to be the uniform decomposition of the interval $[3,5]$ simply by mesh $\varepsilon = 1/N$ with an integer N), then we obtain a comb-like figure F_ε as in Fig. 5.8 Right. The characteristic function $\chi_\varepsilon(x,y)$ of F_ε converges to half the characteristic function χ_Q of the square $Q = \{3 \le x, y \le 5\}$ in the weak topology of $L^2(Q)$. In fact, $F_\varepsilon, \varepsilon = 1/N$, $N = 1, 2, \ldots$ forms a bounded sequence in $L^2(Q)$, hence weakly compact. On the other hand, for any continuous function $\varphi(x,y)$ we have obviously

$$\langle \chi_\varepsilon(x,y), \varphi(x,y) \rangle = \iint_{F_\varepsilon} \varphi(x,y)dxdy \to \frac{1}{2} \iint_{3 \le x, y \le 5} \varphi(x,y)dxdy. \quad (5.39)$$

Since continuous functions are dense in $L^2(Q)$, the weak limit of any subsequence should agree with this fixed function $(1/2)\chi_Q(x,y)$. Thus the sequence itself converges to this function in weak $L^2(Q)$-topology. This implies that F_ε cannot have a strong $L^1(Q)$-limit. For, the strong $L^1(Q)$-convergence would imply the weak $L^2(Q)$-convergence in view of Lebesgue's dominated convergence theorem. But on the other hand, the strong $L^1(Q)$

convergence would imply that the limit function $\chi(x, y)$ is a characteristic function of a measurable subset of Q, because by the dominated convergence theorem we have

$$0 \equiv \iint_Q \chi_\varepsilon(x,y)^2 (1 - \chi_\varepsilon(x,y))^2 dx dy \qquad (5.40)$$

$$\to \iint_Q \chi(x,y)^2 (1 - \chi(x,y))^2 dx dy.$$

Hence $\chi \equiv 0$ or 1 a.e. again. This is a contradiction.

For this projection data set, an arbitrary modification of switching components will give a reconstructed figure consisting of two rectangles of width rate λ and two comb-like regions of width rate $1 - \lambda$ for any $0 < \lambda < 1$.

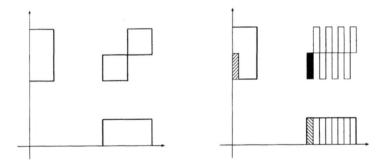

FIGURE 5.8. (Left) Favorable reconstruction. (Right) Reconstruction by Ryser's algorithm.

In examining the convergence of plane figures, several norms are available. The first is the L^1-*norm* in $\mathbf{R}^2$. This is convenient in the sense that the L^1-limit of a sequence of characteristic functions of plane figures is again the characteristic function of a plane figure as was shown above. But this convergence allows a long-living, very thin tail, which is far from the limit figure.

The second one is the *Hausdorff distance*. The Hausdorff distance of two plane sets F, G is defined by

$$\mathrm{dis}_H(F, G) := \max\{\max_{P \in F} \min_{Q \in G} \|P - Q\|, \max_{P \in G} \min_{Q \in F} \|P - Q\|\}. \qquad (5.41)$$

Here $\| \cdot \|$ denotes a norm of the plane. For our purpose, it is more suitable to choose the maximum norm

$$\|(x, y)\| = \max\{|x|, |y|\} \qquad (5.42)$$

than the usual Euclidean one, because for this choice (5.41) gives the maximum breadth of the symmetric difference $F \ominus G$ with respect to x- or

y-coordinate. If $F \subset G$, then the first member of the maximum in (5.41) is superfluous, because it reduces to zero. According to a fundamental theorem of Hausdorff, plane figures (more precisely, compact sets), which are contained inside a fixed rectangle, constitute a compact metric space with respect to the Hausdorff distance. In our case all the approximations may be considered to be contained in a rectangle $Q = [A, B] \times [C, D]$, where the interval $[A, B]$ resp. $[C, D]$ are so chosen that it contains the support of the x- resp. y-projection data. Thus without any further discussion we can conclude that we can find a subsequence from $\{F^\varepsilon\}_{\varepsilon > 0}$, which converges by the Hausdorff metric to a figure F. It is favorable in the sense that it does not allow thin far tail just by the definition of this metric, and this really works well as long as we treat only convex figures (see, e.g., [7]). But unfortunately, for general non-convex sets the convergence by Hausdorff metric does not necessarily imply even the convergence of the area. In fact, in the above example F_ε converges in Hausdorff metric to the square Q, which obviously is not a desired reconstruction. In this sense, the L^2-weak convergence keeps more information because it preserves the value of the integral, hence the area if only the limit is a characteristic function.

Let us now introduce the notion of *Lipschitzian* figures, that is, those surrounded by a finite number of arcs each of which is defined as the graph of a uniformly Lipschits continuous function in some rotated coordinates. As is well-known in elementary integration theory of Riemann-Jordan, such a figure F can be approximated from inside resp. from outside by a union of ε-squares F_I^ε resp. F_O^ε, and the difference of the area remains within $L\varepsilon$, where L is a constant depending only on the Lipschitz continuity and length of the boundary of the figure. More strongly, the Hausdorff distance of two approximations F_I^ε, F_O^ε is estimated by $M\varepsilon$ with a similar constant M. The notion of Lipschitzian figures is also compatible with the projections. Recall that in view of Ascoli-Arzelà's theorem a sequence of functions, which are equi-Lipschitz continuous, makes a relatively compact set in the space of continuous functions. Thus the following notion is useful for us:

Definition 5.1.   A sequence of figures F_n is called *almost equi-Lipschitzian* if there exists another sequence of figures G_n such that $\lambda_2(F_n \ominus G_n)$ tends to 0 and that the boundaries of G_n are made of a finite number of parts each of which is given as the graph of a sequence of equi-Lipschitz continuous functions to some fixed direction.

An almost equi-Lipschizian sequence becomes relatively compact in $L^1(Q)$. Thus if we can construct such a sequence of approximate reconstructions, we can expect at least a solution of continuous reconstruction problem as the limit of an L^1-converging subsequence. Our computer experiments as shown in Section 5.2 suggest that a reconstruction which gives the maximum value to μ_1 in (5.34) might give an almost equi-Lipschitzian sequence when the projection data come from a type 1 Lipschitzian figure. If in addition the maximizer is unique, the limit of any subsequence becomes the same. Hence in that case the sequence itself will converge to that limit. But the order of stability may be weak because the convergence in computer experiments was rather slow. Justification of these are all left open.

In the unique case everything goes well without any assumption on the regularity of the figures, and there is only the stability estimate to be discussed. The following result was given in [9]:

Theorem 5.6.   *Let f_y, f_x, g_y and g_x be non-negative, essentially bounded integrable functions. Assume that (f_y, f_x) and (g_y, g_x) uniquely determine the figures with f and g as the characteristic function, respectively. Then*

$$\|f - g\|_{L^1(\mathbf{R}^2)} \le C \cdot \max\{\|f_y - g_y\|_{L^\infty(\mathbf{R})}, \|f_x - g_x\|_{L^\infty(\mathbf{R})}\}, \qquad (5.43)$$

where C can be taken as follows:

$$
\begin{aligned}
C := \min\{&(9(\|f_x\|_{L^\infty(\mathbf{R})} + \|g_x\|_{L^\infty(\mathbf{R})}) + 3(\|f_y\|_{L^\infty(\mathbf{R})} + \|g_y\|_{L^\infty(\mathbf{R})})), \\
&(9(\|f_y\|_{L^\infty(\mathbf{R})} + \|g_y\|_{L^\infty(\mathbf{R})}) + 3(\|f_x\|_{L^\infty(\mathbf{R})} + \|g_x\|_{L^\infty(\mathbf{R})})), \\
&6(\|f_x\|_{L^\infty(\mathbf{R})} + \|g_x\|_{L^\infty(\mathbf{R})} + \|f_y\|_{L^\infty(\mathbf{R})} + \|g_y\|_{L^\infty(\mathbf{R})})\}.
\end{aligned}
\qquad (5.44)
$$

This not only implies the convergence of the discrete approximative reconstructions to the original continuous one, but also assures the continuous dependence of the reconstructed figure on the projection data. A similar conclusion holds also with respect to the Hausdorff metric if we restrict our consideration to Lipschtzian figures and assume the closeness of the projection data both by L^1 and Hausdorff metrics.

The proof of the above theorem given in [9] is based on the discrete approximation:

Lemma 5.2.   *Suppose that f_y, f_x are two non-negative, essentially bounded integrable functions that determine a measurable plane set F uniquely. Then for any $\varepsilon > 0$ we can find two projection functions g_y, g_x, which are step functions of step width $\delta > 0$ for some $\delta > 0$, and satisfy the uniqueness condition, such that*

$$0 \le f_y - g_y \le \varepsilon, \qquad 0 \le f_y - g_y \le \varepsilon, \qquad (5.45)$$

and that the characteristic functions of the reconstructed figures satisfy

$$\|f - g\|_{L^1(\mathbf{R}^2)} \le \{\|f_y\|_{L^1(\mathbf{R}^2)}) + \|f_x\|_{L^\infty(\mathbf{R})}\}\varepsilon. \qquad (5.46)$$

This Lemma is proved by a kind of induction combined with the approximation of figures from inside.

Lemma 5.3.   *Let f_y, f_x, g_y, g_x be two sets of simple functions that, as projection data, uniquely determine the plane figures F, G, with the characteristic* *functions f, g, respectively. Then for any $\varepsilon > 0$,*

$$\|f_y - g_y\|_{L^\infty(\mathbf{R})} < \varepsilon, \qquad \|f_x - g_x\|_{L^\infty(\mathbf{R})} < \varepsilon \qquad (5.47)$$

implies

$$\|f - g\|_{L^1(\mathbf{R}^2)} \qquad (5.48)$$
$$\leq [4\{\|f_x\|_{L^\infty(\mathbf{R})} + \|g_x\|_{L^\infty(\mathbf{R})}\} + \{\|f_y\|_{L^\infty(\mathbf{R})} + \|g_y\|_{L^\infty(\mathbf{R})}\}]\varepsilon.$$

In fact, without loss of generality we can assume that the subsets of constancy K_j, $j = 1, \ldots, N$, are common to f_y, g_y, by taking the union and the common subdivision of their supports if necessary. Then the uniqueness condition implies that the reconstructed figures can be written in the form

$$F = \bigcup_{j=1}^{N} K_j \times F_j, \qquad G = \bigcup_{j=1}^{N} K_j \times G_j. \qquad (5.49)$$

We have

$$\lambda_1(F_j) - \varepsilon \leq \lambda_1(G_j) \leq \lambda_1(F_j) + \varepsilon, \quad j = 1, \ldots, N. \qquad (5.50)$$

Also, without loss of generality, we can assume that $\lambda_1(F_j)$ are in decreasing order. Then by Theorem 5.1 (1), the uniqueness condition implies that $F_1 \supset F_2 \supset \cdots \supset F_N$. Then $G'_j := \bigcap_{1 \leq k \leq j} G_k$ is also decreasing; hence it uniquely determines a plane figure G' with the projection functions g'_y, g'_x. Employing induction we can show that

$$\lambda_1(F_j) - \varepsilon \leq \lambda_1(G'_j) \leq \lambda_1(F_j) + \varepsilon, \quad j = 1, \ldots, N. \qquad (5.51)$$

Under these preparations we can easily show that

$$\lambda_2(G \setminus G') \leq 2\varepsilon \sum_{j=1}^{N} \lambda_1(K_j) \leq 2\varepsilon\{\|f_x\|_{L^\infty(\mathbf{R})} + \|g_x\|_{L^\infty(\mathbf{R})}\}, \qquad (5.52)$$

and

$$\lambda_2(F \setminus G') = \int \max\{f_x(y) - g'_x(y), 0\}dy \qquad (5.53)$$
$$\leq \int |f_x(y) - g_x(y)|dy + \int \{g_x(y) - g'_x(y)\}dy$$
$$\leq \varepsilon\{\|f_y\|_{L^\infty(\mathbf{R})} + \|g_y\|_{L^\infty(\mathbf{R})}\} + 2\varepsilon\{\|f_x\|_{L^\infty(\mathbf{R})} + \|g_x\|_{L^\infty(\mathbf{R})}\}.$$

Summing these up we obtain the above estimate.

Here is an example of a unique figure and its discretized reconstruction well suggesting the stability of discrete approximation.

134 Akira Kaneko, Lei Huang

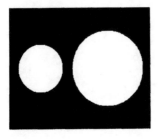 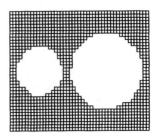

FIGURE 5.9. (Left) Original figure. (Right) Discretized approximate reconstruction by Huang's algorithm.

Acknowledgments

The authors would like to thank Professor Kuba for his hearty encouragement and valuable suggestions. The first author was supported in part by Grant-in-Aid for Scientific Research (No. 07404003), Ministry of Education, Science and Culture.

References

[1] G. G. Lorentz, "A problem of plane measure," *Amer. J. Math.* **71**, 417–426 (1949).

[2] H. J. Ryser, *Combinatorial Mathematics*. (The Math. Association of America, Washington, DC), 1963.

[3] A. Kuba and A. Volčič, "Characterization of measurable plane sets which are reconstructable from their two projections," *Inverse Problems* **4**, 513–527 (1988).

[4] A. Kuba, "Reconstruction of unique binary matrices with prescribed elements," *Acta Cybernetica* **12**, 57–70 (1995).

[5] L. Huang, *The reconstruction of uniquely determined plane sets from two projections in discrete case*. (Preprint Series UTMS **95–29**, Univ. of Tokyo, Tokyo), 1995.

[6] A. Kuba, "The reconstruction of two-directionally connected binary patterns from their two orthogonal projections," *Computer Vision, Graphics and Image Processing* **27**, 249–265 (1984).

[7] R. J. Gardner, *Geometric Tomography*. (Cambridge University Press, Cambridge, UK), 1995.

[8] K. Nakayama, Ch. Kobayashi, and A. Kaneko, *A deterministic algorithm for reconstruction from two projections*. (Preprint Series OCHA-IS **98-2**, Ochanomizu Univ., Tokyo), 1998.

[9] L. Huang and T. Takiguchi, "The reconstruction of uniquely determined plane sets from two projections," *J. Inverse and Ill-Posed Prob.* **6**, 217–242 (1988).

Chapter 6

Reconstruction of Two-Valued Functions and Matrices

Attila Kuba[1]

ABSTRACT   The reconstruction of a two-valued function from its two projections is considered. It is shown that this problem can be transformed into the solved problem of the reconstruction of characteristic functions (i.e., functions with values 0 and 1). Necessary and sufficient conditions are given to decide the existence and the uniqueness of a two-valued function if its projections and the two values are known. These conditions can also be applied if the two values are not given in advance. It is proved that merely the knowledge of the projections (i.e., without the two values) is not enough for the unique reconstruction of a two-valued function. However, on the basis of two given functions it is possible to decide whether they are the projections of a uniquely reconstructible two-valued function. Also the corresponding values can be determined in this way. The reconstruction of two-valued matrices from their row and column sums (projections) is also considered. It is shown that this problem can be transformed into the solved problem of the reconstruction of (0,1)-matrices. In the same way as in the case of two-valued functions, necessary and sufficient conditions are given to decide the existence and the uniqueness of a two-valued matrix if its projections and the two values are known. It is proved that, generally, there is only a finite number of solutions even if the two values are not fixed. Finally, an algorithm is given to reconstruct two-valued matrices from two projections.

6.1   Introduction

Consider an integrable two-variable function on $\mathbf{R}^2$. Its *horizontal* and *vertical projections* are defined by its integrals along each horizontal and vertical line, respectively. The *reconstruction problem* of a function from its two projections can be defined for different classes of functions.

For example, in the case of characteristic functions of measurable plane sets, G. G. Lorentz [1] solved the reconstruction problem when the functions to be reconstructed can only have values 0 and 1. He gave necessary

---

[1]József Attila University, Department of Applied Informatics, Árpád tér 2., H-6720 Szeged, Hungary, E-mail: kuba@inf.u-szeged.hu

and sufficient conditions for function pairs of unique, nonunique or inconsistent projections. Another condition for the existence of a set having given projections can be found in [2]. Characterization results [3], [4] and a reconstruction formula [3] have also been published on unique sets.

This chapter deals with the reconstruction of two-variable functions from their horizontal and vertical projections, when the functions are integrable on a rectangle of the plane and they can take only *two unknown values* (not necessarily 0 and 1). It is shown that this *two-valued reconstruction problem* can be solved by using the results known in the case of characteristic functions. A formula is derived to describe a necessary and sufficient condition on the existence and uniqueness of a two-valued function with the given projection pair as projections. These results show that if the first value is small enough and the second one is great enough then there is a solution of the two-valued reconstruction problem. Furthermore, a method is given to decide whether the given function pair is a unique projection pair with respect to some values. Finally, it is shown that these values of the eventual uniqueness and the corresponding two-valued unique function are computable.

6.2   Characteristic functions

Before starting the discussion of the two-valued reconstruction problem, we summarize the definitions and results that are connected to the reconstruction of the characteristic functions of planar measurable sets and that will be used later in the two-valued reconstruction problem. The same notation will be used as in [5] and [3].

Let F be a measurable plane set having a finite two-dimensional Lebesgue measure. Its characteristic function is denoted by $f(x, y)$. The *horizontal* and *vertical projections* of F (or, equivalently, of f) are defined by

$$[\mathcal{P}_x F](y) = \int_{-\infty}^{\infty} f(x, y) dx \qquad (6.1)$$

and

$$[\mathcal{P}_y F](x) = \int_{-\infty}^{\infty} f(x, y) dy, \qquad (6.2)$$

respectively.

On the basis of the projections, such sets can be divided into two classes. The class of *unique sets* contains the measurable plane sets that are uniquely determined (up to a set of measure zero) by the two projections. Otherwise, the sets belong in the class of *nonunique sets*.

Accordingly, a function pair is *unique/nonunique* if the functions are equal to the projections of a unique/nonunique set almost everywhere (in brief: a.e.). Finally, a function pair is *inconsistent* if there is no measurable plane set that has projections equal to the function pair a.e.

Let $f_x(y)$ and $f_y(x)$ denote the projections of $f(x,y)$. The *second projections*, f_{xy} and f_{yx}, and the *third projections*, f_{xyx} and f_{yxy}, are defined as in Chapter 5 by Kaneko and Huang.

In 1949 G. G. Lorentz gave a characterization theorem of the projections [1] (for a new proof of this theorem see Chapter 5 by Kaneko and Huang in this book). Using the definitions of the second and third projections, we can reformulate the characterization result as follows.

Theorem 6.1.   *Let $f_x(y)$ and $f_y(x)$ be nonnegative integrable functions such that*

$$\int_{-\infty}^{\infty} f_x(\eta)d\eta = \int_{-\infty}^{\infty} f_y(\xi)d\xi. \tag{6.3}$$

(i) f_x and f_y are unique if and only if

$$\int_0^x f_{xy}(\xi)d\xi = \int_0^x f_{yxy}(\xi)d\xi \tag{6.4}$$

for all $x > 0$.

(ii) f_x and f_y are nonunique if and only if

$$\int_0^x f_{xy}(\xi)d\xi \geq \int_0^x f_{yxy}(\xi)d\xi \tag{6.5}$$

for all $x > 0$, and there is an $x > 0$ for which strict inequality holds.

(iii) f_x and f_y are inconsistent if and only if

$$\int_0^x f_{xy}(\xi)d\xi < \int_0^x f_{yxy}(\xi)d\xi \tag{6.6}$$

for some $x > 0$.

6.3   Two-valued functions

Now the definitions and notations necessary for the two-valued reconstruction problem will be introduced.

Let $g(x,y)$ be an integrable function on the rectangle $[0,a] \times [0,b]$, where a and b are positive real numbers. The *horizontal* and *vertical projection* of g are defined as

$$[\mathcal{P}_x g](y) = \int_0^a g(x,y)dx \tag{6.7}$$

and

$$[\mathcal{P}_y g](x) = \int\limits_0^b g(x,y)dy, \qquad (6.8)$$

respectively. Due to Fubini's theorem, the horizontal and vertical projections exist a.e. on the intervals $0 \le y \le b$ and $0 \le x \le a$, respectively, they are integrable and have the same integral on these intervals.

The two-valued reconstruction problem: Let g_x and g_y be integrable functions on $[0,b]$ and $[0,a]$, respectively, such that

$$\int\limits_0^b g_x(\eta)d\eta = \int\limits_0^a g_y(\xi)d\xi. \qquad (6.9)$$

Find a two-valued integrable function $g(x,y)$ on $[0,a] \times [0,b]$ such that

$$\mathcal{P}_x g = g_x \quad \text{and} \quad \mathcal{P}_y g = g_y \qquad (6.10)$$

a.e.

The reconstruction of characteristic functions can be considered as a special case of the two-valued reconstruction problem, where the two values of the functions can be only 0 and 1. Hereafter, let us call the first problem discussed in Section 6.2 as the *(0,1) reconstruction problem*.

As in the case of the (0,1) reconstruction problem, the two-valued functions can be divided into two classes. A two-valued function f_1 is *nonunique* if there is another two-valued function f_2 (i.e. f_1 and f_2 differ from each other on a set having positive measure) such that f_1 and f_2 have the same range and the same two projections. Otherwise, the two-valued function belongs to the class of *unique two-valued functions*.

A function pair is *unique/nonunique with respect to* (shortly: w.r.t.) *two given values* if the functions are equal to the projections of a unique/nonunique two-valued function a.e. having only the given two values. Finally, a function pair is *inconsistent w.r.t. two given values* if there is no function having the given two values and projections equal to the function pair a.e.

We are going to show that each two-valued reconstruction problem can be transformed into a (0,1) reconstruction problem. Let us find a two-valued function $g(x,y)$, as a solution, in the form of

$$g(x,y) = c \cdot f(x,y) + d, \qquad (6.11)$$

where f is a characteristic function of a measurable subset of $[0,a] \times [0,b]$, i.e., $f : [0,a] \times [0,b] \longrightarrow \{0,1\}$, c and d are real numbers.

If $c = 0$ then $g_x(y) = a \cdot d$ and $g_y(x) = b \cdot d$, which is a trivial case. If $c < 0$ then consider the reconstruction of $-g = (-c) \cdot f - d$ from the projections $-g_x$ and $-g_y$. It is clear that if $g = c \cdot f + d$ is a solution of the two-valued reconstruction problem with values d and $c + d$, then $-c \cdot (1 - f) + c + d$ is the same solution with values $c + d$ and d. That is, if we have a solution with a positive c then we can construct the same solution with negative c, and vice versa. Therefore, without loss of generality, it can be supposed that $c > 0$ hereafter.

We are going to define the second and third projections of g (see Fig. 6.1). At the same time we shall give the relations between the projections of f and g.

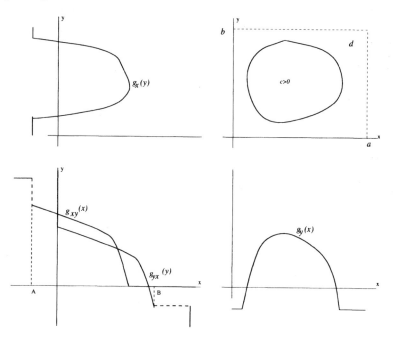

FIGURE 6.1. Projections of the two-valued function $g(x, y)$.

From (6.11) it follows that

$$g_y(x) = c \cdot f_y(x) + bd, \tag{6.12}$$

$$g_x(y) = c \cdot f_x(y) + ad, \tag{6.13}$$

and so

$$f_y(x) = \frac{g_y(x) - bd}{c}, \tag{6.14}$$

$$f_x(y) = \frac{g_x(y) - ad}{c} \tag{6.15}$$

a.e. on the intervals $[0, a]$ and $[0, b]$. Since f_x and f_y should be nonnegative functions, it is necessary that $g_y(x) \geq bd$ and $g_x(y) \geq ad$ on $[0, a]$ and $[0, b]$, respectively. Equivalently, the nonnegativity of the projections f_x and f_y means that d should be small enough, that is,

$$d \leq d_0, \tag{6.16}$$

where

$$d_0 = \min \left\{ \inf_{[0,b]} \left\{ \frac{g_x(y)}{a} \right\}, \inf_{[0,a]} \left\{ \frac{g_y(x)}{b} \right\} \right\}. \tag{6.17}$$

Now let us consider the second projections. They can be defined for f_{xy} and f_{yx} in a similar way:

$$g_{xy}(x) = \lambda_1(\{\eta \mid g_x(\eta) \geq x, \ \eta \in [0, b]\}) \tag{6.18}$$

and

$$g_{yx}(y) = \lambda_1(\{\xi \mid g_y(\xi) \geq y, \ \xi \in [0, a]\}). \tag{6.19}$$

We remark here that the nonnegative functions $g_{xy}(x)$ and $g_{yx}(y)$ are defined on every real value of x and y, respectively, not only for nonnegative values (see Fig. 6.1). Then

$$
\begin{aligned}
f_{yx}(y) &= \lambda_1(\{\xi \mid f_y(\xi) \geq y, \ \xi \in [0, a]\}) \\
&= \lambda_1\left(\left\{\xi \mid \frac{g_y(\xi) - bd}{c} \geq y, \ \xi \in [0, a]\right\}\right) \\
&= \lambda_1(\{\xi \mid g_y(\xi) \geq cy + bd, \ \xi \in [0, a]\}) \\
&= g_{yx}(cy + bd) \tag{6.20}
\end{aligned}
$$

for all $y \geq 0$. Similarly,

$$f_{xy}(x) = g_{xy}(cx + ad) \tag{6.21}$$

for all $x \geq 0$.

Finally, let us take the third projections. The straightforward definition of

$$g_{yxy}(x) = \lambda_1(\{\eta \mid g_{yx}(\eta) \geq x\}) \tag{6.22}$$

is not suitable, because g_{yx} is defined for all real number and so the measure of the set $\{\eta \mid g_{yx}(\eta) \geq x\}$ can be infinite for certain values of x. Instead of this definition, we define the third projection $g_{yxy}(x)$ by using the measure of the difference between the sets $\{\eta \mid g_{yx}(\eta) \geq x\}$ and $\{\eta \mid \eta < 0\}$. More exactly,

$$g_{yxy}(x) = \begin{cases} \lambda_1(\{\eta \mid g_{yx}(\eta) \geq x\} \setminus \{\eta \mid \eta < 0\}), \\ \qquad \text{if} \quad \{\eta \mid g_{yx}(\eta) \geq x\} \supseteq \{\eta \mid \eta < 0\}, \\ -\lambda_1(\{\eta \mid \eta < 0\} \setminus \{\eta \mid g_{yx}(\eta) \geq x\}), \\ \qquad \text{if} \quad \{\eta \mid g_{yx}(\eta) \geq x\} \subset \{\eta \mid \eta < 0\}. \end{cases} \tag{6.23}$$

Two remarks to this definition: Since g_{yx} is a monotone decreasing function there are only two possibilities: $\{\eta \mid g_{yx}(\eta) \geq x\} \supseteq \{\eta \mid \eta < 0\}$ and $\{\eta \mid g_{yx}(\eta) \geq x\} \subset \{\eta \mid \eta < 0\}$. Therefore, the definition is correct. Secondly, if g_y is a nonnegative function, then $\{\eta \mid g_{yx}(\eta) \geq x\} \supseteq \{\eta \mid \eta < 0\}$ for any $x \geq 0$. That is, the new definition would give the same function as the old one for nonnegative values of x.

An analogous definition is given for $g_{xyx}(y)$:

$$g_{xyx}(y) = \begin{cases} \lambda_1(\{\xi \mid g_{xy}(\xi) \geq y\} \setminus \{\xi \mid \xi < 0\}), \\ \qquad \text{if} \{\xi \mid g_{xy}(\xi) \geq y\} \supseteq \{\xi \mid \xi < 0\}, \\ -\lambda_1(\{\xi \mid \xi < 0\} \setminus \{\xi \mid g_{xy}(\xi) \geq y\}), \\ \qquad \text{if} \{\xi \mid g_{xy}(\xi) \geq y\} \subset \{\xi \mid \xi < 0\}. \end{cases} \tag{6.24}$$

We remark here that the nonnegative functions $g_{yxy}(x)$ and $g_{xyx}(y)$ are defined on every nonnegative value of x and y, respectively (see Fig. 6.1). Let $0 \leq x \leq a$, then

$$\begin{aligned} f_{yxy}(x) &= \lambda_1(\{\eta \mid f_{yx}(\eta) \geq x\}) \\ &= \lambda_1(\{\eta \mid g_{yx}(c\eta + bd) \geq x\} \setminus \{\eta \mid \eta < 0\}) \\ &= \begin{cases} \lambda_1(\{\eta \mid g_{yx}(c\eta) \geq x\} \setminus \{\eta \mid \eta < 0\}) - bd, \\ \qquad \text{if} \{\eta \mid g_{yx}(c\eta) \geq x\} \supseteq \{\eta \mid \eta < 0\}, \\ -\lambda_1(\{\eta \mid \eta < 0\} \setminus \{\eta \mid g_{yx}(c\eta) \geq x\}) - bd, \\ \qquad \text{if} \{\eta \mid g_{yx}(c\eta) \geq x\} \subset \{\eta \mid \eta < 0\} \end{cases} \\ &= \frac{1}{c} \cdot g_{yxy}(x) - bd. \end{aligned} \tag{6.25}$$

Similarly,

$$f_{xyx}(y) = \frac{1}{c} \cdot g_{xyx}(y) - ad \tag{6.26}$$

for all $0 \leq y \leq b$.

6.4 Reconstruction of two-valued functions

Our idea is to construct a function $g(x, y) = c \cdot f(x, y) + d$ as a solution of the two-valued reconstruction problem where c, d are real numbers and

f is a characteristic function of a measurable subset of $[0, a] \times [0, b]$. We know from Theorem 6.1 that for given f_x and f_y there is such an $f(x, y)$ on $[0, a] \times [0, b]$, if and only if

$$\int_0^x f_{xy}(\xi)d\xi \geq \int_0^x f_{yxy}(\xi)d\xi \qquad (6.27)$$

for all $x > 0$. From (6.21) and (6.25) it follows that this condition is equivalent to

$$\int_0^x g_{xy}(c\xi + ad)d\xi \geq \int_0^x (\frac{1}{c}g_{yxy}(\xi) - bd)d\xi. \qquad (6.28)$$

After some elementary transformations we get

$$\int_{ad}^{cx+ad} g_{xy}(\xi)d\xi \geq \int_0^x g_{yxy}(\xi)d\xi - bcdx. \qquad (6.29)$$

In order to have shorter expressions, let us introduce the following notations

$$G_{xy}(x) = \int_0^x g_{xy}(\xi)d\xi \qquad (6.30)$$

and

$$G_{yxy}(x) = \int_0^x g_{yxy}(\xi)d\xi. \qquad (6.31)$$

Now we can state the theorem giving the necessary and sufficient conditions of uniqueness, existence, and inconsistency in the case of the two-valued reconstruction problem.

Theorem 6.2.   Let $g_x(y)$ and $g_y(x)$ be integrable functions on intervals $[0, b]$ and $[0, a]$, respectively, such that they have the same finite integrals. Furthermore, let $c > 0$ and d be real numbers.

(i) g_x and g_y are unique w.r.t. d and $c + d$, if and only if

$$G_{xy}(cx + ad) - G_{xy}(ad) = G_{yxy}(x) - bcdx \qquad (6.32)$$

for all $0 \leq x \leq a$.

(ii) g_x and g_y are nonunique w.r.t. d and $c + d$, if and only if

$$G_{xy}(cx + ad) - G_{xy}(ad) \geq G_{yxy}(x) - bcdx \qquad (6.33)$$

for all $0 \leq x \leq a$, and there is an $x > 0$ for which strict inequality holds.

(iii) g_x and g_y are inconsistent w.r.t. d and $c + d$, if and only if

$$G_{xy}(cx + ad) - G_{xy}(ad) \leq G_{yxy}(x) - bcdx \qquad (6.34)$$

for some $0 \leq x \leq a$.

Theorem 6.2 gives answer to the two-valued reconstruction problem if the range of the function to be reconstructed, i.e., $\{d, c + d\}$, is known. What can we say if c and d are unknown?

Theorem 6.3.   *Let $g_x(y)$ and $g_y(x)$ be integrable functions on intervals $[0, b]$ and $[0, a]$, respectively, such that they have the same finite integrals. For any $d \leq d_0$ there is a real number c_0 such that if $c \geq c_0$ then there is a solution having projections $g_x(y)$, $g_y(x)$ and having the range of $\{d, c + d\}$.*

Proof: Let d be a real number such that $d \leq d_0$ where d_0 is given by (6.17). Then consider the functions

$$\bar{g}_x(y) = g_x(y) - ad \qquad \text{and} \qquad \bar{g}_y(x) = g_y(x) - bd. \qquad (6.35)$$

Clearly, there is a two-valued function $g = c \cdot f + d$ on $[0, a] \times [0, b]$ with projections g_x and g_y and with values d and $c + d$ if and only if there is a two-valued function $\bar{g} = c \cdot f$ with projections $\bar{g}_x$ and $\bar{g}_y$ and with values 0 and c. Now we can apply Theorem 6.2 for the functions $\bar{g}_x$ and $\bar{g}_y$ in the special case of $d = 0$. Accordingly, there is such a two-valued function $\bar{g}$ if and only if

$$\bar{G}_{xy}(cx) \geq \bar{G}_{yxy}(x) \qquad (6.36)$$

for all $0 \leq x \leq a$. Since $\bar{g}_{xy}$ and $\bar{g}_{yxy}$ are nonnegative functions, their integral-functions $\bar{G}_{xy}$ and $\bar{G}_{yxy}$ are monotone nonincreasing functions, having inverses $\bar{G}_{xy}^{-1}$ and $\bar{G}_{yxy}^{-1}$, respectively. Then (6.36) is equivalent to

$$\frac{1}{c} \cdot \bar{G}_{xy}^{-1}(y) \leq \bar{G}_{yxy}^{-1}(y). \qquad (6.37)$$

Therefore, the existence of the function g (or equivalently $\bar{g}$) is equivalent to $c \geq c_0$, where

$$c_0 = \max_{y > 0} \{ \frac{\bar{G}_{xy}^{-1}(y)}{\bar{G}_{yxy}^{-1}(y)} \}. \qquad (6.38)$$

Therefore, Theorem 6.3 is proved.   □

As a consequence of Theorem 6.3 consider now how we can reconstruct a two-valued function from two projections. Let $g_x(y)$ and $g_y(x)$ be integrable functions on intervals $[0, b]$ and $[0, a]$, respectively, such that they have the same finite integral. Suppose that the function to be reconstructed has the form $g(x, y) = c \cdot f(x, y) + d$.

Algorithm 6.1.   *For reconstructing a two-valued function $g(x, y)$ from $g_x(y)$ and $g_y(x)$:*
Step 1. Select an arbitrary (small) real number d such that $d \leq d_0$ where d_0 is given by (6.17).

Step 2. Subtract the values ad and bd from the function-pair g_x and g_y, respectively, getting a new function-pair $\bar{g}_x(y) = g_x(y) - ad$ and $\bar{g}_y(x) = g_y(x) - bd$.

Step 3. Select an arbitrary (big) real number c such that $c \geq c_0$ where c_0 is given by (6.38).

Step 4. Divide the function-pair $\bar{g}_x$ and $\bar{g}_y$ by c. In this way we have a newer function-pair $f_x(y) = \bar{g}_x(y)/c$ and $f_y(x) = \bar{g}_y(x)/c$ being the projections of a $(0,1)$-value function $f(x,y)$ according to Theorem 6.3.

Step 5. Reconstruct a $(0,1)$-value function f from the projections f_x and f_y.

Step 6. Construct $g(x,y) = c \cdot f(x,y) + d$.

Remark 6.1.   *The reconstruction algorithm has an interesting special case when we select $c = c_0$. In this case it is possible that for some $\xi \in (0,a)$*

$$\bar{G}_{xy}(c\xi) = \bar{G}_{yxy}(\xi), \tag{6.39}$$

which means that there are sub-rectangles in $[0,a] \times [0,b]$ where all of the solutions $\bar{g}$ have the same values (so-called invariant rectangles, cf. [4]).

Let us see now the question of *uniqueness*. From Theorem 6.2 we know that a function pair $g_x(y)$ and $g_y(x)$ on intervals $[0,b]$ and $[0,a]$, respectively, is unique w.r.t. two unknown values c and d if and only if

$$G_{xy}(cx + ad) - G_{xy}(ad) = G_{yxy}(x) - bcdx \tag{6.40}$$

for all $0 \leq x \leq a$. Taking the derivatives of both sides of the equation, we get that this condition is equivalent to

$$c \cdot g_{xy}(cx + ad) = g_{yxy}(x) - bcd \tag{6.41}$$

for all $0 \leq x \leq a$. That is, in the case of uniqueness the functions g_{xy} and g_{yxy} can be transformed into each other by suitable translations and scaling. If the values c and d are not known then we can compute them from the positions of certain points of the functions g_{xy} and g_{yxy}.

For example, we can find the points where the nonincreasing functions g_{xy} and g_{yxy} starts to decrease and where they starts to be constant. More exactly, we are going to determine two points A and B in the domain of g_{xy} and the corresponding two points A' and B' in the domain of g_{yxy}. Let point A be where g_{xy} starts to decrease ($g_{xy}(x) = b$ on $(-\infty, A]$). There are two cases to find the corresponding point A' depending on the measure of the set $\{x \mid g_y(x) = bd\} = \{x \mid f_y(x) = b\}$:

(i) If $\lambda_1(\{x \mid g_y(x) = bd\}) = 0$ then let A' be the point where g_{yxy} starts, i.e., $A' = 0$.

(ii) If $\lambda_1(\{x \mid g_y(x) = bd\}) > 0$ then let A' be the point where g_{yxy} starts to decrease (in this case $A' > 0$).

Analogously, let point B be where g_{xy} starts to be constant ($g_{xy}(x) = 0$ on $(B, \infty]$). There are two cases to find the corresponding point B' depending on the measure of the set $\{y \mid g_x(y) = ad\} = \{y \mid f_x(y) = a\}$:

(i) If $\lambda_1(\{y \mid g_x(y) = ad\}) = 0$ then let B' be the point where g_{yxy} starts to be constant on $(B', a]$, or, if there is no such interval then let $B' = a$.

(ii) If $\lambda_1(\{x \mid g_x(y) = ad\}) > 0$ then let $B' = a$.

Since we do not know in advance which case we have, we have to test the equality (6.41) for both possible values of A' and B'.

Then according to equation (6.41) points A and B can be transformed onto the points A' and B' by the transformation $cx + ad \longrightarrow x'$, that is,

$$cA + ad = A', \tag{6.42}$$

$$cB + ad = B'. \tag{6.43}$$

From this equation system we get

$$c = \frac{A' - B'}{A - B} \tag{6.44}$$

and

$$d = \frac{AB' - A'B}{A - B}. \tag{6.45}$$

Therefore, from the function pair $g_x(y)$ and $g_y(x)$ it is possible to decide whether there are two values c and d such that $g_x(y)$ and $g_y(x)$ are unique w.r.t. these values. If there are such values then they can be determined by (6.44) and (6.45).

6.5   Two-valued matrices

A discrete version of the two-value reconstruction problem is the reconstruction of *two-valued matrices*. Generally, the *reconstruction problem* of a matrix from its row and column sums can be defined for different classes. For example, in the case of (0,1)-matrices (or binary matrices), there are classical results due to D. Gale [6] and H. J. Ryser [7] giving necessary and sufficient conditions on the existence and uniqueness of (0,1)-matrices. A summary of this combinatorial problem is given by R. A. Brualdi [8]. In 1968 L. Mirsky [9] studied the reconstruction of integral matrices. Generally, the problem of reconstruction of matrices can also be reformulated as solving special linear equation systems. In this context the problem has been studied for several classes of matrices [10] and a reconstruction method based on linear programming has been suggested [11]. Some possible examples of the application of the reconstruction of two-valued matrices can be found in [12] and [13]. In this and the following two sections of the current chapter we discuss the problem of reconstruction of two-valued matrices based on the material in [14].

Let m and n be fixed positive integers. Let $G = (g(i,j))$ denote a real $m \times n$ matrix, i.e., the indices $i \in M$ and $j \in N$, where

$$M = \{1, 2, \dots, m\} \quad \text{and} \quad N = \{1, 2, \dots, n\}. \tag{6.46}$$

We say that the matrix G is *two-valued* if there exist real numbers d and e such that

$$g(i,j) \in \{d, e\} \quad \text{for all} \quad i \in M; \quad j \in N. \tag{6.47}$$

One may assume that $d < e$. Let further $c = e - d$ thus $c > 0$.

The *horizontal* and *vertical projections* are determined by the row sums $g_x(i)$ and column sums $g_y(j)$ of the matrix G. Thus,

$$g_x(i) = \sum_{j=1}^{n} g(i,j); \qquad g_y(j) = \sum_{i=1}^{m} g(i,j). \tag{6.48}$$

It follows that

$$\sum_{i=1}^{m} g_x(i) = \sum_{j=1}^{n} g_y(j) = L \quad \text{(say).} \tag{6.49}$$

In the sequel, we assume that the given vectors g_x, g_y satisfies (6.49).

Let $\mathcal{G}_o = \mathcal{G}_o(g_x, g_y)$ denote the class of matrices having projections g_x and g_y. For example, the matrix $G = (g(i,j)) = (g_x(i) \cdot g_y(j)/L)$ is an element of the class $\mathcal{G}_o(g_x, g_y)$.

The two-valued reconstruction problem for matrices. Given two vectors g_x and g_y, find a two-valued matrix $G \in \mathcal{G}_o(g_x, g_y)$. Specifically, we like to find all pairs $\{d, e\}$ such that (6.47) holds for some $G \in \mathcal{G}_o$.

Definition 6.1. *The pair (c, d) will be said to be admissible w.r.t. the projections g_x and g_y if $\mathcal{G}_o(g_x, g_y)$ contains at least one matrix $G = (g(i,j))$ satisfying (6.47). The set of all such admissible pairs (c, d) is denoted as $W_o = W_o(g_x, g_y)$.*

Consider now the connection between two-valued and binary matrices. To each two-valued matrix we are going to give a binary matrix in the following way. Let $G = (g(i,j))$ be an $m \times n$ two-valued matrix having values d and $e \ (= c + d)$. Then, let

$$f(i,j) = \frac{g(i,j) - d}{c} \qquad \text{for all } i \in M; \ j \in N. \qquad (6.50)$$

Clearly, $f(i,j) \in \{0,1\}$ and its row and column sums, r_i and s_j, respectively, are

$$r_i = \frac{g_x(i) - nd}{c} \qquad \text{and} \qquad s_j = \frac{g_y(j) - md}{c} \qquad (6.51)$$

for all $i \in M$ and $j \in N$. Furthermore,

$$r_i \in N_o \quad \text{and} \quad s_j \in M_o \qquad (6.52)$$

where

$$N_o = \{0, 1, \ldots, n\} \quad \text{and} \quad M_o = \{0, 1, \ldots, m\}. \qquad (6.53)$$

Note that r_i and s_j, respectively, is also equal to the number of elements e in row i of G, and column j of G, respectively. By the way, in view of (6.49) and (6.51), one always has

$$r_1 + \cdots + r_m = s_1 + \cdots + s_n. \qquad (6.54)$$

Definition 6.2.   *The pair (c,d) will be said to be weakly admissible w.r.t. the projections g_x and g_y if (6.52) holds for the numbers r_i (i $\in$ M) and s_j (j $\in$ N) defined by (6.51). The set of all such weakly admissible pairs (c,d) will be denoted as $W = W(g_x, g_y)$.*

It follows from the above remarks that $W_o(g_x, g_y) \subset W(g_x, g_y)$.

From now on, we will assume (without loss of generality) that the given vectors g_x and g_y satisfies

$$g_x(1) \geq g_x(2) \geq \cdots \geq g_x(m) \quad \text{and} \quad g_y(1) \geq g_y(2) \geq \cdots \geq g_y(n). \qquad (6.55)$$

Thus, the r_i and s_j defined by (6.51) will always satisfy

$$r_1 \geq r_2 \geq \cdots \geq r_m \quad \text{and} \quad s_1 \geq s_2 \geq \cdots \geq s_n. \qquad (6.56)$$

Now, we can apply the following existence and uniqueness results due to Gale [6] and Ryser [7].

Lemma 6.1.   *Let r_i (i $\in$ M) and s_j (j $\in$ N) be given integers satisfying $0 \leq r_i \leq n$; $0 \leq s_j \leq m$ and (6.56). Then in order that there exists an $\{0,1\}$-valued $m \times n$ matrix $F = (f(i,j))$ with row sums r_i and column sums s_j, it is necessary and sufficient that*

$$r_1 + r_2 + \cdots + r_t \leq \bar{s}_1 + \bar{s}_2 + \cdots + \bar{s}_t \quad \text{for all} \quad t \in M. \qquad (6.57)$$

Here, $\bar{s}_t$ denotes the number of indices $j = 1, \ldots, n$ with $s_j \geq t$. Moreover, the above $\{0, 1\}$-valued matrix F is unique if and only if

$$\bar{s}_t = r_t \quad \text{for all} \quad t \in M. \tag{6.58}$$

Remark 6.2.   *Lemma 6.1 can be considered as the discrete version of Theorem 6.1, where the vectors r_i, s_j and $\bar{s}_j$ correspond to the functions f_{xy}, f_{yx} and f_{yxy}, respectively.*

Theorem 6.4.   *Let g_x and g_y be given, as in (6.49), and consider a fixed pair (c, d) with $c > 0$. Then the following are equivalent.*

  (i) There exists an $m \times n$ matrix $G = (g(i, j))$ satisfying (6.47) and (6.48).

  (ii) The pair (c, d) is admissible.

  (iii) The pair (c, d) is weakly admissible and the integers r_i and s_j defined by (6.51) satisfy the inequalities (6.57).

Proof: This follows from Lemma 6.1.   □

Corollary 6.1.   *Suppose g_x and g_y are such that $g_y(j)$ is independent of j. Then in order that (c, d) be admissible, it is necessary and sufficient that*

$$r_i = \frac{g_x(i) - nd}{c} \in N_o \quad \text{for all} \quad i \in M, \tag{6.59}$$

in such a way that $r_1 + \cdots + r_m = 0 \pmod{n}$.

Proof: The stated condition is equivalent to the pair (c, d) being weakly admissible. For this weak admissibility requires (6.59) and, moreover, that $s := (g_y(j) - md)/c$ (which is independent of j) be an integer with $0 \leq s \leq m$. And in the presence of (6.59), the latter condition is equivalent to $r_1 + \cdots + r_m = 0 \pmod{n}$, as follows from $ns = \sum_j s_j = \sum_i r_i$.

In view of Theorem 6.4, it thus suffices to show that the condition (6.57) is automatically satisfied in the situation on hand, where in particular $s_j = s$ is independent of j with $s \in \{0, 1, \ldots, m\}$. For, note that $\bar{s}_t = n$ for $1 \leq t \leq s$, while $\bar{s}_t = 0$ for $t > s$. Thus, the right-hand side of (6.57) equals $sn = \sum_i r_i$ when $t \geq s$ and it equals $tn \geq r_1 + \cdots + r_t$ when $1 \leq t \leq s$.   □

Remark 6.3.   *Still assuming that $g_y(j)$ is constant, an easy analysis shows that, for a given pair (c, d), the associated $\{d, e\}$-valued matrix $G = (g(i, j))$ exists uniquely if and only if, for some integer $0 \leq s \leq m$, one has that $g_x(i) = ne$ if $i \leq s$ and $g_x(i) = nd$ if $i > s$. Accordingly, $g(i, j) = e$ if $1 \leq i \leq s$ and $g(i, j) = d$ if $s < i \leq m$. Provided this first projection is nonconstant, that is, $g_x(1) > g_x(m)$, $g_x(i)$ is thus constant except for a single downward jump at $i = s < m$. Specifically, $g_x(i)/n$ equals e for $i \leq s$, and equals d for $i > s$,* *showing that the pair $\{d, e\}$ is fully determined by the projections. In particular, if the vertical projection is constant but not the first then there is at most one uniqueness pair (c, d).*

Let g_x and g_y be given as in (6.49). Let us first handle the case that both projections $g_x(i)$ and $g_y(j)$ are constant. Equivalently, by (6.49), letting $u = L/mn$,

$$g_x(i) = nu \quad \text{for all} \quad i \in M; \qquad g_y(j) = mu \quad \text{for all} \quad j \in M. \qquad (6.60)$$

Theorem 6.5.   *Assume that g_x and g_y are of the special form (6.60). Then in order that $(c, d) \in W_o(g_x, g_y)$ it is sufficient that either $d = u$ (while $c > 0$ is arbitrary) or else $e = c + d = u$. All the (infinitely many) admissible pairs of this special type lead to one and the same matrix G, namely, $G = (g(i, j) = u)$; all (i, j).*

Moreover, there are no other admissible pairs if and only if m and n are relatively prime. Hence, in that case, the latter constant matrix is the only two-valued matrix G having constant projections as in (6.60).

Suppose that instead $(m, n) = k \geq 2$. Thus $m = pk$ and $n = qk$ with p and q as positive integers with $(p, q) = 1$. Then $W_o(g_x, g_y)$ consists of all pairs (c, d) with

$$c > 0, \quad d = u - hc/k, \quad \text{thus} \quad e = u + (k - h)c/k, \qquad (6.61)$$

where $h \in \{0, 1, \ldots, k\}$. Any corresponding matrix G with projections (6.60) and $g(i, j) \in \{d, e\}$ would have precisely $r = hq$ elements e in each row (of length $n = kq$) and further $s = hp$ elements e in each column (of length $m = kp$).

Proof: The first assertion follows immediately from the observation that $\mathcal{G}_o$ contains the 1-valued $m \times n$ matrix $G = (g(i, j) = u,$ all $i, j)$. Next consider an arbitrary matrix $G = (g(i, j))$ with constant projections as in (6.60) and such that $g(i, j) \in \{d, e\}$ for all i, j. In view of (6.51), each row of G contains r elements e and each column of G contains s elements e, with r and s as integers such that

$$r = n(u - d)/c; \quad s = m(u - d)/c \quad \text{and} \quad 0 \leq r \leq n; \ 0 \leq s \leq m. \qquad (6.62)$$

Thus, $mr = ns$ thus $pr = qs$. But $(p, q) = 1$, hence, $r = hq$; $s = hp$ with $h \in \{0, 1, \ldots, k\}$. If $h = 0$ then $r = s = 0$ thus $g(i, j) = d$ for all i, j necessarily with $d = u$. Similarly, if $h = k$ then $r = kq = n$ and $s = kp = m$ thus $g(i, j) = e$ for all i, j, necessarily with $e = u$. Thus both of these cases merely yield the constant matrix $G = (g(i, j) = u)$.

Let us finally turn to the remaining case $1 \leq h \leq k - 1$. It requires that $k = (m, n) \geq 2$. It follows from (6.62) that presently d and e are of the form

(6.61), where $c > 0$ is arbitrary. Note that $d < u < e$. In order to show that this pair (c, d) is indeed admissible, we must show that matrices G as described in the last part of Theorem 6.5 do exist. One way is to select any subset A of $\{0, 1, \ldots, k-1\}$ of size $|A| = h$ and to define $g(i, j) = e$ if $i + j \in A \pmod{k}$ and $g(i, j) = d$, otherwise. $\square$

From now on, we assume that at least one of the projections $g_x(i)$ and $g_y(j)$ is nonconstant. We claim that then there are only finitely many admissible pairs (c, d). More precisely, not only $W_o(g_x, g_y)$ is finite but also the (larger) set $W(g_x, g_y)$ consisting of all weakly admissible pairs (c, d).

By definition, see (6.52) and (6.51), a pair (c, d) (with $c > 0$) is weakly admissible if and only if there exist integers

$$r_i \in N_0 \quad (i \in M); \qquad s_j \in M_0 \quad (j \in N), \qquad (6.63)$$

such that

$$\begin{aligned} cr_i + nd &= g_x(i) \quad \text{(for all } i \in M); \\ cs_j + md &= g_y(j) \quad \text{(for all } j \in N). \end{aligned} \qquad (6.64)$$

Thus, if $1 \leq h < i \leq m$ then $r_h = r_i$ if and only if $g_x(h) = g_x(i)$. And if $1 \leq j < k \leq n$ then $s_j = s_k$ if and only if $g_y(j) = g_y(k)$. Similarly, $mr_i - ns_j$ has exactly the same sign as $mg_x(i) - ng_y(j)$, (for each $i \in M$; $j \in N$).

Suppose the vertical projection is nonconstant. Thus, there exist indices $1 \leq j < k \leq n$ with $g_y(j) \neq g_y(k)$, thus $g_y(j) > g_y(k)$, thus $s_j > s_k$. But then

$$cs_j + md = g_y(j); \qquad cs_k + md = g_y(k) \qquad (6.65)$$

together imply that

$$c = \frac{g_y(j) - g_y(k)}{s_j - s_k} > 0; \qquad d = \frac{g_y(k)s_j - g_y(j)s_k}{m(s_j - s_k)}. \qquad (6.66)$$

Here, s_j and s_k are integers with $0 \leq s_k < s_j \leq m$ thus the denominator $q = s_j - s_k$ satisfies $q \in M_0$. Consequently, c itself can gave at most m different values. Moreover, there can be no more than $\binom{m+1}{2}$ different admissible pairs (c, d). This bound is sharp, see Example 6.1 later. As to condition (6.66), it would be sufficient to consider only the case where both $k = j + 1$ and $g_y(j) > g_y(j + 1)$. If so then both right-hand sides in (6.66) are automatically independent of j and k.

Similarly, for each pair h, i with $1 \leq h < i \leq m$ and $g_x(h) \neq g_x(i)$,

$$c = \frac{g_x(h) - g_x(i)}{r_h - r_i} > 0; \qquad d = \frac{g_x(i)r_h - g_x(h)r_i}{n(r_h - r_i)}. \qquad (6.67)$$

Here, $0 \le r_i < r_h \le n$. Thus c can have at most n different values and, moreover, there are at most $\binom{n+1}{2}$ admissible pairs (c, d). Similarly,

$$c = \frac{mg_x(i) - ng_y(j)}{mr_i - ns_j}; \qquad d = \frac{-g_x(i)s_j + g_y(j)r_i}{mr_i - ns_j}, \qquad (6.68)$$

each time that $i \in M$ and $j \in N$ are such that $mg_x(i) \neq ng_y(j)$, thus $mr_i \neq ns_j$.

A geometrical picture of $W = W(g_x, g_y)$ arises when one interprets (6.64) as a collection of straight half lines in the (c, d)-plane. Let $K(\alpha, \beta)$ denote the half line defined by

$$K(\alpha, \beta) = \{(c, d) : c > 0; \; d = \alpha - \beta c\}. \qquad (6.69)$$

It has intercept α and slope $-\beta$. From (6.63), (6.64), the pair (c, d) is weakly admissible if and only if:

(i) For each $i \in M$, (c, d) belongs to the (fan shaped) union $U(i)$ of half lines $K(g_x(i)/n, r/n)$ with $r = r_i$ running through $\{0, 1, \ldots, n\}$.

(ii) For each $j \in N$, (c, d) belongs to the union $V(j)$ of the half lines $K(g_y(j)/m, s/m)$ with $s = s_j$ running through $\{0, 1, \ldots, m\}$.

Correspondingly, $W = W(g_x, g_y)$ could also be defined as the intersection

$$W = U(1) \cap U(2) \cap \cdots \cap U(m) \cap V(1) \cap V(2) \cap \cdots \cap V(m). \qquad (6.70)$$

From the above analysis, any two among the $m + n$ fans $U(i)$ and $V(j)$ $(i \in M; j \in N)$ have a finite (but nonempty) intersection if and only if those fans have different intercepts.

By the way, in the excluded case that both projections $g_x(i)$ and $g_y(j)$ are constant, one has $g_x(i)/n = g_y(j)/n = u$, for all $i \in M; j \in N$, that is, all intercepts above are equal. Hence, in this case W is equal to the union of all half lines $K(u, z)$ with $z \in Z$, where $Z = \{0, 1/n, 2/n, \ldots, n/n\} \cap \{0, 1/m, 2/m, \ldots, m/m\}$. If $(m, n) = 1$ then simply $Z = \{0, 1\}$. In general, $Z = \{0, 1/k, 2/k, \ldots, k/k\}$ where $k = (m, n)$. Thus W has exactly the same form (6.61) as W_o.

That is, in the case of constant projections, all weakly admissible pairs (c, d) are even admissible. In fact, this same property already holds when just one of the projections is constant, see Corollary 6.1 (and its proof).

6.6   Reconstruction of two-valued matrices

For the construction of all two-valued $m \times n$ matrices $G = (g(i, j))$ having given projections $g_x(i)$ $(i \in M)$ and $g_y(j)$ $(j \in N)$, the following algorithm can be applied. The input to this algorithm are any vectors g_x and g_y as in (6.49) that satisfies both (6.48) and (6.55).

Algorithm 6.2.   *For reconstructing a two-valued matrix G.*

1. *Determine the set W of all weakly admissible pairs (c,d), either using (6.70) or else using (6.63), (6.64). The two values on hand are d and $e = c + d$.*

2. *For each $(c,d) \in W$ do steps 3, 4, 5 and 6.*

3. *Compute the numbers $r_i(c,d)$ and $s_j(c,d)$ from (6.51). These numbers satisfy (6.52) precisely because $(c,d) \in W$.*

4. *Check condition (6.57). Here, $\bar{s}_t$ denotes the number of $j \in N$ with $s_j \geq t$. If it fails to hold then (c,d) is inadmissible. That is, there does not exist any $\{d, e = c + d\}$-valued matrix G having projections $g_x(i)$ and $g_y(j)$. Therefore, continue by considering the next pair $(c,d) \in W$.*

5. *Since (6.57) holds, we know that (c,d) is indeed admissible. Equivalently, there exists at least one $\{0,1\}$-valued $m \times n$ matrix $F = (f(i,j))$ having row sums r_i $(i \in M)$ and column sums s_j $(j \in N)$. If desired, determine all such F. An easy construction of one such F is given by Ryser's [7] method.*

6. *For each F obtained in Step 5, output the $m \times n$ matrix $G = (g(i,j))$ with $g(i,j) = d$ or $e = c + d$, respectively, depending on whether $f(i,j) = 0$ or 1, respectively.*

Let the given vectors g_x and g_y be as in (6.49) and (6.55), and suppose we did located a single pair $(c_o, d_o) \in W(g_x, g_y)$, $(c_o > 0)$. That is, the numbers

$$g_x^o(i) = \tfrac{g_x(i) - nd_o}{c_o} \quad (i \in M);$$
$$g_y^o(j) = \tfrac{g_y(j) - md_o}{c_o} \quad (j \in N) \tag{6.71}$$

satisfy $g_x^o(i) \in N_0$ and $g_y^o(j) \in M_0$. Equivalently, $(1,0) \in W(g_x^o, g_y^o)$ where g_x^o and g_y^o (a linear transform of g_x and g_y) are defined by

$$g_y^o = (g_x^o(1), g_x^o(2), \ldots, g_x^o(m)); \quad g_y^o = (g_y^o(1), g_y^o(2), \ldots, g_y^o(n)). \tag{6.72}$$

One easily verifies the equivalence

$$(c,d) \in W(g_x^o, g_y^o) \quad \text{if and only if} \quad (c_o c, c_o d + d_o) \in W(g_x, g_y), \tag{6.73}$$

and also the analogous equivalence for the pair $W_o(g_x^o, g_y^o)$, $W_o(g_x, g_y)$. This shows that it is no great loss of generality to assume that $(1,0) \in W(g_x, g_y)$.

From now on, in this section, we will assume that indeed $(1,0) \in W(g_x, g_y)$. Equivalently,

$$g_x(i) \in N_0 \quad (i \in M); \qquad g_y(j) \in M_0 \quad (j \in N). \tag{6.74}$$

One wants to find all $(c,d) \in W(g_x, g_y)$. From (6.66) and (6.67), the components c and d will always be rational numbers.

Lemma 6.2. *Suppose that (6.74) holds and let $(c,d) \in W(g_x, g_y)$.*

(i) If $g_x(i) - g_x(i+1) = t > 0$ then $c = t/h$ for some $h \in N$.

(ii) If $g_y(j) - g_y(j+1) = t > 0$ then $c = t/h$ for some $h \in M$.

(iii) Moreover,

$$c \geq \frac{g_x(1) - g_x(m)}{n}; \qquad c \geq \frac{g_y(1) - g_y(n)}{m}. \tag{6.75}$$

Proof: Immediate from (6.66) and (6.67).   □

In the following illustrations, we restrict ourselves to the special case

$$m = n; \qquad g_x(j) = g_y(j) \quad \text{for all } j \in N. \tag{6.76}$$

This naturally forces that $r_j = s_j$, see (6.51). While g_x and g_y are now determined by the vector $g_y^* = (g_y(1), \ldots, g_y(n))$. Here, the $g_y(j)$ are given *integers* such that

$$0 \leq g_y(n) \leq \cdots \leq g_y(2) \leq g_y(1) \leq n \qquad \text{and} \qquad g_y(1) - g_y(n) > 0. \tag{6.77}$$

From (6.63) and (6.64), $(c,d) \in W(g_x, g_y)$ if and only if

$$s_j = s_j(c,d) := \frac{g_y(j) - nd}{c} \in N_0 \qquad \text{for all } j \in N. \tag{6.78}$$

Thus, $s_j > s_k$ if and only if $g_y(j) > g_y(k)$. We also write $s^* = (s_1, s_2, \ldots, s_n)$ and $\bar{s}^* = (\bar{s}_1, \ldots, \bar{s}_n)$. Here, $\bar{s}_t$ denotes the number of indices $j = 1, \ldots, n$ with $s_j \geq t$. From Theorem 6.4, if $(c,d) \in W_0(g_x, g_y)$, then $(c,d) \in W_0(g_x, g_y)$ if and only if

$$s_1 + s_2 + \cdots + s_t \leq \bar{s}_1 + \bar{s}_2 + \cdots + \bar{s}_t \quad \text{for } t = 1, \ldots, n. \tag{6.79}$$

Example 6.1.   Suppose that

$$g_y(j) = w + 1 \quad \text{for} \quad 1 \leq j \leq k; \qquad g_y(j) = w \quad \text{for} \quad k < j \leq n, \tag{6.80}$$

where $1 \leq k < n$ and w are given integers. From Lemma 6.2, if $(c, d) \in W(g_x, g_y)$ then $c = 1/h$ for some $h \in N$. From (6.78) and (6.80), the s_j on hand must be such that

$$s_j = p \quad \text{if} \quad 1 \leq j \leq k; \qquad s_j = q \quad \text{if} \quad k < j \leq n, \qquad (6.81)$$

with p and q as integers such that $0 \leq q < p \leq n$. There are precisely $\binom{n+1}{2}$ such pairs (p, q). In fact, $(c, d) \in W(g_x, g_y)$ if and only if the pair of equations

$$w + 1 - nd = pc; \qquad w - nd = qc, \qquad (6.82)$$

hold for some choice of the integers $0 \leq q < p \leq n$. In which case

$$c = \frac{1}{p - q}; \qquad d = \frac{pw - q(w + 1)}{n(p - q)}. \qquad (6.83)$$

We conclude that $W(g_x, g_y)$ consists of precisely $\binom{n+1}{2}$ pairs (c, d), namely, one for each choice of the pair (p, q) with $0 \leq q < p \leq n$.

We next want to determine which of these pairs $(c, d) \in W(g_x, g_y)$ even belong to $W_o(g_x, g_y)$. We thus must check condition (6.79). Here, in view of (6.81),

$$\begin{aligned} \bar{s}_t &= n \quad \text{if} \quad 1 \leq t \leq q; \\ \bar{s}_t &= k \quad \text{if} \quad q < t \leq p; \\ \bar{s}_t &= 0 \quad \text{if} \quad p < t \leq n. \end{aligned} \qquad (6.84)$$

As a check, one has $\sum \bar{s}_t = \sum s_j$ since $qn + (p - q)k = kp + (n - k)q$. In verifying condition (6.79), it is important to pay attention to the slope of the function

$$z(t) = (\bar{s}_1 + \bar{s}_2 + \cdots + \bar{s}_t) - (s_1 + s_2 + \cdots + s_t), \qquad (6.85)$$

$(t = 0, 1, \ldots, n; z(0) = z(n) = 0)$. Usually, $z(t)$ is unimodal (first up and then down) in which case it its obvious that $z(t) \geq 0$ for all t. The only exception is the case $q < k < p$. Then $z(t)$ has an up-down-up-down behavior with a local minimum at $t = k$. Hence, in this case $(c, d) \in W_o(g_x, g_y)$ if and only if $z(k) \geq 0$. In this way we find that (c, d) as in (6.83) belongs to $W_o(g_x, g_y)$ if and only if

$$kp \leq k^2 + (n - k)q \quad \text{whenever} \quad q < k < p. \qquad (6.86)$$

As an illustration, suppose $m = n = 3$ with both projections equal to $g_x^* = g_y^* = (2, 1, 1)$. Thus, have here the case $k = 1$ and $w = 1$. The possible pairs (p, q) are $(3, 0)$, $(2, 0)$, $(1, 0)$, $(3, 1)$, $(2, 1)$ and $(3, 2)$. Hence, using (6.83), the weakly admissible pairs (c, d) are given by

$$\left(\frac{1}{3}, \frac{1}{3}\right); \ \left(\frac{1}{2}, \frac{1}{3}\right); \ \left(1, \frac{1}{3}\right); \ \left(\frac{1}{2}, \frac{1}{6}\right); \ (1, 0) \quad \text{and} \quad \left(1, -\frac{1}{3}\right), \qquad (6.87)$$

respectively. Presently, (6.86) requires that $p \leq 1 + 2q$ whenever $q < 1 < p$. Equivalently, if $q = 0$ then $p = 1$. This rules out the (p, q) pairs $(3, 0)$ and $(2, 0)$. Consequently, $W_o(g_x, g_y)$ consists of the four pairs $(1, 0); (1, \frac{1}{3}); (1, -\frac{1}{3}); (\frac{1}{2}, \frac{1}{6})$.

The corresponding pairs $(d, e) = (d, c + d)$ are $(0, 1)$; $(\frac{1}{3}, \frac{4}{3})$; $(-\frac{1}{3}, \frac{2}{3})$; $(\frac{1}{6}, \frac{2}{3})$. The two (c, d) pairs $(1, 0)$ and $(\frac{1}{2}, \frac{1}{6})$ satisfy $\bar{s}_t = s_t$, for all t, and thus (by Lemma 6.1) are uniqueness pairs in that each yields only a single solution G.

Example 6.2. Choose $m = n = 8$ and take both projections equal to

$$g_x^* = g_y^* = (5, 5, 5, 5, 5, 4, 4, 3). \tag{6.88}$$

Suppose $(c, d) \in W(g_x, g_y)$. It follows from Lemma 6.2 that $c = 1/h$ for some $h \in N$ and also that $c \geq 2/8 = 1/4$, thus, $c \in \{1/4, 1/3, 1/2, 1\}$. From (6.78), the associated integers s_j must be such that $s_j = x$ for $1 \leq j \leq 5$; $s_6 = s_7 = y$ while $s_8 = z$. Here, x, y, z are integers such that $0 \leq z < y < x \leq 8$. In addition

$$x = (5 - 8d)/c; \qquad y = (4 - 8d)/c; \qquad z = (3 - 8d)/c. \tag{6.89}$$

Eliminating d, this implies that $x - y = y - z = 1/c$; hence, $y = (x + z)/2$. In particular, x and z must be of the same parity. Moreover,

$$c = \frac{2}{x - z}; \qquad d = \frac{3x - 5z}{8(x - z)}. \tag{6.90}$$

There are exactly 15 possible pairs (x, z), namely, $(8, 0)$; $(8, 2)$; $(8, 4)$; $(8, 6)$; $(7, 1)$; $(7, 3)$; $(7, 5)$; $(6, 0)$; $(6, 2)$; $(6, 4)$; $(5, 1)$; $(5, 3)$; $(4, 0)$; $(4, 2)$; $(3, 1)$, showing that $W(g_x, g_y)$ consists of 15 pairs (c, d). Three of these pairs do not belong $W_o(g_x, g_y)$, namely, when (x, z) equals $(8, 0)$; $(8, 2)$ or $(7, 1)$. The first has

$$s^* = (8, 8, 8, 8, 8, 4, 4, 0) \quad \text{thus} \quad \bar{s}^* = (7, 7, 7, 7, 5, 5, 5, 5), \tag{6.91}$$

and thus fails condition (6.79) for most t. The pair $(x, z) = (8, 2)$ has

$$s^* = (8, 8, 8, 8, 8, 5, 5, 2) \quad \text{thus} \quad \bar{s}^* = (8, 8, 7, 7, 7, 5, 5, 5) \tag{6.92}$$

and thus fails to satisfy (6.79). Finally, the pair $(x, z) = (7, 1)$ has

$$s^* = (7, 7, 7, 7, 7, 4, 4, 1) \quad \text{thus} \quad \bar{s}^* = (8, 7, 7, 7, 5, 5, 5, 0), \tag{6.93}$$

and thus (barely) fails (6.79). On the other hand, the pair $x = 6$ and $z = 0$ has $c = \frac{1}{3}$ and $d = \frac{3}{8}$ while $s^* = (6, 6, 6, 6, 6, 3, 3, 0)$ thus $\bar{s}^* = (7, 7, 7, 5, 5, 5, 0, 0)$, which do satisfy condition (6.79). In fact, this is the only pair $(c, d) \in W_o(g_x, g_y)$ with $c = \frac{1}{3}$. The set $W_o(g_x, g_y)$ contains four pairs in $W_o(g_x, g_y)$ with $c = \frac{1}{2}$ and seven pairs with $c = 1$. Altogether $|W_o(g_x, g_y)| = 1 + 4 + 7 = 12$.

6.7 Uniqueness in the case of two-valued matrices

Let g_x and g_y be fixed vectors as in (6.49) and (6.55). We further assume that each of the projections $g_x(i)$ ($i \in M$) and $g_y(j)$ ($j \in N$) is nonconstant.

Definition 6.3.   *A pair (c, d) with $c > 0$ is said to be g_x, g_y-uniqueness pair (or simply a uniqueness pair) if $(c, d) \in W_o(g_x, g_y)$ and further $\mathcal{G}_o(g_x, g_y)$ contains precisely one matrix $G = (g(i, j))$ satisfying (6.47).*

Theorem 6.6.   *In order that (c, d) be a uniqueness pair, it is necessary and sufficient that $(c, d) \in W(g_x, g_y)$ and that, moreover,*

$$r_t = \bar{s}_t \qquad \text{for all} \quad t = 1, .., m. \tag{6.94}$$

Remark 6.4.   *As usual, the r_i and s_j are defined by (6.51) and satisfy (6.52) and (6.56). The $\bar{s}_t$ and ρ_t are as defined as in Lemma 6.1.*

Proof: Assume that $(c, d) \in W(g_x, g_y)$, (as is clearly necessary). Equivalently, the r_i and s_j defined by (6.51) do satisfy (6.52). The pair (c, d) belongs to $W_o(g_x, g_y)$ precisely when there exists at least one matrix $G \in \mathcal{G}_o(g_x, g_y)$ satisfying (6.47). From Theorem 6.4, this is true if and only if (6.57) holds. By Lemma 6.1, in order that (c, d) be a uniqueness pair, that is, in order that the latter matrix G be unique, it is necessary and sufficient that (6.94) holds. Note that (6.94) implies (6.57).   □

In the following we shall apply the idea used by Wang for reconstructing unique (0,1)-matrices [16]. Let $F = (f(i, j))$ be a $\{0, 1\}$-valued $m \times n$ matrix. A row of F is said to be *full* if it only contains elements 1. Similarly for a full column, empty row or empty column. Analogously suppose $G = (g(i, j))$ satisfies $g(i, j) \in \{d, e\}$ for all i, j (with $c = e - d > 0$). Then the i-th row of G can be said to be full when $g(i, j) = e$ for all j and empty if $g(i, j) = d$ for all j. Similarly for columns.

Lemma 6.3.   *Let F be a $\{0, 1\}$-valued matrix that is uniquely determined by its row sums r_i together with its column sums s_j. Equivalently, the r_i and s_j satisfy (6.94). Then F has either a full row or else an empty column, but not both. Thus,*

$$\text{either} \quad r_1 = n \quad \text{or} \quad s_n = 0. \tag{6.95}$$

Similarly, F has either a full column or else an empty row but not both. Thus,

$$\text{either} \quad s_1 = m \quad \text{or} \quad r_m = 0. \tag{6.96}$$

Remark 6.5.   *Each of these properties leads to an inductive type of characterization of such a unique matrix F. Deleting all full rows (assuming there is at least one) the resulting matrix F' must again be a uniqueness matrix but now without any full row. Hence, F' must have one or more empty columns. Deleting all such empty columns leads to a new uniqueness matrix F''. And so on.*

Proof: If $s_n > 0$ then $\bar{s}_1 = n$, hence, $r_1 = \bar{s}_1 = n$. Here, we used the criterion (6.94) for uniqueness. A more satisfying proof is as follows. Suppose F has neither any full row nor any empty column. Thus if $f(i_o, j_o) = 1$ then $f(i_o, j_1) = 0$ for some $j_1 \neq j_o$, which in turn implies that $f(i_1, j_1)$ for some $i_1 \neq i_o$. And so on. Sooner or later some point (i, j) is visited for the second time, showing that a so-called bad cycle exists, which in turn contradicts the uniqueness of F.   □

Theorem 6.7.   *There are at most two g_x, g_y-uniqueness pairs. In fact, a uniqueness pair (c, d) must have one of the forms (6.99) and (6.101).*

Remark 6.6.   *If one projection is constant but not the other then there is at most one uniqueness pair, as follows from Remark 6.3.*

For the moment consider the case that both projections are constant. Then by Theorem 6.5, there exist infinitely many uniqueness pairs (d, e), specifically, those for which either $d = u$ or else $e = c + d = u$. Nevertheless, all these uniqueness pairs (d, e) lead to one and the same matrix G, namely, the "constant" matrix G having $g(i, j) = u$ for all i, j. In order that there exist admissible pairs that are not uniqueness pairs, it is necessary and sufficient that $k = (m, n) \geq 2$. Namely, these are precisely the pairs of the form (6.17) having $h \in \{1, 2, ..., k - 1\}$.

Definition 6.4.   *Let $p_x > 0$ be the number of indices $i \in M$ with $g_x(i) = g_x(1)$. Similarly, let $q_x > 0$ be the number of indices $i \in M$ with $g_x(i) = g_x(m)$. Here, $p_x + q_x \leq m$, since $g_x(i)$ $(i \in M)$ is nonconstant.*
Let $p_y > 0$ and $q_y > 0$ be the analogous quantities relative to the vertical projection $g_y(j)$. One has $p_y + q_y \leq n$ since $g_y(j)$ is nonconstant. Note that these positive integers p_x, p_y, q_x and q_y are fixed, and known to an observer who only knows g_x and g_y.

Proof: (of Theorem 6.7) Let (c, d) be a fixed uniqueness pair, and let the r_i and s_j be as in Theorem 6.6. Thus there exists a unique $\{0, 1\}$-valued matrix F having the r_i as row sums and the s_j as column sums. Either $r_1 = n$ or $s_n = 0$, but not both, as follows from Lemma 6.3.

First suppose $r_1 = n$. In view of (6.62), one has that

$$r_j = n \quad \text{for} \quad 1 \leq i \leq p_x; \qquad r_i < n \quad \text{for} \quad p_x < i \leq n. \qquad (6.97)$$

Equivalently, F has precisely p_x full rows, thus, $s_j \geq p_x$ for all j. Let F' denote the matrix obtained from $F = (f(i, j))$ by dropping those full rows. This new matrix F' must again be an uniqueness matrix (relative to its projections). Since F' has no full rows, it must have empty columns. As is easily seen, this is equivalent to $s_n = p_x$. In view of (6.51), this leads to the equations

$$n = r_1 = \frac{g_x(1) - nd}{c} \quad \text{and} \quad p_x = s_n = \frac{g_y(n) - md}{c}. \qquad (6.98)$$

Solving for c and d, one obtains that

$$c = \frac{mg_x(1) - ng_y(n)}{n(m - p_x)}, \qquad d = \frac{ng_y(n) - p_x g_x(1)}{n(m - p_x)}. \tag{6.99}$$

Next consider the case $s_n = 0$. Again using (6.62), it follows that F has q_y empty columns. It follows that $r_i \leq n - q_y$ for all $i \in M$. Dropping those empty columns, one arrives at a new uniqueness matrix F' without any empty column. But then F' must have a full row, which is equivalent to $r_1 = n - q_y$. By (6.51), this leads to the equations

$$n - q_y = r_1 = \frac{g_x(1) - nd}{c} \qquad and \qquad 0 = s_n = \frac{g_y(n) - md}{c}. \tag{6.100}$$

Solving for c and d, this yields that

$$c = \frac{mg_x(1) - ng_y(n)}{m(n - q_y)}; \qquad d = \frac{g_y(n)}{m}. \tag{6.101}$$

We conclude that (c, d) cannot possibly a uniqueness pair unless it has one of the forms (6.99) and (6.101). This proves Theorem 6.7. We will refrain from deriving analogous formulae for a uniqueness pair (c, d) when instead we use the fact that either $s_1 = m$ or $r_m = 0$. □

Example 6.3.   Let $m = n = 3$, $g_x = (2, 1, 0)$, and $g_y = (2, 1, 0)$. Thus $p_x = q_y = 1$. Here (6.99) gives $c = 1$; $d = (0 - 2)/6 = -\frac{1}{3}$ yielding the potential pair $(1, -\frac{1}{3})$ while (6.101) yields the potential pair $(c, d) = (1, 0)$. One can easily check that each of these two pairs is a uniqueness pair and that further $W_o(g_x, g_y)$ and even $W(g_x, g_y)$ contains no other pairs (c, d). Thus, in this example, there are precisely two two-valued 3×3 matrices G having the given projections, as follows.

2	1	1	0		2	2/3	2/3	2/3
1	1	0	0		1	2/3	2/3	-1/3
0	0	0	0		0	2/3	-1/3	-1/3

$$\tag{6.102}$$

	2	1	0		2	1	0

Acknowledgment

This work was supported by the Hungarian Ministry of Education Grant FKFP 0908.

References

[1] G. G. Lorentz, "A problem of plane measure," *Amer. J. Math* **71**, 417-426 (1949).

[2] H. G. Kellerer, "Masstheoretische Marginalprobleme," *Math. Annalen* **153**, 168-198 (1964).

[3] A. Kuba and A. Volčič, "Characterization of measurable plane sets which are reconstructable from their two projections," *Inverse Problems* **4**, 513-527 (1988).

[4] P. C. Fishburn, J. C. Lagarias, J. A. Reeds, and L. A. Shepp, "Sets uniquely determined by projections on axes," *Discrete Mathematics* **91**, 149-159 (1991).

[5] A. Kuba, "Reconstruction of measurable plane sets from their two projections taken in arbitrary directions," *Inverse Problems* **7**, 101-107 (1991).

[6] D. Gale, "Theorem on flows in networks," *Pacific. J. Math.* **7**, 1073-1082 (1957).

[7] H. J. Ryser, "Combinatorial properties of matrices of zeros and ones," *Canad. J. Math.* **9**, 371-377 (1957).

[8] R. A. Brualdi, "Matrices of zeros and ones with fixed row and column sum vectors," *Linear Algebra and Its Applications* **33**, 159-231 (1980).

[9] L. Mirsky, "Combinatorial theorems and integral matrices," *J. Comb. Theory* **5**, 30-44 (1968).

[10] R. Aharoni, G. T. Herman, and A. Kuba, "Binary vectors partially determined by linear equation system," *Discrete Math.* **171**, 1-16 (1997).

[11] P. C. Fishburn, P. Schwander, L. A. Shepp, and J. Vanderbei, "The discrete Radon transform and its approximate inversion via linear programming," *Discrete Appl. Math.* **75**, 39-61 (1997).

[12] S. K. Chang and C. K. Chow, "The reconstruction of three-dimensional objects from two orthogonal projections and its application to cardiac cineangiography," *IEEE Trans. Comp.* **C-22**, 18-28 (1973).

[13] G. P. M. Prause and D. G. W. Onnasch, "Binary reconstruction of the heart chambers from biplane angiographic image sequence," *IEEE Trans. Medical Imaging* **15**, 532-559 (1996).

[14] J. H. B. Kemperman and A. Kuba, "Reconstruction of two-valued matrices from their two projections," *Int. J. Imaging Systems and Technology* **9**, 110-117 (1998).

[15] A. Kuba and A. Volčič, "The structure of the class of non-uniquely reconstructible sets," *Acta Sci. Szeged* **58**, 363-388 (1993).

[16] Y. R. Wang, "Characterization of binary patterns and their projections," *IEEE Trans. Comput.* **C-24**, 1032-1035 (1995).

Chapter 7

Reconstruction of Connected Sets from Two Projections

Alberto Del Lungo[1]
Maurice Nivat[2]

ABSTRACT The problem of reconstructing a two-dimensional discrete set from its projections has been studied in discrete mathematics and applied in several areas. It has some interesting applications in image processing, electron microscopy, statistical data security, biplane angiography and graph theory. This chapter presents the computational complexity results of the problem of reconstructing a set from its horizontal and vertical projections with respect to some classes of sets on which some connectivity constraints are imposed. We show that this reconstruction problem can be solved in polynomial time in a class of discrete sets, and is NP-complete otherwise.

7.1   Introduction

The inverse problem of reconstructing a discrete set from its projections has been studied from many authors. This study is motived by some interesting applications in image processing [1], statistical data security [2], biplane angiography [3] and graph theory [4]. Moreover, the problem is of primary importance in reconstructing three-dimensional crystals from two-dimensional projections taken by an electron microscope [5–8]. The classical and most studied case is the reconstruction of a two-dimensional discrete set from its horizontal and vertical projections. This problem is equivalent to the reconstruction of a binary matrix from its row and column sums. Ryser [9], and subsequently Chang [10], showed that the problem can be solved in time $O(nm)$, where n and m denote the sizes of the matrix. We refer the reader to an excellent survey on the binary matrices with given row and column sums by Brualdi [11]. In some cases, a lot of discrete sets have the same orthogonal projections. Therefore, the horizontal and vertical

[1]Università di Firenze, Dipartimento di Sistemi e Informatica (DSI), Via Lombroso 6/17, 50134, Firenze, Italy, E-mail: dellungo@dsi.unifi.it

[2]Université Denis Diderot, Laboratoire d'Informatique, Algorithmique, Fondements et Applications (LIAFA), 2, place Jussieu 75251 Paris Cedex 05, France, E-mail: Maurice.Nivat@liafa.jussieu.fr

projections do not provide sufficient information for unique reconstruction. We can reduce the ambiguity by furnishing some properties of the set to be reconstructed a priori (for example: convexity, connection, symmetries); the algorithms can then take advantage of this information to reconstruct the set [12, 13]. The reconstruction of these special sets has been posed in several applications [3, 14].

The aim of this chapter is to present the computational complexity results of the problem of reconstructing a set from its horizontal and vertical projections with respect to some classes of sets on which some connectivity constraints are imposed. In particular, we take the following three connectivity constraints into consideration: *horizontally convex* (or *h*-convex), *vertically convex* (or *v*-convex) and *4-connectivity* (or polyomino). We show that this reconstruction problem can be solved in polynomial time, if the three properties are all verified by the discrete set. In this case the set is called *convex polyomino*. At the same time, we prove that it is NP-complete to reconstruct a discrete set verifying just one or two of the three properties. Table 7.1 illustrates a summary of these complexity results.

	h and v-convex	h-convex	v-convex	no restric.
Polyomino	P	NP-comp.	NP-comp.	NP-comp.
No restriction	NP-comp.	NP-comp.	NP-comp.	P

TABLE 7.1. The computational complexity of discrete set reconstruction.

The chapter is organized as follows. Section 2 introduces some notations and formulates the problem. Section 3 presents the NP-completeness of the problem on some classes of sets. The final Section 4 describes an algorithm that reconstructs a convex polyomino starting out from its horizontal and vertical projections, in polynomial time.

7.2   Preliminaries

A *discrete set* is a finite subset of the integer lattice $\mathbb{Z}^2$ defined up to a translation; it can be represented by a binary matrix or a set of *cells* (unitary squares), as shown in Fig. 7.1. In this chapter, we represent the discrete sets by means of the sets of cells and we number their rows and columns starting from the left-upper corner. Without the restriction of generality, we can suppose that the discrete sets to be studied have non-empty rows for $i = 1, 2, \ldots, m$ and non-empty columns for $j = 1, 2, \ldots, n$. The positive integers m and n are the number of rows and columns of set, respectively. The cell (i, j) is the intersection of the i-th row with the j-th column.

Let S be a discrete set. Let us denote the vector of *horizontal projection*

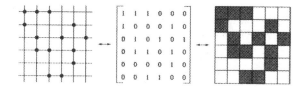

FIGURE 7.1. Correspondence among a discrete set, a binary matrix, and a set of cells.

(or row projection) by $H = (h_1, h_2, \ldots, h_m)$, where $h_i \geq 1$ is the number of cells of S in the i-th row, $1 \leq i \leq m$, and the vector of *vertical projection* (or column projection) by $V = (v_1, v_2, \ldots, v_n)$, where $v_j \geq 1$ is the number of cells of S in the j-th column, $1 \leq j \leq n$ (see Fig. 7.2).

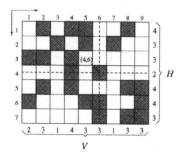

FIGURE 7.2. A discrete set and its horizontal and vertical projections.

We now introduce some definitions that allow us to characterize discrete sets. The *4-neighbors* of (i, j) are the cells $(i-1, j)$, $(i, j-1)$, $(i, j+1)$, and $(i+1, j)$. A sequence of cells (i_0, j_0), $(i_1, j_1), \ldots, (i_n, j_n)$ is called *lattice path* if (i_{k-1}, j_{k-1}) is a 4-neighbor of (i_k, j_k) for all $k = 1, 2, \ldots, n$. A *polyomino* S is a discrete set in which for any pair of cells of S there exists a lattice path in S connecting them (see Fig. 7.3), and we say that S has the property p. These sets are well-known combinatorial objects [15] and are called *4-connected sets* in discrete geometry and computer vision. A discrete set is

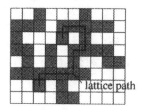

FIGURE 7.3. A polyomino.

horizontally convex (or *h-convex*) if its rows are 4-connected. Analogously, it is *vertically convex* (or *v-convex*) if its columns are 4-connected. We indicate these properties by h and v, respectively. A discrete set is *convex* if its columns and rows are 4-connected (i.e., it has the properties h and v). Figure 7.4 shows some discrete sets having the above-mentioned geometric properties.

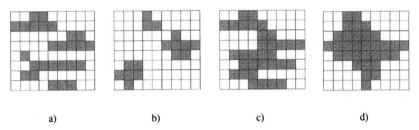

a)   b)   c)   d)

FIGURE 7.4. a) An h-convex set. b) A convex set. c) An h-convex polyomino. d) A convex polyomino.

Let $p_1, p_2, \ldots, p_{k-1}$ and p_k be some geometric properties. We denote the class of discrete sets having the properties $p_1, p_2, \ldots, p_{k-1}$ and p_k by $(p_1, p_2, \ldots, p_k)$. For instance, the class of convex polyominoes has the properties p, h and v, and so we denote this class by (p, h, v).

We are going to define the problem of reconstructing a discrete set from its horizontal and vertical projections. Let $H = (h_1, h_2, \ldots, h_m) \in \mathbb{N}^m$ and $V = (v_1, v_2, \ldots, v_n) \in \mathbb{N}^n$ ($\mathbb{N}$ denotes the set of positive integers). The pair (H, V) is said to be *satisfiable* in the class $(p_1, p_2, \ldots, p_k)$ if there is at least one set S of $(p_1, p_2, \ldots, p_k)$ having horizontal and vertical projections equal to H and V. We can also say that S *satisfies* (H, V) in $(p_1, p_2, \ldots, p_k)$. We deduce that, if (H, V) is satisfiable in $(p_1, p_2, \ldots, p_k)$, then:

$$1 \le h_i \le n, \ \text{ for each } i \in \{1, \ldots, m\},$$
$$1 \le v_j \le m, \ \text{ for each } j \in \{1, \ldots, n\}, \tag{7.1}$$
$$\sum_{i=1}^{m} h_i = \sum_{j=1}^{n} v_j.$$

Consequently, if S satisfies (H, V), S is contained in the the discrete rectangle $R = \{(i, j) : 1 \le i \le m, 1 \le j \le n\}$ (see Fig. 7.2). Our reconstruction problem can be formulated as follows.

Problem. Reconstructing a Set from its Horizontal and Vertical Projections (*RSHVP*)
Instance. Two vectors $H = (h_1, \ldots, h_m) \in \mathbb{N}^m$ and $V = (v_1, \ldots, v_n) \in \mathbb{N}^n$, and the class $(p_1, p_2, \ldots, p_k)$ of discrete sets.
Question. Is the pair (H, V) satisfiable in $(p_1, p_2, \ldots, p_k)$?

Ryser [9], and subsequently Chang [10] solved the problem on the class $(\emptyset)$, that is, without extra restrictions imposed onto the combinatorial structure of the sets. They gave an exact combinatorial characterization of the projections (H, V) that correspond to a set. Both authors derived a fast algorithm that, starting out with $V \in \mathbb{N}^n$ and $H \in \mathbb{N}^m$ affirm the existence of a set satisfying (H, V) in time $O(nm)$. In the following sections, we study the *RSHVP* problem on the classes of discrete sets having some of the following properties: p (polyomino), h (horizontally convex) and v (vertically convex).

7.3 Intractability results

The central purpose of this section is to show that the *RSHVP* problem on the classes of discrete sets having just one or two of the properties p, h, and v is NP-complete.

7.3.1 The complexity of RSHVP on (h), (p, h), (v), and (p, v)

We are going to prove that the *RSHVP* problem on the class of vertically convex polyominoes is NP-complete. This result is from [16]. Let us examine the following NP-complete problem (see [17]).

Problem. Numerical Matching with Target Sums (*NMTS*)
Instance. Disjoint sets $X = \{x_1, x_2, \ldots, x_n\}$ and $Y = \{y_1, y_2, \ldots, y_n\}$, each containing n elements, a function $s : X \cup Y \to \mathbb{N}$ polynomial in n, and a vector $V = (v_1, v_2, \ldots, v_n) \in \mathbb{N}^n$.
Question. Can set $X \cup Y$ be partitioned into n disjoint sets $A_1, A_2, \ldots, A_n$ such that: $\forall j \in \{1, \ldots, n\}$ $A_j = \{x, y\}$ with $x \in X$ and $y \in Y$, and $s(x) + s(y) = v_j$?

Theorem 7.1. *RSHVP on class (p, v) is NP-complete.*

Proof: It is easy to see that *RSHVP* on (p, v) belongs to NP. We now give a polynomial time reduction from *NMTS* to *RSHVP*. Let an arbitrary instance of *NMTS* be given. We must construct two vectors $H' \in \mathbb{N}^m$ and $V' \in \mathbb{N}^n$ in such a way that (H', V') is satisfiable in (p, v) if and only if the *NMTS* instance has a solution. Assuming that $u_j = s(x_j)$ and $d_j = s(y_j)$, for $1 \leq j \leq n$, two vectors of positive integers $U = (u_1, u_2, \ldots, u_n)$ and $D = (d_1, d_2, \ldots, d_n)$ are obtained from X and Y. Each element u_j (d_j) is associated with a column containing u_j (d_j) cells. We join these columns as shown in Fig. 7.5(a). We define (H', V') (i.e., the *RSHVP* instance) as follows:

- $H' = (h_1', h_2', \ldots, h_m')$, where h_i' is the number of cells in the i-th row of the polyomino in Fig. 7.5(b),

- $V' = V$.

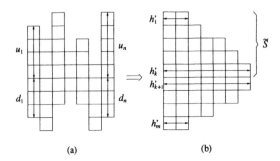

(a)   (b)

FIGURE 7.5. a) The vertically convex polyomino obtained from the columns associated to U and D. b) Its horizontal projection.

Since the number m of rows is such that:

$$m = \max U + \max D = \max\{s(x) : x \in X\} + \max\{s(y) : y \in Y\}, \qquad (7.2)$$

and since the function s is polynomial in n and the number of columns is equal to n, (H', V') can be constructed in polynomial time in the size of the given *NMTS* instance. It is worth noting that there is a $k \in \{1, \ldots, m\}$ such that $h'_k = h'_{k+1} = n$, because the elements of U and D are positive integers (see Fig. 7.5(b)). Let us assume that there is a vertically convex polyomino S satisfying (H', V'). Since $h'_k = h'_{k+1} = n$, we have that the rows k and $(k+1)$ of S are n long. Moreover, S is vertically convex and so we can associate a vector $U' = (u'_1, u'_2, \ldots, u'_n) \in \mathbb{N}^n$ to the columns of S made up of its first k rows and a vector $D' = (d'_1, d'_2, \ldots, d'_n) \in \mathbb{N}^n$ to the columns of S made up of the subsequent $m-k$ rows (see Fig. 7.6(a)). S satisfies (H', V') and so its j-th column is v'_j long,

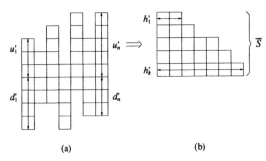

(a)   (b)

FIGURE 7.6. a) A vertically convex polyomino that satisfies (H', V'). b) Its partial horizontal projection.

and therefore vectors U' and D' are such that $u'_j + d'_j = v_j$ for each $j \in \{1, \ldots, n\}$. We now prove that U' and D' are a permutation of U and D, respectively. Let $\bar{S}$ be the polyomino obtained from the columns associated to U' lined up according to their decreasing length (see Fig. 7.6(b)). Since S satisfies (H', V'), the length of the i-th row of $\bar{S}$ is equal to h'_i. Let us examine the polyomino $\tilde{S}$ obtained by the columns associated to U lined up according to their decreasing length (see Fig. 7.5(b)). According to our definition of H', the length of the i-th row of $\tilde{S}$ coincides with h'_i and so $\bar{S} = \tilde{S}$. As a result, U' is a permutation of U, and similarly, D' is a permutation of D. Therefore, there is a permutation σ of U and a permutation ρ of D such that $u_{\sigma(j)} + d_{\rho(j)} = v_j$, for $j = 1, 2, \ldots, n$. Consequently, $\{A_1, A_2, \ldots, A_n\}$ such that $A_j = \{x_{\sigma(j)}, y_{\rho(j)}\}$ for $j \in \{1, \ldots, n\}$, is a solution of the *NMTS* instance.

Vice versa, let us assume that the *NMTS* instance has solution. There is a permutation σ of U and a permutation ρ of D such that $u_{\sigma(j)} + d_{\rho(j)} = v_j$ for $j = 1, 2, \ldots, n$. By joining the columns related to $\sigma(U)$ to $\rho(D)$ as shown in Fig. 7.7, we obtain a vertically convex polyomino that satisfies (H', V'). Therefore, *NMTS* $\propto$ *RSHVP* on (p, v) and the Theorem is proved. $\qquad\square$

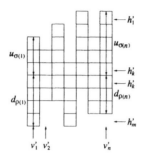

FIGURE 7.7. A vertically convex polyomino obtained by joining the columns related to $\sigma(U)$ and $\rho(D)$.

By symmetry, *RSHVP* on (p, h) is NP-complete. By proceeding in the same way, we can prove that *NMTS* $\propto$ *RSHVP* on (v). In other words, we have:

Theorem 7.2.   *RSHVP on classes (h), (v) and (p, h) is NP-complete.*

7.3.2   The complexity of RSHVP on (p) and (h, v)

We prove that the *RSHVP* problem on the class of polyominoes is NP-complete. This result has been established by Woeginger [18], and we are going to describe his reduction. Let us take the following version of the NP-complete *3-PARTITION* problem into consideration (see [17]).

Problem. *3-PARTITION*
Instance. A set of positive integers $A = \{a_1, a_2, \ldots, a_{3k}\}$ and a positive integer b such that $\sum_{i=1}^{3k} a_i = k(2b + 1)$ and $(2b + 1)/4 < a_i < (2b + 1)/2$, for each $i \in \{1, \ldots, 3k\}$.
Question. Does there exist a partition of A into k disjoint 3-element sets $\{A_1, A_2, \ldots, A_k\}$ such that $\sum_{a_i \in A_j} a_i = 2b + 1$ for each $j \in \{1, \ldots, k\}$?

Theorem 7.3.   *RSHVP on class (p) is NP-complete.*

Proof: It is easy to see that *RSHVP* on (p) belongs to NP. We now give a polynomial time reduction from *3-PARTITION* to *RSHVP*. Let an arbitrary instance of *3-PARTITION* be given. We must construct two vectors $H' \in \mathbb{N}^m$ and $V' \in \mathbb{N}^n$ in such a way that (H', V') is satisfiable in (p) if and only if the *3-PARTITION* instance has solution. By setting $m = (2b + 2)k + 1$ and $n = 12k$ we define (H', V') as follows:

- H' is made up of $3k$ blocks each with four elements, where the i-th block is $1, a_i + 1, 2, n$, that is:

$$H' = (1, a_1 + 1, 2, n, 1, a_2 + 1, 2, n, \ldots, 1, a_{3k} + 1, 2, n). \qquad (7.3)$$

- V' starts with $v_1' = m$, followed by k identical blocks. Every block has $2b + 2$ elements and it is equal to

$$(3k, 3k + 2, \underbrace{3k + 1, \ldots, 3k + 1}_{(b-1)-\text{ times}}, 3k + 2, \underbrace{3k + 1, \ldots, 3k + 1}_{(b-1)-\text{ times}}, 3k + 2). \qquad (7.4)$$

Let us assume that there is a polyomino S satisfying (H', V'). We say that the rows $4i - 3, 4i - 2, 4i - 1$ and $4i$ of S constitute the i-th *r-block* R_i, for $1 \le i \le 3k$, and that the columns from $(2b + 2)(j - 1) + 2$ to $(2b + 2)j + 1$ of S form the j-th *c-block* C_j, for $1 \le j \le k$ (see Fig. 7.8). Since $h_{4i}' = n$, the lowest row of R_i is n long. Therefore, this is the position of $3k$ cells of S in every column. Since every c-block C_j starts with a column of length $3k$, the cells of S in the column $(2b+2)(j-1)+2$, with $1 \le j \le k$, are exactly at the intersection with the row $4i$, with $1 \le i \le 3k$. Moreover, $v_1' = m$ and so the first column of S is m long, and this fixes the position of the single cell of S in the row $4i - 3$, and the position of one of the two cell of S in the row $4i - 1$, with $1 \le i \le 3k$. The reader can check these properties by using the polyomino in Fig. 7.8.

Let us now take the second row of R_i into consideration (i.e., $(4i - 2)$-th row of S). We are going to prove that the $a_i + 1$ cells of S in this row are two disjoint sets: one single cell is in the first column, and a_i cells form a 4-connected set completely contained within one c-block (see Fig. 7.8). From the previous discussion it follows that the first column contains a cell of the $(4i - 2)$-th row of S and there is no cell of this row in the second column. We now assume that there are two further 4-connected set in the $(4i - 2)$-th row of S. From the definition of polyomino we deduce that these two sets have to be connected to the rest of polyomino. The $(4i - 3)$-th row of S contains a single cell in the first column and so these connections are obtained by means of the $(4i - 1)$-th row. Since $h_{4i-1}' = 2$, this row contains only two cells of S, one in the first column, and another one that can only connect a single 4-connected set in $(4i - 2)$-th row to the rest of polyomino. Hence, the $(4i-2)$-th row contains a 4-connected set made up of a_i cells. If this set is contained in two adjacent c-blocks C_j and C_{j+1}, it

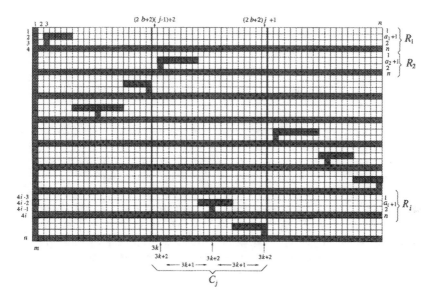

FIGURE 7.8. A polyomino that satisfies (H', V').

has to cross the first column of C_{j+1}. From the above discussion we have that there is no cell of S at the intersection of this column with the $(4i - 2)$-th row. Consequently, the 4-connected set with a_i cells is completely contained within one c-block.

Let us now define a partition $\{A_1, A_2, \ldots, A_k\}$ of $A = \{a_1, a_2, \ldots, a_{3k}\}$. Element a_i belongs to A_j if and only if the 4-connected set of length a_i in the $(4i - 2)$-th row belongs to C_j. The cell that connects the set of length a_i to the rest of polyomino is in a column containing $3k + 2$ cells of S (see Fig. 7.8). Since C_j has three columns containing $3k + 2$ cells, there are three "connecting" cell in C_j. Consequently, A_j is made up of three elements of A. The intersection of C_j with R_i contains $(2b + 2)$ cells (in the $(4i)$-th column) or $(2b + 2) + 1 + a_i$ cells $(2b + 2$ in the $(4i)$-th column, a single connecting cell in the $(4i - 1)$-th column and a_i in the $(4i - 2)$-th column). C_j contains $(3k + 1)(2b + 2) + 2$ cells and so:

$$(3k + 1)(2b + 2) + 2 = 3k(2b + 2) + \sum_{a_i \in A_j} (a_i + 1), \tag{7.5}$$

Since $|A_j| = 3$, we deduce that: $\sum_{a_i \in A_j} a_i = 2b + 1$. Therefore, $\{A_1, A_2, \ldots, A_k\}$ is a solution of the *3-PARTITION* instance.

Vice versa, let us assume that the *3-PARTITION* instance has solution. We have to reconstruct a polyomino S satisfying (H', V'). From $v'_1 = m$ and $h'_{4i} = n$, for $1 \leq i \leq 3k$, we obtain that the cells in the first column and in the $(4i)$-th row, with $1 \leq i \leq 3k$, belong to S. Let $A_j = \{a_{i_1}, a_{i_2}, a_{i_3}\}$ be the j-th triple in the solution of the *3-PARTITION* instance. We reconstruct S in the following way:

- $(4i_1 - 2, j) \in S$, with $(2b + 2)(j - 1) + 3 \leq k \leq (2b + 2)(j - 1) + a_{i_1} + 2$,

- $(4i_2-2, j) \in S$, with $(2b+2)(j-1)+a_{i_1}+3 \le k \le (2b+2)(j-1)+a_{i_1}+a_{i_2}+2$,

- $(4i_3 - 2, j) \in S$, with $(2b + 2)(j - 1) + a_{i_1} + a_{i_2} + 3 \le k \le (2b + 2)j + 1$.

Moreover, we put in S the three "connecting" cells: $(4i_1 - 1, (2b + 2)(j - 1) + 3), (4i_2 - 1, (2b + 2)(j - 1) + b + 3)$ and $(4i_3 - 1, (2b + 2)j + 1)$. We repeat this procedure for every triple in the solution of the *3-PARTITION* instance. It is easy to verify that the resulting set S is a polyomino that satisfies (H', V'). □

Let us now take the class of convex sets into consideration. *RSHVP* on (h, v) has been studied by Kuba [13]. He proposed a reconstruction algorithm with an exponential worst-case time complexity. Subsequently, Woeginger [18] showed that this problem is NP-complete. Again the proof is a reduction from *3-PARTITION*.

Theorem 7.4.   *RSHVP on class (h, v) NP-complete.*

Proof: Let an arbitrary instance of *3-PARTITION* be given. We must construct two vectors $H' \in \mathbb{N}^m$ and $V' \in \mathbb{N}^n$ in such a way that (H', V') is satisfiable in (h, v) if and only if the *3-PARTITION* instance has solution. We define (H', V') as follows:

- H' is made up of $3k$ blocks, where the i-th block is $0, a_i$, that is:
$$H' = (0, a_1, 0, a_2, \dots, 0, a_{3k-1}, 0, a_{3k}). \qquad (7.6)$$

- V' is made up of k identical blocks. Every block has $2b + 2$ elements and it is equal to
$$(0, \underbrace{1, 1, \dots, 1}_{(2b+1)- \text{ times}}). \qquad (7.7)$$

We can show that (H', V') is satisfiable in (h, v) if and only if the *3-PARTITION* instance has solution. The proof is very similar to that one of Theorem 7.3. □

Remark 7.1.   We wish to point out that a convex set is a collection of disjoint convex polyominoes (see Fig. 7.4(b)). Quite surprisingly, as shown in the following section, *RSHVP* on the class of convex polyominoes can be solved in polynomial time.

7.4 Reconstruction of convex polyominoes

The aim of this section is to describe an algorithm that decides whether or not there is a convex polyomino whose horizontal and vertical projections are given by two assigned vectors (H, V). If there is at least one convex polyomino having these projections, the algorithm reconstructs one of them in $O(n^3 m^3(n + m))$ time. Therefore, we show that the *RSHVP* problem on the class of convex polyominoes can be solved in polynomial time. This result is from [16, 19]. We begin by introducing the geometrical concept of median. We show that if the discrete set is a convex polyomino, the medians belong to the set. By extending this geometric property, we can deduce some operations for the reconstruction. Then, we are able to define the algorithm.

7.4.1   The medians

Let S be a discrete set having horizontal and vertical projections equal to $H = (h_1, h_2, \ldots, h_m) \in \mathbb{N}^m$ and $V = (v_1, v_2, \ldots, v_n) \in \mathbb{N}^n$. We introduce the following notation: $A = \sum_{i=1}^{m} h_i = \sum_{j=1}^{n} v_j$ and

$$H_0 = 0 \text{ and } H_k = \sum_{i=1}^{k} h_i, \text{ for } k = 1, \ldots, m, \qquad (7.8)$$

$$V_0 = 0 \text{ and } V_k = \sum_{j=1}^{k} v_j, \text{ for } k = 1, \ldots, n. \qquad (7.9)$$

The i-th row of S is said to be a *median row* if: $H_{i-1} \le \frac{A}{2} \le H_i$. Analogously, the j-th column of S is said to be a *median column* if: $V_{j-1} \le \frac{A}{2} \le V_j$. The *median* of S is the intersection of a median row and a median column. Since there can be no more than two median rows and two median columns, S has 1, 2, or 4 medians. We use this definition of median because, if S is a convex polyomino, the medians belong to S, while this is not so if S is not a convex polyomino (see Fig. 7.9).

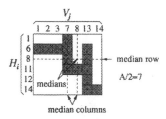

FIGURE 7.9. The medians of a discrete set.

We now prove that the medians of a convex polyomino S belong to S. Let (i, j) be a cell in the discrete rectangle $R = \{(i, j) : 1 \le i \le m, 1 \le j \le n\}$ containing S. This cell defines four sub-rectangles:

$$NW(i, j) = \{(h, k) \in R : 1 \le h \le i \text{ and } 1 \le k \le j\}, \qquad (7.10)$$

$$SW(i,j) = \{(h,k) \in R : i \leq h \leq n \text{ and } 1 \leq k \leq j\}, \qquad (7.11)$$
$$SE(i,j) = \{(h,k) \in R : i \leq h \leq n \text{ and } j \leq k \leq m\}, \qquad (7.12)$$
$$NE(i,j) = \{(h,k) \in R : 1 \leq h \leq i \text{ and } j \leq k \leq m\}, \qquad (7.13)$$

(see Fig. 7.10). If (i,j) does not belong to S, the intersection of a subrectangle with S is the empty set. For example, the cell (i,j) in Fig. 7.10 does not belong to S, and the rectangle having an empty intersection with S is $SW(i,j)$. Consequently,

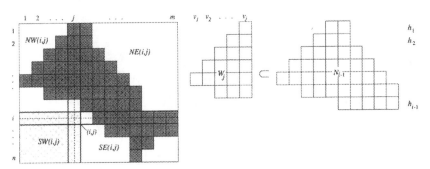

FIGURE 7.10. The cell (i,j) does not belong to S and $SW(i,j) \cap S = \emptyset$.

Lemma 7.1.   *Let (i,j) be a cell of the rectangle R containing a convex polyomino S. The cell (i,j) belongs to S if and only if $SW(i,j) \cap S \neq \emptyset$, $NE(i,j) \cap S \neq \emptyset$, $NW(i,j) \cap S \neq \emptyset$ and $SE(i,j) \cap S \neq \emptyset$.*

Moreover:

Lemma 7.2.   *Let (i,j) be a cell of the rectangle R containing a convex polyomino S satisfying (H,V).*

1. *If $V_j \geq H_{i-1}$, then $SW(i,j) \cap S \neq \emptyset$.*

2. *If $H_i \geq V_{j-1}$, then $NE(i,j) \cap S \neq \emptyset$.*

3. *If $H_i \geq A - V_j$, then $NW(i,j) \cap S \neq \emptyset$.*

4. *If $A - V_{j-1} \geq H_{i-1}$, then $SE(i,j) \cap S \neq \emptyset$.*

Proof: Let W_j be the first j columns of S and let N_{i-1} be its first $i-1$ rows. If $SW(i,j) \cap S = \emptyset$, then $W_j \subset N_{i-1}$ (see Fig. 7.10). Since the number of cells in W_j is V_j and the number of cells in N_{i-1} is H_{i-1}, it follows that if $SW(i,j) \cap S = \emptyset$, then $V_j < H_{i-1}$. Therefore, if $V_j \geq H_{i-1}$, then $SW(i,j) \cap S \neq \emptyset$. By proceeding in the same way for $NW(i,j)$, $SE(i,j)$ and $NE(i,j)$ it follows the other statements of the Lemma. $\square$

From Lemmas 7.1 and 7.2 we obtain the following proposition.

Proposition 7.1.   *Let (i,j) be a cell of the rectangle R containing a convex polyomino S satisfying (H,V). If*

$$V_j \geq H_{i-1}, \quad H_i \geq V_{j-1}, \quad H_i \geq A - V_j, \quad and \quad A - V_{j-1} \geq H_{i-1}, \qquad (7.14)$$

then (i,j) belongs to S.

This proposition allows us prove that:

Theorem 7.5.   *If S is a convex polyomino, the medians belong to S.*

Proof: Let (i,j) be a median of S. Since (i,j) is the intersection of a median row and a median column, we have: $H_{i-1} \leq A/2 \leq H_i$, and $V_{j-1} \leq A/2 \leq V_j$. It follows that: $V_j \geq H_{i-1}$, $H_i \geq V_{j-1}$, $H_i \geq A - V_j$, $A - V_{j-1} \geq H_{i-1}$, and, from the previous proposition, we deduce that (i,j) belongs to S. $\qquad\qquad\square$

Fig. 7.11 shows some convex polyominoes and their medians.

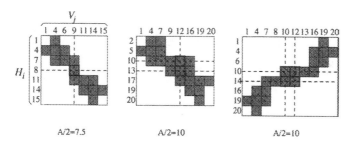

FIGURE 7.11. Some convex polyominoes and their medians.

7.4.2   The spine and its reconstruction

We want to reconstruct a convex polyomino S from its projections (H,V). Its medians belong to S and can be determined by means of the partial sums H_i and V_j. Therefore, we can determine 1, 2, or 4 cells that belong to S. We denote the set of medians by M and we want to find out if we can extend this useful property to obtain a set E such that $M \subseteq E \subseteq S$. We define E as the set of cells (i,j) of R satisfying the four conditions (7.14). From Proposition 7.1 and the definition of median it follows that: $M \subseteq E \subseteq S$. Unfortunately, E often has almost the same size as M. In Fig. 7.12, for example, M and E are made up of one and three cells, respectively. If we want E to grow bigger, we have to impose some conditions on the shape of S and we therefore introduce the concept of *foot*. Let $[S,S']$ $([N,N'], [E,E'], [W,W'])$ be the intersection of the boundary of S with the lower

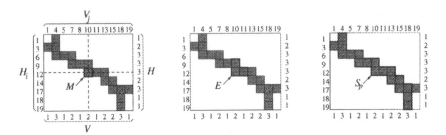

FIGURE 7.12. The sets M, E and S_p of a convex polyomino.

(upper, right, left) side of R. The segment $[S, S']$ is the base of a set made up of h_m consecutive columns of S, called *foot* of S and denoted by P_S. Moreover, $\{s_1, \ldots, s_2\}$ are the positions of the columns of P_S. We define the three other feet P_N, P_E and P_W of S in the same way by referring to the intersections $[N, N']$, $[E, E']$, $[W, W']$. The positions of P_N, P_E, and P_W are $\{n_1, \ldots, n_2\}$, $\{e_1, \ldots, e_2\}$ and $\{w_1, \ldots, w_2\}$, respectively (see Fig. 7.13).

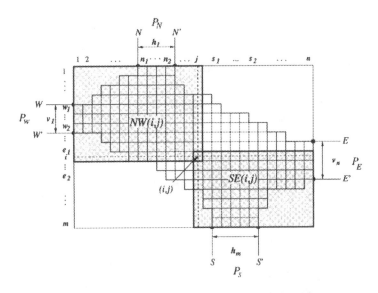

FIGURE 7.13. The feet of a convex polyomino.

Proposition 7.2. *Let (i, j) be a cell of the rectangle R containing a convex polyomino S satisfying (H, V).*

- *If $n_1 \leq j \leq s_2$, $V_j \geq H_{i-1}$ and $H_i \geq V_{j-1}$, then $(i, j) \in S$.*

- *If $s_1 \leq j \leq n_2$, $H_i \geq A - V_j$ and $A - V_{j-1} \geq H_{i-1}$, then $(i, j) \in S$.*

- *If $w_1 \leq i \leq e_2$, $V_j \geq H_{i-1}$ and $H_i \geq V_{j-1}$, then $(i, j) \in S$.*

- *If $e_1 \leq i \leq w_2$, $H_i \geq A - V_j$ and $A - V_{j-1} \geq H_{i-1}$, then $(i,j) \in S$.*

Proof: We assume that $n_1 \leq s_2$ (i.e., P_N is to the left of P_S). For each cell (i,j) such that $n_1 \leq j \leq s_2$, we have $NW(i,j) \cap S \neq \emptyset$ and $SE(i,j) \cap S \neq \emptyset$ (see Fig. 7.13). Hence, from Lemmas 7.1 and 7.2, it follows that, if $V_j \geq H_{i-1}$ and $H_i \geq V_{j-1}$, then (i,j) belongs to S. By proceeding in the same way with $s_1 \leq n_2$ and with P_W and P_E, it follows the other statements of the proposition. □

The *spine* of S, denoted by S_p, is the union of E with the set of cells (i,j) in R verifying at least one of the following conditions:

- $(n_1 \leq j \leq s_2$ or $w_1 \leq i \leq e_2)$ and $V_j \geq H_{i-1}$, $H_i \geq V_{j-1}$,

- $(s_1 \leq j \leq n_2$ or $e_1 \leq i \leq w_2)$ and $H_i \geq A - V_j$, $A - V_{j-1} \geq H_{i-1}$.

From Propositions 7.1 and 7.2 we can deduce that $S_p \subseteq S$. Therefore, if we know the foot positions of S, we can determine the set S_p belonging to S by means of (H,V). Figures 7.12 and 7.14 illustrates S_p, and it is worth noting that there is only one cell of S that does not belong S_p in Fig. 7.12.

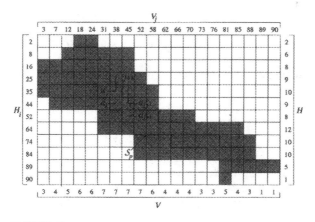

FIGURE 7.14. The spine of a convex polyomino.

Let us now establish a property of the feet. From the definition of convex polyomino, it follows that two pairs of consecutive feet have a non-empty intersection (see Fig. 7.15). In fact, if $P_N \cap P_W = \emptyset$ and $P_N \cap P_E = \emptyset$, we obtain a vertical disconnection. Therefore,

$$(P_N \cap P_W \neq \emptyset \wedge P_S \cap P_E \neq \emptyset) \vee (P_N \cap P_E \neq \emptyset \wedge P_S \cap P_W \neq \emptyset). \quad (7.15)$$

The spine and the feet have the following property.

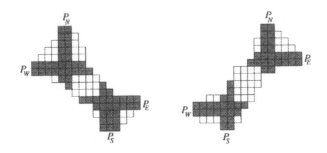

FIGURE 7.15. Foot positions.

Proposition 7.3. *Let R be the rectangle containing a convex polyomino S. The union of the spine with the feet of S is a polyomino having at least one cell in each row and column of R.*

Proof: We assume that P_N is to the left of P_S (i.e., $n_1 \leq s_2$). Let NS be the set of cells (i, j) of R such that $n_1 \leq j \leq s_2$, $V_j \geq H_{i-1}$ and $H_i \geq V_{j-1}$. There are two row indexes d_j and u_j such that:

$$V_j \geq H_{i-1} \text{ for each } i \leq d_j, \text{ and } V_j < H_{d_j}, \tag{7.16}$$

$$H_i \geq V_{j-1} \text{ for each } i \geq u_j, \text{ and } H_{u_j-1} < V_{j-1}. \tag{7.17}$$

Since $V_j \geq H_{i-1}$ and $H_i \geq V_{j-1}$ if and only if $u_j \leq i \leq d_j$, the j-th column of NS is 4-connected and (u_j, j) and (d_j, j) are the upmost and lowest cells of this column, respectively (see fig. 7.14). If $n_1 \leq j+1 \leq s_2$ and d_{j+1}, u_{j+1} are the row indexes related to the $(j+1)$-th column, we have that:

$$H_{u_j-1} < V_{j-1} < V_j \leq H_{u_{j+1}}, \tag{7.18}$$

$$H_{u_{j+1}-1} < V_j < H_{d_j}, \tag{7.19}$$

$$H_{d_j-1} \leq V_j < V_{j+1} < H_{d_{j+1}}. \tag{7.20}$$

It follows that $u_j \leq u_{j+1} \leq d_j \leq d_{j+1}$. Since $u_j \leq d_j$, NS has at least one cell in the j-th column. From $u_j \leq u_{j+1} \leq d_j$ we deduce that NS is a polyomino. Consequently, the set $NS \cup P_N \cup P_S$ is a polyomino having at least one cell in each row of R.

We assume that P_W is to the north of P_E (i.e., $w_1 \leq e_2$). Let WE be the set of cells (i, j) of R such that $w_1 \leq i \leq e_2$, $V_j \geq H_{i-1}$ and $H_i \geq V_{j-1}$. By proceeding in the same way, we can prove that $WE \cup P_W \cup P_E$ is a polyomino having at least one cell in each column of R. From the condition (7.15) it follows that $NS \cup P_N \cup P_S$ and $WE \cup P_W \cup P_E$ have a non-empty intersection. The spine S_p is equal to $NS \cup WE$ and so the set $S_p \cup P_N \cup P_S \cup P_W \cup P_E$ is a polyomino having at least one cell in each row and column of R. We proceed in the same way with all the other cases. $\qquad \square$

The reader can check this property by using H_i and V_j shown in Fig. 7.14.

7.4.3   The reconstruction algorithm

In this section, we define a greedy algorithm that decides whether or not
there is a convex polyomino S satisfying a pair of assigned vectors (H, V).
The first step of the algorithm is to check if (H, V) verifies the condition (7.1). If so, we go on to construct the feet of S. The algorithm chooses
a position of the four feet so that condition (7.15) is satisfied. In this case, we
say that the four feet determine an *allowed foot configuration*. P_N is made
up of h_1 columns and so it can have $n - h_1 + 1$ possible positions. The number of possible positions for P_S, P_W and P_E is equal to $n - h_m + 1, m - v_1 + 1$
and $m - v_n + 1$, and, therefore, the number of allowed foot configurations is
not greater than $(n - h_1 + 1)(n - h_m + 1)(m - v_1 + 1)(m - v_n + 1) \leq n^2 m^2$.
Moreover, to decide if a foot position is an allowed foot configuration involves a computational cost of $O(n + m)$.

Let Q be an allowed foot configuration. We attempt to construct a convex
polyomino S satisfying (H, V) and such that $Q \subseteq S$. We call *kernel* any set
α of cells such that $Q \subseteq \alpha \subseteq S$, and we call *shell* any set β of cells such that
$S \subseteq \beta \subseteq R$, where R is the rectangle containing S. Assuming that $\alpha := Q$
and $\beta := R$, the basic idea of the algorithm consists in reducing the shell
and expanding the kernel by means of some operations. If S exists, the
reconstruction algorithm stops when $\alpha = S = \beta$. If S does not exist, the
reconstruction fails, that is, the operations produce a kernel α and a shell β
such that $\alpha \not\subseteq \beta$. In this case, there is no convex polyomino having its feet in
position Q that satisfies (H, V), and so the algorithm is performed starting
from another allowed foot configuration. Since we know the position of the
four feet of S, we can determine the spine S_p by means of (H, V). From
Proposition 7.2 it follows that $S_p \subseteq S$, and so we can expand the kernel
by putting S_p into α (i.e., $\alpha := \alpha \cup S_p$). The operation of determining
S_p from the known foot position is called *partial sum operation* and its
computational cost is $O(nm)$. Moreover, from Proposition 7.3 we deduce
that α is a polyomino having at least one cell in each column and row of R.
We now determine a further expansion of kernel and reduction of shell by
means of *filling operations* that take advantage of the convexity constraints.

The filling operations

Let us define the filling operations on the rows. We introduce the following
notations:

- R_i, α_i, β_i indicate the i-th row of R, the cells of α and β belonging to
  the i-th row of R, respectively (i.e., $\alpha_i = \alpha \cap R_i$ and $\beta_i = \beta \cap R_i$).

- $l(\alpha_i) = \min\{j \mid (i, j) \in \alpha_i, \ 1 \leq j \leq n\}$ and $r(\alpha_i) = \max\{j \mid (i, j) \in$
  $\alpha_i, \ 1 \leq j \leq n\}$ (i.e., $(i, l(\alpha_i))$ and $(i, r(\alpha_i))$ are the leftmost and
  rightmost cells in α_i, respectively).

Since there is at least one cell of α in each row of R, we have $\alpha_i \neq \emptyset$. There
are two kinds of filling operations: *connecting* and *coherence operations*.

Kernel expansion connecting operation $\oplus$ *on* R_i

$$\oplus(\alpha_i) = \{(i,j) \mid l(\alpha_i) \le j \le r(\alpha_i)\}.$$

Kernel expansion coherence operation $\otimes$ *on* R_i

If β_i is 4-connected (i.e., $\beta_i = \{(i,j) \mid j_1 \le j \le j_2\}$ for some j_1 and j_2), then $\otimes(\alpha_i) = \alpha_i \cup \{(i,j) \mid l(\alpha_i) \le j \le j_1 + h_i - 1$ or $j_2 - h_i + 1 \le j \le r(\alpha_i)\}$; else $\otimes(\alpha_i) = \alpha_i$.

Shell reduction connecting operation $\ominus$ *on* R_i

Let $(i,k) \notin \beta_i$. If $k < l(\alpha_i)$, we get $\ominus(\beta_i) = \beta_i - \{(i,j) \mid j \le k\}$, while if $k > r(\alpha_i)$, we get $\ominus(\beta_i) = \beta_i - \{(i,j) \mid j \ge k\}$.

Shell reduction coherence operation $\odot$ *on* R_i

$$\odot(\beta_i) = \beta_i - \{(i,j) \mid j \le r(\alpha_i) - h_i \text{ or } j \ge l(\alpha_i) + h_i\}.$$

The filling operations on the columns are defined analogously. Figure 7.16 shows a row on which the filling operations are performed. We assume that the cells inserted in the kernel by $\oplus$ and $\otimes$ are dark gray-colored, while the cells eliminated from the shell by $\ominus$ and $\odot$ are light gray-colored.

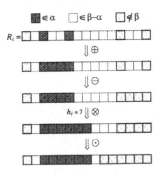

FIGURE 7.16. An example of using the filling operations.

The algorithm performs the filling operations on rows and columns in the following order $\oplus, \ominus, \otimes, \odot$ and sets $\alpha := \oplus(\alpha), \beta := \ominus(\beta), \alpha := \otimes(\alpha)$ and $\beta := \odot(\beta)$ at each row or column. If there is a convex polyomino S that satisfies (H,V) and such that $Q \subseteq S$, by performing the filling operations on rows and columns we obtain α and β such that: $Q \subseteq \alpha \subseteq S \subseteq \beta \subseteq R$. Therefore, if by performing the filling operations we obtain $\alpha \not\subseteq \beta$ (i.e., the cells put into the kernel by $\oplus$ and $\otimes$ do not belong to the shell or the cells eliminated from the shell by $\ominus$ and $\odot$ belong to the kernel), there is no convex polyomino S that satisfies (H,V) and such that $Q \subseteq S$. In this case, the attempts to reconstruct fail and the algorithm stops, chooses a different allowed foot configuration and repeats the whole procedure on this new foot position. If the previous situation does not occur, the algorithm produces α and β such that $\alpha \subseteq \beta$ and they cannot be further changed by the filling operations. We are going to prove that α and β are two convex polyominoes. We know that there is at least one cell of α in each row and column of R and so it is easy to prove that:

Proposition 7.4.   *Let us perform the filling operations on R_i in the following order:* $\oplus, \ominus, \otimes, \odot$. *If we obtain α_i, β_i such that $\alpha_i \subseteq \beta_i$, then α_i, β_i are invariant with respect to the filling operations and 4-connected, that is:* $\alpha_i = \{(i,j) \,|\, l(\alpha_i) \leq j \leq r(\alpha_i)\}$ *and* $\beta_i = \{(i,j) \,|\, l(\beta_i) \leq j \leq r(\beta_i)\}$. *Moreover:*

$$r(\alpha_i) - l(\beta_i) + 1 = r(\beta_i) - l(\alpha_i) + 1 = h_i. \tag{7.21}$$

The same properties hold when $\oplus, \ominus, \otimes$, and $\odot$ are performed on the columns. In Fig. 7.16, the cells of kernel are $\alpha_i = \{(i,3),(i,6)\}$ and by performing the filling operations, we obtain: $\alpha_i = \{(i,j) \,|\, 3 \leq j \leq 8\}$, $\beta_i = \{(i,j) \,|\, 2 \leq j \leq 9\}$ and $r(\alpha_i) - l(\beta_i) + 1 = r(\beta_i) - l(\alpha_i) + 1 = h_i = 7$. From Proposition 7.3, we deduce that the initial configuration of the kernel (i.e., $\alpha = Q \cup Sp$) is a polyomino having at least one cell in each row and column of R. From Proposition 7.4, it follows that if α and β are invariant with respect to the filling operations and such that $\alpha \subseteq \beta$, the rows and columns of α and β are 4-connected. Consequently, α and β are two convex polyominoes (see Fig. 7.17).

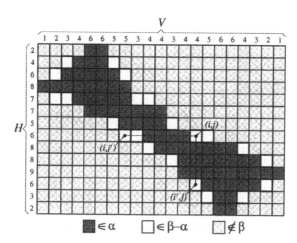

FIGURE 7.17. Invariant α and β with respect to the filling operations and $\alpha \subset \beta$.

Remark 7.2.   *From property (7.21) we have that:*

$$l(\alpha_i) - l(\beta_i) = r(\beta_i) - r(\alpha_i), \tag{7.22}$$

that is, the number of $\beta_i - \alpha_i$ cells on the left of α_i coincides with the number of cells on the right of α_i. Moreover, since $\alpha_i \subseteq \beta_i$, we obtain that:

$$r(\alpha_i) - l(\alpha_i) + 1 \le h_i \le r(\beta_i) - l(\beta_i) + 1. \tag{7.23}$$

In the example of Fig. 7.16, we have $l(\alpha_i) - l(\beta_i) = r(\beta_i) - r(\alpha_i) = 1$ and $6 \le h_i \le 8$.

We now want to calculate the time required for constructing α and β invariant with respect to the filling operations. The algorithm performs the four operations on all the rows and columns of R and repeats this procedure until α and β cannot undergo any further changes. Performing $\oplus, \ominus, \otimes$, and $\odot$ on a row (column) involves a constant computational cost. Therefore, every time these operations are performed on all the rows and columns, $O(n + m)$ operations are performed. The procedure is repeated less than nm times because it always inserts at least one cell in α or eliminates at least one cell from β. Since the number of cells of R is equal to nm, the procedure cannot be repeated more than nm times. Consequently, α and β are constructed in time $O(nm(n + m))$. In case of failure, that is, the algorithm generates α and β such that $\alpha \not\subseteq \beta$, the computational cost is still $O(nm(n + m))$.

2-Satisfiability problem

Let us assume that the algorithm produce a kernel α and a shell β invariant with respect to the filling operations and such that $\alpha \subseteq \beta$.

If $\alpha = \beta$, then α is a convex polyomino satisfying (H, V) and so $S = \alpha$.

Example 7.1.   Let (H, V) be the pair of vectors in Fig 7.14. We choose the following foot configuration: P_N is in columns $\{4, 5\}$, P_W is in rows $\{3, 4, 5\}$, P_S is in column $\{16\}$ and P_E is in row $\{11\}$. By performing the partial sum operation and the filling operations, we obtain α and β that cannot be further changed by these operations and such that: $\alpha = \beta$. Therefore, we get a convex polyomino $S = \alpha$ that satisfies (H, V).

If $\alpha \subset \beta$, then $\beta - \alpha \ne \emptyset$ (see Fig. 7.17). In this case, $\beta - \alpha$ is a set of *indeterminated cells* and we are not yet able to say that there is a convex polyomino S that satisfies (H, V). In fact, Figs. 7.17 and 7.18 show two pairs of vectors from which we obtain α and β invariant with respect to the filling operations and $\alpha \subset \beta$. A convex polyomino satisfying the pair in Fig. 7.17 does not exist, and there are two convex polyominoes satisfying the pair in Fig. 7.18. Therefore, in order to establish the existence of S, another operation has to be performed. We define *evaluation v* of $\beta - \alpha$ as a coloring of the indeterminated cells such that every cell of $\beta - \alpha$ is dark or light gray; we denote $v(\alpha)$ the new kernel obtained. Determining the existence of S is thus linked to determining the existence of an evaluation

v of $\beta - \alpha$ for which $v(\alpha)$ is a convex polyomino that satisfies (H, V). We know that α and β are two convex polyominoes. From Proposition 7.4, we can easily deduce that:

Corollary 7.1. *Let α and β be invariant with respect to the filling operations and such that $\alpha \subset \beta$. Assuming that $(i, j) \in \beta_i - \alpha_i$, we have:*

- *if $l(\beta_i) \leq j \leq l(\alpha_i) - 1$, then $(i, j + h_i) \in \beta_i - \alpha_i$,*

- *if $r(\alpha_i) + 1 \leq j \leq r(\beta_i)$, then $(i, j - h_i) \in \beta_i - \alpha_i$.*

Let $(i, j) \in \beta_i - \alpha_i$, with $l(\beta_i) \leq j < l(\alpha_i)$. From Corollary 7.1, it follows that $(i, j+h_i) \in \beta_i - \alpha_i$. If cell (i, j) become dark (light) gray, by performing the coherence operations on R_i, the cell $(i, j + h_i)$ become light (dark) gray. For example, if the cell $(i, 2)$ of the row in Fig. 7.16 become dark gray, the cell $(i, 9)$ has to be light gray. The same holds for the columns. Therefore, there is a relationship between the indeterminated cells caused by the coherence operations. If $(i, j) \in \beta - \alpha$, there are two cells $(i, j'), (i', j) \in \beta - \alpha$ such that $|j - j'| = h_i, |i - i'| = v_j$. If (i, j) is dark (light) gray, $(i, j'), (i', j)$ are light (dark) gray. The reader can check this property by using α and β in Fig. 7.17. This similarity allows us to introduce the following definition. We call *graph on $\beta - \alpha$* the graph $G = (V, E)$ such that:

- $V = \beta - \alpha$,

- $((i, j), (i', j')) \in E$ iff $(i = i'$ and $|j - j'| = h_i)$ or $(j = j'$ and $|i - i'| = v_j)$.

G is a graph whose vertices are the indeterminated cells and:

    - the degree of each vertex is equal to 2,
    - if $((i, j), (i', j')) \in E$, then $(i, j) \neq (i', j')$;
    - every component of G contains an even number of vertices.

Therefore, G is a cycle or a union of disjoint cycles, each of which contains at least 4 vertices. Fig. 7.18 shows an example of graph on $\beta - \alpha$ made up of three disjoint cycles. Determining a cycle in G requires a linear time with respect to the number of its vertices. Since the cycles are disjoint, the time required for constructing G is $O(nm)$. Every vertex of the graph is a cell of $\beta - \alpha$ that can be colored dark or light gray and so the vertex can assume two different states. We can say that $(i, j) \in V$ has value "1" or "0" depending on how (i, j) is colored. We assume that 1 (0) is for the dark (light) gray. If $(i, j) \in V$ has value $x \in \{0, 1\}$, the values of the vertices belonging to the cycle containing (i, j) are univocally determined by x. In fact, if $((i, j), (i', j))$ and $((i, j), (i, j')) \in E$, the value of (i', j) and (i, j') is $\bar{x}$. Consequently, a cycle in G can only assume two states and the number of vertices having value "1" is equal to the number of vertices having

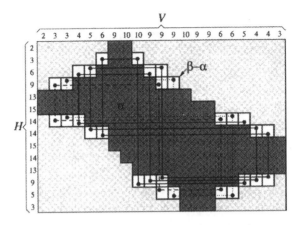

FIGURE 7.18. Graph on $\beta - \alpha$ made up of three disjoint cycles.

value "0". We indicate the cycles of G by $\{(V_1, E_1), (V_2, E_2), \ldots, (V_k, E_k)\}$. Assuming that $(i, j) \in V_h$, we label the cell with the Boolean variable x_h and, starting out from (i, j), we go cross the cycle labelling the vertices x_h or $\bar{x}_h$, according to whether the number of edges between the corresponding vertex and (i, j) is even or odd. The labelling can be done during the construction of the graph (see Fig. 7.19). By assigning some values to

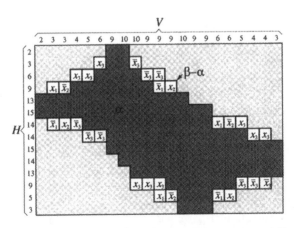

FIGURE 7.19. Possible states of the cycles of G.

the Boolean variables $x_1, x_2, \ldots, x_k$, we obtain an evaluation of the cycles because each assignment determines the state of a cycle. An evaluation of the cycles coincides with an evaluation v of $\beta - \alpha$ and it therefore originates a kernel $v(\alpha)$ that satisfies (H, V). Therefore:

Proposition 7.5.   *There is a convex polyomino S that satisfies (H, V) and such that $Q \subset S$ if and only if there is an evaluation v of the cycles of G for* *which $v(\alpha)$ is a convex polyomino.*

Consequently, determining the existence of S is linked to determining an evaluation v such that the rows and columns of α are 4-connected. Let us now take the following set of indeterminated cells into consideration.

$$W(\beta - \alpha) = \{(i,j) \in \beta - \alpha \mid 1 \le i \le m, \ l(\beta_i) \le j \le l(\alpha_i)\}. \qquad (7.24)$$

This set is made up of the cells in $\beta - \alpha$ that are to the west of P_N and P_S. Let R_i be a row containing cells of $W(\beta - \alpha)$. The number of cells in $W(\beta_i - \alpha_i)$ is $p = l(\alpha_i) - l(\beta_i)$. Let us cross over R_i from left to right and denote the Boolean variables associated to the cells of $W(\beta_i - \alpha_i)$ by $Z = (z_1, z_2, \ldots, z_p)$, where $z_i \in \{x_1, \bar{x}_1, \ldots, x_k, \bar{x}_k\}$. An evaluation v of the cycles of G determines an evaluation of Z and therefore of $W(\beta_i - \alpha_i)$. The evaluation v originates a connected row $v(\alpha_i)$ if and only if there is an integer $q \in \{1, \ldots, (p+1)\}$ such that:

$$z_h = \begin{cases} 0 & \text{if } h < q \\ 1 & \text{if } h \ge q \end{cases} \qquad (7.25)$$

If this condition holds, then v labels the cells in $W(\beta_i - \alpha_i)$ as follows:

$$R_i = 0 \ldots 0 \, z_1 \ldots z_{q-1} z_q \ldots z_p \, 1 \ldots 1 \, \bar{z}_1 \ldots \bar{z}_{q-1} \bar{z}_q \ldots \bar{z}_p \, 0 \ldots 0,$$
$$v(R_i) = 0 \ldots 0 \, 0 \ldots 0 \, 1 \ldots 1 \, 1 \ldots 1 \, 1 \ldots 1 \, 0 \ldots 0 \, 0 \ldots 0.$$

and therefore $v(\alpha_i)$ is 4-connected. Vice versa, if $v(\alpha_i)$ is 4-connected, the condition (7.25) obviously holds. We say that an evaluation v of the cycles of G is *connected* on R_i if the values assumed by the elements of Z verify the condition (7.25).

Lemma 7.3. *An evaluation v of the cycles of G is connected on R_i if and only if the values assumed by the elements of Z satisfy the following collection F of clauses over X:*

$$F_i = (\bar{z}_1 \vee z_2) \wedge (\bar{z}_2 \vee z_3) \wedge \ldots \wedge (\bar{z}_{p-1} \vee z_p). \qquad (7.26)$$

Proof: Let v be a connected evaluation on R_i. Since the condition (7.25) holds, given clause $\bar{z}_{h-1} \vee z_h$, there are three possibilities:
- if $h < q$, then $z_{h-1} = 0$ and $z_h = 0$,
- if $h = q$, then $z_{h-1} = 0$ and $z_h = 1$,
- if $h > q$, then $z_{h-1} = 1$ and $z_h = 1$.
In each case, $\bar{z}_{h-1} \vee z_h$ is equal to 1 and so F is equal to 1.
   Vice versa, if the values of the elements of Z satisfy F, $\bar{z}_{h-1} \vee z_h = 1$ for each $h \in \{2, \ldots, p\}$. If the evaluation v is not connected on R_i, there is at least one $q \in \{2, \ldots, p\}$ such that $z_{q-1} = 1$ and $z_q = 0$. But this means that $\bar{z}_{q-1} \vee z_q = 0$, and so v is connected on R_i. $\qquad \square$

By using the same procedure for the columns we determine a clause collection C over $X = \{x_1, x_2, \ldots, x_k\}$ made up of clauses containing two
variables. Therefore, if the kernel and the shell obtained by the filling operations are such that $\alpha \subset \beta$, the problem of determining the existence
of a convex polyomino that satisfies (H, V) is linked to the 2-Satisfiability
problem (also referred to as 2SAT [17]). The 2SAT problem can be solved
in linear time with respect to the number of clauses of C and variables of
X (see [20]). The number of variables of X coincides with the number of
cycles of G and is therefore less than $nm/4$. The number of clauses of F^i
is less than $n/2$ and so the number of clauses of C is less than nm. As a
result, the time needed to find out if there is an assignment of values to the
variables of X that satisfies C is less than $O(nm)$. Moreover, the number of
operations needed for constructing C is less than nm. Therefore, if we start
out with α and β invariant with respect to the filling operations and $\alpha \subset \beta$,
then we can find out if (H, V) is satisfiable in (p, h, v) in time $O(nm)$.

As a summary we can describe the reconstruction algorithm as follows.

Input: Two vectors $H \in \mathbb{N}^m$, $V \in \mathbb{N}^n$;
Output: a convex polyomino that satisfies (H, V) **or** a message that
there is no such set;
1. check if (H, V) verifies the condition (7.1);
2. compute H_i, V_j for $i = 1, \ldots, m$ and $j = 1, \ldots, n$;
3. repeat
        3.1. choose an allowed foot configuration getting Q;
        3.2. $\alpha := Q$;
        3.3. perform partial sum operation;
        3.4. $\alpha := \alpha \cup S_p$;
        3.5. $\beta := R$;
        3.6. repeat
                3.6.1. perform the filling operations;
        until $\alpha \not\subset \beta$ **or** α, β are invariants;
        3.7. if $\alpha = \beta$ **then** $S = \alpha$ is a solution;
        3.8. if $\alpha \subset \beta$ **then** link our problem to **2SAT**;
until there is a convex polyomino S that satisfies (H, V) **or** all the
foot configurations have been examined.

In this algorithm, we have to examine all the allowed foot configurations
at most (i.e., $O(n^2 m^2)$ positions). Performing the partial sums operation
on the columns and rows involves a computational cost of $O(nm)$. The
complexity of the filling operations procedure is $O(nm(n+m))$. If necessary,
we link our problem to 2SAT problem and the complexity of this procedure
is $O(nm)$. Consequently:

Theorem 7.6.   *RSHVP on (p, h, v) can be solved in time $O(n^3 m^3 (n + m))$.*

Acknowledgments

The authors would like to thank E. Barcucci and R. Pinzani for their helpful discussions.

References

[1] A. R. Shliferstein and Y. T. Chien, "Switching components and the ambiguity problem in the reconstruction of pictures from their projections," *Pattern Recognition* **10**, 327-340 (1978).

[2] R. W. Irving and M. R. Jerrum, "Three-dimensional statistical data security problems," *SIAM Journal of Computing* **23**, 170-184 (1994).

[3] G. P. M. Prause and D. G. W. Onnasch, "Binary reconstruction of the heart chambers from biplane angiographic image sequence," *IEEE Trans. Medical Imaging* **15**, 532-559 (1996).

[4] R. P. Anstee, "Invariant sets of arcs in network flow problems," *Discrete Applied Mathematics* **13**, 1-7 (1986).

[5] P. Fishburn, P. Schwander, L. Shepp, and R. J. Vanderbei, "The discrete Radon transform and its approximate inversion via linear programming," *Discrete Applied Mathematics* **75**, 39-61 (1997).

[6] R. J. Gardner, P. Gritzmann, and D. Prangenberg, "On the computational complexity of reconstructing lattice sets from their X-rays," *Technical Report 970.05012, Techn. Univ. München, Fak. f. Math., München*, (1997).

[7] C. Kisielowski, P. Schwander, F. H. Baumann, M. Seibt, Y. Kim, and A. Ourmazd, "An approach to quantitative high-resolution transmission electron microscopy of crystalline materials," *Ultramicroscopy* **58**, 131-155 (1995).

[8] P. Schwander, C. Kisielowski, M. Seibt, F. H. Baumann, Y. Kim, and A. Ourmazd, "Mapping projected potential, interfacial roughness, and composition in general crystalline solids by quantitative transmission electron microscopy," *Physical Review Letters* **71**, 4150-4153 (1993).

[9] H. J. Ryser, "Combinatorial properties of matrices of zeros and ones," *Canad. J. Math.* **9**, 371-377 (1957).

[10] S. K. Chang, "The reconstruction of binary patterns from their projections," *Communications ACM* **14**, 21-24 (1971).

[11] R. A. Brualdi, "Matrices of zeros and ones with fixed row and column sum vectors," *Linear Algebra and Applications* **33**, 159-231 (1980).

[12] A. Del Lungo, "Polyominoes defined by two vectors," *Theoretical Computer Science* **127**, 187-198 (1994).

[13] A. Kuba, "The reconstruction of two-directionally connected binary patterns from their two orthogonal projections," *Computer Vision, Graphics, and Image Processing* **27**, 249-265 (1984).

[14] S. K. Chang and C. K. Chow, "The reconstruction of three-dimensional objects from two orthogonal projections and its application to cardiac cineangiography," *IEEE Trans. on Computers* **22**, 18-28 (1973).

[15] S. W. Golomb, *Polyominoes*, Revised and Expanded Edition, (Princeton University Press, Princeton, NJ), 1994.

[16] E. Barcucci, A. Del Lungo, M. Nivat, and R. Pinzani, "Reconstructing convex polyominoes from horizontal and vertical projections," *Theoretical Computer Science* **155**, 321-347 (1996).

[17] M. R. Garey and D.S. Johnson, *Computers and intractability: A guide to the theory of NP-completeness*, (Freeman, New York), 1979.

[18] G. J. Woeginger, "The reconstruction of polyominoes from their orthogonal projections," *Technical Report SFB-65, TU Graz, Graz* (1996).

[19] E. Barcucci, A. Del Lungo, M. Nivat, and R. Pinzani, "Medians of polyominoes: a property for the reconstruction," *International Journal of Imaging Systems and Technology* **8**, 69-77 (1998).

[20] B. Aspvall, M. F. Plass, and R. E. Tarjan, "A linear-time algorithm for testing the truth of certain quantified Boolean formulas," *Information Processing Letters* **8**, 121-123 (1979).

Part II

Algorithms

Chapter 8

Binary Tomography Using Gibbs Priors

Samuel Matej[1]
Avi Vardi[2]
Gabor T. Herman[3]
Eilat Vardi[4]

ABSTRACT   The problem of reconstructing a binary image (usually an image in the plane and not necessarily on a Cartesian grid) from a few projections translates into the problem of solving a system of equations, which is very underdetermined and leads in general to a large class of solutions. It is desirable to limit the class of possible solutions, by using appropriate prior information, to only those which are reasonably typical of the class of images which contains the unknown image that we wish to reconstruct. One may indeed pose the following hypothesis: if the image is a typical member of a class of images having a certain distribution, then by using this information we can limit the class of possible solutions to only those which are close to the given unknown image. This hypothesis is experimentally validated for the specific case of a class of binary images defined on the hexagonal grid, where the probability of the occurrence of a particular image of the class is determined by a Gibbs distribution and reconstruction is to be done from the three natural projections. Another case for which the hypothesis is tested is reconstruction, from the three projections, of semiconductor surface phantoms defined on the square grid. The time-consuming nature of the stochastic reconstruction algorithm is ameliorated by a preprocessing step that discovers image locations at which the value is the same in all images having the given projections; this reduces the search space considerably. We discuss, in particular, a linear-programming approach to finding such "invariant" locations.

[1]University of Pennsylvania, Department of Radiology, Medical Image Processing Group, Blockley Hall, Fourth Floor, 423 Guardian Drive, Philadelphia, PA 19104-6021, USA, E-mail: matej@mipg.upenn.edu

[2]SAS Institute, R4218, Cary, NC 27513, USA, E-mail: avvard@wnt.sas.com

[3]University of Pennsylvania, Department of Radiology, Medical Image Processing Group, Blockley Hall, Fourth Floor, 423 Guardian Drive, Philadelphia, PA 19104-6021, USA, E-mail: gabor@mipg.upenn.edu

[4]Technion - Technical Institute of Israel, P.O. Box 41, Haifa 32000, Israel, E-mail: seilat@techst02.technion.ac.il

8.1   Introduction

It is typical of many *binary tomography* applications that only a few projections are available [1, 2]. The corresponding system of equations is very underdetermined and leads typically to a large class of solutions. It is desirable to reduce the class of possible solutions to only those that are reasonably "close" to the unknown measured/scanned image. Appropriate prior information on the image may be useful for this task [3]. In addition to the inherent information in binary tomography that there are only two possible values, *Gibbs priors* [4, 5] describing the local behavior/character of the image can also provide useful information. We pose the hypothesis that, for certain *Gibbs distributions*, knowledge that the image is a random element from the distribution is sufficient for limiting the class of possible solutions to only those that are close to the given unknown image.

Binary images can be described in many applications by the following simplified characterization: a set of *objects* — "white" regions of similar shapes — are located in a "black" background. (We adopt the convention that 1 represents white and 0 represents black.) This can be easily translated into Gibbs distributions by using a set of configurations of neighboring image elements and assigning a value (an indicator of the likelihood of occurrence) to each of these configurations. The most natural configurations for the aforementioned characterization are small uniform groups of black or white image elements, together with configurations containing edges and corners. Each Gibbs distribution produces a class of images: randomly selected members of the class will have certain similarities to each other (e.g., they will contain a similar number of objects, which are of similar size and "convexity"). A sample image from a given Gibbs distribution can be generated using the Metropolis algorithm [4, 6].

The most natural tessellation of the plane for the case of three projections is the one into identical hexagons. Since an affine transformation of the plane will insure that the three lines for which the projections are known are at 60° to each other and that the sampling distance on each line is the same; we may assume that the tessellation of the plane is into regular hexagons and that the projections are sampled so that each hexagon contributes to one and only one of the sampled values of each projection and the line to whose integral it contributes goes through the center of the hexagon. The collection of all such hexagon centers is referred to as the hexagonal grid (see Fig. 3.1).

For images defined on the hexagonal grid, the description of a Gibbs distribution can be done in a straightforward way. In the hexagonal grid, an image is composed of picture elements of hexagonal shape (*hexels*). Every hexel has six neighbors and is sharing with each of them one side; thus the abovementioned "configurations" consist of the various possible arrangements of the six black and white neighbors of a black or white hexel.

In our work the image is defined to be spatially limited to a large hexagonal support, but in principle the image support can be of any shape. The hexagonal grid has three natural projections that are at 60° to each other. A projection is defined as a data set, which for every line (in a set of parallel lines each of which goes through hexel centers and is perpendicular to hexel sides), tells us how many white hexels are intersected by that line. This information needs to be specified only for those lines that intersect the support of the image. In this chapter we are testing the posed hypothesis for the reconstruction of binary images defined on the hexagonal grid from the three natural projections.

Another type of test presented in this chapter is motivated by the task of reconstructing semiconductor surface layers from a few projections. Fishburn *et al.* [2] designed three test phantoms, defined on the square grid, for assessing the suitability of binary tomography for this task. These phantoms have been recently used in the binary tomography literature by the several other researchers (see, e.g., [7] and other chapters in this book). The common experience reported by these researchers is that knowing the horizontal, vertical and one diagonal projection is not sufficient for exact recovery of such phantoms. In this chapter we show that our algorithm, which makes use of an appropriate Gibbs prior, correctly recovers the test phantoms of [2] from these three projections.

The following section introduces Gibbs distributions, discusses their definition either using a look-up table or using typical configurations on the hexagonal grid, and describes the Metropolis algorithm for sampling such distributions. The reconstruction algorithm based on the given projection data and the Gibbs prior is presented in the third section. The results of the experimental study for images on the hexagonal grid are discussed in the fourth section. The fifth section discusses our approach to finding invariant elements (elements that have the same value in all binary images satisfying the three projections); the purpose of this is to reduce the search space of the time-consuming stochastic reconstruction algorithms. The results of the tests based on the semiconductor surface phantoms defined on the square grid are presented in the sixth section. The final section presents our conclusions.

8.2   Gibbs distributions on the hexagonal grid

Local properties of a given binary image ω defined on H hexels (each hexel is indexed by an integer h, $1 \leq h \leq H$, and $\omega(h)$ is either black or white) can be characterized by a Gibbs distribution of the form

$$\Pi(\omega) = \frac{1}{Z} e^{\beta \sum_{h=1}^{H} I_h(\omega)} , \qquad (8.1)$$

where $\Pi(\omega)$ is the probability of occurrence of the image ω, Z is the normalizing factor, which insures that Π is a probability density function; i.e., that the sum of $\Pi(\omega)$ over all possible binary images is 1, β is a parameter defining the "peakedness" of the Gibbs distribution (this is one of the parameters controlling the appearance of the typical images), and $I_h(\omega)$ is the "local energy function" for the hexel indexed by h, $1 \leq h \leq H$. The local energy function is defined in such a way that it encourages certain local configurations, such as uniform white or black clusters of hexels and configurations forming edges or corners. Each of these configurations can be encouraged to a different extent by assigning to them a specific value. For an image defined on the hexagonal grid we have adopted the convention that the local energy function at a hexel depends only on its color and those of its six neighbors. Thus, the color of a particular hexel influences only the value of the local energy function of itself and that of its six neighbors.

Appropriate definition of the local energy function plays an important role in successful image recovery. The definition should reflect the characteristics of a typical image of the particular application area. There are many possible ways of defining the local energy function. One of them is to use a look-up table that contains a value for each possible configuration. (In our case, there are 128 possible configurations.) Given an ensemble of typical images for a particular application, the look-up table can be created by counting the number of times each particular configuration appears in the images. The usefulness of the resulting prior depends on the size of this ensemble (the larger, the better) and on how representative the images in the ensemble are for the application area. (An example of this approach applied to the reconstruction of images defined on the square grid is presented in Section 8.6). Another way of defining the local energy function is based on predefining an image model containing several free parameters characterizing specific image features. Values of the free parameters can be determined as those that best experimentally fit an ensemble of typical images of the particular application area.

To demonstrate the ideas of this chapter we have chosen a particular image model by considering only the following features: convex white corners, edges, uniform black regions and uniform white regions. This model is sufficient for many, but clearly not for all, classes of binary images. For our chosen model, the local energy at hexel h can be calculated by inspecting its neighbors in a cyclical (e.g., clockwise) order. The local energy function $I_h(\omega)$ is defined to have one of following values:

k_1 – for convex white corner – the hexel h is white and three consecutive neighbors are white (the rest are black) or the hexel h is black and five consecutive neighbors are black;

k_2 – for edge – four of consecutive neighbors are of the same color as the hexel h;

k_3 – for uniform black region – h and all its neighbors are black;

k_4 – for uniform white region – h and all its neighbors are white;

0 – otherwise,

where k_i are specific constants (parameters) characterizing (together with the parameter β) the particular Gibbs distribution. For the purpose of defining the local energy for those hexels that are at the image boundary, the image is considered to be surrounded by black background hexels. We adopt the convention of specifying a particular Gibbs distribution as $k_1\_k_2\_k_3\_k_4\_b$ (e.g., 4_12_12_12_1.21), where $b = e^{\beta}$. Four examples of random images from different Gibbs distributions are shown in Fig. 8.1. We have observed that, unless k_3 and k_4 are equal, it is hard to define a distribution whose typical images have some large features without being almost totally black or white. Parameter k_1, which controls the number of convex white vertices, has an influence on the size of the image objects. Obviously, k_2 controls the "edginess" of the image. For example, the only difference in the parameters for the two bottom images in Fig. 8.1 is in k_2; giving a higher value to it on the left indeed results in a more "edgy" image.

A sample image from a given Gibbs distribution can be generated using a sufficiently long run of the Metropolis algorithm [4]; see also Subsection 3.1.3, of this book. In one step of this algorithm a random hexel from the image ω_1 is selected and its color is inverted, resulting in the image ω_2. The algorithm then explores the resulting change in the image probability, based on the given Gibbs distribution. The fact that we are interested only in the change of the probability, and not in its actual value, makes the calculations practically possible (the calculation of the coefficient Z, which is eliminated by this, would require an extremely long time). Another substantial simplification is due to the fact that the change of one hexel at index h_1 influences the local energy values only in the set $N(h_1)$, which contains itself and its six neighbors. Consequently, the change of the probability has to be calculated only over the seven hexels $h \in N(h_1)$. The change of the image probability is calculated as the ratio

$$p = \frac{\Pi(\omega_2)}{\Pi(\omega_1)} = b^{\sum_{h \in N(h_1)} [I_h(\omega_2) - I_h(\omega_1)]} . \tag{8.2}$$

If $p \geq 1$ then the algorithm accepts the image ω_2, otherwise the change is accepted with probability p (and, hence, the image ω_1 is retained with probability $1 - p$). This algorithm samples (in the limit) the distribution Π (see, e.g., [4, Chapter 8]).

8.3   Reconstruction algorithms

Assume that we are given the three natural projections of a hexagonal image, which is a sample from a known Gibbs distribution. (In our experimental study the known Gibbs prior is used for the sample image generation.) Then, a reconstruction algorithm for finding an image consistent with the data in the three projections (i.e., a *feasible image*) can be expanded by the

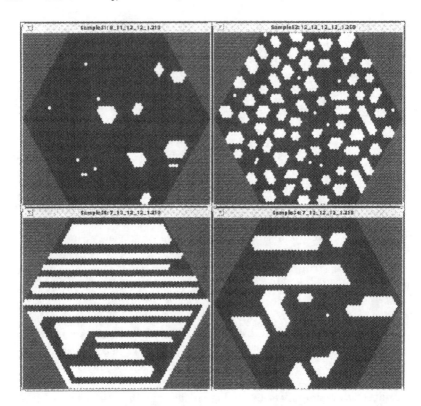

FIGURE 8.1. Examples showing random images from different Gibbs distributions using parameters: 9_11_12_12_1.21 (top-left), 12_12_12_12_1.25 (top-right), 7_13_12_12_1.21 (bottom-left), 7_12_12_12_1.21 (bottom-right). (Note that the only difference in the parameters for the two bottom images is in the "edge" parameter k_2; giving a higher value to it on the left indeed results in a more "edgy" image.)

additional requirement that the reconstructed image should also be a typical sample from the given Gibbs distribution. We use a modified Metropolis algorithm in which the search for a likely image is altered to take also into account the effect of replacing ω_1 by ω_2 on the consistency with the given projection data. Roughly speaking, if the data inconsistency is increased or decreased, then the change is discouraged or encouraged, respectively. The relative influence of the data inconsistency is controlled by a parameter α ($\alpha \geq 0$). To be exact, the Metropolis algorithm is modified by replacing in each step the p of (8.2) by

$$p' = b\left\{\sum_{h \in N(h_1)}[I_h(\omega_2) - I_h(\omega_1)]\right\} - \alpha\left\{F_{h_1}(\omega_2) - F_{h_1}(\omega_1)\right\}, \qquad (8.3)$$

where

$$F_{h_1}(\omega) = |d_{h_1}(\omega) - m_{h_1}|, \qquad (8.4)$$

$$d_{h_1}(\omega) = \sum_{i=1}^{3} d_{h_1}^i(\omega), \tag{8.5}$$

$$m_{h_1} = \sum_{i=1}^{3} m_{h_1}^i, \tag{8.6}$$

$d_{h_1}^i(\omega)$ is the number of white hexels in image ω on the line going in the direction i through the hexel h_1 and $m_{h_1}^i$ is the value of the corresponding item in the given projection data.

Additional information for reconstruction algorithms can be derived from the so-called *invariant hexels*. A hexel is invariant if it has a unique color in all feasible images. We implemented a computationally very inexpensive approach that finds (for the image class used in our study) sufficiently many invariant hexels for the successful recovery of images from projection data. We refer to this as the *brute force approach*; in a later section we discuss a more sophisticated approach (involving linear programming) for finding additional invariant hexels. The projection data are the input to the brute force approach. Initially the image is totally black and all hexels are considered free (i.e., not yet prescribed). The brute force approach repeatedly cycles through the data (lines and projections), at each step updating the image as follows:

- if in the current image the number of white hexels on the given line matches that in the projection data, then all free hexels on that line are prescribed to be black;

- if in the current image the total number of white and free hexels on the given line matches the number of white hexels for that line in the projection data, then all free hexels on that line are prescribed to be white.

This procedure is repeated until no changes are detected for a whole cycle through the data.

Clearly, the hexels, which are prescribed to be black or white by the brute force approach, have to be black or white, respectively, in any feasible image. In our reconstruction algorithms we start with an image in which the prescribed hexels have the appropriate color and in the process of the algorithms the color of a prescribed hexel is not altered.

We refer as **Algorithm 1** to the following procedure. Start with an image in which a random color (black or white) is assigned to the free hexels at the end of the brute force approach. In a typical step, the current image ω_1 is altered by randomly picking one such free hexel and changing its color to obtain the image ω_2. Then ω_2 may, or may not, replace ω_1 as determined by the Metropolis principle with p' defined as in (8.3). Such a procedure is guided preferentially toward images that have relatively large probability, as defined by (8.1), and are at the same time not too inconsistent with the projection data. The procedure is run for a "long time" (see below) and at its termination we select as its output that image from the sequence produced by it which has the maximum probability (8.1).

We observed that Algorithm 1 can get "stuck" at some "local optimum" during the iterative process. This can happen, for example, if the algorithm arrives at a feasible image ω such that the change in any hexel would result in a p' whose value is less than 1 and a large number of hexels would have to be changed in ω to obtain a feasible image ω' such that $\Pi(\omega') > \Pi(\omega)$. (A specific instance of this is illustrated in the next section.) In such a situation Algorithm 1 is likely to remain in the vicinity of ω for extremely many steps; i.e., be stuck for all practical purposes. One possible remedy is to utilize additional prior information, such as information on the typical size of the objects in the image. If such information is available, then the size of the image objects can be tested at regular intervals and those objects which are untypically small can be removed (i.e., all hexels which are in that object are set to black). Similarly, small connected black regions surrounded by white hexels can be removed (by setting all hexels in them to white). This can considerably speed-up the algorithm by making a relatively large change to the image, which in Algorithm 1 could only be achieved by a long sequence of low-probability steps. We refer to the modified Metropolis algorithm with this additional feature as **Algorithm 2**. Its output is specified similarly to that of Algorithm 1.

8.4   Experimental study

In our experimental study we investigated the actual benefit of prior information for binary image reconstruction. The images were defined on the hexagonal grid and were restricted to a hexagon-shaped region with six sides of 30 hexels each; consequently in our experiments $H=2,611$. Since computer displays work with square image rasters, in the displays of our images (such as in Fig. 8.1) the hexels are approximated by a nearly hexagonal-shaped group of raster pixels.

The particular Gibbs parameters were selected based on the following criteria: typical images from the resulting Gibbs distribution should be obtainable within a reasonable time (within 300,000 iterations as described later) and they should contain only a few relatively large objects of reasonable convexity. Sample images from various Gibbs distributions were generated using the Metropolis algorithm. To insure that the algorithm has been run long enough to provide a typical sample of the distribution, we made the following experiment. We initialized the Metropolis algorithm with two different images: with a blank black image and with a completely white image. Then we ran both cases until they both stabilized with images of similar energy, as defined by (8.1), and similar number of white hexels. The process of stabilization takes many iterations, typically more than 100,000, for those Gibbs distributions that resulted in sample images that appeared to us to be reasonably structured in interesting ways (see Fig. 8.1). As a result of the way we implemented the random picking of hexels, the number of steps per iteration of the Metropolis algorithm varies from iteration to iteration. (It is such that, for any free hexel, the probability that the hexel is picked during an iteration is larger than the probability of the alternative.) In general, by decreasing the parameter b the images stabilize faster but have a more chaotic character (due to the less "peaked" nature of the Gibbs distribution). By increasing the value of b, the changes during the Metropolis algorithm appear to be slower and, for a large b, the algorithm has difficulty moving away from the uniform images to a typical sample.

For various sets of Gibbs parameters, the above-described process was repeated several times with different seeds of the random number generator (function *drand48* from the Unix C library). Based on the criteria described above, we selected the Gibbs distribution 4_12_12_12_1.18 for further experiments. For these parameters, we observed that we need 300,000 iterations of the Metropolis algorithm to be confident that the generated images are typical samples from the Gibbs distribution.

For the selected Gibbs distribution we generated 30 sample images to which we refer as "original images." For each original image we calculated the three projections. The brute force approach was sufficient to completely recover the original image in 9 cases. In the remaining 21 cases the behavior of the algorithms was as follows.

In 8 cases Algorithm 1 was completely successful in the sense that it reproduced the original image (or an image that differed from the original only at one hexel) typically within less than 3,000 iterations, at which point the image remained stable. (In all our experiments α was chosen to be 16; this choice results in giving slightly more importance to the desirability of changing the color of an isolated white hexel than to the desirability of improving consistency with the given data for all three projections.) Three examples are depicted in the Fig. 8.2. The original images, which were identical to the resulting images of Algorithm 1 (with the exception of a single hexel difference in the first and third image), are on the left. The starting images (images obtained by the brute force method) are on the right. The black and white regions in the starting images contain prescribed black and white image hexels, respectively. The gray regions are containing hexels for which the brute force method did not indicate invariance and, consequently, in which Algorithm 1 was further applied.

In the remaining 13 cases the original image was not reproduced during 300,000 iterations of Algorithm 1. Furthermore, the probability, as described by (8.1), of each of the images produced by Algorithm 1 was substantially lower than the probability of the original image. To be more exact, we define the energy difference for any of the reconstructions ω_r

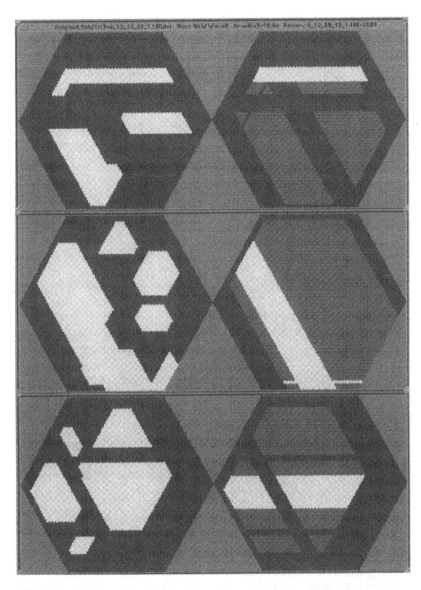

FIGURE 8.2. Three examples of images successfully recovered by Algorithm 1 are shown. The original images, which were essentially identical to the output images of Algorithm 1, appear on the left. The results of the brute force approach, which provided the starting images for Algorithm 1, are represented on the right. The black and white regions contain the hexels prescribed to be black, respectively white, by the brute force approach. The gray regions contain the free hexels; only the free hexels are changed by Algorithm 1.

produced by Algorithm 1, when the original image is ω_o, as

$$\sum_{h=1}^{H}[I_h(\omega_o) - I_h(\omega_r)] \, . \qquad (8.7)$$

In the 13 cases under discussion this number was always positive. Among all the images produced by Algorithm 1, the image ω_r that minimizes (8.7) is its output. In Fig. 8.3 we plot the image difference (the number of hexels at which the output ω_r differs from ω_o) against the energy difference, defined by (8.7). Thus the energy difference is approximately proportional to the image difference. This supports our claim that by increasing the Gibbs probability we get closer to the correct solution. (For the 8 successful cases, both the energy difference and the image difference were zero.)

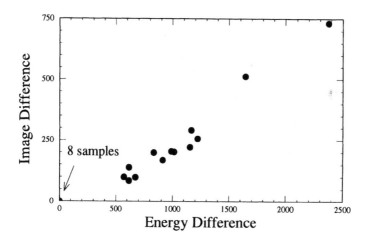

FIGURE 8.3. Correlation between the energy difference, defined by (8.7), and the image difference (the number of hexels at which the reconstruction by Algorithm 1 differs from the original).

Experiments with Algorithm 1 showed a strong correlation between the energy difference and the difference from the original image. However, for the cases in which we were not able to reduce the energy difference to zero, the question remained: would it be possible to get the correct solution by altering the algorithm so that it reduces the energy difference to zero? Algorithm 2 answered this question quite satisfactorily. In our implementation of the algorithm, we checked the sizes of connected regions at every 1,000 iterations. If the number of hexels in a connected white or black region was less than 30 (such a small size would be very atypical for the selected Gibbs prior), then the region was set to the opposite color. We tested this version of Algorithm 2 at least twice (two or three times with different seeds of the random generator) for each of the image samples. Using the algorithm, we were able to essentially recover the original image in all but one case (we obtained either exactly the original image or an image that differed from the original at one hexel). In the single case in which we did not succeed, we were not able to get even close to reducing the energy difference to zero and to recovering the original image; Algorithm 2 with the selected parameters had not enough power to move away from a local optimum. We tested Algorithm 2 also by starting from the image at which Algorithm 1 got stuck. Again, we were able to recover the original image in all but one case. (In one additional case we had to increase the tested region size to 55 to be able to move from the local optimum.)

We observed that the size of the nonprescribed region was the factor influencing the success and speed of the algorithms. In the image that was not recovered by Algorithm 2, only a few hexels along the boundaries of the image were prescribed by the brute force approach.

Examples of three of the cases that were solved, within 300,000 iterations, by Algorithm 2 (but not by Algorithm 1) are in the Fig. 8.4. The images with the minimum energy difference during the execution of Algorithm 1 (small black disks at the energy differences 572, 1220, and 1644 in Fig. 8.3) are on the left and the results of Algorithm 2 are on the right. Two of these images are identical to the original image and one (the first image) differs from the original at one hexel. It is interesting to note that the result of Algorithm 1 shown in the first row on the left is a feasible image; i.e., it satisfies the projection data. The small regions differing from the original image represent a switching set (changing the colors of all of the hexels in the switching set does not change the three natural projections). After this image was obtained by Algorithm 1, it did not have enough power to move from this local optimum. On the other hand, this was obviously a simple task for Algorithm 2.

To summarize, for the 30 random images from the Gibbs distribution 4_12_12_12_1.18, the correct solution was found in 9 cases by the brute force approach, in 8 cases by Algorithm 1, and in 12 cases by Algorithm 2. There was only one case where our approach failed to recover the original image within one hexel difference. We repeated the whole experiment described in this section for another Gibbs distribution, namely 7_13_12_12_1.175 (one whose typical elements tend to have long "edgy" objects, as will be illustrated in the next section). In this case the brute force approach by itself was not sufficient to identify any of the 30 random images, but they were all correctly recovered using our overall approach.

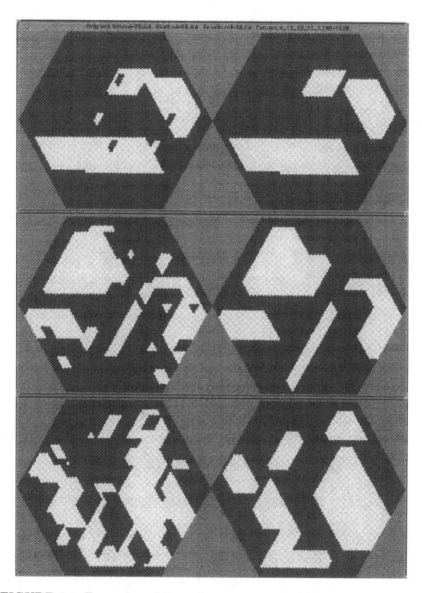

FIGURE 8.4. Examples of three images recovered by the Algorithm 2 are shown on the right. Corresponding minimum energy difference images, as produced by the Algorithm 1, are shown on the left.

8.5   Finding additional invariant elements

Clearly, the finding of invariant elements is a worthwhile endeavor. In the first instance, those are the only elements whose value is definitely determined by the projections; hence their color is the only absolutely reliable information about the unknown binary image. Furthermore, the more invariant elements we find, the smaller is the search space of the stochastic reconstruction algorithms described in the previous sections and, consequently, they are likely to perform more reliably and faster. In this section we introduce a method that can identify elements whose invariance is not discovered by the brute force approach.

Let I be the number of free hexels at the end of the brute force method and let us reindex them by integers i, $1 \leq i \leq I$. We make use of the following notation. For any I-dimensional vector d of 0s and 1s, we use ω_d to denote the image in which the hexels prescribed by the brute force approach have those prescribed values and the ith free hexel is given the value d_i. Let J be the number of integration lines in the projections that contain at least one of these hexels; we index these lines by integers j, $1 \leq j \leq J$.

Let c be a fixed I-dimensional vector of 0s and 1s such that if we assign to each free hexel i the value c_i, then ω_c is a feasible image. (We discuss below how we find such a vector c.) We define $I \times J$ integers as follows: for $1 \leq i \leq I$ and $1 \leq j \leq J$,

$$
m_{i,j} = \begin{cases} 1, & \text{if the } i\text{th free hexel lies on the } j\text{th line and } c_i = 1, \\ -1, & \text{if the } i\text{th free hexel lies on the } j\text{th line and } c_i = 0, \\ 0, & \text{otherwise.} \end{cases}
$$

$$(8.8)$$

Lemma 8.1.   *For any I-dimensional vector d of 0s and 1s such that ω_d is a feasible image, we have that, for $1 \leq j \leq J$,*

$$
\sum_{c_i=1} c_i m_{i,j} - \sum_{c_i=0} c_i m_{i,j} = \sum_{d_i=1} d_i m_{i,j} - \sum_{d_i=0} d_i m_{i,j} \tag{8.9}
$$

(The notation $\sum_{c_i=1}$ indicates summing over those free hexels for which $c_i = 1$.)

Proof: For any line for which projection data are collected, there are three kinds of hexels. Those that are prescribed by the brute force approach are invariant and so must have the same color in the feasible images ω_c and ω_d. For the free hexels the c_i can be 1 (in which case $m_{i,j} = 1$) or the c_i can be 0 (in which case $m_{i,j} = -1$) and so the left side of (8.9) is the contribution of the free hexels in ω_c to the jth line and the right side of (8.9) is the contribution of the free hexels in ω_d to the jth line. Since both ω_c and ω_d are feasible, these contributions must be the same.   □

We call a pair (y, z) of a J-dimensional real-valued vector y and an I-

dimensional real-valued vector z *acceptable* if they satisfy the inequalities:

$$\sum_{j=1}^{J} m_{i,j} y_j + z_i \leq 0, \quad \text{for } 1 \leq i \leq I, \tag{8.10}$$

$$0 \leq z_i \leq 1, \quad \text{for } 1 \leq i \leq I. \tag{8.11}$$

The importance of this concept is due to the following theorem, whose proof is based on some ideas originally presented in [8].

Theorem 8.1. *If (y^*, z^*) is an acceptable pair such that for any acceptable pair (y, z)*

$$\sum_{i=1}^{I} z_i \leq \sum_{i=1}^{I} z_i^* , \tag{8.12}$$

then, for every k for which $z_k^* > 0$, the hexel k is invariant (and hence its value is c_k).

Proof: It follows from (8.10) and (8.11) that

$$\sum_{j=1}^{J} m_{i,j} y_j^* \leq 0, \quad for \ \ 1 \leq i \leq I, \tag{8.13}$$

and, since $z_k^* > 0$, that

$$\sum_{j=1}^{J} m_{k,j} y_j^* < 0 . \tag{8.14}$$

Let d be any I dimensional vector such that ω_d is feasible. We need to show that $d_k = c_k$.

Consider the equality that can be trivially proved to be valid by rearranging its terms:

$$\sum_{c_i=1} \left((c_i - d_i) \sum_{j=1}^{J} m_{i,j} y_j^* \right) + \sum_{c_i=0} \left((d_i - c_i) \sum_{j=1}^{J} m_{i,j} y_j^* \right) =$$
$$\sum_{j=1}^{J} \left(\left[\sum_{c_i=1} c_i m_{i,j} - \sum_{c_i=0} c_i m_{i,j} \right] - \left[\sum_{c_i=1} d_i m_{i,j} - \sum_{c_i=0} d_i m_{i,j} \right] \right) y_j^* . \tag{8.15}$$

The right-hand side of this equation has value 0, since all the terms in the outer sum have value 0 by Lemma 8.1. On the left-hand side, the second item of each product is nonpositive by (8.13) and is negative in case $i = k$ by (8.14). Since the first item of each product on the left-hand side is nonnegative, the sum can only be 0 if $d_k = c_k$.   □

Finding such a (y^*, z^*) can be efficiently done by using linear programming [9]. However, the $m_{i,j}$s of (8.8) are defined in terms of the vector c.

We now discuss how to find the vector c having the desired properties. Clearly, it is sufficient to find any feasible image. We do this by using a tabu search [10], which is a popular heuristic for combinatorial optimization problems.

The tabu search produces a sequence of images; our aim is to produce a feasible image. In all the images, values prescribed by the brute force approach will be retained. Initially, all other hexels are randomly assigned a value of 0 or 1.

For any image ω, we use $S(\omega)$ to denote the sum of the absolute differences between the line integrals in the projection data and the corresponding line integrals for ω. Clearly, ω is feasible if, and only if, $S(\omega)$ is zero. In any single step of the tabu search we first identify that subset of hexels (from the set of hexels that are free at the end of the brute force approach) for which switching the color of that hexel would result in the smallest possible value of $S(\omega)$. (Note that this maybe larger than the value of $S(\omega)$ without switching, since ω maybe such that switching the color of any hexel increases the value of $S(\omega)$.) We select a further subset of this subset of hexels by choosing those that have the highest number of neighbors and are of opposite color. Finally, we randomly select a single hexel from this subset. Switching the color of this hexel appears to be desirable, in the sense that it provides a maximal consistency with the projection data and at the same time aims toward local uniformity, which is a common characteristic of the Gibbs distributions in which we are interested. However, an algorithm consisting of a sequence of such switches is likely to cycle without ever reaching a feasible image.

Tabu search prevents this by the introduction of a so-called *tabu list* into the algorithm. This is a queue of fixed length. We set (based on a small set of preliminary experiments) the queue size to be 43, which is approximately the average number of image hexels in one line. When the color of a hexel is switched during the tabu search, a new entry is put on top of the tabu list (causing an element to be released from its bottom). The element that is entered contains the index of the hexel that has just been switched and the smaller of the values of $S(\omega)$ just before and just after the switch. The effect of the tabu list on the tabu search as described in the previous paragraph is that the color of the selected hexel will not be switched if the index of the hexel is in the tabu list, unless the resulting $S(\omega)$ is smaller than the value stored with that index in the tabu list.

For all the 60 random samples from the two different Gibbs distributions that we have discussed at the end of the last section, tabu search succeeded to find an image consistent with the three natural projections of the sample image. The results of this and the consequent use of linear programming to identify additional invariant hexels is illustrated in Figs. 8.5 and 8.6 for the two Gibbs distributions.

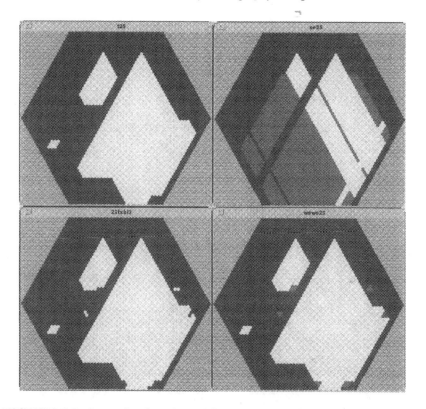

FIGURE 8.5. A randomly selected image from the Gibbs distribution 4_12_12_12_1.18 is shown on the top left. The output of the brute force method is illustrated on the top right, with gray indicating the location of the hexels remaining free at the end of the brute force approach. A feasible image, obtained from the projections using tabu search, is on the bottom left. Additional invariant hexels, both white and black, obtained by linear programming can be seen in the bottom right image.

8.6   Gibbs prior definition using a look-up table

The Gibbs priors can also be obtained based on counting the number of occurrences of each possible local configuration (configuration of picture elements in a small window) in an ensemble of images which are representative for the given application. As discussed in the Section 8.2, the frequency (histogram) of occurrences can be stored in a look-up table. To illustrate this approach we employed the three test phantoms of Fishburn et al. [2] (see Figs. 12.3, 12.4, and 12.5), which are defined on the square grid. The projection data (line sums through the picture element centers) were collected from three views; two orthogonal views along the Cartesian axes in the plane, plus a diagonal view at $45°$ (view of the direction $(1, 1)$

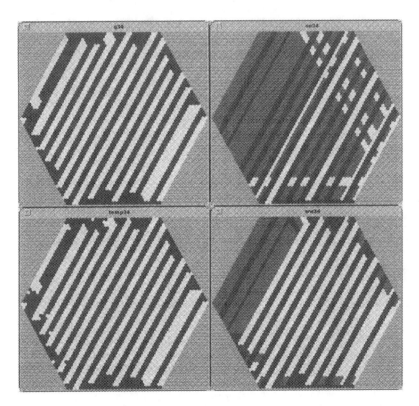

FIGURE 8.6. A randomly selected image from the Gibbs distribution 7_13_12_12_1.175 is shown on the top left. The output of the brute force method is illustrated on the top right, with gray indicating the location of the hexels remaining free at the end of the brute force approach. A feasible image, obtained from the projections using tabu search, is on the bottom left. Additional invariant hexels, both white and black, obtained by linear programming can be seen in the bottom right image.

in [2]) in agreement with other papers in this book. We defined the local area as the 3 × 3 neighborhood of a given pixel, leading to a look-up table having 512 entries. The images used to generate the look-up table were symmetrical versions (around the vertical axis) of the three phantoms. The symmetrical versions were used in order to make this test more realistic; i.e., to avoid using of the same images in the Gibbs prior calculation and in the reconstruction.

The reconstruction was initialized similarly to our previous experiments. The starting images contained randomly generated white (one) and black (zero) pixels in those locations which were not determined by the brute force approach to be invariant, and in the rest of the locations they contained the determined invariant color. Phantom 2 was fully determined by the brute force approach. Consequently, only Phantoms 1 and 3 (Fig. 8.7, top left and bottom left images) were used for the reconstruction tests. Results of the brute force algorithm are shown on the right in the Fig. 8.7, with * representing the undetermined (free) locations in the phantoms.

Images were reconstructed using Algorithm 1 (described in Section 8.3). $I_h(\omega)$ in (8.3) was defined as $\log(q + 1)$, where q represents occurrence frequency (in the ensemble of the representative images) of the given local configuration at the pixel h in the image ω. The value of $\log(q + 1)$ is stored, for each configuration, in the look-up table at the corresponding table address representing the given configuration. The parameters b and α were selected to be $b = 1.40$ and $\alpha = 7.50$, based on a small preliminary study. For both phantoms we were able to find the correct solution (the original image) in a short time. Namely, we needed on average about 50 iterations for Phantom 1 (containing 467 free positions after the brute force algorithm) and about 190 iterations for Phantom 3 (containing 1,013 free pixels). Here, one iteration consists of the K Metropolis tests (tries to change a randomly selected free pixel), where K is the number of free locations in the image. The averages are based on ten random runs of the Algorithm 1. We reemphasize that in each of the random runs the phantom was recovered exactly.

8.7 Conclusions

We have shown how Gibbs priors can be defined and used in binary reconstruction problems when images are defined on the hexagonal or on the square grid. Experimental tests were done for the case when data are known for three projections. A modified Metropolis algorithm based on the known Gibbs prior proved to provide a good tool to move the reconstruction process toward the correct solution when the projection data by themselves were not sufficient to find such a solution. However, sometimes this algorithm got stuck at a local optimum and, in such cases, more complex techniques (using additional prior information such as the typical size of the objects) are needed. Our experiments suggest that if an algorithm is able to maximize the Gibbs probability subject to feasibility, then it is likely to be able to (nearly) recover a random sample from the Gibbs distribution. This supports our hypothesis posed in the introduction, namely that if an image is a typical member of a class of images having a certain Gibbs distribution, then by using this information we can limit the class of possible solutions to only those which are close to the given unknown image. We have also shown how linear programming can be used to find invariant image elements.

```
 1    .................................00000       ...............................................
 2    .................................00          ...............................................
 3    ................11...............o.o          .....•••••••••••••••••••••••••••••••••••••••....
 4    ...............1111..............o..o         ....•••••••••••••••••••••••••••••••••••••••••...
 5    ...11...........1111..........1..o...o        ....•••••••••••••••••••••••••••••••••••••••••...
 6    ...1111.........1111............111.....      ....1•••••••••••••••••••••••••••••••••••••••••..
 7    ...11111........1111111........11111....      ..•1•••••••••••••••••••••••••••••••••••••••••...
 8    ..1111111.......1111111........11111....      ..•1•••••••••••••••••••••••••••••••••••••••••...
 9    ..11111111...1111111...111....11111111...     ..•1•••••••••••••••••••••••••••••••••••••••••...
10    ..11111111111..1111111111111111....11111111.. ..•1•••••••••••••••••••••••••••••••••••••••••...
11    ..111111111111111111111111111...11111111..    ..•1•••••••••••••••••••••••••••••••••••••••••...
12    ..11111111111111111111111111111.11111111..    ..•1•••••••••••••••••••••••••••••••••••••••••...
13    ..1111111111111111111111111111111111111..     ..111111111111111111111111111111111111111111..
14    ..11111111111111111111111111111111111111..    ..111111111111111111111111111111111111111111..
15    ..11111111111111111111111111111111111111..    ..111111111111111111111111111111111111111111..
16    ..11111111111111111111111111111111111111..    ..111111111111111111111111111111111111111111..
17    ..11111111111111111111111111111111111111..    ..111111111111111111111111111111111111111111..
18    ..11111111111111111111111111111111111111..    ..111111111111111111111111111111111111111111..
19    ..11111111111111111111111111111111111111..    ..111111111111111111111111111111111111111111..
20    ..11111111111111111111111111111111111111..    ..111111111111111111111111111111111111111111..
21    ..11111111111111111111111111111111111111..    ..111111111111111111111111111111111111111111..
22    ..11111111111111111111111111111111111111..    ..111111111111111111111111111111111111111111..
23    ..11111111111111111111111111111111111111..    ..111111111111111111111111111111111111111111..
24    ..11111111111111111111111111111111111111..    ..111111111111111111111111111111111111111111..
25    ..11111111111111111111111111111111111....     ..111111111111111111111111111111111111111....
26    ..111111111111111111......11111111.....       ..•1•••••••••••••••••••••••...••••••••......
27    ..111.....                                    ..•1•••••••••••••••••••••••...••••••••......
28    ...............................               ...............................................
29    ...............................               ...............................................


 1    ...............................               ...............................................
 2    ...............................               ...............................................
 3    ...............1...............               ....•••••••••••••••••••••••••••••••••••••••....
 4    ...............11..............                ....•••••••••••••••••••••••••••••••••••••••....
 5    ...........11..1111.........1..........        ...•••••••••••••••••••••••••••••••••••••••••...
 6    ...11.......111..11111.......111..11111111..   ..•••••••••••••••••••••••••••••••••••••••••••..
 7    ...111....11111111111.....111111111111111..    ..•••••••••••••••••••••••••••••••••••••••••••..
 8    ...1111..1111111111111.....1111111111111111..  ..•••••••••••••••••••••••••••••••••••••••••••..
 9    ..11111111111111111111...1111111111111111..    ..•••••••••••••••••••••••••••••••••••••••••••..
10    ..11111111111111111111.1111111111111111..      ..•••••••••••••••••••••••••••••••••••••••••••..
11    ..11111111111111111111111111111111111111..     ..111111111111111111111111111111111111111111..
12    ..11111111111111111111111111111111111111..     ..111111111111111111111111111111111111111111..
13    ..11111111111111111111111111111111111111..     ..111111111111111111111111111111111111111111..
14    ..11111111111111111111111111111111111111..     ..111111111111111111111111111111111111111111..
15    ..11111111111111111111111111.1111111111..      ..•••••••••••••••••••••••••••••••••••••••••••..
16    ..11111111111111111111111111..11111111..       ..•••••••••••••••••••••••••••••••••••••••••••..
17    ..11111111111111111111111111..11111111..       ..•••••••••••••••••••••••••••••••••••••••••••..
18    ..11111111111111111111111111...11111111..      ..•••••••••••••••••••••••••••••••••••••••••••..
19    ...11111111111111111111111....11111111..       ..•••••••••••••••••••••••••••••••••••••••••••..
20    ...11111111111111111111111....11111111..       ..•••••••••••••••••••••••••••••••••••••••••••..
21    ...11111111111111111111111....11111111..       ..•••••••••••••••••••••••••••••••••••••••••••..
22    ...11111111111111111111......11111111..        ..•••••••••••••••••••••••••••••••••••••••••••..
23    ...11111111111111111111.......11111111..       ..•••••••••••••••••••••••••••••••••••••••••••..
24    ...11111111111111....11.........11111111..     ..•••••••••••••••••••••••••••••••••••••••••••..
25    ....1....1111111..........1111111..            ..•••••••••••••••••••••••••••••••••••••••••••..
26    ........1111111.............1111..             ..•••••••••••••••••••••••••••••••••••••••••....
27    .........111111..................1....         ..•••••••••••••••••••••••••••••••••••••......
28    .........111111....................            ..•••••••••••••••••••••••••••••••••••••......
29    .........111111....................            ..•••••••••••••••••••••••••••••••••••••......
30    .........111111....................            ..•••••••••••••••••••••••••••••••••••••......
31    .........1..11.....................            ..•••••••••••••••••••••••••••••••••••••......
32    .........1.........................            ..•••••••••••••••••••••••••••••••••••••......
33    .........1.........................            ..•••••••••••••••••••••••••••••••••••••......
34    .........1.........................            ..•••••••••••••••••••••••••••••••••••••......
35    ...................................            ...............................................
36    ...................................            ...............................................
```

FIGURE 8.7. Phantom 1 (top left) and Phantom 3 (bottom left) of [2] and the corresponding outputs of the brute force algorithm (right side). On the left, . and 1 represent values zero and one, respectively, in the phantom and o shows the three directions of the projection line sums. On the right, . and 1 represent invariant zeros and ones that are found by the brute algorithm and * represent locations that were not determined by the brute force algorithm and hence are accessed by the reconstruction algorithm.

In order to solve practical problems, such as the recovery of the shape of cardiac ventricles in cineangiography [1] or the details of a crystal from transmission electron micrographs [2], two essential further steps have to be taken. The first is to produce an appropriate Gibbs prior that models the ensemble of images in the particular application area. The approaches mentioned in [3,5] may well be applicable here. The second is to take care of the fact that, in practice, projection data are likely to be only approximated by measurements. Essential use has been made in this work of the exactness of the projection data. (This is so especially in producing the prescribed black and white hexels. Note that the brute force approach can be modified to handle projection data for which there is no feasible image, but in this case the same hexel may be prescribed to be either black or white depending on the order in which the data are accessed.) The extension of this approach to noisy measurements is an important research direction.

Acknowledgments

This work was supported by the National Science Foundation Grant DMS-9612077 and by the National Institutes of Health Grants HL-28438 and CA-54356.

References

[1] S.-K. Chang and C. K. Chow, "The reconstruction of three-dimensional objects from two orthogonal projections and its application to cardiac cineangiography," *IEEE Trans. on Computers* **22**, 18-28 (1973).

[2] P. Fishburn, P. Schwander, L. Shepp, and R. J. Vanderbei, "The discrete Radon transform and its approximate inversion via linear programming," *Discrete Applied Mathematics* **75**, 39-61 (1997).

[3] M. T. Chan, G. T. Herman, and E. Levitan, "A Bayesian approach to PET reconstruction using image-modeling Gibbs priors: Implementation and comparison," *IEEE Trans. Nucl. Sci.* **44**, 1347-1354 (1997).

[4] G. Winkler, *Image Analysis, Random Fields and Dynamic Monte Carlo Methods* (Springer-Verlag, Heidelberg), 1995.

[5] E. Levitan, M. Chan, and G. T. Herman, "Image-modeling Gibbs priors," *Graph. Models Image Proc.* **57**, 117-130 (1995).

[6] N. Metropolis, A. W. Rosenbluth, M. N. Rosenbluth, A. H. Teller, and E. Teller, "Equations of state calculations by fast computing machines," *J. Chem. Phys.* **21**, 1087-1092 (1953).

[7] G. T. Herman and A. Kuba (Eds.), "Special Issue on Discrete Tomography," *Int. J. Imaging Syst. and Technol.* **9**, No. 2/3, 1998.

[8] R. Aharoni, G. T. Herman, and A. Kuba, "Binary vectors partially determined by linear equation systems," *Discrete Mathematics* **171**, 1-16 (1997).

[9] S. Wright, *Primal-Dual Interior-Point Methods* (SIAM, Philadelphia), 1997.

[10] C. Reeves, *Modern Heuristic Techniques for Combinatorial Problems* (John Wiley and Sons, New York), 1993.

Chapter 9

Probabilistic Modeling
of Discrete Images

Michael T. Chan[1]
Gabor T. Herman[2]
Emanuel Levitan[3]

ABSTRACT We present a methodology for constructing probabilistic models of discrete images using Gibbs distributions. The method differs from previous approaches in that the formulation is suited for the modeling of discrete images, and hence readily applicable to discrete tomography problems. Second, the distribution is "image-modeling" in the sense that random samples drawn from the distribution are likely to share important characteristics of the images in the application area. We propose a technique to estimate parameters of the model, based not only on local characteristics of the images, but also on their global properties. Using it as image priors in a Bayesian framework, we apply the model to the problems of recovering discrete images corrupted by additive Gaussian noise and discrete tomographic reconstruction. We demonstrate the usefulness of the proposed model and compare its effectiveness with previous approaches.

9.1 Introduction

Gibbs distributions, which are the joint distributions of Markov random fields (MRFs), are at the essence of statistical mechanics. The use of these distributions as prior image models in a Bayesian framework have been found efficacious in many image processing problems such as segmentation, noise removal, restoration and reconstruction since the appearance of [1,2].

One design variable of a Gibbs model is the order of the neighborhood. Although we do have some freedom in choosing the order of the neighborhood, many of the previously proposed Gibbs priors typically exploit only pairwise interactions of nearest pixel neighbors. The use of higher order in-

---

[1]Rockwell Science Center, 1049 Camino Dos Rios, Thousand Oaks, CA 91360, USA. E-mail: mtchan@risc.rockwell.com

[2]Department of Radiology, University of Pennsylvania, Philadelphia, PA 19104, USA. E-mail: gabor@mipg.upenn.edu

[3]Faculty of Medicine, Technion, Haifa 31096, Israel. Retired. E-mail: rpremnl@technion.ac.il

teractions has not been very much investigated. Most pairwise-interacting models have mainly a smoothing effect on the recovered images. It has been observed that randomly sampled images from the distributions specified by such priors have typically a uniform appearance [1,3] and do not share important characteristics of the images used in the application area; they cannot be described as "image-modeling" and are often inadequate in a statistical sense.

In this chapter, we present an approach to model discrete images probabilistically using image-modeling Gibbs distributions. The global property we choose to model for our demonstration is that images are composed of piecewise-homogeneous regions. For illustration purposes, images used in the experiments here have four gray levels although the number can be arbitrary. The potential function of the Gibbs model is defined in a local neighborhood in which 3×3 pixel cliques as well as pair cliques are used to model respectively the continuity of borders around image regions and the homogeneity within individual regions. The resulting model has the property that random image configurations generated (e.g., by Gibbs sampler) from the governing distribution indeed exhibit properties shared by images with piecewise homogeneous regions. Image-modeling Gibbs distributions which are intended for the modeling of other desired global properties may have to be specifically designed, perhaps using other types of local pixel interactions. The model we present here can be viewed as a special case of the model in [4] where the number of gray levels can be more than just a few.

The main reason for applying the Bayesian approach to image reconstruction is to reduce the imperfection of the reconstructed images caused by noise in the measurements. The approach has been employed in the the image reconstruction literature by a number of researchers [5–10] using a variety of continuous priors. Our formulation here is particularly suited for modeling discrete images. In this chapter, we investigate the advantages of using image-modeling Gibbs priors over using other priors [1].

To avoid misunderstanding, we emphasize the most essential aspect of the proposed approach: the image-modeling prior is useful if the distribution defined by it reflects some important aspects of the ensemble of images that we are likely to come across in a particular application area. Consequently, different priors have to be created for different types of images. In this chapter we demonstrate the approach and its performance on a particular family of images; to obtain similarly good results for another class of images, the techniques presented in this chapter should be used to design an image-modeling prior that is appropriate for that class.

9.2 Image-modeling distributions for discrete images

We describe how an image-modeling distribution useful for our application area is constructed. The global property of the class of images we wish to model is that images are composed of piecewise homogeneous regions. We do this by including the information on both the homogeneity of regions and the continuity of border structures in a probabilistic way. A statistical model of images is characterized by its joint probability function. For a Markov random field image model this is given by the Gibbs distribution [11]:

$$\Pi(X) = \frac{1}{Z} e^{-\beta H(X)}. \tag{9.1}$$

Here $X = (x_1, \cdots, x_N)$ is an image of N pixels in which x_n denotes the gray value of the nth pixel. $H(X)$ is called the *energy function* or the *Hamiltonian* and is represented as a weighted sum of clique potentials (as defined more precisely below), β is the scaling constant and Z is a normalizing factor. In the terminology of statistical mechanics, β is the inverse of the *temperature* and Z is the *partition function*. Desired properties of images are incorporated into the model via the design of an appropriate energy function. The gray values of the pixels in X can assume any integral value in $[0, M-1]$ where M is the number of gray levels. We begin defining our model by writing the energy function as

$$H(X) = H_1(X) + H_2(X). \tag{9.2}$$

The first term, which models homogeneity, is

$$H_1(X) = -\left(\sum_{C \in \mathcal{C}_+} \lambda_1 \Phi_C(X) + \sum_{C \in \mathcal{C}_\times} \lambda_2 \Phi_C(X) \right)$$

$$\tag{9.3}$$

with

$$\Phi_{\{j_1, j_2\}}(X) = \begin{cases} \exp(-\frac{(x_{j_1} - x_{j_2})^2}{2\delta^2}) & \text{if } \delta > 0 \\ I(x_{j_1} - x_{j_2}) & \text{otherwise,} \end{cases} \tag{9.4}$$

where $\mathcal{C}_+$ denotes the set of all horizontal and vertical pair cliques, $\mathcal{C}_\times$ denotes that of the diagonal ones, and $I(.)$ denotes the binary indicator function. The coefficients λ_1 and λ_2 control the strengths of each type of interaction and δ is a non-negative parameter which (together with λ_i) controls the degree of homogeneity. The second term, which models the borders between regions, is

$$H_2(X) = - \sum_{C \in \mathcal{C}_{3 \times 3}} (\kappa_1 I_C^1(X) + \kappa_2 I_C^2(X) + \kappa_3 I_C^3(X)), \tag{9.5}$$

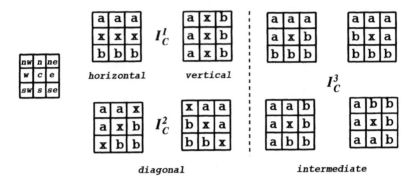

FIGURE 9.1. Pictorial clique potential definition for borders in different orientations. Pixels labeled by 'a' and 'b' have "dissimilar" gray levels. Pixels labeled by 'x' in a clique all have gray levels "similar" to those labeled by either 'a' or 'b'. The legend on the left defines the pixel indices used in equation (9.6).

where $\mathcal{C}_{3\times3}$ denotes the set of all cliques with 3×3 of blocks of pixels and

$$
I_C^1(X) = \begin{cases}
1, & \text{if } |x_k - x_c| \leq \delta \;\; \forall k \in \{w, nw, n, ne, e\} \\
& \text{and } |x_k - x_s| \leq \delta \;\; \forall k \in \{sw, se\} \text{ and } |x_n - x_s| > \Delta, \\
1, & \text{if } |x_k - x_c| \leq \delta \;\; \forall k \in \{w, sw, s, se, e\} \\
& \text{and } |x_k - x_n| \leq \delta \;\; \forall k \in \{nw, ne\} \text{ and } |x_n - x_s| > \Delta, \\
1, & \text{if } |x_k - x_c| \leq \delta \;\; \forall k \in \{s, sw, w, nw, n\} \\
& \text{and } |x_k - x_e| \leq \delta \;\; \forall k \in \{se, ne\} \text{ and } |x_e - x_w| > \Delta, \\
1, & \text{if } |x_k - x_c| \leq \delta \;\; \forall k \in \{s, se, e, ne, n\} \\
& \text{and } |x_k - x_w| \leq \delta \;\; \forall k \in \{sw, nw\} \text{ and } |x_e - x_w| > \Delta, \\
0, & \text{otherwise.}
\end{cases}
$$

$$(9.6)$$

(I_C^2 and I_C^3 are similarly defined as depicted in Fig. 9.1.) The subscripts c, n, e, s, w (denoting center, north, east, south, and west, respectively) are used to index the pixels in a 3×3 clique. The first case in (9.6), for example, is depicted in Fig. 9.1 by the left clique labeled "horizontal" in which the pixels labeled by 'x' have gray levels "similar" to those labeled by 'a'. Each term models borders in a particular set of orientations and the coefficients κ_1, κ_2 and κ_3 control the strength of each type of interaction. δ is as defined in (9.4) and Δ (with $\Delta \geq \delta$) represents the expected magnitude of the border. Note that by using 3×3 cliques, borders at intermediate orientations can also be modeled; see I_C^3 in Fig. 9.1. Both δ and Δ are introduced here so that our model can be generalized to suit modeling of images with arbitrary number of gray levels. For the examples in this section involving images with four gray levels, setting both Δ and δ to zero is most appropriate.

9.3 Parameter estimation

We believe that the determination of model parameters is best performed based on uncorrupted images for which we intend to build a model. We understand, however, that in situations where the original image is not available, we may have to resort to methods which estimate parameters of the prior models involved from observed data as in [12, 13], Here we assume that a representative sample of the class of images is available. In the following section, we discuss a methodology for choosing the values of the parameters so as to ensure that the resulting distribution is an image-modeling distribution. (For us here, that means one which shares the characteristics of piecewise homogeneous images.)

9.3.1 Isotropic considerations

To encourage spatially isotropic interaction in the modeling of homogeneity, we set $\lambda_2 = \frac{1}{\sqrt{2}}\lambda_1$. For the "border elements," on the other hand, we set $\frac{1}{2}\kappa_3 = \kappa_2 = \kappa_1$. The factor $\frac{1}{2}$ comes from the fact that vertical, horizontal, and diagonal border elements always appear in pairs at the border between two regions (at least for idealized straight borders). As indicated earlier, the parameters Δ and δ are typically predetermined based on some prior knowledge about the difference in gray levels between adjacent regions and the number of levels of quantization in the images. Furthermore, without loss generality, we set $\lambda_1 = 1$, whereas the remaining two parameters κ_1 and β are to be estimated.

9.3.2 Combining global and local characteristics

We describe a parameter estimation technique based on the ideas presented in [14]. In addition to *maximum pseudo-likelihood* (MPL) estimation [1] of β, an essential component of the method is a search mechanism to find the value of the parameter (κ_1 here) giving rise to models from which random images generated have structural features similar to that of a given data image (which is assumed to be a representative image from the application area). The consideration of global properties in selecting parameter values is important to the construction of image-modeling distributions. This has been previously done by visual comparison, which works reasonably well [14]. Here, we present a technique to automate this by comparing the data image with images generated from a model based on a metric which reflects the structural characteristics in the images. Examples of intuitive metrics appropriate for our model could include mean cluster size and mean radius of gyration of clusters [15]. Here we choose to use

$$G(X) = \kappa_1^{-1} H_2(X). \tag{9.7}$$

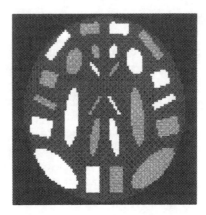

FIGURE 9.2. A mathematical phantom with four gray levels.

To be more specific, the two parameters, namely κ_1 and β, are determined as follows:

1. Begin with a small initial guess of κ_1.

2. With the current κ_1, estimate β using the MPL method.

3. Generate random sample images from the corresponding distribution and estimate $E[G(X)|\beta, \kappa_1]$ from the images by Monte Carlo methods (e.g., using the Gibbs Sampler [2]).

4. Check if
$$| E[G(X)| \beta, \kappa_1] - G(X^*) |= 0, \qquad (9.8)$$

   where X^* is the data image, is approximately satisfied. Stop if (9.8) is satisfied to a desirable degree of accuracy.

5. Increment κ_1 by a small constant step and go to Step 2.

(Although the updating rule in Step 5 can be replaced by something more sophisticated, we have used the above simple rule for the purpose of illustrating the method.) Note that with the isotropic considerations in Section 9.3.1 (with $\frac{1}{2}\kappa_3 = \kappa_2 = \kappa_1$), G as defined above does not depend on the values of the parameters of the model and hence its value for the data image is constant. The constraint (9.8) is a global one, since it requires the computation of a metric which is a function of the whole image. The determination of κ_1 is important in our model, because too large a value would introduce undesirably many borders in the images.

Figure 9.2 shows a 95×95 mathematical phantom with which we will illustrate the parameter estimation procedure. The phantom is based on a typical slice in a computerized overlay atlas of the average anatomy in twenty-six axial slices of the brain [16], which is used to evaluate the activity in various neurological structures of the brain based on images produced by

κ_1	$\hat{\beta}$	$E[G]$	$\mathrm{Var}[G]$
0.90	0.9730	-0.0292	0.0119^2
0.92	0.9679	-0.1038	0.0086^2
0.94	0.9629	-0.1732	0.0164^2
0.96	0.9580	-0.2404	0.0091^2
0.98	0.9533	-0.2800	0.0124^2
1.00	0.9486	-0.3073	0.0115^2
Data Image	—	-0.1964	—

TABLE 9.1. For the different values of κ_1, the right three columns show the corresponding MPL estimates of β, the estimated averages $E[G]$, and the variance $\mathrm{Var}[G]$.

positron emission tomography. Although the four gray levels we have used in the phantom here do not truly reflect the typical relative activities in the various regions, the geometry of the regions are properly represented.

With $\triangle$ and δ set to zero, we began the process with $\kappa_1 = 0.90$ (in Step 1) and we updated κ_1 by incrementing its value by 0.02 (in Step 5). In Table 9.1 we tabulate the MPL estimate $\hat{\beta}$ of the model for a range of values of κ_1.

Also shown in the table are the corresponding means and variances of the quantity G estimated using Monte Carlo methods for the different values of the parameters. A total of 5000 sweeps of the Gibbs Sampler were used in each case. The first 2500 sweeps were skipped to make sure that convergence is reached and 10 images (sampled 250 sweeps apart) from the rest were used for the estimation of $E[G]$.

Note that as κ_1 was gradually increased, the value of G was also increased in magnitude. The optimal estimate of the parameters are given by $(\kappa_1, \beta) = (0.94, 0.963)$. Figure 9.3 shows random images from the Gibbs distribution with values of the parameters shown in Table 9.1. Upon visual inspection, the sample images of the resulting model do exhibit characteristics similar to the data image. [4] Another observation we can make is that the shapes of regions and the borders around the regions indeed do not have a specific orientational preference (as we have intended).

9.4 Recovering images corrupted by additive noise

In this section, we investigate the usefulness of the prior in actual problems and compare its performance with that of another prior previously

---

[4]We should emphasize that it is only a random sample from the prior distribution. Therefore it does not necessarily resemble an image of, for example, a particular brain slice, although they may (and are supposed to) share similar global structural properties.

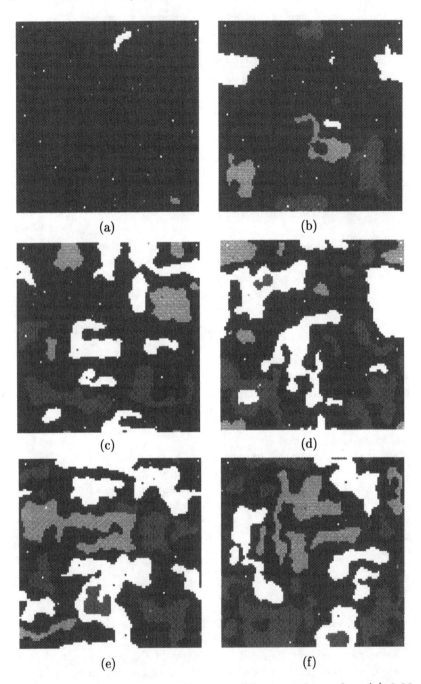

FIGURE 9.3. Random realizations at different values of κ_1 (a) 0.90 (b) 0.92 (c) 0.94 (d) 0.96 (e) 0.98 (f) 1.00. They are generated using the Gibbs Sampler for 10,000 sweeps. There are four gray levels in the images.

proposed. Here we consider the problem of recovering images corrupted by additive Gaussian noise. With a noise degradation model in terms of a likelihood function, one approach to the problem is to use the maximum likelihood criterion. A more desirable alternative is to incorporate into the estimation process a prior distribution of the images. According to Bayes' theorem, the posterior distribution of the images is given by

$$P(X|Y) = \frac{\Pi(X)L(Y|X)}{P(Y)} \tag{9.9}$$

where $\Pi(X)$ is characterized by distribution (9.1), $P(Y)$ is the probability of the measurements Y, and the likelihood function is given by

$$L(Y|X) = \frac{1}{\sqrt{2\pi\sigma^2}^N} \exp(-\sum_i^N \frac{(y_i - x_i)^2}{2\sigma^2}) \tag{9.10}$$

with σ denoting the standard deviation of the noise.

Using the Maximum a Priori probability (MAP) criterion, the problem can now be formulated as the optimization problem:

$$\max_X \Pi(X)L(Y|X) \tag{9.11}$$

($P(Y)$ is dropped, since it is independent of X). Equivalently, the above reduces to the global minimization problem:

$$\min_X \left[\sum_i^N \frac{(y_i - x_i)^2}{2\sigma^2}) + \beta H(X) \right]. \tag{9.12}$$

The above minimization is difficult with our prior because of the non-convexity of $H(X)$. One approach is to use the Gibbs Sampler in conjunction with simulated annealing (SA) [2]. In this scheme, the pixels in the image are visited one at a time and are updated based on the conditional distribution at each site. Because of the Markovian properties of the prior, the computation of the conditional distribution is local and is not computationally demanding.

In the first experiment, we use the image with which the parameters of our prior model were estimated as the test image itself. Gaussian noise with $\sigma = 0.7$ was added to the original image in Fig. 9.4(a). Three different estimates of the original were obtained using three different methods: the ML method (in this case obtained simply by rounding the pixel values in the noisy image to the nearest gray level in [0,3]), the MAP method using a pairwise-interacting prior (i.e., with κ_i set to 0, which is equivalent to the model in [1]), and the MAP method using the proposed image-modeling prior. The results are shown in Figs. 9.4(b), (c), and (d), respectively. A range of values for β was tried for the pairwise-interacting prior and the

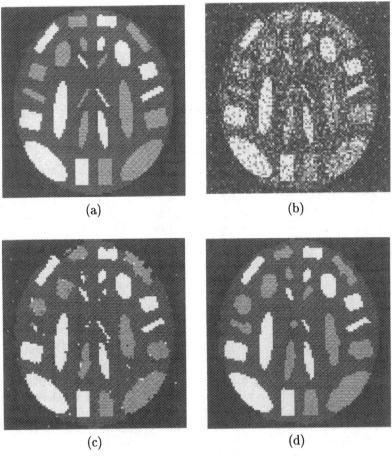

(a)   (b)

(c)   (d)

FIGURE 9.4. (a) Phantom 1. (b) ML estimate (39.28%). (c) MAP estimate using a pairwise-interacting prior (5.76%). (d) MAP estimate using the image-modeling prior (2.95%). The values in parentheses are misclassification errors. There are four gray levels in the images.

Misclassification Error

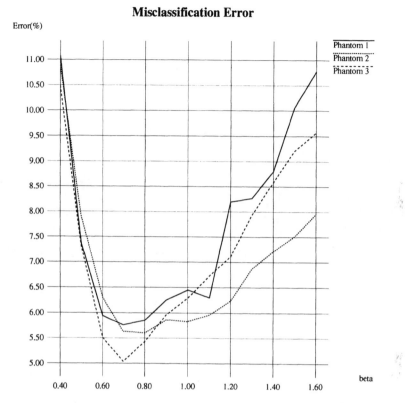

FIGURE 9.5. Variation of misclassification error as a function of β in images restored using a pairwise-interacting prior.

reconstruction with the smallest misclassification error (corresponding to β = 0.7, see Fig. 9.5) was shown. We observe that the image-modeling prior gave qualitatively better results — the shapes and borders of the regions were better reconstructed. Similar conclusions can be drawn based on the misclassification errors.

In the second experiment, we tested our model using two other phantom images different from the one we have used to estimate the prior model. Although different, they have similar characteristics as they correspond to some other planes of the brain. The corresponding results are shown in Figs. 9.6 and 9.7.

Again, the values of β used in the pairwise-interacting prior were the ones that gave the smallest misclassification errors. (The optimal values were 0.8 and 0.7, respectively; again see Fig. 9.5.) Again, our approach gave the best results from both qualitative and quantitative points of view. A summary of the misclassification error is given in Table 9.2.

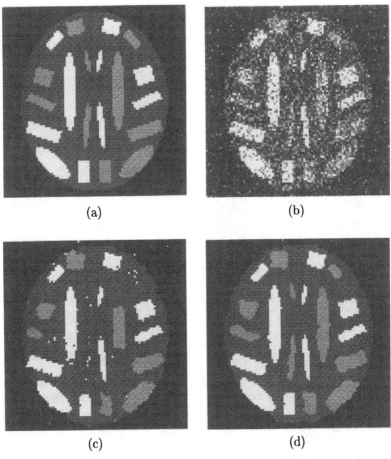

FIGURE 9.6. (a) Phantom 2. (b) ML estimate (38.38%). (c) MAP estimate using a pairwise-interacting prior (5.60%). (d) MAP estimate using the image-modeling prior (2.76%). The values in parentheses are misclassification errors. There are four gray levels in the images.

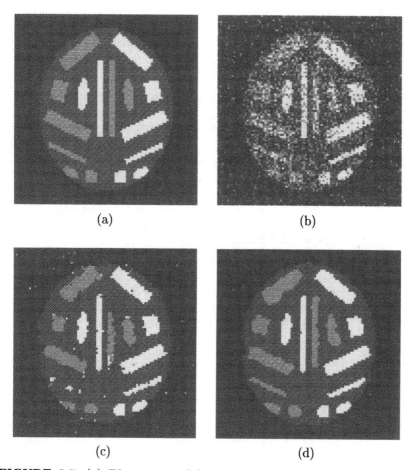

FIGURE 9.7. (a) Phantom 3. (b) ML estimate (35.50%). (c) MAP estimate using a pairwise-interacting prior (5.04%). (d) MAP estimate using the image-modeling prior (2.40%). The values in parentheses are misclassification errors. There are four gray levels in the images.

	Expt. 1	Expt. 2	Expt. 3
ML	39.28%	38.38%	35.30%
MAP (pairwise-interacting prior)	5.76%	5.60%	5.04%
MAP (image-modeling prior)	2.95%	2.76%	2.40%

TABLE 9.2. Misclassification errors of the restored images shown in Figs. 9.4, 9.6, and 9.7, respectively.

9.5   Adaptation to discrete tomographic reconstruction

Here we look at adapting the technique employed in the previous section to Positron Emission Tomography (PET). The MAP approach has been employed in the PET image reconstruction literature by a number of researchers [5–10] using a variety of priors. Our interest here is to investigate the usefulness of image-modeling Gibbs distributions as priors using a discrete formulation, in which the pixel values are represented by 8-bit quantities, i.e., integers in [0,255].

9.5.1   The posterior model and optimization criteria

The formulation of Bayesian reconstruction model is very similar to that described in Section 9.4. The posterior distribution has the same form as (9.11) except that the likelihood function is replaced by [17]

$$L(Y|X) = \prod_{i=1}^{I} \frac{(\sum_j^J l_{ij} x_j)^{y_i} exp(-\sum_j^J l_{ij} x_j)}{y_i!} \tag{9.13}$$

where l_{ij} is related to the probability of detecting a pair of coincidence along the ith line (out of a total of I lines) as a result of a positron annihilation occurred in the jth pixel (out of a total of J pixels). Figure 9.8 illustrates the geometry of the measurement process.

One approach to obtain an MAP estimate is again to use the Gibbs Sampler in conjunction with simulated annealing (SA) [2]. This time, however, the conditional distribution is no longer local because the likelihood function is not. Each time the conditional distribution is to be calculated say at pixel j, the relative change of the posterior energy has to be evaluated for all possible values of $x_j \in [0, 255]$. Running SA is therefore computationally infeasible. Deterministic approaches based on mean field approximations of various models have been found to produce good solutions in shorter times for certain problems [9,18,19], but they are not directly applicable to our image prior. Other directions which one can explore to find the MAP solution to this problem have been proposed elsewhere [20].

With the MAP criterion for estimation described above, the solution is defined by the mode of the posterior distribution. An alternative criterion

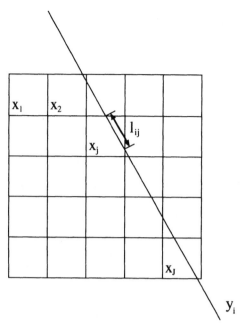

FIGURE 9.8. The geometry of data collection for a single line. The expected number of coincidences per unit length in the j pixel is x_j. The actual number of coincidences counted for the ith line is y_i. The length of intersection of the ith line with the jth pixel is l_{ij}.

is the Minimum Mean Square Error (MMSE) criterion, in which case the solution is defined by the mean of the posterior distribution given by [21]:

$$E[X|Y] = \sum P(X|Y) \cdot X. \tag{9.14}$$

A stochastic approach based on Monte Carlo methods can be used by sampling the posterior distribution using the Gibbs Sampler. The iterates $X^{(r)}$ form a Markov chain with the asymptotic distribution (9.9). The ergodicity of the chain guarantees that an ergodic average will converge to the MMSE estimate [2], the value of which in practice can be estimated by calculating the average of K samples $\{X^{(r)} : r = K'+k \times R$ for $k = 1, \ldots, K\}$ for some large enough values of R and K'. K' needs to be sufficiently large to ensure that the sampling process has converged, whereas R also needs to be large enough so that the sample $X^{(r)}$'s are sufficiently uncorrelated. Again this sampling process is computationally expensive because of the involvement of the likelihood function (9.13), whose local neighborhood structure has a large spatial extent. In the sections below, we focus primarily on MMSE estimation as we found it to be more accurate than MAP estimation in the experiments performed here.

9.5.2 An approximate two-step reconstruction approach

To alleviate the computational burden discussed above, we propose to two-step method for the problem. The basic idea is to consider the output of a classical image reconstruction technique as a degraded version of the original image and to apply a Bayesian approach to estimate from it the original image (based on a model of noise and on our image-modeling Gibbs distribution as the prior). Such an approach is computationally much less expensive than direct Bayesian estimation based on the original measured data. The two-step reconstruction procedure can be summarized as follows:

1. Perform a reconstruction using a fast algorithm to produce X';

2. Perform a Bayesian restoration of X' to produce X''.

This procedure is partly motivated by the fact that a number of fast algorithms for the PET image reconstruction problem do exist, and they produce images whose noise properties are understood to some extent [22]. The standard *Filtered Backprojection* algorithm (FBP) [23] is employed here, which produce an initial estimate X' – Step 1 of the procedure.

In Step 2 of the procedure, we improve the image X' by viewing the problem as an image restoration problem (without making direct use of the measurements Y). This requires a noise model which is dependent on the reconstruction algorithm used in Step 1. For FBP, a Gaussian model has been found to work reasonably well [24]. The noise model takes the form:

$$L'(X'|X) = \prod_{j=1}^{J} \frac{1}{\sqrt{2\pi\sigma^2}} \exp\left(-\frac{(x'_j - x_j - \mu(x_j, x_{\partial j}))^2}{2\sigma^2}\right), \qquad (9.15)$$

where σ is the effective standard deviation of the noise, and μ, the bias at each pixel, is a third order polynomial, which is dependent on the original pixel value and those of its closest neighbors. We refer you to [24] for the details on how the parameters of (9.15) can be estimated from appropriate training data. By replacing Y and $L(Y|X)$ in (9.11) with X' and $L'(X'|X)$ respectively, Step 2 can be solved using the same procedure used in Section 9.4. One difference though is that the number of gray levels allowed here is substantially larger. The parameters of the corresponding image-modeling Gibbs distribution would need to be estimated using a sample image with the same number of gray levels. Although the parameter estimation procedure described in Section 9.3.2 is applicable here, the number of iterations of the sampling procedure required (in the third step) is substantially larger because the configuration space (or the set of all possible images) is also much larger. Here, it suffice to mention that some heuristics were used to speed up the process and we refer the you to [24] for a discussion on that.

Regarding the sampling process used the reconstruction procedure of Step 2, the speed of convergence is also slower in general because of the increased number of gray levels involved. To speed up the process, we used a slightly modified Gibbs sampler described in [25], which assumes that images are smoothly varying, or more precisely, locally-bounded. This requirement is relatively mild and the modified Gibbs sampler is quite applicable in our case.

9.5.3 Experimental results

We simulated the measurement process of PET imaging using the mathematical brain phantom in Fig. 9.9(a) under the same conditions as those described in [26] (involving 3,000,000 coincidence counts, 300×151 projections with independent Poisson noise). The phantom, an 8-bit image with gray values quantized in the range [0,255], consists of an elliptical background (gray level equals 100) with elliptical and rectangular blobby features (the gray level inside each is either 195 or 200). Although there are only a few primary gray levels, there are intermediate values at the borders which represent partial volumes. The two-step reconstruction procedure was applied using the FBP algorithm (whose output is shown in Fig. 9.9(b)). We performed a total of 500 sweeps of the algorithm at constant temperature $T_k = 1.0$. After the first 250 sweeps images subsequently generated every other 25 sweeps (for a total of 10 samples) were averaged.

In the first experiment, we used the image with which we estimated our Gibbs prior as the test image itself. Figure 9.10(c) shows the final MMSE estimate obtained using a pairwise-interacting prior, whereas Fig. 9.10(d) is obtained by using our prior. The value of β used in the pairwise-interacting prior were the one that gave the smallest mean-square error. It can be observed that the proposed model did a better job especially at the smaller regions where the spatial supports are small.

To avoid any confusion, we shall say that although there are few primary gray levels in the original, we have no knowledge which gray levels were the primary ones in the phantom in the reconstruction process. There is a finite probability for each pixel to take on any of the 256 gray values during reconstruction, but many of them were highly unlikely under the influence of both the image prior and the likelihood function. If one would inspect the reconstructed images closely, one can expect to see a smooth variation in gray levels in the reconstructed regions, each with some overall mean plus some variation.

In the second experiment, we tested our model using another phantom different from the one we used to estimate the prior model. Although the phantom was different, it has similar characteristics as it correspond to another planes of the brain. The projection data were generated in a manner similar to the way in which the projection data were generated in the previous experiment. The only difference was that the total simulated counts were different since the total activities in the different planes were not the same and we were keeping the scan time effectively constant. Figure 9.10

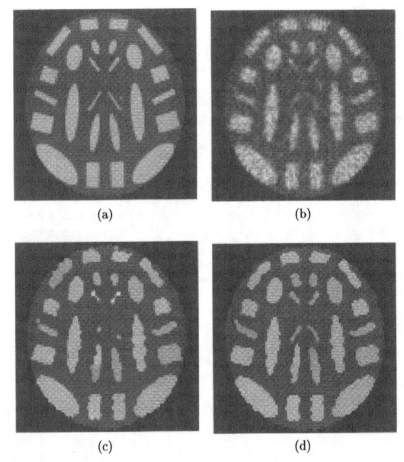

(a)   (b)

(c)   (d)

FIGURE 9.9. (a) Original phantom image. (b) Reconstructed image using FBP. (c) MMSE estimate with the pairwise-interacting prior (MSE=208.4). (d) MMSE estimate with the proposed prior (MSE=180.3). The images are quantized in the range [0,255] and the primary gray levels in the original were 0, 100, 195, and 200.

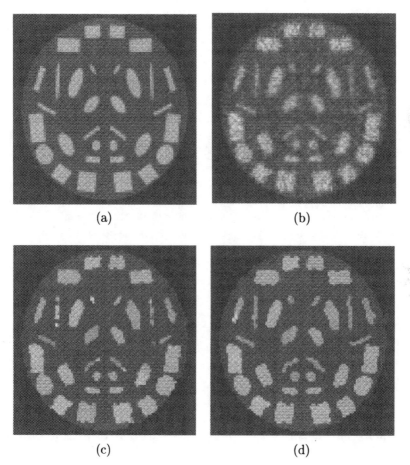

(a)   (b)

(c)   (d)

FIGURE 9.10. (a) Original phantom image. (b) Reconstructed image using FBP. (c) MMSE estimate with the pairwise-interacting prior (MSE=177.6). (d) MMSE estimate with the proposed prior (MSE=171.1). The images are quantized in the range [0,255] and the primary gray levels in the original were 0, 100, 195, and 200. Here, neither the image-modeling prior nor the noise model for the FBP stage were tuned to the phantom.

shows the original image, FBP reconstruction, and reconstructions obtained using the two different priors. Again, the value of β used in the pairwise-interacting prior was the one that gave the smallest mean-square error. We observe again that the image-modeling prior give qualitatively better results; the shapes and borders of the regions were better reconstructed. Similar conclusions are drawn based on the mean-square errors. Note that neither the prior nor the noise model were tuned to the image here, so the posterior model did exhibit some level of robustness.

9.6   Conclusions

We presented a methodology to construct probabilistic models of discrete images using Gibbs distributions. We also proposed a technique to estimate parameters of the model based not only on local characteristics of the images, but also on their global properties. We showed that the resulting distribution thus estimated is "image-modeling" in the sense that random samples from it are likely to share important characteristics — such as piecewise homogeneity — of the images of the application area. We demonstrated that, for the problem of recovery images corrupted by additive Gaussian noise, one can do better with image-modeling priors than using some other Gibbs priors that have been advocated in the literature. Finally we applied the proposed prior to PET using a discrete formulation. A two-step reconstruction procedure was proposed to relieve some of the additional computational burden. The results demonstrated the efficacy of the image-modeling prior.

Acknowledgments

This work was supported by NIH grant HL-28438 and NSF grant DMS-96127077.

References

[1] J. Besag, "On the statistical analysis of dirty pictures (with discussion)." *Journal of the Royal Statistical Society Series B* **48**, 259-302 (1986).

[2] S. Geman and D. Geman, "Stochastic relaxation, Gibbs distributions, and the Bayesian restoration of images," *IEEE Transactions on Pattern Analysis and Machine Intelligence* **6**, 721-741 (1984).

[3] A. J. Gray, J. W. Kay, and D. M. Titterington, "An empirical study of the simulation of various models used for images," *IEEE Transactions on Pattern Analysis and Machine Intelligence* **16**, 507-512, 1994.

[4] M. T. Chan, G. T. Herman, and E. Levitan, "A Bayesian approach to PET reconstruction using image-modeling Gibbs priors: Implementation and comparison," *IEEE Transactions on Nuclear Science* **44**, 1347–1354 (1997).

[5] S. Geman and D. McClure, "Statistical methods for tomographic image reconstruction," In *Proceedings of the 46th Session of the ISI, Bulletin of the ISI*, volume 52, pp. 5-21, 1987.

[6] P. Green, "Bayesian reconstructions from emission tomography data using a modified EM algorithm," *IEEE Transactions on Medical Imaging* **9**, 84–93 (1990).

[7] G. T. Herman, A. R. De Pierro, and N. Gai, "On methods for maximum a posteriori image reconstruction with a normal prior," *Journal of Visual Communication and Image Representation* **3**, 316–324 (1992).

[8] R. Leahy and X. Yan, "Incorporation of anatomical MR data for improved functional imaging with PET," In *12th International Conference on Information Processing in Medical Imaging*, pp. 105-120, 1990.

[9] M. Lee, A. Rangarajan, I. G. Zubal, and G. Gindi, "A continuation method for emission tomography," *IEEE Transactions on Nuclear Science* **40**, 2049–2058 (1993).

[10] E. Levitan and G. T. Herman, "A maximum a posteriori probability expectation maximization for image reconstruction in emission tomography," *IEEE Transactions on Medical Imaging* **6**, 185–192 (1987).

[11] J. Besag, "Spatial interactions and the statistical analysis of lattice systems (with discussion)," *Journal of the Royal Statistical Society Series B* **36**, 192–236 (1974).

[12] V. E. Johnson, W. H. Wong, X. Hu, and C. T. Chen, "Image restoration using Gibbs priors: Boundary modeling, treatment of blurring, and selection of hyperparameter," *IEEE Transactions on Pattern Analysis and Machine Intelligence* **13**, 413–425 (1991).

[13] Z. Zhou, R.M. Leahy, and E.U. Mumcuoglu, "Maximum likelihood hyperparameter estimation for Gibbs priors from incomplete data with applications to PET," In R. Di Paola Y. Bizais, and C. Barillot, *Information Processing in Medical Imaging* (Kluwer Academic Publishers, Dordrecht, The Netherlands), pp. 39–52, 1995.

[14] E. Levitan, M. Chan, and G. T. Herman, "Image-modeling Gibbs priors," *Graphical Models and Image Processing* **57**, 117–130 (1995).

[15] H. Gould and J. Tobochnik, *An Introduction to Computer Simulation Methods: Application to Physical Systems (Part 2)* (Addison-Wesley Publishing Company, Reading, MA), 1988. Chapter 12.

[16] A. Alavi, R. Dann, J. Chawluk, J. Alavi, M. Kushner, and M. Reivich, "Positron emission tomography imaging of regional cerebral glucose metabolism," *Seminars in Nuclear Medicine* **16**, 2–34 (1986).

[17] L. Shepp and Y. Vardi, "Maximum likelihood reconstruction in emission tomography," *IEEE Transactions on Medical Imaging* **1**, 113–121 (1982).

[18] D. Geiger and F. Girosi, "Parallel and deterministic algorithms from MRF's: Surface reconstruction," *IEEE Transactions on Pattern Analysis and Machine Intelligence* **13**, 401–412 (1991).

[19] J. Zerubia and R. Chellappa, "Mean field annealing using compound Gauss-Markov random fields for edge detection and image estimation," *IEEE Transactions on Neural Networks* **4**, 703–709 (1993).

[20] G. T. Herman, M. Chan, Y. Censor, E. Levitan, R. M. Lewitt, and T. K. Narayan, "Maximum a posteriori image reconstruction from projections," In S. E. Levinson and L. Shepp, *Image Models (and their Speech Model Cousins)*, (Springer-Verlag, New York), pp. 53–89, 1996.

[21] A. Papoulis, *Probability, Random Variables, and Stochastic Processes*, Second Edition (McGraw-Hill, New York), 1984.

[22] D. W. Wilson and B. M. W. Tsui, "Noise properties of filtered-backprojection and ML-EM reconstructed emission tomographic images," *IEEE Transactions on Nuclear Science* **40**, 1198–1203 (1993).

[23] S. W. Rowland, "Computer implementation of image reconstruction formulas," In G. T. Herman, *Image Reconstruction from Projections: Implementation and Applications*, (Springer-Verlag, Berlin), pp. 9–79, 1979.

[24] M. T. Chan, G. T. Herman, and E. Levitan, "Bayesian image reconstruction using image-modeling Gibbs priors," *International Journal of Imaging Systems and Technology* **9**, 85–98 (1998).

[25] C. Yang, "Efficient stochastic algorithms on locally bounded image space," *CVGIP: Graphical Models and Image Processing* **55**, 494–506 (1993).

[26] J. Browne and G. T. Herman, "Computerized evaluation of image reconstruction algorithms," *International Journal of Imaging Systems and Technology* **7**, 256–267 (1996).

Chapter 10

Multiscale Bayesian Methods for Discrete Tomography

Thomas Frese[1]
Charles A. Bouman[2]
Ken Sauer[3]

ABSTRACT Statistical methods of discrete tomographic reconstruction pose new problems both in stochastic modeling to define an optimal reconstruction, and in optimization to find that reconstruction. Multiscale models have succeeded in improving representation of structure of varying scale in imagery, a chronic problem for common Markov random fields. This chapter shows that associated multiscale methods of optimization also avoid local minima of the log a posteriori probability better than single-resolution techniques. These methods are applied here to both segmentation/reconstruction of the unknown cross sections and estimation of unknown parameters represented by the discrete levels.

10.1   Introduction

The reconstruction of images from projections is important in a variety of problems including tasks in medical imaging and non-destructive testing. Perhaps, the reconstruction technique most frequently used in commercial applications is convolution backprojection (CBP) [1]. While CBP works well for reconstruction problems with a complete set of projections having high signal-to-noise ratio (SNR), special cases benefit from alternative algorithms that can better model the imaging geometry and measurement process. These cases arise, for example, in low-dosage medical imaging [2], non-destructive testing of materials with widely varying densities [3] and applications with limited-angle projections [4] or hollow projections [5]. In such cases, statistical and discrete-valued methods can substantially im-

---

[1]Purdue University, Department of Electrical and Computer Engineering, West Lafayette, IN 47907-1285, USA, E-mail: frese@ecn.purdue.edu

[2]Purdue University, Department of Electrical and Computer Engineering, West Lafayette, IN 47907-1285, USA, E-mail: bouman@ecn.purdue.edu

[3]University of Notre Dame, Department of Electrical Engineering, 275 Fitzpatrick Hall, Notre Dame, IN 46556-5637, USA, E-mail: sauer@nd.edu

prove the reconstruction quality by incorporating important prior information about both the imaging system and the object being imaged. Discrete reconstruction methods are based on the assumption that the object being imaged is composed of a discrete set of materials each with uniform properties. Therefore, an ideal reconstruction should only contain pixel or voxel values from a corresponding set of discrete levels. In this case, the problem of reconstruction reduces to one of determining the specific levels present in a reconstruction and then classifying each pixel to one of these discrete levels. Discrete reconstruction methods impose a very strong constraint on the reconstruction process, and therefore can substantially improve reconstruction quality.

Early methods for discrete-valued reconstruction focused on reconstructions of binary arrays from only the horizontal and vertical projections [6]. The deterministic projections were treated as a system of linear equations. Attention was particularly paid to the ambiguity of reconstructions formulated in the context of switching components [6, 7]. Algorithms for unambiguous reconstruction were developed by assuming object constraints such as connectedness in 2D [8] or convexity in 3D [9]. In addition, these concepts were extended to four or more projection angles including the analysis of the ambiguity problem [7, 10]. However, all of these techniques assume deterministic projection measurements and do not perform optimally under high noise conditions.

A second approach to discrete-valued reconstruction detects parameterized objects directly in the projection domain. This strategy is applicable when the objective is to detect specific objects or regions such as tumors in medical imaging or material defects in non-destructive testing. Rossi and Willsky [11] introduced this approach by performing maximum likelihood (ML) estimation of the location of a single object in the imaging plane. This concept was later extended to a three-dimensional parameterization supporting multiple objects per plane [12]. Here, constrained objects in 3D are formed as a combination of basic cylinders whose parameters are estimated as part of the reconstruction. A review of object parameterization methods as well as a new algorithm for the approximate reconstruction of compact objects modeled by polyhedral shapes is given in Chapter 14 by A. Mohammad-Djafari and C. Soussen in this book. Parameterized object reconstruction methods are specifically designed for low SNR conditions. However, they rely on a priori knowledge about shape characteristics of the objects in the cross section. These methods are therefore not applicable in cases where such information is unavailable or the objects in the cross section cannot easily be parameterized.

In this work, we focus on discrete-valued reconstruction from noisy projections using statistical methods. Statistical methods model the random nature of the physical data collection process, then seek the solution that best matches the probabilistic behavior of the data. Consequently, statistical methods can improve performance considerably in cases of low

SNR. Statistical approaches also easily incorporate special geometries such as limited- or missing-angle projection measurements. Common statistical techniques incorporate implicit information about desired characteristics of the reconstruction without explicit modeling of objects in the cross section.

A statistical method that is well suited for tomographic reconstruction is Bayesian maximum *a posteriori* (MAP) estimation. Bayesian methods in general have been shown to improve performance in many emission and transmission tomography problems [13–16] as well as in image restoration tasks [17, 18]. Bayesian MAP estimation reconstructs the image as a tradeoff between matching the projection data and regularizing the solution by a prior probability distribution. The regularization imposed by the prior reflects assumed characteristics of feasible reconstructions. Due to this regularization, the MAP estimation problem is well-posed and avoids the high noise sensitivity frequently encountered in maximum likelihood (ML) estimation.

Priors for Bayesian reconstruction methods are often chosen to impose smoothness constraints on the reconstruction to eliminate high-frequency noise. A prior model that has generally proven to be useful in the tomographic setting is the Markov random field (MRF) image model [13–15, 19, 20]. Chapter 9 by M. T. Chan, G. T. Herman, and E. Levitan in this book presents a new MRF for modeling image prior distributions and describes methods for estimating the MRF's parameters. These parameter estimation techniques allow the model to be adapted to the specific characteristics of an ensemble of images. Importantly, the Bayesian estimate is computed directly from the convolution backprojection reconstruction, rather than from the original projection data. This approach has the advantage of reducing computation.

In contrast, we use a simple discrete MRF model [21, 22, 33], and instead focus on the computational difficulties resulting from direct Bayesian reconstruction from the tomographic data. In order to solve this optimization problem, we employ multiscale algorithms to both reduce computation and improve convergence to the global minimum. In addition, we introduce a method for estimating the densities of the discrete regions as part of the reconstruction process. This is important because precise knowledge of these discrete densities is required for accurate Bayesian reconstruction.

The MAP reconstruction itself can be formulated as an optimization problem, which can be solved using a number of different techniques. The expectation-maximization (EM) algorithm, suitable for ML reconstruction [23], has been adopted for MAP estimation with Gaussian priors [24–27]. Extensions of these models to more general MRF priors were proposed in [14, 15, 28, 29]. However, application of the EM algorithm for MAP estimation is difficult and usually suffers from slow convergence.

Instead of using EM techniques, we focus on the direct optimization of the MAP equation. We adopt a pixel-wise update method known as iterative coordinate descent (ICD) [16, 30], which maximizes the MAP criterion by iteratively updating each pixel of the image. The discrete version of ICD used here essentially implements the iterated conditional modes (ICM) technique introduced by Besag [22]. However, while ICM was designed for image restoration tasks, the ICD algorithm is specifically designed for the tomographic reconstruction problem resulting in dramatically improved computational efficiency.

In addition to solving the optimization problem, the discrete-valued reconstruction requires knowledge of the density or emission rate levels in the cross section. In practice, exact information about these discrete levels is often unavailable. In such cases it is desirable to estimate the densities or emission rates as part of the reconstruction. In Section 10.5, we discuss our method to estimate these discrete classes concurrently with the reconstruction process. We show how the class estimation can be formulated as a continuous-valued tomographic reconstruction problem with the number of points equal to the number of classes.

Finally, we extend our reconstruction method to a multiresolution algorithm. Multiresolution techniques achieve performance improvements in a variety of imaging problems [31, 32] including image segmentation [33, 34] and continuous-valued tomographic reconstruction [35]. Multiresolution algorithms reconstruct the image at different resolutions, typically progressing from coarse to fine scale. The coarse scale solutions serve as initialization or prior information for reconstructions at finer scales. Due to the improved initialization and the higher SNR at coarse scale, multiresolution algorithms are typically more robust with respect to local minima. In addition, local pixel interactions at coarse scale are equivalent to large scale interactions at fine scale. This combined with the low computational complexity at coarse scale makes multiscale algorithms very efficient.

The multiscale algorithm presented here is a straightforward extension of our fixed-scale algorithm. The reconstruction is performed in a coarse-to-fine fashion by initializing each resolution level with the interpolated reconstruction of the next coarser level. The reconstructions at each level are computed using the fixed-resolution method. Our experimental results demonstrate that this multiscale algorithm is less prone to being trapped in local minima and in many cases, computationally more efficient than the fixed-resolution version.

10.2 Stochastic data models for tomography

In this section, we will develop the statistical framework for MAP reconstruction in computed tomography. Our framework is applicable to both transmission and emission measurements and supports general imaging geometries. The models presented here are based on the exact Poisson statistics of the photon measurements. Computationally more efficient but

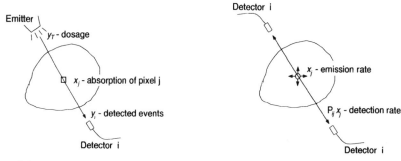

(a) Transmission setup   (b) PET emission setup

FIGURE 10.1. Physical setup for transmission and positron emission tomography (PET). In transmission tomography (a), photons are induced into the cross section. After attenuation by the absorptive material, detectors measure the remaining photon rates. In positron emission tomography (b), the cross section contains a radioisotope and is surrounded by a ring of detectors. If two detectors register photons at the same time, a pixel emission is assumed to have occurred on the projection line between them.

approximate models can be obtained by using a Taylor expansion of the likelihood function [16, 30].

In transmission tomography, the objective is to measure photon attenuation for different projections through a cross section of absorptive material. An illustration of the physical setup is shown in Fig. 10.1(a). The cross section is surrounded by a ring of photon emitters and detectors. The emitters induce a calibrated photon rate y_T directed along certain angular and parallel projections. After attenuation by the absorptive material, the photon rates are measured by the detector opposite the respective emitter. The photon rates measured by the detectors are not direct measurements of attenuation. Instead they are noisy photon counts that can be modeled as Poisson-distributed random variables.

In order to write the probability density for the Poisson measurements, define X as the N-dimensional vector of attenuation densities of the pixels in raster order. Let Y denote the vector of photon counts for all M projections at different angles and parallel offsets. Furthermore, let P_{ij} correspond to the length of intersection between the jth pixel and the ith projection. Then P is the matrix of elements P_{ij} and P_{i*} denotes the vector formed by its ith row. Given these assumptions, the photon count Y_i, corresponding to projection i, is Poisson distributed with mean $y_T \exp(-P_{i*}x)$. The distribution of the Y_i may then be written as

$$\mathcal{P}(Y = y|x) = \prod_{i=1}^{M} \frac{\exp(-y_T e^{-P_{i*}x})(y_T e^{-P_{i*}x})^{y_i}}{y_i!}. \qquad (10.1)$$

We use upper-case letters for random variables and lower-case letters for particular realizations. Taking the logarithm of (10.1), we obtain the log-likelihood

$$\text{(transmission)} \quad L(y|x) = \log \mathcal{P}(Y = y|x) =$$

$$\sum_{i=1}^{M} \left(-y_T e^{-P_{i*}x} + y_i(\log y_T - P_{i*}x) - \log(y_i!) \right). \tag{10.2}$$

In emission tomography, no dosage is induced into the cross section. Instead, the image plane contains some photon-emitting material. A physical setup for the specific example of positron emission tomography (PET) is shown in Fig. 10.1(b). In this case, the cross section contains a radioactive isotope. Recombination of positrons in the radioisotope results in emission of gamma rays in two opposite directions. These gamma rays are detected by a ring of detectors around the cross section. If two detectors register photons at the same time, this is counted as an emission on the projection line between them. In the following, we will develop the statistical model for the general emission case.

The objective in emission tomography is to reconstruct the emission rates of all pixels in the image plane. Again, the photon detections can be modeled as Poisson distributed random variables. In order to emphasize the similarity to the transmission problem, we will use the same notation, but interpret x as the vector of emission rates for all N pixels and Y as the observed photon counts. We define P_{ij} as the probability that an emission from pixel j is registered by the ith detector pair. The photon counts Y are then Poisson distributed with parameter $P_{i*}x$ which yields the distribution

$$\mathcal{P}(Y = y|x) = \prod_{i=1}^{M} \frac{\exp(-P_{i*}x)(P_{i*}x)^{y_i}}{y_i!}. \tag{10.3}$$

The log-likelihood is therefore given by

$$\text{(emission)} \quad L(y|x) = \log \mathcal{P}(Y = y|x) =$$

$$\sum_{i=1}^{M} \left(-P_{i*}x + y_i \log(P_{i*}x) - \log(y_i!) \right). \tag{10.4}$$

The log-likelihood functions for both the transmission and the emission case have the form

$$\log \mathcal{P}(Y = y|x) = - \sum_{i=1}^{M} f_i(P_{i*}x) \tag{10.5}$$

where $f_i(\cdot)$ are convex and differentiable functions. This common form will lead to similar methods of solving these two problems. In the following, we will write all equations for the emission case; however, all methods apply analogously to the transmission case.

For the emission problem, maximum likelihood (ML) estimation of x from y yields the optimization problem

$$\hat{x}_{ML} = \arg\min_x \sum_{i=1}^{M} (P_{i*}x - y_i \log(P_{i*}x)) \ . \tag{10.6}$$

For low signal-to-noise-ratio medical imaging problems, the ML estimate has well-documented shortcomings [36–38]. Noise and sampling limitations can produce high-frequency noise in the ML reconstruction that is not present in the original cross section. It is therefore desirable to regularize tomographic inversion by some means. Maximum *a posteriori* probability (MAP) estimation addresses this problem by treating the original image as a random field, X, with prior distribution, $p(x)$. Again, we use a lower-case x to denote a particular realization of the random vector X. The prior distribution regularizes the optimization problem so that a unique solution always exists [39]. The logarithm of the *a posteriori* distribution of X given Y may be computed using Bayes' formula.

$$L_p(x|y) \stackrel{\triangle}{=} \log \mathcal{P}(X = x|Y = y)$$
$$= L(y|x) + \log p(x) - \log \mathcal{P}(Y = y) \tag{10.7}$$

The maximum *a posteriori* (MAP) estimate is then the value of $\hat{x}$, which maximizes the *a posteriori* density given the observations y

$$\hat{x} = \arg\max_x L_p(x|y) \tag{10.8}$$
$$= \arg\max_x \{L(y|x) + \log p(x)\}$$
$$= \arg\max_x \{L(y,x)\} \ .$$

The last equation indicates that the MAP estimate also maximizes the log of the joint distribution, $L(y,x) = \log \mathcal{P}(X = x, Y = y)$.

The MAP estimate has been shown to substantially improve performance in many image reconstruction and estimation problems. While computation of the exact MAP estimate is computationally intractable for the discrete problem, approximate solutions can be obtained with reasonable complexity as outlined in the next section. We will treat only the MAP estimation problem, since the ML estimate is the special case of a constant prior distribution.

10.3   Markov random field prior models

While the likelihood term $L(y|x)$ in the MAP equation (10.8) is determined by the physics of the data collection process, the prior distribution is selected by the experimenter to model desired characteristics of typical reconstructions. Most commonly, the prior models are chosen to reflect the high correlation of adjacent pixels. A model that has proven particularly useful is the Markov random field (MRF) [40]. Similar to a Markov chain in one dimension, the 2D MRF limits pixel interactions to a local neighborhood of pixels. This localization allows for efficient optimization of the MAP equation.

In order to write the equations for the MRF prior, we first need to define the concept of a neighborhood. If i denotes a single pixel location, we will denote its neighborhood by ∂i. This neighborhood can consist of any set of pixels $\{k : k \neq i\}$ satisfying the symmetry property that $i \in \partial k \Rightarrow k \in \partial i$. Given this definition, a MRF is a random field that has the property

$$p(x_i|x_j, j \neq i) = p(x_i|x_{\partial i}). \tag{10.9}$$

In other words, the prior conditional probability of a pixel value depends only on a local neighborhood of pixels. Under some weak technical conditions, a random field is a MRF if and only if it has a probability distribution corresponding to a Gibbs distribution [40,41]. This result, which is known as the Hammersley-Clifford theorem, may be used to express the likelihood function $\log p(x)$. While the theory of MRF's is quite extensive [42–44], we will restrict ourselves to a simple model based on at most an 8-point neighborhood.

Since we are interested in discrete-valued tomographic reconstruction, we assume that each pixel takes on a value from a set $\mathcal{E}$ of K discrete emission rates. We then apply a discrete MRF prior model that is frequently used in segmentation problems [21, 22, 33]. The model encourages neighboring locations to have the same states or, in our case, emission rates. To define the model, we must first define two simple functions, $t_1(x)$ and $t_2(x)$. Function $t_1(x)$ is the number of horizontally and vertically neighboring pixel pairs with different emission rates in x, and $t_2(x)$ is the number of diagonally neighboring pixel pairs with different emission rates in x. The discrete density function for $x \in \mathcal{E}^N$ is then assumed to be of the form

$$\log p(x) = -(\beta_1 t_1(x) + \beta_2 t_2(x)) + \log(Z) \tag{10.10}$$

where Z is an unknown constant called the partition function. The regularization parameters β_1 and β_2 weight the influence of the prior in comparison to the likelihood term. Larger values of β_1 and β_2 assign higher cost to local pixel differences, which will result in a smoother reconstruction. Based on the geometry of the 8-point neighborhood, β_2 is often chosen as $\beta_2 = \beta_1/\sqrt{2}$. In the following, we will often write β for β_1 and assume $\beta_2 = \beta_1/\sqrt{2}$.

Substituting the prior (10.10) into the MAP and likelihood equations

(10.8) and (10.4) for the emission case, we obtain the optimization criterion

$$\hat{x} = \arg \max_{x \in \mathcal{E}^N} \left\{ \sum_{i=1}^{M} (-P_{i*}x + y_i \log(P_{i*}x)) \right.$$

$$\left. -(\beta_1 t_1(x) + \beta_2 t_2(x)) \right\}. \tag{10.11}$$

10.4   Optimization techniques

In order to compute the MAP reconstruction, we must perform the optimization of (10.11). Gradient methods such as steepest descent or conjugate gradient optimization are not directly applicable, since the discrete prior (10.10) is non-differentiable.

A method that is well suited for the MAP optimization is a discrete version of iterative coordinate descent (ICD) [16,30]. The ICD method sequentially updates each pixel of the image. With each update, the current pixel is chosen to maximize the posterior probability (10.11). Therefore, the discrete ICD algorithm essentially implements the well-known ICM optimization introduced by Besag [22]. However, while ICM was originally developed for image restoration tasks, the ICD implementation is specifically designed for the tomographic reconstruction problem. The ICD algorithm takes advantage of the sparse structure of the forward projection matrix P to dramatically speed-up the optimization. Furthermore, ICD initializes the optimization with the convolution backprojection instead of the ML initialization used by ICM. The ML estimate is not a good initialization for tomographic reconstruction problems and, since the pixel likelihoods are not independent, the ML estimate is computationally expensive to compute. The convolution backprojection, in comparison, is inexpensive to compute and captures most of the low-spatial frequency behavior of the reconstruction. This makes the CBP a suitable initialization, especially since coordinate-wise update methods have slow convergence for low spatial frequencies and fast convergence for high-spatial frequencies. In the following, we will show how the ICD can be used to efficiently compute the MAP estimate.

Let $v_1(z, x_{\partial j})$ be the number of horizontal and vertical neighbors of x_j, which do not have emission rate z, and $v_2(z, x_{\partial j})$ be the number of diagonal neighbors of x_j, which do not have emission rate z. Then, the maximization of the MAP equation with respect to pixel x_j can be written as

$$x_j^{n+1} = \arg \min_z \{ -L(y|X_j = z, X_k = x_k^n, k \neq j)$$

$$+ (\beta_1 v_1(z, x_{\partial j}) + \beta_2 v_2(z, x_{\partial j})) \}. \tag{10.12}$$

In our notation, x^n is the image containing all previous pixel updates. Thus, the reconstruction x^{n+1} differs from x^n only at pixel j. A full update of the reconstruction requires N applications of (10.12).

Computation of the log-likelihood $L(y|z, x^n)$ using (10.4) for each pixel update would still lead to prohibitive computational complexity. This can be avoided by using only the change in the log-likelihood

$$\Delta L(z) = \sum_{i \in \mathcal{I}_j} \left(-P_{ij}z + y_i \log(P_{i*}x^n + P_{ij}(z - x_j^n)) \right) - y_i \log(P_{i*}x^n))$$

(10.13)

where I_j is the set of projections i intersecting pixel x_j, i.e., $\mathcal{I}_j = \{i : P_{ij} \neq 0 , 1 \leq i \leq M\}$. Leaving out the terms that are constant with respect to z, the update equation for x_j can then be written as

$$x_j^{n+1} = \arg\min_z \left\{ \sum_{i \in \mathcal{I}_j} (P_{ij}z - y_i \log(P_{i*}x^n + P_{ij}(z - x_j^n))) \right.$$

$$\left. + (\beta_1 v_1(z, x_{\partial j}) + \beta_2 v_2(z, x_{\partial j})) \right\}. \quad (10.14)$$

Assuming a reasonably small set $\mathcal{E}$ of K possible emission rates, the minimization can be carried out by trying all $z \in \mathcal{E}$ and selecting the one that minimizes (10.14). We store the M-dimensional state vector $S = Px$ between iterations. After a pixel x_j is updated, the components of S can be efficiently updated using

$$S_i^{n+1} = S_i^n + P_{ij}(x_j^{n+1} - x_j^n). \quad (10.15)$$

This update is necessary only for the components $i \in \mathcal{I}_j$ since for all other projections $P_{ij} = 0$.

In order to assess the computational complexity of the reconstruction, we first define M_0 as the average number of projections passing through a single pixel

$$M_0 = \frac{1}{N} \sum_{j=1}^{N} |\mathcal{I}_j| . \quad (10.16)$$

The computational cost for a pixel update is then on the order of KM_0 operations. The complexity of a full update of the reconstruction is therefore NKM_0. This is quite reasonable, considering that due to the sparsity of P, M_0 is typically small compared to M, i.e., $M_0 \ll M$. In cases where K is large, it might be desirable to reduce computation by using a global second-order approximation to the likelihood functions (10.2) and (10.4) as described in [16, 30]. Using these techniques, computation for a single pixel update can be reduced to order $K + M_0$, resulting in $N(K + M_0)$ complexity for a full reconstruction update.

10.5   Estimation of discrete levels

So far, we have assumed the set $\mathcal{E}$ of discrete emission rates or densities to be known. In practice, however, the exact emission rates corresponding to different regions in the cross section may not be known. Even if a good initial guess is available, the accuracy of the emission rates is critical for the reconstruction. For illustration, assume that the emission rate of a particular region is over-estimated by some amount. For projections y_i, which pass through this region, the forward projected reconstruction $P_{i*}x$ will be larger than the measured photon count, i.e., $P_{i*}x > y_i$. To compensate for this mismatch, the reconstruction algorithm may misclassify large numbers of pixels. Therefore, it is desirable to estimate the discrete emission rates as part of the reconstruction algorithm.

In this section, we show how the emission rates can be estimated concurrently with the reconstruction. We implement ML estimation of the emission rates by iteratively updating entire regions of pixels with equal emission rates [45]. We will show that this estimation is equivalent to a continuous valued tomographic ML reconstruction problem with K pixels. The updates of the emission rates will be performed between each full ICD update of the reconstruction.

Let $\theta_1 \ldots \theta_K$ denote the discrete emission rates so that $\mathcal{E} = \{\theta_1, \ldots, \theta_K\}$. Changing a single emission rate θ_k is equivalent to changing all pixels in the reconstruction that are classified to have emission rate θ_k. If we define a region as the collection of all pixels with the same emission rate, we obtain K different regions in the reconstruction. Analogous to the projection matrix P for individual pixels, we can now define a projection matrix Q for the regions. Given the region geometries, we can compute the entry Q_{ik} as the probability that an emission from the kth region is registered by the ith detector.

Assuming knowledge of Q, the likelihood for the emission rates can be computed analogously to the pixel likelihoods in (10.2) and (10.4). The resulting optimization problem is equivalent to a continuous-valued reconstruction with K pixels and projection matrix Q.

In practice, direct computation of Q from the geometry of the regions would be computationally involved and difficult to update. Instead, we can obtain an expression for the entries of Q by adding the contributions of all pixels in a region. We can rewrite the i'th forward projection $P_{i*}x$ as follows

$$P_{i*}x = \sum_{j=1}^{N} P_{ij}x_j = \sum_{k=1}^{K} \left(\theta_k \sum_{\{j:x_j=\theta_k\}} P_{ij} \right)$$

$$= \sum_{k=1}^{K} \theta_k Q_{ik} \quad = \quad Q_{i*}\theta \qquad (10.17)$$

where

$$Q_{ik} = \sum_{\{j:x_j=\theta_k\}} P_{ij}. \tag{10.18}$$

For the emission case, this yields the likelihood function

$$\log \mathcal{P}(Y = y|\theta) = \sum_{i=1}^{M} \left(-Q_{i*}\theta + y_i \log(Q_{i*}\theta) - \log(y_i!)\right). \tag{10.19}$$

This log-likelihood function is clearly of the same form as (10.4), except that the discrete-valued N-component vector x is replaced by the continuous-valued K-component vector θ. Also, the new projection matrix Q is of size $M \times K$ instead of $M \times N$. Thus, maximum likelihood estimation of θ is equivalent to a continuous-valued tomographic ML reconstruction with K pixels.

Since θ is continuous valued, the optimization of (10.19) is different from the discrete case. In general, all methods proposed for continuous-valued tomographic reconstruction can be applied. Again, we will use ICD optimization since it is easily implemented with constraints such as positivity of the emission rates. The ICD update equation of the θ_k is analogously to (10.14) given by

$$\theta_k^{n+1} = \arg\min_{v \geq 0} \left\{ \sum_{i \in \tilde{I}_k} (Q_{ik}v - y_i \log(Q_{i*}\theta^n + Q_{ik}(v - \theta_k^n))) \right\} \tag{10.20}$$

where $v \geq 0$ enforces the non-negativity of the emission rates and $\tilde{I}_k$ is defined as $\tilde{I}_k = \{i : Q_{ik} \neq 0 , \ 1 \leq i \leq M\}$. Since the cost function in (10.20) is well approximated by a quadratic, the optimization can be efficiently implemented using Newton's method.

Let ϕ_1 and ϕ_2 be the first and second derivatives of the log-likelihood function evaluated at the current emission rate θ_k. The Newton update for minimization of (10.20) is then given by

$$\theta_k' = \max\left\{\theta_k - \frac{\phi_1}{\phi_2}, \ 0\right\} \tag{10.21}$$

where the derivatives ϕ_1 and ϕ_2 are computed as

$$\phi_1 = \sum_{i \in \tilde{I}_k} Q_{ik}\left(1 - \frac{y_i}{Q_{i*}\theta}\right) \tag{10.22}$$

$$\phi_2 = \sum_{i \in \tilde{I}_k} y_i \left(\frac{Q_{ik}}{Q_{i*}\theta}\right)^2. \tag{10.23}$$

The Newton updates (10.21)-(10.23) are repeatedly applied until $|\phi_1| < \epsilon$. For our experimentation, we have found an accuracy of $\epsilon = 0.001$ to be sufficient. For efficient computation, we store and update the same state vector $S = Px = Q\theta$ as in the discrete MAP reconstruction (10.15). If θ_k^n is updated to θ_k^{n+1}, S can be updated as

$$S_i^{n+1} = S_i^n + Q_{ik}(\theta_k^{n+1} - \theta_k^n) \qquad (10.24)$$

for all $i \in \tilde{I}_k$.

In order to assess computational complexity, we define H as the average number of Newton-iterations per class update (10.20). Furthermore, we use the number of projections M as a bound for the size of the sets $\tilde{I}_k$. Computation of a single emission rate θ_k then requires on the order of MH multiplies and divides. Typically, only a few Newton-iterations are necessary to obtain sufficient accuracy $(H < 2)$. The computational complexity of updating the ML estimate of θ is then KMH. Note that KMH is typically small in comparison to a complete update of the discrete reconstruction x of order NKM_0.

The iterations for the estimation of θ can be performed between full reconstruction updates. Each time a pixel changes during the reconstruction, the new Q matrix can be obtained as follows: If $x_j^n = \theta_k$ and $x_j^{n+1} = \theta_l$, then

$$Q'_{ik} = Q_{ik} - P_{ij}$$
$$Q'_{il} = Q_{il} + P_{ij} \qquad (10.25)$$

for all projections $i \in I_j$. This recursion results in a computationally efficient algorithm since it avoids recomputing Q using (10.18) after each reconstruction update.

In order to apply the estimation of the emission rates as described above, it is necessary to obtain initial values for the estimates of θ_k. In practice, initial values for the θ_k can be extracted from the convolution backprojection reconstruction. One possibility is to extract the initial θ_k manually by taking the average value of approximately uniform regions in the CBP. This ensures that the estimated emission rates correspond to the regions of interest in the reconstruction and minimizes chances of the estimation getting trapped in local minima.

If, on the other hand, a fully unsupervised algorithm is desired, clustering techniques can be applied to the CBP reconstruction to estimate the initial emission rates θ_k. To do this, we used a clustering method based on Gaussian mixture models and the EM algorithm [46]. This method used the Rissanen criterion to estimate both the number of clusters K as well as the mean emission rate of each cluster. These estimates were then used to initialize the estimation of the emission rates, which resulted in a fully unsupervised reconstruction algorithm.

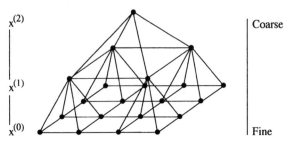

$x^{(2)}$

$x^{(1)}$

$x^{(0)}$

Coarse

Fine

FIGURE 10.2. Illustration of multiresolution structure. Shown are pixels in three different resolution levels. We assume a quadtree structure in which each coarse-scale pixel corresponds to four pixels at the next finer scale.

10.6   Multiscale approaches

We now extend the previous results to a multiresolution framework. Multiresolution algorithms reconstruct the cross section at different resolutions, typically starting at coarse resolution and progressing to the desired finest resolution. Figure 10.2 illustrates the multiresolution structure used in our algorithm. We assume a quadtree model in which each coarse scale pixel corresponds to four pixels at the next finer scale. Each resolution level is half the size of the next finer level in each direction and therefore contains only $1/4^{th}$ the number of pixels. The small number of pixels at coarse scales implies lower computational complexity at these levels.

Compared to the fixed-scale reconstruction, the multiscale approach has several significant advantages. While at first, reconstructing the cross section at several resolutions might seem like additional overhead, the multiscale algorithm has substantially faster convergence behavior. The fixed-scale ICD reconstruction algorithm updates one pixel at a time using a prior that only depends on a small pixel neighborhood. As a result, propagation of information per iteration is limited, which results in slow convergence for low spatial frequencies. The multiscale version of the algorithm improves this by first reconstructing the image at coarse resolutions where local interactions are equivalent to large-scale propagation at fine resolutions. The coarse-scale reconstructions then serve as an initialization for the finer reconstructions. Since the coarse reconstructions already contain the large-scale behavior of the solution, substantially fewer iterations are necessary at the finer scales. This, combined with the fact that the coarse-scale reconstructions are of low complexity, makes the multiscale algorithm very efficient. In addition to increased efficiency, the multiresolution algorithm is more robust with respect to local minima in the optimization. This increased robustness holds for both the reconstruction and the estimation of the emission rates.

10.7 Multiscale MRF

The multiscale MRF model is a straightforward generalization of the fixed-resolution model in section 10.3. For the multiresolution case, we essentially use the fixed-scale algorithm for each resolution level and use the result to initialize the next finer level [33].

Let $x^{(n)}$ denote the reconstruction at resolution n, where $n = 0$ is the finest resolution and $n = L - 1$ is the coarsest resolution. In order to calculate the log-likelihood function for level n, we simply compute a new projection matrix $P^{(n)}$, which incorporates the larger pixel size at level n. The matrix $P^{(n)}$ is of dimension $M \times 4^{-n} N$. The log-likelihood for the emission case is then given by

$$L^{(n)}(y|x^{(n)}) = \sum_{i=1}^{M} \left(-P_{i*}^{(n)} x^{(n)} + y_i \log(P_{i*}^{(n)} x^{(n)}) - \log(y_i!) \right). \quad (10.26)$$

This yields the MAP equation

$$\hat{x}^{(n)} = \arg\min_{x^{(n)}} \left\{ -L^{(n)}(y|x^{(n)}) + \beta_1^{(n)} t_1(x^{(n)}) + \beta_2^{(n)} t_2(x^{(n)}) \right\}. \quad (10.27)$$

The remaining question is how to choose the coarse-resolution parameters $\beta_1^{(n)}$ and $\beta_2^{(n)}$. An intuitive approach is to choose these parameters so that the cost functions for any two adjacent resolutions are equal when the finer reconstruction $x^{(n-1)}$ equals the coarser reconstruction $x^{(n)}$ [33]. This assumes that the finer reconstruction $x^{(n)}$ is constant on blocks of 2 by 2 pixels.

Let I denote the operator, which interpolates by a factor of two using pixel-replication. The equality of adjacent levels can then be written as $x^{(n-1)} = I x^{(n)}$. We now observe that a horizontal or vertical pixel difference in $x^{(n)}$ results in two horizontal or vertical plus two diagonal differences in the pixel-replicated $I x^{(n)}$, and one diagonal pixel difference in $x^{(n)}$ yields one diagonal pixel difference in $I x^{(n)}$. Therefore, $x^{(n-1)} = I x^{(n)}$ implies

$$t_1^{(n-1)} = 2 t_1^{(n)}$$
$$t_2^{(n-1)} = 2 t_1^{(n)} + t_2^{(n)}. \quad (10.28)$$

Consequently, the fine- and coarse-resolution cost functions will be equal if

$$\beta_1^{(n)} = 2(\beta_1^{(n-1)} + \beta_2^{(n-1)})$$
$$\beta_2^{(n)} = \beta_2^{(n-1)} \quad (10.29)$$

for all resolutions n. By using these parameters, minimization of (10.27) corresponds to the minimization of the original MAP equation (10.11) under the constraint that the solution be constant on the appropriately sized blocks.

Coarse-resolution minimization using the parameters given by (10.29) will effectively minimize (10.11) if the correct segmentation is approximately block constant. However, this recursion for the parameters has an undesirable property. It implies that the MRF models for coarser resolution segmentations should have progressively higher spatial correlation, or alternatively, finer resolution segmentations should have lower correlation. This, of course, runs counter to normal assumptions of spatial coherence in images, and will tend to cause insufficient spatial correlation at finer resolutions or excessive correlation at coarse resolutions. A more reasonable approach is to assume that the spatial correlation is independent of the resolution since this avoids the problem of excessive correlation at coarse resolutions. Also, this assumption is appropriate when prior information is unavailable about the likely scale of regions in the image. Therefore, in all experimentation, we will fix the parameters of the MRF as a function of scale

$$\beta_1^{(n)} = \beta_1$$
$$\beta_2^{(n)} = \beta_2. \tag{10.30}$$

The L level Multiresolution MAP reconstruction algorithm may then be summarized as follows:

1. Compute CBP and estimate initial emission rates θ.

2. Classify CBP pixels into discrete emission rates θ_k using thresholding. Decimate the result $(L-1)$-times to initialize $x^{(L-1)}$. Set $n = L - 1$.

3. Compute reconstruction $x^{(n)}$ using the following method:

    (a) Update $x^{(n)}$ using one full pass of discrete ICD algorithm.
    (b) If no pixel change occurs, goto 4.
    (c) Perform six full updates of discrete levels θ, goto (a).

4. If $n = 0$ stop.

5. Initialize $x^{(n-1)}$ with pixel-replicated $x^{(n)}$.

6. Set $n = n - 1$, goto 3.

The parameters β_1 and β_2 can be chosen manually to achieve the amount of regularization desired.

10.8 Computational complexity

Table 10.1 compares the computational complexity for one full update of the reconstruction to one update of the emission rates θ. The complexity of the reconstruction update NKM_0 depends on the number of pixels

	Reconstruction Update	Emission Rate Update
Fixed Scale	NKM_0	KMH
Multiscale	$4^{-n}NKM_0^{(n)} \approx 2^{-n}NKM_0$	KMH

N	Number of pixels in the reconstruction
K	Number of discrete emission rates θ_k
M	Number of projections
$M_0^{(n)}$	Average number of projections intersecting a pixel at scale n, $M_0 = M_0^{(0)}$
H	Average number of Newton iterations for update of single θ_k

TABLE 10.1. Computational complexity for reconstruction and emission rate updates. While the complexity of the reconstruction is a function of the resolution n, the cost for the estimation of θ is constant. For the overall reconstruction, the time spent on estimation of θ is typically less than 10% of total execution time.

N and, therefore, on the resolution of the reconstruction. In the multiresolution framework, each level contains $1/4^{th}$ of the number of pixels of the next finer level. The reconstruction complexity at scale n is therefore $4^{-n}NKM_0^{(n)}$, where $M_0^{(n)}$ replaces M_0. Due to the larger pixel size at coarse resolution, more projections intersect each coarse-scale pixel and $M_0^{(n)}$ increases with n. In order to compare the complexities for different scales, we can approximate $M_0^{(n)}$ as follows: As the size of a pixel doubles in each direction, we assume that the number of parallel projections intersecting the pixel at each angle doubles. The cost of a reconstruction update at scale n is therefore approximately $2^{-n}NKM_0$. Assuming that the multiscale reconstruction performs the same number of iterations at each scale as the fixed resolution algorithm, the multiscale overhead is bounded by a factor of 2. In most real applications, however, the multiscale algorithm performs considerably fewer computationally expensive iterations at fine scale than the fixed-scale method.

The complexity of the emission rate update is not a function of resolution. To obtain a bound on the computational cost, we assume that all M projections intersect each region. Since the number of Newton iterations per class update H is usually small, the upper bound KMH for the emission rate update is small in comparison to the cost NKM_0 for a reconstruction update at finest or fixed scale. At coarse resolutions, however, the complexity for the emission rate update may become comparable to the cost for a reconstruction update. Again, the advantage of the multiscale method is that the emission rates often converge after the reconstruction of the coarser scales. Therefore, fewer iterations for reconstruction and emission rate estimation are necessary at finer scale.

In practice, the total cost of the emission rate estimation is usually small compared to that of the reconstruction updates. Performing six updates of θ between full reconstruction updates, we find that the cost of the emission rate updates is typically less than 10% of the total execution time. In addition, the multiscale algorithm is typically faster than the fixed-resolution method.

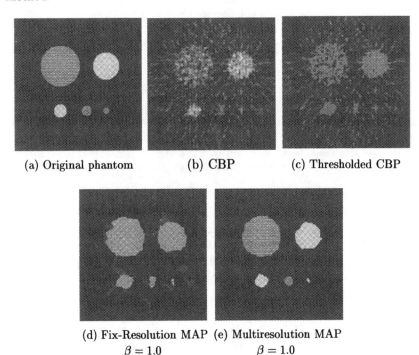

(a) Original phantom   (b) CBP   (c) Thresholded CBP

(d) Fix-Resolution MAP (e) Multiresolution MAP
$\beta = 1.0$ $\beta = 1.0$

FIGURE 10.3. Results for synthetic cross section. Shown in (a) is the original cross section. The continuous-valued CBP (b) contains considerable noise, which is still present in the thresholded version (c), using the thresholds determined by unsupervised clustering. The fixed-resolution algorithm (d), gets trapped in a local minimum resulting in class estimates close to the initialization. The multiresolution algorithm (e) estimates the classes correctly and achieves higher reconstruction performance.

10.9   Results

Reconstructions using the fixed- and multiscale-algorithms on synthetic data are shown in Fig. 10.3. Figure 10.3(a) shows the original cross section of size 192 by 192 pixels where each pixel is of both width and height 3.13mm. The cross section contains pixels with three different emission

	Em.-Rate θ_1	Em.-Rate θ_2	Em.-Rate θ_3
Original Phantom	0.001	0.05	0.1
CBP Clustering	0.0005	0.0108	0.04
Fixed-Res. MAP	0.0007	0.0105	0.0632
Multires. MAP	0.0010	0.0512	0.1028

TABLE 10.2. Original and estimated emission rates for synthetic cross section. While the fixed-scale algorithm gets trapped near the clustering initialization, the multiscale method estimates the emission rates quite accurately. All units are in mm^{-1}.

	Multi-Resolution	Fixed-Resolution
Phantom I	27	59
Phantom II	349	404

TABLE 10.3. CPU-time in seconds for fixed- and multiresolution algorithms. Both algorithms were run until convergence and terminated when no pixel change occurred in a discrete reconstruction update.

rates as shown in Table 10.2. The projection data was calculated at 16 evenly spaced angles each with 192 parallel projections. The projection beam was assumed to be infinitely thin. The data samples where formed by Poisson random variables with the appropriate means.

Figure 10.3(b) shows the convolution backprojection (CBP) reconstruction using a generalized Hamming filter weighted by a Gaussian envelope. The CBP reconstruction was used to obtain initial values for the emission rates θ. The unsupervised clustering routine using a Gaussian mixture model applied to the CBP reconstruction identified three clusters with mean emission rates $\theta = [0.005, 0.0108, 0.04]$. The clustering result consists of two classes with very low emission rates corresponding to background pixels and only one class with higher emission rate corresponding to the discs in the foreground. A first, discrete-valued reconstruction can be obtained by thresholding the CBP reconstruction using the midpoints between the emission rates determined by the clustering routine. The resulting thresholded CBP is shown in Fig. 10.3(c). In addition to the errors in class estimates, the result contains noise and aliasing effects. Figure 10.3(d) shows the fixed-resolution MAP reconstruction using $\beta = 1.0$ where we assume that $\beta_1 = \beta$ and $\beta_2 = \beta/\sqrt{2}$. The fixed-resolution reconstruction was initialized to the thresholded CBP reconstruction and the class estimates were initialized to the clustering result. While the reconstruction is less noisy than the thresholded CBP, the estimation of emission rates is trapped in a local minimum close to the initial values from the clustering result. This results in the classification of all 5 discs into the same class of emission rates.

The reconstruction result using the multiscale algorithm with $L = 5$

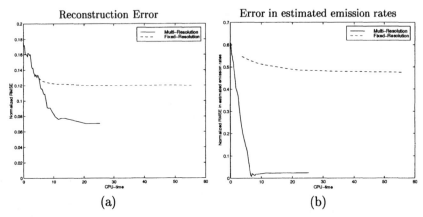

FIGURE 10.4. Comparison of convergence for the fixed- and multiresolution MAP reconstructions of Fig. 10.3(d)-(e). Shown in (a) is the normalized reconstruction error as a function of CPU-time. The multiscale algorithm converges considerably faster than the fixed-resolution method. This is partly due to the fast convergence of the emission rate estimates in the multiscale case (b). The multiresolution algorithm achieves lower final error in estimation and reconstruction.

resolution levels and $\beta = 1.0$ is shown in Fig. 10.3(e). The algorithm was initialized as in the fixed-scale case. The estimated emission rates using the multiscale technique are very close to the true values as shown in Table 10.2. This results in correct classification of the 4 larger discs in the cross section. Only the smallest disc is misclassified to a smaller area but higher emission rate than in the original phantom. This is not surprising, considering the high level of noise and the small size of the disc, which practically eliminates it from coarser resolution levels. For $\beta = 1.0$, there is essentially no high-frequency noise in the reconstruction. Overall, the quality of the multiscale reconstruction is superior to the fixed-scale MAP reconstruction and the thresholded CBP. The multiscale method is particularly robust with respect to the estimation of the emission rates.

In addition to the superior reconstruction quality, the multiresolution method is faster than the fixed-scale algorithm. Table 10.3 shows the execution times for both the fixed- and multiresolution reconstructions (Phantom I). Both algorithms were run until convergence and terminated when no pixel change occurred in a discrete reconstruction update. While the multiscale method terminated after 25 seconds, the fixed-scale method needed 56 seconds to converge. Figure 10.4 compares the error convergence of the two algorithms. Figure 10.4(a) shows the reconstruction error as a function of CPU-time. The reconstruction error is calculated as normalized root mean

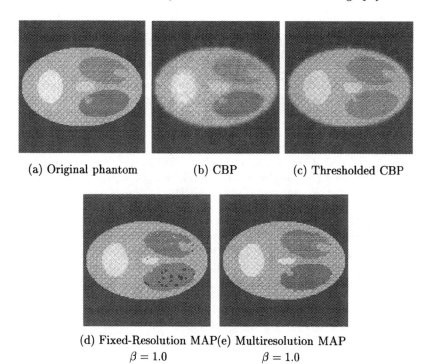

(a) Original phantom   (b) CBP   (c) Thresholded CBP

(d) Fixed-Resolution MAP (e) Multiresolution MAP
$\beta = 1.0$ $\beta = 1.0$

FIGURE 10.5. Results for second synthetic cross section. The clustering only identifies 2 out of 7 classes correctly as reflected in the thresholded CBP (c). The fixed-resolution algorithm (d) estimates 3 of 7 classes correctly, and fails to divide the two gray ovals on right into two distinct classes, which results in compensation artifacts. The multiresolution algorithm (e) performs better, estimating 5 out of seven classes correctly. Neither algorithm divides the bright left and center spot into two distinct classes. Both also miss the emission rate of the small patch within the lower right oval.

square error, i.e.,

$$E = \sqrt{\frac{\sum_{j=1}^{N}(\hat{x}_j - x_j)^2}{\sum_{j=1}^{N} x_j^2}} \tag{10.31}$$

where x denotes the true cross section and $\hat{x}$ denotes the current estimate of the cross section. In the multiscale case, $\hat{x}$ is computed by interpolating $x^{(n)}$ using pixel replication. The multiscale algorithm converges considerably faster and achieves lower final reconstruction error than the fixed-resolution method. We also observed that the multiscale method achieves larger posterior likelihood, confirming that the fixed-scale algorithm gets trapped in a local minimum.

The difference in convergence speed and final reconstruction error between the fixed- and multiscale algorithm is reflected in the convergence

	θ_1	θ_2	θ_3	θ_4	θ_5	θ_6	θ_7
Orig. Phantom	0.001	1.2	1.6	2.0	2.4	3.2	3.6
CBP Clustering	0.0005	0.028	0.094	0.307	**1.606**	**2.359**	3.335
Fixed-Res. MAP	**0.001**	0.028	0.094	0.338	1.445	**2.403**	**3.574**
Multires. MAP	**0.001**	0.144	0.336	**1.211**	**1.602**	**2.404**	**3.578**

TABLE 10.4. Original and estimated emission rates for second synthetic cross section. Bold-faced numbers represent emission rates that were estimated within a reasonable tolerance of their true values. Both, the fixed- and multiscale algorithm were initialized to the emission rates determined by the clustering algorithm. All units are in mm^{-1}.

behavior of the emission rate estimates. Figure 10.4(b) shows the convergence of the normalized root mean square error of the emission rate estimates. For the multiscale algorithm, the θ are essentially converged after only a few coarse-scale iterations. This reduces the number of computationally expensive iterations at finer scales, thereby accelerating overall convergence substantially.

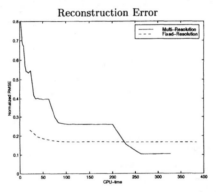

FIGURE 10.6. Error convergence for fixed- and multiresolution MAP reconstructions of the second phantom. While the multiscale error at coarser scales is comparably high, convergence at each resolution is rapid. Again, the multiresolution algorithm terminates earlier and achieves lower final reconstruction error than the fixed-resolution method.

Results for a second synthetic cross section are shown in Fig. 10.5. The original cross section in Fig. 10.5(a) contains 7 discrete levels of emission rates. The size of the phantom is 128 by 128 pixels where each pixel is of both width and height 1.56mm. The projection data was calculated at 128 evenly spaced angles, each with 128 parallel projections. Again, the data samples were obtained as Poisson random variables with the appropriate mean. Figure 10.5(b) shows the convolution backprojection that is blurred and contains considerable amounts of noise. The clustering routine was used to obtain initial values for the emission rates. Due to the high noise in the CBP reconstruction the number of clusters was not estimated but manually set to seven. As shown in Table 10.4, the clustering only identified 2 out of the 7 classes within a reasonable tolerance of their true values. The thresholded CBP shown in Fig. 10.5(c) shows that the two gray ovals on the right are erroneously classified to have the same emission rate. Similarly, the bright patch on the left is set to the same emission rate as the center spot. In addition, the small patch within the gray oval on the lower right is misclassified. Figure 10.5(d) shows the reconstruction using the fixed-resolution algorithm. As before, the emission rates were initialized to the cluster means and the reconstruction was initialized to the thresholded CBP. As indicated in Table 10.4, the fixed-resolution algorithm terminates with class estimates close to the initial cluster values. While the background level of 0.001 is now correctly estimated, the emission rate for the two gray ovals with original rates 1.2 and 1.6 has moved between the two values to $\theta_5 = 1.4458$. Notice that the overestimation of the lower right oval yields a mismatch between observed projection counts y and the forward projected reconstruction Px. Since the pixel values x within the oval are too large, we obtain $P_{i*}x > y_i$ for many projections intersecting this region. To compensate for this, the reconstruction algorithm inserts a pattern of black spots into the region, which lowers the average projection count. Analogously, the gray oval on the upper right contains white spots to compensate underestimation of the emission rate 1.6 by 1.4458. Effects such as these result from the algorithm's being trapped in local minima of the MAP cost function. This is particularly critical for fixed-resolution reconstructions that include the estimation of emission rates.

The multiscale algorithm is less prone to being trapped in local minima. For this phantom, 5 out of 7 emission rates are estimated correctly. The reconstruction as shown in Fig. 10.5(e) contains little noise and classifies the two gray ovals correctly. However, the left and center bright regions with emission rates 3.6 and 3.2 are still both classified as having a single emission rate of 3.5783. This can be improved by initializing the emission rates closer to their true values. In general, by varying the initial estimate for the emission rates, it is often possible for the fixed-scale algorithm to obtain reconstructions comparable to the multiscale reconstruction. However, the fixed-resolution algorithm is less robust with respect to the emission rate estimation and close initialization does not guarantee a comparable reconstruction.

In almost all cases, with and without estimation of emission rates, the multiresolution algorithm is faster than the fixed-resolution method. As shown in Table 10.3 (Phantom II), the multiscale algorithm terminates after 349 seconds compared to 404 seconds for the fixed-resolution method. Figure 10.6 compares the error convergence for the fixed and multiscale reconstructions of the second phantom. The multiscale error at coarse scales is comparably high since the coarse-scale reconstructions cannot account for

	Multi-Resolution	Fixed-Resolution
Phantom I	6.48% (1.75/27s)	1.64% (0.97/59s)
Phantom II	8.70% (30.37/349s)	2.77% (11.21/404s)

TABLE 10.5. Percentage of CPU-time used for estimation of emission rates. In all cases, the complexity for estimating θ is smaller than 10% of the total execution time. Shown in brackets are the CPU-times for estimating θ over the total execution times in seconds.

the phantom's fine structure. However, the multiscale algorithm converges rapidly at each scale, resulting in lower total execution time. Again, the multiresolution algorithm achieves lower final reconstruction error.

Finally, we examine the computational complexity of the estimation of emission rates in relation to the overall complexity of the algorithms. Table 10.5 shows the percentage of CPU-time used for the estimation of θ. For all reconstructions, six full updates of θ were performed between full reconstruction updates. In all cases, the emission rate updates make up less than 10% of the total CPU-time. The percentages are smaller for the fixed-resolution algorithm than for the multiresolution algorithm. Since the fixed-resolution algorithm performs more computationally expensive iterations at fine scale, the relative cost for reconstruction updates is higher than for the multiscale method. Added over all resolutions, however, the multiscale algorithm performs more iterations than the fixed-scale method. Since an iteration at any scale includes a fixed-cost update of θ, the multiscale method spends more absolute time on estimating the emission rates. This may be reduced by introducing a convergence criteria for the emission rate updates instead of running a fixed number of iterations between reconstruction updates.

In conclusion, the results indicate that the multiresolution algorithm can achieve reconstruction results superior to the fixed-scale method. It is particularly robust with respect to the initialization of emission rates. Furthermore, the multiscale method is typically faster than the fixed-resolution algorithm. For both algorithms, the computational cost for estimating the emission rates is small in comparison to the reconstruction complexity.

10.10   Conclusion

In this work, we have described a fixed- and multiscale method for discrete-valued Bayesian reconstruction. The multiscale MRF reconstruction algorithm is a straightforward extension of the fixed-scale model. Interaction between resolution levels is obtained by initialization of each reconstruction with the previous coarser reconstruction. The algorithm includes an efficient method for estimating the discrete emission rates. The quality of the multiresolution reconstructions is significantly better than thresholded CBP reconstructions. In comparison to a fixed-scale MAP reconstruction, the multiresolution method is less prone to local minima and converges faster.

Acknowledgment

This work was supported by the National Science Foundation under Grant MIP97-07763.

References

[1] G. Herman, *Image Reconstruction from Projections: The Fundamentals of Computerized Tomography* (Academic Press, New York), 1980.

[2] G. C. McKinnon and R. H. T. Bates, "Towards imaging the beating heart usefully with a conventional CT scanner," *IEEE Trans. on Biomedical Engineering* **BME-28**, 123–127 (1981).

[3] J. G. Sanderson, "Reconstruction of fuel pin bundles by a maximum entropy method," *IEEE Trans. on Nuclear Science* **NS-26**, 2685–2688 (1979).

[4] T. Inouye, "Image reconstruction with limited-angle projection data," *IEEE Trans. on Nuclear Science* **NS-26**, 2666–2684 (1979).

[5] G. H. Glover and N. J. Pelc, "An algorithm for the reduction of metal clip artifacts in CT reconstruction," *Med. Phys.* **8**, 799–807 (1981).

[6] S. K. Chang, "The reconstruction of binary patterns from their projections," *Communications of the ACM* **14**, 21–25 (1971).

[7] A. Shliferstein and Y. T. Chien, "Switching components and the ambiguity problem in the reconstruction of pictures from their projections," *Pattern Recognition* **10**, 327–340 (1978).

[8] A. Kuba, "The reconstruction of two-directionally connected binary patterns from their two orthogonal projections," *Comput. Vision Graphics and Image Process.* **27**, 249–265 (1984).

[9] S. K. Chang and C. K. Chow, "The reconstruction of three-dimensional objects from two orthogonal projections and its application to cardiac cineangiography," *IEEE Trans. on Computers* **C-22**, 18–28 (1973).

[10] M. Soumekh, "Binary image reconstruction from four projections," *Proc. of IEEE Int'l Conf. on Acoust., Speech and Sig. Proc.*, (IEEE, New York City NY), pp. 1280–1283, 1988.

[11] D. J. Rossi and A. S. Willsky, "Reconstruction from projections based on detection and estimation of objects – parts I and II: Performance analysis and robustness analysis," *IEEE Trans. on Acoustics, Speech, and Signal Processing* **ASSP-32**, 886–906 (1984).

[12] Y. Bresler, J. A. Fessler, and A. Macovski, "A Bayesian approach to reconstruction from incomplete projections of a multiple object 3D domain," *IEEE Trans. on Pattern Analysis and Machine Intelligence* **11**, 840–858 (1989).

[13] S. Geman and D. McClure, "Bayesian image analysis: An application to single photon emission tomography," *Proc. Statist. Comput. sect. Amer. Stat. Assoc.*, Washington, DC, pp. 12–18, 1985.

[14] T. Hebert and R. Leahy, "A generalized EM algorithm for 3-D Bayesian reconstruction from Poisson data using Gibbs priors," *IEEE Trans. on Medical Imaging* **8**, 194–202 (1989).

[15] P. J. Green, "Bayesian reconstruction from emission tomography data using a modified EM algorithm," *IEEE Trans. on Medical Imaging* **9**, 84–93 (1990).

[16] K. Sauer and C. A. Bouman, "A local update strategy for iterative reconstruction from projections," *IEEE Trans. on Signal Processing* **41**, 534–548 (1993).

[17] B. Hunt, "Bayesian methods in nonlinear digital image restoration," *IEEE Trans. on Computers* **C-26**, 219–229 (1977).

[18] S. Geman and D. Geman, "Stochastic relaxation, Gibbs distributions and the Bayesian restoration of images," *IEEE Trans. on Pattern Analysis and Machine Intelligence* **PAMI-6**, 721–741 (1984).

[19] S. Geman and D. McClure, "Statistical methods for tomographic image reconstruction," *Bull. Int. Stat. Inst.* **LII-4**, 5–21 (1987).

[20] C. A. Bouman and K. Sauer, "A generalized Gaussian image model for edge-preserving MAP estimation," *IEEE Trans. on Image Processing* **2**, 296–310 (1993).

[21] H. Derin, H. Elliot, R. Cristi, and D. Geman, "Bayes smoothing algorithms for segmentation of binary images modeled by Markov random fields," *IEEE Trans. on Pattern Analysis and Machine Intelligence* **PAMI-6**, 707–719 (1984).

[22] J. Besag, "On the statistical analysis of dirty pictures," *Journal of the Royal Statistical Society B* **48**, 259–302 (1986).

[23] L. Shepp and Y. Vardi, "Maximum likelihood reconstruction for emission tomography," *IEEE Trans. on Medical Imaging* **MI-1**, 113–122 (1982).

[24] H. Hart and Z. Liang, "Bayesian image processing in two dimensions," *IEEE Trans. on Medical Imaging* **MI-6**, 201–208 (1987).

[25] Z. Liang and H. Hart, "Bayesian image processing of data from constrained source distributions–I: Non-valued, uncorrelated and correlated constraints," *Bull. Math. Biol.* **49**, 51–74 (1987).

[26] G. T. Herman and D. Odhner, "Performance evaluation of an iterative image reconstruction algorithm for positron emission tomography," *IEEE Trans. on Medical Imaging* **10**, 336–346 (1991).

[27] G. T. Herman, A. R. De Pierro, and N. Gai, "On methods for maximum a posteriori image reconstruction with normal prior," *J. Visual Comm. Image Rep.* **3**, 316–324 (1992).

[28] T. Hebert and S. Gopal, "The GEM MAP algorithm with 3-D SPECT system response," *IEEE Trans. on Medical Imaging* **11**, 81–90 (1992).

[29] A. De Pierro, "A modified expectation maximization algorithm for penalized likelihood estimation in emission tomography," *IEEE Trans. on Medical Imaging* **14**, 132–137 (1995).

[30] C. A. Bouman and K. Sauer, "A unified approach to statistical tomography using coordinate descent optimization," *IEEE Trans. on Image Processing* **5**, 480–492 (1996).

[31] M. R. Luettgen, W. C. Karl, and A. S. Willsky, "Efficient multiscale regularization with applications to the computation of optical flow," *IEEE Trans. on Image Processing* **3**, 41–63 (1994).

[32] F. Heitz, P. Perez, and P. Bouthemy, "Multiscale minimization of global energy functions in some visual recovery problems," *Comput. Vision Graphics and Image Process.* **59**, 125–134 (1994).

[33] C. A. Bouman and B. Liu, "Multiple resolution segmentation of textured images," *IEEE Trans. on Pattern Analysis and Machine Intelligence* **13**, 99–113 (1991).

[34] C. A. Bouman and M. Shapiro, "A multiscale random field model for Bayesian image segmentation," *IEEE Trans. on Image Processing* **3**, 162–177 (1994).

[35] S. S. Saquib, C. A. Bouman, and K. Sauer, "A non-homogeneous MRF model for multiresolution Bayesian estimation," *Proc. of IEEE Int'l Conf. on Image Proc.*, (IEEE, Lausanne Switzerland), pp. 445–448, 1996.

[36] D. Snyder and M. Miller, "The use of sieves to stabilize images produced with the EM algorithm for emission tomography," *IEEE Trans. on Nuclear Science* **NS-32**, 3864–3871 (1985).

[37] E. Veklerov and J. Llacer, "Stopping rule for the MLE algorithm based on statistical hypothesis testing," *IEEE Trans. on Medical Imaging* **MI-6**, 313–319 (1987).

[38] T. Hebert, R. Leahy, and M. Singh, "Fast MLE for SPECT using an intermediate polar representation and a stopping criterion," *IEEE Trans. on Nuclear Science* **35**, 615–619 (1988).

[39] A. Tikhonov and V. Arsenin, *Solutions of Ill-Posed Problems* (Winston and Sons, New York), 1977.

[40] J. Besag, "Spatial interaction and the statistical analysis of lattice systems," *Journal of the Royal Statistical Society B* **36**, 192–236 (1974).

[41] R. Kindermann and J. Snell, *Markov Random Fields and their Applications* (American Mathematical Society, Providence), 1980.

[42] R. Kashyap and R. Chellappa, "Estimation and choice of neighbors in spatial-interaction models of images," *IEEE Trans. on Information Theory* **IT-29**, 60–72 (1983).

[43] D. Pickard, "Inference for discrete Markov fields: The simplest nontrivial case," *Journal of the American Statistical Association* **82**, 90–96 (1987).

[44] R. Dubes and A. Jain, "Random field models in image analysis," *Journal of Applied Statistics* **16**, 131–164 (1989).

[45] K. Sauer and C. Bouman, "Bayesian estimation of transmission tomograms using segmentation based optimization," *IEEE Trans. on Nuclear Science* **39**, 1144–1152 (1992).

[46] C. A. Bouman, "Cluster: an unsupervised algorithm for modeling Gaussian mixtures." Available from http://www.ece.purdue.edu/~bouman, 1997.

Chapter 11

An Algebraic Solution for Discrete Tomography

Andrew E. Yagle[1]

ABSTRACT Discrete tomography is the problem of reconstructing a binary image defined on a discrete lattice of points from its projections at only a few angles. It has applications in X-ray crystallography, in which the projections are the number of atoms in the crystal along a given line, and nondestructive testing. The 2D version of this problem is fairly well understood, and several algorithms for solving it are known, most of which involve discrete mathematics or network theory. However, the 3D problem is much harder to solve. This chapter shows how the problem can be recast in a purely algebraic form. This results in: (1) new insight into the number of projection angles needed for an almost surely unique solution; (2) non-obvious dependencies in projection data; and (3) new algorithms for solving it. We then present an explicit formula for reconstructing a finite-support object from a finite number of its discrete projections over a limited range of angles, again making extensive use of the discrete Fourier transform in doing so. We compute the object directly as a linear combination of the projections. The well-known ill-posedness of the limited-angle tomography problem manifests itself in some very large coefficients in these linear combinations; these coefficients, which are computed off-line, provide a direct sensitivity measure of the reconstruction samples to the projections samples. The discrete nature of the problem implies that the projections must also take on integer values; this means noise can be rejected. This makes the formula practical.

11.1 Introduction

11.1.1 Applications

In the version of the discrete tomography problem, which is the subject matter of this chapter, we have an object defined on a discrete lattice of points and taking on only two possible known values, which without loss of generality can be taken to be zero and one. We also have projection data

---

[1]The University of Michigan, Dept. of Electrical Engineering and Computer Science, Ann Arbor MI 48109-2122, USA, E-mail: aey@eecs.umich.edu

at the same number of angles as the dimension of the problem (i.e., two angles for the 2D problem and three angles for the 3D problem). These projections are various sums of the object pixels (zero or one) along the principal axes of the lattice. The goal is to reconstruct the binary image from its projections. Note that since the projections are sums of zeros and ones, they are integers; this allows error correction and elimination of noise known to be less than 0.5 in absolute value.

This problem arises in X-ray tomography, where possible atom locations in the unit cell of a crystal are defined on a discrete lattice. The presence of an atom at a specific location corresponds to a pixel value of one at that location; the absence of an atom corresponds to a pixel value of zero. The X-ray measurements are related to the number of atoms along a specific direction, i.e., the sum of the pixel values along that line. Measurements are usually only available along three or so orthogonal directions. The goal is to reconstruct the locations in the unit cell occupied by atoms, i.e., reconstruct the pixel (zero or one) at each lattice point.

This problem also arises in nondestructive testing, in which the goal is to determine flaws (inclusions, bubbles, or hollow regions) inside a block of otherwise homogeneous material. In this case the zero or one pixel values correspond to presence or absence of material at a specific location, or to the presence of a different material at some location. If the absorption at a specific location can take on two possible values, these can easily be transformed into zero and one.

11.1.2 Discussion

The discrete tomography problem is clearly more difficult than the usual tomography problem, since the number of angles is so small. It is clear that the restriction of pixel values to zero or one must be exploited in order to obtain a unique solution. This suggests the use of discrete mathematics, and many algorithms for the 2D problem use this approach. The 3D case has proven to be much more intractable than the 2D case.

Our approach is to reformulate the problem in the discrete Fourier transform (DFT) domain. We also employ the Agarwal-Cooley convolution mapping in the reformulation. This yields four advantages:

1. Insight into the number of projection angles required for an almost surely unique solution.

2. Insight into hidden dependencies in the projection data.

3. New approaches and algorithms for solving the 3D problem.

4. An explicit formula for the 2D problem with several view angles, which avoids even the solution of a linear system of equations.

For a good picture of the state of the art in discrete tomography, both theory and applications, see the 1998 special issue of the *International Journal of Imaging Systems and Technology* on discrete tomography, or [1]. We present small numerical examples in which the reader can follow details, rather than simply providing a large object and noting that the algorithms successfully reconstructed it.

11.2   Problem formulation and nonuniqueness

11.2.1   Problem formulation

The 3D discrete tomography problem can be formulated as follows. Let $x(i_1, i_2, i_3) = 0$ or 1 for $1 \leq i_j \leq M_j, 1 \leq j \leq 3$ for some integers M_1, M_2, M_3. The $M_1 \times M_2 \times M_3$ 3D discrete tomography problem is to reconstruct $x(i_1, i_2, i_3)$ from its projections

$$p_1(i_2, i_3) = \sum_{i_1=1}^{M_1} x(i_1, i_2, i_3);$$

$$p_2(i_1, i_3) = \sum_{i_2=1}^{M_2} x(i_1, i_2, i_3); \tag{11.1}$$

$$p_3(i_1, i_2) = \sum_{i_3=1}^{M_3} x(i_1, i_2, i_3).$$

It is not at all clear that this can be done uniquely. Note that if $M_1 = M_2 = M_3 = M$ then we have $3M^2$ equations in M^3 unknowns, so the problem seems to be underdetermined. In fact, we will demonstrate dependencies even among the $3M^2$ projection values we do have.

11.2.2   Nonuniqueness

The 2D version of this problem, which is defined analogously to (11.1), does have a well-known ambiguity. Let $\{i_a, i_b, j_a, j_b\}$ be four indices such that

$$x(i_a, j_a) = x(i_b, j_b) = 1; \quad x(i_a, j_b) = x(i_b, j_a) = 0. \tag{11.2}$$

In (11.2) we can exchange "0" and "1" without affecting any of the projections. The likelihood of a quadruple $\begin{bmatrix} 1 & 0 \\ 0 & 1 \end{bmatrix}$ occurring somewhere in a 2D object of substantial size is high (note that the rows and columns need not adjoin each other). Such an exchange is what is referred to as a rectangular 4-switch in Chapter 3 by Kong and Herman in this book. Every such quadruple creates an ambiguity in the 2D discrete tomography problem.

The 3D version of this ambiguity is more involved. Let $\{i_a, j_a, k_a, i_b, j_b, k_b\}$ be six unequal indices such that

$$x(i_a, j_a, k_a) = x(i_a, j_b, k_b) = x(i_b, j_a, k_b) = x(i_b, j_b, k_a) = 1; \quad (11.3)$$
$$x(i_a, j_a, k_b) = x(i_b, j_b, k_b) = x(i_b, j_a, k_a) = x(i_a, j_b, k_a) = 0.$$

In (11.3) we can again exchange "0" and "1" without affecting any of the projections (11.1) (in 3D this time). The likelihood of an octuple consisting of two parallel quadruples $\begin{bmatrix} 1 & 0 \\ 0 & 1 \end{bmatrix}$ and $\begin{bmatrix} 0 & 1 \\ 1 & 0 \end{bmatrix}$ is again high, due to the great number of such octuples. Each such octuple creates an ambiguity [2].

Why does this happen? We now provide some insight. The material that follows seems to be new.

11.3   Reformulation and insights using the DFT

11.3.1   Reformulation using the DFT

The condition $x(i_1, i_2, i_3) = 0, 1$ can be written as

$$x^2(i_1, i_2, i_3) - x(i_1, i_2, i_3) = x(i_1, i_2, i_3)(x(i_1, i_2, i_3) - 1) = 0. \quad (11.4)$$

Taking the $(M_1 \times M_2 \times M_3)$-point 3D DFT, defined as [3]

$$X(k_1, k_2, k_3) = \sum_{i_1, i_2, i_3} x(i_1, i_2, i_3) e^{\frac{-j2\pi(i_1 k_1 + i_2 k_2 + i_3 k_3)}{M_1 M_2 M_3}}, \quad j = \sqrt{-1}, \quad (11.5)$$

of (11.4) and using the discrete convolution theorem [3] gives

$$X(k_1, k_2, k_3) * * * X(k_1, k_2, k_3) = (M_1 M_2 M_3) \cdot X(k_1, k_2, k_3), \quad (11.6)$$

where $* * *$ denotes the 3D cyclic convolution of order (M_1, M_2, M_3) [3]:

$$X(k_1, k_2, k_3) * * * Y(k_1, k_2, k_3) =$$

$$\sum_{k_1'=1}^{M_1} \sum_{k_2'=1}^{M_2} \sum_{k_3'=1}^{M_3} X(k_1', k_2', k_3') \cdot Y((k_1 - k_1'), (k_2 - k_2'), (k_3 - k_3')), \quad (11.7)$$

in which periodic extensions of $Y(k_1, k_2, k_3)$ have been taken.

Furthermore, using the projection-slice theorem [3], knowledge of the projections (11.1) amounts to knowledge of

$$\begin{aligned} P_1(k_2, k_3) &= X(0, k_2, k_3); \\ P_2(k_1, k_3) &= X(k_1, 0, k_3); \\ P_3(k_1, k_2) &= X(k_1, k_2, 0), \end{aligned} \quad (11.8)$$

where $P_i(\cdot)$ are the obvious 2D DFTs of (11.1).

11.3.2 Ambiguity insights using the DFT

It is now immediately clear why the ambiguity noted above occurs. First, consider the 2D case. We can clearly add any term of the form

$$\left(e^{j2\pi i_a k_1/M_1} - e^{j2\pi i_b k_1/M_1}\right)\left(e^{j2\pi j_a k_2/M_2} - e^{j2\pi j_b k_2/M_2}\right) \tag{11.9}$$

to $X(k_1, k_2)$, without altering the given projection data, since the term is zero if either $k_1 = 0$ or $k_2 = 0$. Expanding this gives the ambiguity (11.2).

In the 3D case this term becomes

$$\left(e^{j2\pi i_a k_1/M_1} - e^{j2\pi i_b k_1/M_1}\right)\left(e^{j2\pi j_a k_2/M_2} - e^{j2\pi j_b k_2/M_2}\right)\left(e^{j2\pi k_a k_3/M_3} - e^{j2\pi k_b k_3/M_3}\right). \tag{11.10}$$

Expanding this term gives the ambiguity (11.3).

It is clear that other such ambiguities can be obtained by adding up several such terms. While this is not a great insight, it does suggest that the Fourier transform may be an insightful approach to discrete tomography.

11.3.3 Relation to phase retrieval

Using this formulation, there is an interesting relation between discrete tomography and the dual of the *phase retrieval problem* of reconstructing a finite-support object from the square of the magnitude of its DFT (hence the term "phase retrieval (from magnitude)"), or, equivalently, from its autocorrelation (convolution of the object with its reflection). For more details on these terms see [3].

Reformulate the discrete tomography problem so that each object value is ±1 instead of 0, 1. This reformulated discrete tomography problem is related to the *dual* of the phase retrieval problem, as follows:

1. In phase retrieval we know the object is zero beyond its borders; in discrete tomography we know $X(k_1, k_2, k_3)$ on the borders $k_1 = 0$, $k_2 = 0$, and $k_3 = 0$.

2. In phase retrieval we know the autocorrelation of the object; in discrete tomography we know the correlation of $X(k_1, k_2, k_3)$ with itself (this is zero unless $k_1 = k_2 = k_3 = 0$).

3. In phase retrieval we know the square of the Fourier magnitude; in discrete tomography we know the square of each object value is unity.

11.3.4 Agarwal-Cooley fast convolution

Assume without loss of generality that M_1, M_2, M_3 are relatively prime (we can let these be three consecutive integers with M_2 even; the discrete tomography problem can obviously be zero-padded). Since M_1, M_2, M_3 are relatively prime, we can map the 3D cyclic convolution in (11.6) into a 1D cyclic convolution of order $(M_1 M_2 M_3)$ [3]. This yields

$$X(k) * X(k) = (M_1 M_2 M_3) \cdot X(k), \qquad (11.11)$$

where $X(k)$ maps to $X(k_1, k_2, k_3)$ using a residue number system mapping. This implies we know $X(k)$ for all k that are multiples of M_1, M_2 or M_3.

From this formulation of the discrete tomography problem we observe:

1. The problem can be formulated as a system of $M_1 M_2 M_3$ simultaneous quadratic equations in $(M_1 - 1)(M_2 - 1)(M_3 - 1)$ unknowns with $M_1 M_2 M_3 - (M_1 - 1)(M_2 - 1)(M_3 - 1)$ known values from the projections. For example, the $2 \times 2 \times 2$ problem actually has only $(2 - 1)^3 = 1$ unknown, and the $3 \times 3 \times 3$ problem actually has only $(3 - 1)^3 = 8$ unknowns (and $3^3 - 8 = 19$ known values).

2. This is not at all apparent from (11.1), in which we seem to have $M_1 M_2 + M_1 M_3 + M_2 M_3$ equations and known values in $M_1 M_2 M_3$ unknowns, each being zero or one. The redundancy in the projections is not all obvious. One that is obvious is

$$\sum_{i_2, i_3} p_1(i_2, i_3) = \sum_{i_1, i_3} p_2(i_1, i_3) = \sum_{i_1, i_2} p_3(i_1, i_2). \qquad (11.12)$$

   Using the algebraic formulation, the numbers of both knowns and unknowns are reduced.

3. From (11.11) it is clear $x(n) = DFT^{-1}\{X(k)\} = 0, 1$. We thus have a 1D discrete problem in which we are given $X(k)$ at integer multiples of three numbers M_1, M_2, M_3. Now consider the 2D $M_1 \times M_2$ discrete tomography problem. We can again use the Agarwal-Cooley convolution mapping to obtain (11.11), only now we know $X(k)$ for all integer multiples of M_1 and M_2.

4. Although it is clear we have more data in the 3D problem than in the 2D problem, our formulation shows *explicitly* where this extra data shows up. The extra values of $X(k)$ present in the Agarwal-Cooley 1D formulation of the 3D problem are sufficient for a unique solution.

11.4   Solution using DFT reformulation

11.4.1   Solving for $X(k_1, k_2, k_3)$

Inserting the known values of $X(k)$ (using (11.8)) into (11.6) (or the 1D version (11.11)) yields a system of simultaneous quadratic equations

$$X(k_1, k_2, k_3) * * * X(k_1, k_2, k_3) = (M_1 M_2 M_3) \cdot X(k_1, k_2, k_3), \qquad (11.13)$$

in which the number of equations $M_1 M_2 M_3$ exceeds the number of unknowns $(M_1 - 1)(M_2 - 1)(M_3 - 1)$.

Unlike (11.1), this system of equations can be solved using well-established techniques, such as gradient/steepest-descent methods, or homotopy (continuation) methods for solving systems of simultaneous polynomial equations. Note that the projection information is built into the system of equations, which are self-contained.

11.4.2 Linear systems of equations for $X(k_1, k_2, k_3)$

If we are given more than three view angles, the simultaneous quadratic equations may have a subset of equations that are entirely linear in the unknown $X(k_1, k_2, k_3)$. In general, about $2M/3$ view angles are needed for this; more precisely, we need the number of known $X(k_1, k_2, k_3)$ to exceed twice the number of unknown $X(k_1, k_2, k_3)$. For example, for the $8 \times 8 \times 8$ problem, if we are given the six view angles corresponding to $k_1 = 0$, $k_2 = 0$, $k_3 = 0$, $k_1 = k_2$, $k_1 = k_3$, $k_2 = k_3$, we get 296 known values and 216 unknown values, so it almost happens.

If the number of view angles (excluding the vertical) equals the size of the problem, then we don't even need to solve a linear system of equations. Instead, we can extrapolate the unknown $X(k_1, k_2, k_3)$ directly from the known values (see below).

11.4.3 Solving for $x(i_1, i_2, i_3)$

Inserting (11.5) into (11.6) directly would, after much algebra, reduce to (11.4), which is not helpful. But once the known $X(0, k_2, k_3), X(k_1, 0, k_3)$, $X(k_1, k_2, 0)$ have been inserted into (11.6), the subsequent insertion of (11.5) into (11.6) results in a system of $M_1 M_2 M_3$ simultaneous quadratic equations in $M_1 M_2 M_3$ unknowns $x(i_1, i_2, i_3)$. This equation is

$$\sum_{\substack{i_1,i_2,i_3 \\ j_1,j_2,j_3}} C\binom{i_1,i_2,i_3}{j_1,j_2,j_3} x(i_1,i_2,i_3)x(j_1,j_2,j_3) = \sum_{i_1,i_2,i_3} D(i_1,i_2,i_3)x(i_1,i_2,i_3),$$

(11.14)

where $C(\cdot)$ and $D(\cdot)$ are complicated functions of the given $X(k_1, k_2, k_3)$ and the complex exponentials appearing in (11.5).

Like (11.1), (11.14) is a system of equations in the unknowns $x(i_1, i_2, i_3)$. But there are two major advantages of (11.14) over previous formulations:

1. The advantage of (11.14) over (11.1) is that there are as many equations as unknowns. Hence gradient or other methods may be used on (11.14), but not on (11.1).

2. The advantage of (11.14) over (11.11) is that while both are systems of simultaneous quadratic equations, in (11.14) the unknowns are known

to be either zero or one! This is clearly helpful, even if gradient or other continuous methods are being used.

Thus (11.14) combines the best parts of (11.1) and (11.11).

We can do even better than (11.14). Since we know some $X(k_1, k_2, k_3)$, we can write (11.5) as a linear system of equations, partition it, and use Schur complements to eliminate some of the $x(i_1, i_2, i_3)$ as variables. This yields an overdetermined system of simultaneous quadratic equations of the same size as (11.11) (with known values of $X(k_1, k_2, k_3)$ inserted), but with a subset of the $x(i_1, i_2, i_3)$ as variables. This is a smaller problem than (11.14). The Schur complements can then be used to recover the other values of $x(i_1, i_2, i_3)$.

11.5   Illustrative examples

11.5.1 $2 \times 2 \times 2$ general problem

We consider the general $2 \times 2 \times 2$ 3D problem to illustrate the points made above. The general $2 \times 2 \times 2$ 3D image can be depicted as

$$
\begin{matrix}
a & \cdots & b & & \\
\vdots & \ddots & & \ddots & \\
e & & c & \cdots & d \\
& \ddots & \vdots & & \vdots \\
& & g & \cdots & h
\end{matrix}
\qquad (11.15)
$$

where the hidden pixel has value f, and each of a, b, c, d, e, f, g, h equals either 0 or 1. The projections from the top, left side, and front are:

$$
\begin{bmatrix} a+e & b+f \\ c+g & d+h \end{bmatrix}; \quad
\begin{bmatrix} a+b & c+d \\ e+f & g+h \end{bmatrix}; \quad
\begin{bmatrix} a+c & b+d \\ e+g & f+h \end{bmatrix},
\qquad (11.16)
$$

respectively. We seem to have $3(2^2) = 12$ equations in $2^3 = 8$ unknowns. This suggests we can solve the problem as an overdetermined linear system of equations. However, from (11.6) and (11.8) it is clear that we actually have only 7 independent equations in 8 unknowns (we are missing $X(1, 1, 1)$). Hence the problem is underdetermined if we do not make use of the fact that the value of each pixel is either 0 or 1.

11.5.2 $2 \times 2 \times 2$ general solution

Using the given projection data in (11.8) and inserting into (11.6) yields 8 equations in the single $((2-1)^3 = 1)$ unknown $X(1, 1, 1)$:

$$2(a + b + c + d + e + f + g + h)X(1,1,1)$$
$$+2[(a-c)+(b-d)+(e-g)+(f-h)][(a-e)-(b-f)+(c-g)-(d-h)]$$
$$+2[(a-b)+(c-d)+(e-f)+(g-h)][(a-e)-(c-g)+(b-f)-(d-h)]$$
$$+2[(a-e)+(b-f)+(c-g)+(d-h)][(a-c)-(b-d)+(e-g)-(f-h)]$$
$$= 8X(1,1,1) = 8[(a-c)-(b-d)-((e-g)-(f-h))], \qquad (11.17)$$

which can easily be verified. We can then quickly determine $x(i_1, i_2, i_3)$ using an inverse 3D DFT.

The ambiguity noted in (11.3) appears in (11.17) as follows. Suppose $a + b + c + d + e + f + g + h = 4$ and the three products of bracketed terms sum to zero. It is not difficult to see that these are in fact equivalent to (11.3). Then (11.17) reduces to $8X(1,1,1) = 8X(1,1,1)$, which of course is true for any $X(1,1,1)$. Then $X(1,1,1)$ is not uniquely determined, and the solution to (11.15) is nonunique.

Equation (11.14) does not pay off for so small a problem. But the modified version of (11.14) has a single unknown (any one of the $x(i_1, i_2, i_3)$), which can be solved quickly. We then have 7 linear equations (the 7 known $X(k_1, k_2, k_3)$) in 7 unknowns (the other 7 $x(i_1, i_2, i_3)$), which can be solved easily.

11.5.3 $3 \times 3 \times 3$ example

Now consider the $3 \times 3 \times 3$ problem in which all of the object values are unity, except at the center. For convenience, reindex so that the center object value is at the origin. Then $x(0,0,0) = 0$ and $x(i_1, i_2, i_3) = 1$ if any of i_1, i_2 or i_3 is nonzero.

The projections and their 2D 3×3 DFTs are, respectively,

$$p_1 = p_2 = p_3 = \begin{bmatrix} 3 & 3 & 3 \\ 3 & 2 & 3 \\ 3 & 3 & 3 \end{bmatrix}; \quad DFT = \begin{bmatrix} -1 & -1 & -1 \\ -1 & 26 & -1 \\ -1 & -1 & -1 \end{bmatrix}. \qquad (11.18)$$

So $X(0,0,0) = 26$ and $X(k_1, k_2, k_3) = -1$ if any of k_1, k_2 or k_3 is nonzero.

We may choose a subset of 8 entirely linear equations in the 8 unknowns $X(1,1,1)$, $X(2,2,2)$, $X(2,1,1)$, $X(1,2,1)$, $X(1,1,2)$, $X(1,2,2)$, $X(2,1,2)$, $X(2,2,1)$ from the system of $3^3 = 27$ simultaneous quadratic equations in $(3-1)^3 = 8$ unknowns (11.6) as

$$\begin{bmatrix} 26 & -1 & -1 & -1 & -1 & -1 & -1 & -1 \\ -1 & 26 & -1 & -1 & -1 & -1 & -1 & -1 \\ -1 & -1 & 26 & -1 & -1 & -1 & -1 & -1 \\ -1 & -1 & -1 & 26 & -1 & -1 & -1 & -1 \\ -1 & -1 & -1 & -1 & 26 & -1 & -1 & -1 \\ -1 & -1 & -1 & -1 & -1 & 26 & -1 & -1 \\ -1 & -1 & -1 & -1 & -1 & -1 & 26 & -1 \\ -1 & -1 & -1 & -1 & -1 & -1 & -1 & 26 \end{bmatrix} \begin{bmatrix} X(1,1,1) \\ X(2,2,2) \\ X(2,1,1) \\ X(1,2,1) \\ X(1,1,2) \\ X(1,2,2) \\ X(2,1,2) \\ X(2,2,1) \end{bmatrix} = \begin{bmatrix} -19 \\ -19 \\ -19 \\ -19 \\ -19 \\ -19 \\ -19 \\ -19 \end{bmatrix},$$

$$(11.19)$$

where $-19 = 3^3(-1) - 26(-1) - (3^3 - 2 - 7)(-1)(-1)$. Solving this linear system of equations results in

$$X(1,1,1) = X(2,2,2) = X(2,1,1) = X(1,2,1) = X(1,1,2) \quad (11.20)$$
$$= X(1,2,2) = X(2,1,2) = X(2,2,1) = -1,$$

from which $x(i_1, i_2, i_3)$ can be computed using a 3D inverse DFT.

11.6   Closed-form solution to limited-angle discrete tomography

11.6.1   Introduction

The limited-angle tomography problem of reconstructing an object from its projections (Radon transform) over a limited range of angles has applications in medical imaging and industry. Without some a priori information about the object, it cannot be reconstructed uniquely from a limited angular range of projections [4]. A priori information about the object that has been used to achieve a unique reconstruction includes finite support, upper and lower bounds on pixel values, and closeness to a reference function.

In the discrete tomography problem, we have an object defined on a discrete lattice of points and taking on only discrete values. We also have projection data at only a finite number of angles, corresponding to various sums of the discrete values. In the problem considered here, the object is assumed to have support only at integer-valued coordinates (discrete lattice) and the object values are restricted to integers. Then the projections become various sums of these integers, and they are thus integers themselves. This is a valuable property, since additive noise in the projections can be eliminated if the noise is known to be less than 0.5 in absolute value. Here "integer" may of course be scaled to multiples of any small number.

Our new method provides the following advantages over previous approaches:

1. The solution of a large, ill-posed linear system of equations is avoided, eliminating error due to computational noise (round-off error).

2. It is not an iterative algorithm, whose requirement of reprojection at each iteration can lead to consistency problems in the reconstruction.

3. It greatly reduces the computational load, which can be reduced even further very simply by parallelization (iterative algorithms cannot be parallelized over iteration number).

The limited-angle tomography problem is known to be ill-conditioned, i.e., a small perturbation of the data can produce a large change in the reconstructed object. This is manifested in our formula by the large values of some of the coefficients in the linear combinations, which provide a direct sensitivity measure. It also means that any noise in the projection data will result in a wrong (possibly very wrong) reconstruction. But since the object is defined on an integer lattice and the object values are restricted to integers, projections are also restricted to integers. So small amounts of noise can be eliminated in the projections by rounding, and the formula can be used with confidence.

11.6.2 Limited-angle and discrete tomography

Limited-angle tomography

The limited-angle tomography problem is defined as the reconstruction of an object $f(x, y)$ from its Radon transform (projections) $p(t, \theta)$, defined as

$$p(t, \theta) = \int \int f(x, y)\delta(t - x \cos\theta - y \sin\theta)dx\, dy, \qquad (11.21)$$

where we are given the projections $p(t, \theta)$ over only a limited (i.e., less than 180 degrees) range of θ. This means that we cannot used filtered backprojection, the usual procedure for reconstruction from projections.

Using the projection-slice theorem [3], the 1D Fourier transform $P(k, \theta) = \mathcal{F}\{p(t, \theta)\}$ of the projections equals the 2D Fourier transform $F(k_x, k_y) = \mathcal{F}\mathcal{F}\{f(x, y)\}$ of the object, along a slice in the Fourier plane (k_x, k_y) passing through the origin at angle θ to the k_x axis. Hence, in the limited-angle tomography problem we know $F(k_x, k_y)$ in a "bowtie" region, and the limited-angle problem is really a 2D extrapolation problem.

Discrete-tomography formulation

We now make the following two assumptions about $f(x, y)$. First, we assume it can be written as a *finite* sum of weighted impulses with singularities at integer-valued coordinates: $f(x, y) = \sum \sum f(i, j)\delta(x - i)\delta(y - j)$. Note the usual Radon transform results (projection-slice theorem) still hold. Second, we assume that $f(x, y)$ can only take on integer values, so the line integral (11.21) becomes sums of various values of $f(i, j)$ and also becomes integer valued. Of course, "integer" can be replaced by "integer multiple of any small number e." We can still use the DFT by taking periodic extensions, as usual. In fact, the Fourier transform becomes the discrete-time Fourier transform (DTFT): $F(k_x, k_y) = DTFT[f(i, j)]$, which in turn becomes the DFT when periodic extensions are taken.

If the slope of the projections is an irrational number, then each $f(i, j)$ appears separately in the projections, making the reconstruction trivial. This is clearly not in the spirit of discrete tomography, so slopes are restricted to $M + 1$ rational values so each projection is a sum of several values of $f(i, j)$. Here $M = MIN[M_1, M_2]$, where $f(i, j)$ has finite $M_1 \times M_2$-point support. The problem is then to reconstruct $f(i,j)$ from various sums of its values.

The observation noise in the projections is assumed to be less than 0.5 in absolute value. This allows immediate error correction in the projections by rounding, and thus removes the problems caused by the poor conditioning of the problem.

It is clear that we can set up a linear system of $M_1 M_2$ or more equations in $M_1 M_2$ unknowns whose solution is $f(i,j)$. The problem is that this linear system of equations is: (1) very large (order several thousand); (2) not sparse; and (3) ill-conditioned (even apart from being very large) due to the close spacing of the angles. While we could still try to solve this linear system of equations, a closed-form solution would save a tremendous amount of storage and computation, and would also avoid computational roundoff error incurred in solving a large system of equations. We now show how to obtain such a closed-form solution.

11.7   An explicit formula for bandwidth extrapolation

11.7.1   Basic idea

We now quickly summarize the results of [5], which presents a fast algorithm for exact extrapolation of a discrete-time periodic band-limited signal from its known values in an interval having the same length as the bandwidth of the signal.

We consider the discrete-discrete band-limited extrapolation problem: Given $2M + 1$ consecutive values of a discrete-time periodic sequence $x(n)$ with period N whose discrete Fourier transform (DFT) $X(k)$ is known to be zero for $M < |k| \leq N/2$, determine the other values of $x(n)$. Note that while simultaneous time limitation and band limitation is impossible for the continuous-time problem, it is entirely possible in the discrete-discrete problem, since periodic extensions are made in both time and frequency.

If $x(n)$ is band-limited in the sense given in the previous paragraph, then its N-point DFT $X(k)$ satisfies $X(k)S(k) = X(k)$ for any $S(k)$ such that $S(k) = 1$ if $|k| \leq M$. We make the following choice for $S(k)$ ($Z_k = e^{\frac{j2\pi k}{N}}$):

$$S(k) = 1 + \prod_{i=-M}^{M} (Z_k - Z_i) = \sum_{n=1}^{2M+1} c(n) Z_k^n. \qquad (11.22)$$

The inverse DFT of $X(k)S(k) = X(k)$ becomes

$$x(n) = \sum_{i=1}^{2M+1} c(i) x(n - i). \qquad (11.23)$$

This shows that the unknown $x(n)$ can be computed from the $2M + 1$ consecutive known values of $x(n)$, without solving a system of equations, without even a division! The $c(n)$ can be computed ahead of time.

What if we are given *non-consecutive* but equally spaced values of $x(n)$? For example, we might be given $2M+1$ values $\{x(0), x(3), x(6), x(9)\ldots\}$. In this case, we simply modify (11.22) to $S(k) = 1 + \prod(Z_k^3 - Z_i^3) = \sum c(n) Z_k^{3n}$. Then (11.23) is clearly an autoregression that only uses every third value of $x(n)$, as desired. Note that now $S(k) = 1$ not only at $Z_k = Z_i$ but also at $Z_k = Z_i e^{\pm j 2\pi/3}$, but this will not correspond to an *integer* k unless N is a multiple of 3.

For a 2D signal $x(n_1, n_2)$ band-limited in frequencies k_1 and k_2 *separately* (as well as jointly), we may apply the 1D algorithm to extrapolate first in the n_1 direction, and then in the n_2 direction. The well-known ill-posedness of the band-limited extrapolation problem manifests itself in the large values of the coefficients.

11.8 Application to tomography

11.8.1 Discussion of application

We now show how this extrapolation formula applies to limited-angle discrete tomography. We assume we are given the projections at $M + 1$ angles $\{arctan(k/L), |k| \leq M/2\}$ for some L. Note that these angles are not exactly evenly spaced in θ (but they are close to evenly spaced if $L >> M$). More important, the slopes are rational numbers, as required in the problem formulation. By the projection-slice theorem, this means that we are given $F(k_x, k_y)$ along the slices $k_y = k_x(k/L)$ for $|k| \leq M/2$. We assume for convenience of presentation that $f(i, j)$ has support $M_2 \times M$, where $M \leq M_2$; otherwise simply exchange i and j in the sequel.

Sample $F(k_x, k_y)$ on a *concentric squares raster*:

$$F(m, n) = F(k_x = 2\pi \frac{m}{N}, \quad k_y = k_x \frac{n}{L} = 2\pi \frac{mn}{NL}). \tag{11.24}$$

Spacing between samples in k_y increases with $|k_x|$.

It should be clear from the projection-slice theorem that these samples can all be obtained from the given projections of $f(i, j)$. Note that the projections at angle $arctan(k/L)$ of $f(i, j)$ (defined on a rectangular lattice) will be nonzero only at integer multiples of some Δ, and that there are only a finite number of such nonzero values. This means that the DFT can be used to compute samples along each slice.

We are then faced with the problem of extrapolating the rest of $F(k_x, k_y)$ from the samples $F(m, n)$. To do this, define $\hat{f}(m, j)$ as the N-point 1D DFT in i of the object $f(i, j)$, for each integer $0 \leq j \leq N - 1$ (note that $\hat{f}(m, j)$ is a "half-2D-DFT"). Then $F(m, n)$ can be computed from $\hat{f}(m, j)$

by computing the 1D DFT of order NL/m in j of $\hat{f}(m,j)$. Note that the order of this transform *varies with m*.

Since the samples $f(i,j)$ of the object are nonzero only for $|j| < M/2$, $\hat{f}(m,j)$ is nonzero only for $|j| < M/2$. Now fix m. Since we have M samples in n of $F(m,n)$, the 1D DFT of $\hat{f}(m,j)$, we can extrapolate in n the samples of $F(m,n)$. We can repeat this for each m, and in so doing compute $F(k_x, k_y)$ *everywhere* on a sampled grid. This sampled grid will include as a subset a rectangular grid, from which $f(i,j)$ can be computed using a 2D DFT.

11.8.2 Comments

Since the spacing between the samples in k_y *depends on* k_x by $k_y = k_x(k/L)$, the DFT length used for extrapolation will also vary with m. This is not a problem since the extrapolations are all performed in parallel. After the extrapolations are complete, we then need to upsample or downsample the variable spacing samples in k_y so that they all have the same length. This operation consists of an inverse DFT followed by a DFT of different order. Then a simple inverse DFT yields the samples $f(i,j)$.

11.8.3 Summary of procedure

OBJECT: $f(i,j)$ is
1. defined for integer values of i,j;
2. nonzero only for $|i| \le M_2/2, |j| \le M/2$;
3. restricted to taking on integer values.

DATA: Radon transform at limited range of $M+1$ discrete angles $\{arctan(k/L), |k| \le M/2\}$.

These sums of various values of $f(i,j)$ are
restricted to taking on integer values; so that
noise less than 0.5 can be eliminated by rounding.

PROCEDURE:
1. Compute DFT of projections. This yields $F(k_x, k_y)$ sampled on $k_y = k_x(k/L), |k| \le M/2$.

Samples of this *variably sampled* $F(k_x, k_y)$ are $F(m,n)$.
If NL is the least common multiple of $1, 2 \ldots M/2$:

2. For each m, extrapolate $F(m,n)$ in n from given values $\{F(m,n), |n| \le M/2\}$ using 1D extrapolation coefficients based on an NL/m-order DFT.

3. Then compute DFT^{-1} of order NL/m and DFT of order N (downsample) for each m. Then compute 2D DFT^{-1} to obtain sampled $f(x,y)$.

4. If $NL/m = N_1/N_2$ is not an integer, extrapolate $F(m,n)$ in n. This will produce N_1 different values of $F(m,n)$ before they repeat.
Compute DFT^{-1} of order N_1 and downsample the interpolated half-transform $\hat{f}(m,j)$. Then proceed.

This procedure is illustrated by the numerical example to follow. More details and references are available in [6].

11.9   A simple, illustrative numerical example

We present a simple numerical example. This example is intended to be illustrative, demonstrating how the algorithm works and confirming that it does indeed reconstruct the object perfectly. The operation of the algorithm on larger-sized objects should then be apparent. A few comments on numerical implementation for large objects are given later.

11.9.1   Problem statement

The 3×5 object is

$$
\begin{matrix}
 &   & 1 & 2 & 3 &   &   \\
3 & 4 & 5 & 6 & 7 . &   &   \\
 &   & 7 & 8 & 9 &   &   \\
\end{matrix}
\qquad (11.25)
$$

Its vertical projections are $\{3, 12, 15, 8, 7\}$, its NE-SW projections are $\{4, 6, 15, 14, 16\}$, and its NW-SE projections are $\{10, 8, 15, 12, 10\}$. The goal is to reconstruct the pixel values from the projections at these three angles.

Since the pixel values are all integers, the discrete projections, which are various sums of the pixel values, are also all integers. Any additive noise less than 0.5 can therefore be eliminated by rounding. We omit this here since it is quite obvious.

Note that for an object with rectangular support, the corner pixels can always be found directly from projections at any angle other than zero or 90 degrees, since the endpoints of the set of projections at any such angle pass *only* through a single corner pixel. Since this is misleading (it makes the problem look larger than it really is), we have set the four corner pixels of the object to zero.

The problem could of course be solved directly by solving the linear system of equations

$$
\begin{bmatrix} 12 \\ 15 \\ 18 \\ 4 \\ 6 \\ 15 \\ 14 \\ 16 \\ 10 \\ 8 \\ 15 \\ 12 \\ 10 \end{bmatrix}
=
\begin{bmatrix}
1 & 0 & 0 & 0 & 1 & 0 & 0 & 0 & 1 & 0 & 0 \\
0 & 1 & 0 & 0 & 0 & 1 & 0 & 0 & 0 & 1 & 0 \\
0 & 0 & 1 & 0 & 0 & 0 & 1 & 0 & 0 & 0 & 1 \\
1 & 0 & 0 & 1 & 0 & 0 & 0 & 0 & 0 & 0 & 0 \\
0 & 1 & 0 & 0 & 1 & 0 & 0 & 0 & 0 & 0 & 0 \\
0 & 0 & 1 & 0 & 0 & 1 & 0 & 0 & 1 & 0 & 0 \\
0 & 0 & 0 & 0 & 0 & 0 & 1 & 0 & 0 & 1 & 0 \\
0 & 0 & 0 & 0 & 0 & 0 & 0 & 1 & 0 & 0 & 1 \\
0 & 0 & 1 & 0 & 0 & 0 & 0 & 1 & 0 & 0 & 0 \\
0 & 1 & 0 & 0 & 0 & 0 & 1 & 0 & 0 & 0 & 0 \\
1 & 0 & 0 & 0 & 0 & 1 & 0 & 0 & 0 & 0 & 1 \\
0 & 0 & 0 & 0 & 1 & 0 & 0 & 0 & 0 & 1 & 0 \\
0 & 0 & 0 & 1 & 0 & 0 & 0 & 0 & 1 & 0 & 0
\end{bmatrix}
\begin{bmatrix} x_1 \\ x_2 \\ x_3 \\ x_4 \\ x_5 \\ x_6 \\ x_7 \\ x_8 \\ x_9 \\ x_{10} \\ x_{11} \end{bmatrix},
\qquad (11.26)
$$

which is 13 equations (the projections) in 11 unknowns (the pixel values) having solution

$$[x_1, x_2, x_3, x_4, x_5, x_6, x_7, x_8, x_9, x_{10}, x_{11}] = [1, 2, 3, 3, 4, 5, 6, 7, 7, 8, 9]. \qquad (11.27)$$

The method to follow is a closed-form solution to this linear system of equations.

11.9.2   Extrapolation equations

We use an 8×8 2D DFT. Because $f(i,j)$ has support in j $|j| \leq 1$ we have $M = 1$. We will need the extrapolation coefficients for both $N = 8$ and $N = 4$. For clarity, we use the z-transform instead of the DFT [3]; the relation between these is $S_N(z = e^{j2\pi k/N}) = S(k)$ for $S(k)$ defined as above. The extrapolation coefficients $c(i)$ turn out to be:

$$S_{N=4}(z) = 1 + \prod_{i=-1}^{1} (z - e^{-j2\pi i/4}) = z^3 - z^2 + z;$$

$$S_{N=8}(z) = 1 + \prod_{i=-1}^{1} (z - e^{-j2\pi i/8}) = z^3 - 2.414z^2 + 2.414z; \qquad (11.28)$$

$$S_{N=8;skip\,3}(z) = 1 + \prod_{i=-1}^{1} (z^3 - e^{-j2\pi 3i/8}) = z^9 + 0.414z^6 - 0.414z^3.$$

The $c(i)$ are simply the coefficients of these polynomials.

By the projection-slice theorem we immediately know the 8×8-point DFT $F(m,n)$ of $f(i,j)$ at the points shown in the figure below. We now show how to extrapolate the unknown values of $F(m,n)$, denoted by a $*$.

15	$*$	$*$	$*$	$*$	$*$	$*$	$*$
$*$	$15-10\sqrt{2}$ $-j2\sqrt{2}$	$*$	$*$	$*$	$*$	$*$	$15-10\sqrt{2}$ $+j(12-4\sqrt{2})$
$*$	$*$	$-5-4j$	$*$	$*$	$*$	$-5-8j$	$*$
$*$	$*$	$*$	$15+10\sqrt{2}$ $-j2\sqrt{2}$	$*$	$15+10\sqrt{2}$ $-j(12+4\sqrt{2})$	$*$	$*$
-5	$15-15\sqrt{2}$ $-j(4-3\sqrt{2})$	$5+6j$	$15+15\sqrt{2}$ $+j(4+3\sqrt{2})$	55	$15+15\sqrt{2}$ $-j(4+3\sqrt{2})$	$5-6j$	$15-15\sqrt{2}$ $+j(4-3\sqrt{2})$
$*$	$*$	$*$	$15+10\sqrt{2}$ $+j(12+4\sqrt{2})$	$*$	$15+10\sqrt{2}$ $+j2\sqrt{2}$	$*$	$*$
$*$	$*$	$-5+8j$	$*$	$*$	$*$	$-5+4j$	$*$
$*$	$15-10\sqrt{2}$ $-j(12-4\sqrt{2})$	$*$	$*$	$*$	$*$	$*$	$15-10\sqrt{2}$ $+j2\sqrt{2}$
15	$*$	$*$	$*$	$*$	$*$	$*$	$*$

$$(11.29)$$

11.9.3 Extrapolation of unknown $F(m,n)$

Consider the column $m = 1$ of $F(m,n)$. We have the three consecutive values $F(1,1), F(1,0), F(1,-1)$. Using (11.28), we can then compute

$$F(1,2) = 2.414\begin{pmatrix} 15+10\sqrt{2} \\ -j(12+4\sqrt{2}) \end{pmatrix} - 2.414\begin{pmatrix} 15+15\sqrt{2} \\ -j(4+3\sqrt{2}) \end{pmatrix}$$

$$+ \begin{pmatrix} 15+10\sqrt{2} \\ +j2\sqrt{2} \end{pmatrix} = \begin{pmatrix} 5+5\sqrt{2} \\ -j(10+7\sqrt{2}) \end{pmatrix} ; (11.30)$$

$$F(1,3) = 2.414\begin{pmatrix} 5+5\sqrt{2} \\ -j(10+7\sqrt{2}) \end{pmatrix} - 2.414\begin{pmatrix} 15+10\sqrt{2} \\ -j(12+4\sqrt{2}) \end{pmatrix}$$

$$+ \begin{pmatrix} 15+15\sqrt{2} \\ -j(4+3\sqrt{2}) \end{pmatrix} = \begin{pmatrix} -5 \\ -j(8+4\sqrt{2}) \end{pmatrix} ; (11.31)$$

$$F(1,4) = 2.414\begin{pmatrix} -5 \\ -j(8+4\sqrt{2}) \end{pmatrix} - 2.414\begin{pmatrix} 5+5\sqrt{2} \\ -j(10+7\sqrt{2}) \end{pmatrix}$$

$$+ \begin{pmatrix} 15+10\sqrt{2} \\ -j(12+4\sqrt{2}) \end{pmatrix} = \begin{pmatrix} -5-5\sqrt{2} \\ +j(-4+\sqrt{2}) \end{pmatrix} .(11.32)$$

Now consider the column $m = 2$. Now we have only every other value of $F(2,n) : F(2,2), F(2,0), F(2,-2)$. But since we are using an 8×8-point 2D DFT and $8/2 = 4$ is an integer, we can simply use the $N = 4$ extrapolation coefficients from (11.28). We then have

$$F(4,2) = F(2,2) + (-1)F(2,0) + F(2,-2) \qquad (11.33)$$
$$= (-5-8j) - (5-6j) + (-5+4j) = -15+2j.$$

How do we get the *other* values? Take a 4-point inverse 1D DFT of the four known values of $F(2,n)$. This amounts to downsampling in frequency, but due to the zero padding of the original problem the resulting $\hat{f}(2,j)$ will not be aliased (it will simply be repeated). Then take $\hat{f}(2,j)$, discard the repetition, and take an 8-point 1D DFT, yielding $F(2,n)$.

Now consider the column $m = 3$. Now we have only every third value of $F(3,n)$: $F(3,3), F(3,0), F(3,-3)$. We can use the method discussed above for non-consecutive values. Using the extrapolation coefficients from (11.28), we compute $F(3,-2) = F(3,6)$ as

$$F(3,6) = 0.414 \begin{pmatrix} 15 - 10\sqrt{2} \\ j(12 - 4\sqrt{2}) \end{pmatrix} - 0.414 \begin{pmatrix} 15 - 15\sqrt{2} \\ j(4 - 3\sqrt{2}) \end{pmatrix} \quad (11.34)$$

$$+ \begin{pmatrix} 15 - 10\sqrt{2} \\ j2\sqrt{2} \end{pmatrix} = \begin{pmatrix} 5 - 5\sqrt{2} \\ +j(10 - 7\sqrt{2}) \end{pmatrix}.$$

Other values of $F(3,n)$ can be computed similarly (note that they won't be computed in increasing order in n, but this hardly matters).

All of these DFT values can be confirmed to be correct by simply computing the 8×8 2D DFT of the image $f(i,j)$.

11.9.4   Application to large images

It is apparent that this procedure can be applied to arbitrarily large images. The parallelizability of the extrapolations becomes important in this case, since significant computation time can be saved if this can be done.

Although the algorithm is exact, roundoff error must be avoided. The extrapolation coefficients become very large for large problems, and even though $f(i,j)$ is known to take on only integer values, care must be taken that sufficient precision be retained so that multiplication of the known DFT values by the (large) extrapolation coefficients, followed by an inverse DFT, still yields numbers that are close to integers. This requires precise computation of the DFT values from the (given) integer-valued discrete projections. Fortunately, precise computation of the DFT using the fast Fourier transform is not a significant problem. Multiple precision may be necessary if MATLAB or a similar algorithm package is employed.

11.10   Conclusion

We have shown that an algebraic approach to the binary discrete tomography problem leads to several interesting insights into the problem, including the well-known ambiguities associated with the problem. It also leads to purely algebraic algorithms for solving the problem, which appear to be more tractable than the combinatorical approaches usually employed. If a sufficient number of view angles is available, then the problem reduces to a linear system of equations in $X(k_1, k_2, k_3)$. The number of view angles is fewer than the number required for the total number of projection values to equal the total number of unknowns, i.e., the binary nature of the object is being used.

In the special case where the number of view angles equals the problem size, we have provided a closed-form solution of the limited-angle discrete tomography problem. This solution applies an explicit formula for bandwidth extrapolation to the limited-angle discrete tomography problem. It avoids the solution of an ill-conditioned system of equations (with its attendant roundoff error) and also avoids time-consuming iterative algorithms. It provides direct control over all variables in the problem, and shows explicitly the sensitivity of the solution to variations in the data.

By restricting the values of $f(x, y)$ to integers (discrete tomography), the projections are also restricted to integer values. This permits elimination of small amounts of additive noise in the projection data. Since the problem is very ill-conditioned, noise-free projection data is very important. The discrete tomography formulation allows the formula to be used with confidence.

It is interesting to note that the discrete nature of this problem is what makes this closed-form solution possible. Although N can be made arbitrarily large to simulate a continuous Radon transform, the discrete perspective is still needed to obtain the solution, showing the value of discrete tomography.

Acknowledgments

This work was presented at the Workshop on Discrete Tomography held in Szeged, Hungary, in August 1997. The author would like to thank Dr. Gabor Herman for introducing him to this topic, Dr. Attila Kuba for his hospitality in Szeged, and both of them for their efforts in organizing the workshop. Portions of this work have appeared in [6]-[8].

References

[1] P. M. Salzberg, "Binary tomography on lattices," *Congressus Numeratium* **111**, 185-192 (1995).

[2] S. K. Chang and Y. R. Wang, "Three-dimensional object reconstruction from orthogonal projections," *Pattern Recognition* **7**, 167-176 (1975).

[3] D. Dudgeon and R. M. Mersereau, *Multidimensional Digital Signal Processing*, (Prentice-Hall, Englewood Cliffs, NJ), 1984.

[4] K. C. Tam and V. Perez-Mendez, "Tomographical imaging with limited angle input," *J. Opt. Soc. Am. A.* **71**, 582-592 (1981).

[5] H. Soltanian-Zadeh and A. E. Yagle, "A fast algorithm for extrapolation of discrete-time periodic band-limited signals," *Signal Processing* **33**, 183-196 (1993).

[6] A. E. Yagle, "An explicit closed-form solution to the limited angle discrete tomography problem for finite-support objects," *Int. J. Imaging Syst. and Technol.* **9**, 174-180 (1998).

[7] A. E. Yagle, "An algebraic solution to the 3-D discrete tomography problem," in *Proc. 1998 IEEE International Conference on Image Processing*, (IEEE, Piscataway, NJ), to appear in 1999.

[8] A. E. Yagle, "An explicit closed-form solution to the limited angle discrete tomography problem for finite-support objects," in *Proc. 1998 IEEE International Conference on Image Processing*, (IEEE, Piscataway, NJ), to appear in 1999.

Chapter 12

Binary Steering of Nonbinary Iterative Algorithms

Yair Censor[1]
Samuel Matej[2]

ABSTRACT *Existing algorithms for binary image reconstruction that can handle two-dimensional problems are mainly of a combinatorial nature. This has, so far, hindered their direct application to fully three-dimensional binary problems. This chapter proposes a steering scheme by which nonbinary iterative reconstruction algorithms can be steered towards a binary solution of a binary problem. Experimental studies show the viability of this approach.*

12.1 Introduction: Problem definition, approach, and motivation

Let $Ax = b$ be a system of linear equations representing the fully discretized model of a two-dimensional image reconstruction from projections problem. The vector $x = (x_j)_{j=1}^n \in \mathbf{R}^n$, in the n-dimensional Euclidean space, is the *image vector* whose j-th component x_j has the value of the uniform grayness at the j-th pixel. The vector $b = (b_i)_{i=1}^m \in \mathbf{R}^m$ is the *measurements vector* whose i-th component b_i is the value of the i-th line integral through the unknown image. The $m \times n$ *projection matrix* A is a 0-1 matrix having its i-th row and j-th column element a_j^i equal to zero if the i-th ray does not intersect the j-th pixel, and equal to one if it does. The *Binary Reconstruction Problem* is to find a 0-1 vector x^* that is an acceptable approximation to a solution of the system $Ax = b$.

There is a large body of literature on this problem and renewed current interest, see, e.g., Herman and Kuba [1]. Due to their mainly combinatorial nature, existing algorithms for this problem, such as Chang [2], do not lend themselves to extension to three-dimensional problems of binary

---

[1]University of Haifa, Department of Mathematics, Mt.Carmel, Haifa 31905, Israel, E-mail: yair@mathcs2.haifa.ac.il

[2]University of Pennsylvania, Department of Radiology, Medical Image Processing Group, Blockley Hall, Fourth Floor, 423 Guardian Drive, Philadelphia, PA 19104-6021, USA, E-mail: matej@mipg.upenn.edu

reconstruction.

The adoption of *nonbinary* iterative image reconstruction algorithms such as ART, MART, EM, and others (see, e.g., Bauschke and Borwein [3], Censor and Zenios [4], Byrne [5,6], or Herman [7]) to binary reconstruction is problematic because such algorithms do not preserve the binary nature of the iterates even if initialized at a binary vector x^0. This difficulty exists in Vardi and Lee [8, Section I(A), point 6], and in Fishburn *et al.* [9] where simple thresholding is used.

On the other hand, the temptation to apply nonbinary algorithms exists because there is an abundance of such algorithms that have proven their usefulness in nonbinary image reconstruction problems. Moreover, they could, technically speaking, be extended without hindrance to three-dimensional problems, which are harder then two-dimensional problems from the point of view of computational complexity and thus cause combinatorial algorithms to be much more involved, see, e.g., Gritzmann *et al.* [10]. Therefore, if the route that we propose here will be successful for two-dimensional binary reconstruction problems then it will also be immediately applicable to three-dimensional problems.

Our approach to rely on nonbinary iterative image reconstruction algorithms (for fully discretized image reconstruction problems) has its roots in, and is inspired by, the work of Herman [11]. The *binary steering mechanism* we propose here extends and replaces the ad hoc steps devised there by Herman.

Nonbinary iterative reconstruction algorithms of various kinds (asymptotically) solve (depending on the relevant solution concept), or find good approximate solutions of, the linear system of equations of the form $Ax = b$. Several of these algorithms have been shown to perform very efficiently, handle linear inequalities, treat nonnegativity constraints, generate acceptable approximations even in the inconsistent case (i.e., when there exists no nonnegative solution of the system of equations), lend themselves to parallel computations, or have other favorable features.

These algorithms can solve fully discretized real three-dimensional image reconstruction problems because such problems can be modeled into, admittedly much bigger, systems of linear equations.

We present a *mathematical mechanism* that, when used in conjunction with any nonbinary iterative reconstruction algorithm, will steer to acceptable approximate solutions of the binary reconstruction problem.

12.2   The steering mechanism

The iterative nonbinary reconstruction algorithms that are considered here are of the general form described in Fig. 12.1.

In a typical iterative step the algorithm first calculates a quantity called

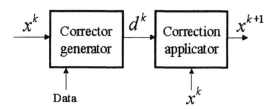

FIGURE 12.1. General structure of an iterative step of a nonbinary iterative image reconstruction algorithm.

corrector, which is then applied to the current iterate. In sequential reconstruction algorithms like ART, ART2, ARM, ART3, MART, etc. (see, e.g., Herman [12], Censor and Zenios [4]), the corrector d^k is a vector whose components are applied to the current iterate x^k in one of several possible ways (addition in ART, componentwise multiplication in MART, etc.) to obtain the next iterate x^{k+1}. The proposed *binary steering mechanism* consists of two additional operations that we describe next.

Given a real number x and two real parameters α and β such that $0 \le \alpha < \beta \le 1$ we define $\tilde{x}$ by

$$\tilde{x} = \begin{cases} 0, & \text{if } x \le \alpha, \\ 1, & \text{if } x \ge \beta, \\ x, & \text{otherwise,} \end{cases} \qquad (12.1)$$

and we say that $\tilde{x}$ is the *(partial) binarization of x with respect to the pair (α, β)*. Applying this notion to a sequence of vectors leads to the next definition.

Definition 12.1. *Let $\{x^k\}_{k \ge 0}$ be a sequence of vectors $x^k = (x_j^k)_{j=1}^n \in \mathbf{R}^n$ and let $\alpha = \{\alpha_k\}_{k \ge 0}$, $\beta = \{\beta_k\}_{k \ge 0}$ and $\{t_k\}_{k \ge 0}$ be three real sequences such that $0 \le \alpha_k < t_k$, $\alpha_k < \alpha_{k+1}$, $t_k < \beta_k \le 1$, and $\beta_{k+1} < \beta_k$, for $k \ge 0$, where t_k is a threshold at the given iteration k. The sequence $\{\tilde{x}^k\}_{k \ge 0}$ defined, for $k \ge 0$ and $j = 1, 2, \ldots, n$, by*

$$\tilde{x}_j^k = \begin{cases} 0, & \text{if } x_j^k \le \alpha_k, \\ 1, & \text{if } x_j^k \ge \beta_k, \\ x_j^k, & \text{otherwise,} \end{cases} \qquad (12.2)$$

is called the (partial) sequential binarization of $\{x^k\}_{k \ge 0}$ with respect to the pair of sequences (α, β) and the threshold sequence $\{t_k\}_{k \ge 0}$.

As will be seen below, we binarize each iterate x^k prior to feeding it to the nonbinary iterative algorithm, of the form of Fig. 12.1, at hand. After the iteration has been performed, a conflict might arise between x^k and the output y^k of the nonbinary iterative algorithm (see Fig. 12.2). The meaning of the term *conflict* here and the manner in which this conflict is dealt with become clear from the next definition.

Definition 12.2.   *Given two real numbers x and y, two real parameters α and β such that $0 \leq \alpha < t$ and $t < \beta \leq 1$, where t is a given threshold, and a fixed ϵ, $0 < \epsilon < 0.1$, we define z by*

$$
z = \begin{cases}
t - \epsilon, & \text{if } x \leq \alpha \text{ and } y \geq t, \\
t + \epsilon, & \text{if } x \geq \beta \text{ and } y \leq t, \\
y, & \text{otherwise},
\end{cases}
\tag{12.3}
$$

and we say that z settles the conflict between x and y with respect to the pair (α, β), the threshold t, and ϵ.

Actually we use this notion for sequences via the following definition.

Definition 12.3.   *Let there be given two vector sequences $\{x^k\}_{k \geq 0}$ and $\{y^k\}_{k \geq 0}$, and two real sequences $\alpha = \{\alpha_k\}_{k \geq 0}$ and $\beta = \{\beta_k\}_{k \geq 0}$, a sequence $\{t_k\}_{k \geq 0}$ of threshold values, having the same properties as in Definition 12.1, and a fixed ϵ with $0 < \epsilon < 0.1$. The sequence $\{z^k\}_{k \geq 0}$, defined for $k \geq 0$ and $j = 1, 2, \ldots, n$, by*

$$
z_j^k = \begin{cases}
t_k - \epsilon, & \text{if } x_j^k \leq \alpha_k \text{ and } y_j^k \geq t_k, \\
t_k + \epsilon, & \text{if } x_j^k \geq \beta_k \text{ and } y_j^k \leq t_k, \\
y, & \text{otherwise},
\end{cases}
\tag{12.4}
$$

is said to settle sequentially the conflict between $\{x^k\}_{k \geq 0}$ and $\{y^k\}_{k \geq 0}$ with respect to the pair (α, β), the threshold sequence $\{t_k\}_{k \geq 0}$, and ϵ.

With the above definitions we describe our proposed steering mechanism which is depicted in Fig. 12.2, here the two middle boxes with the corrector generator and the correction applicator are the same as those in Fig. 12.1. The steering mechanism consist of adding to any such nonbinary algorithm the *Binarizer* and the *Conflict settler* as explained next.

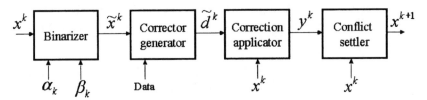

FIGURE 12.2. Binary steering of the nonbinary algorithm is accomplished by additional operations of binarization and conflict settlement.

Each iteration of the overall process begins with a *(partial) binarization* of the current iterate x^k to form $\tilde{x}^k$. As iterations proceed the values α_k keep increasing and the values of β_k decrease so that more and more components fit into the desired binary 0-1 nature of the vector. The corrector $\tilde{d}^k$ is based on $\tilde{x}^k$, not on the original x^k, but it is applied by the *correction applicator* to x^k itself (not to $\tilde{x}^k$). If the resulting y^k has a component y_j^k that is larger or equal to the current threshold value t_k, while its previous value x_j^k was below α_k, then we say that there is a conflict and we prefer not to make a binary decision about this component but rather "settle the conflict" by allowing x_j^k to be only as much as $t_k - \epsilon$. A similar argument explains the rest of (12.4).

When a predetermined iteration index K has been reached or the iterations are stopped at K due to some other stopping criterion then a final thresholding is used to define the final (approximate) solution $x^* = (x_j^*)_{j=1}^n$ by

$$x_j^* = \begin{cases} 0, & \text{if } x_j^K \leq 0.5, \\ 1, & \text{if } x_j^K > 0.5. \end{cases} \tag{12.5}$$

12.3 Experimental study

In the experimental results presented here we use a fixed threshold value $t_k = 0.5$, for all $k \geq 0$, and the value $\epsilon = 0.05$. We constructed the sequence α_k by the formula $\alpha_k = (k/K)t_k$, where k is the iteration index, K is the predetermined number of iterations at which the reconstruction is stopped, and we define $\beta_k = 1 - (k/K)(1 - t_k)$, for $k \geq 0$. The nonbinary iterative reconstruction algorithm that we use is the fully simultaneous Cimmino algorithm; see, e.g., Gastinel [13] or Censor and Zenios [4]. Starting from an arbitrary $x^0 \in \mathbf{R}^n$, given a current iterate x^k, Cimmino's algorithm calculates the next iterate x^{k+1} by

$$x^{k+1} = x^k + \lambda_k \left(\sum_{i=1}^m w_i^k \frac{b_i - \langle a^i, x^k \rangle}{\|a^i\|^2} a^i \right). \tag{12.6}$$

In this formula $\|\cdot\|$ and $\langle \cdot, \cdot \rangle$ are the Euclidean norm and the inner product in $\mathbf{R}^n$, respectively, m is the number of views, a^i is the i-th column of A^T (the transpose of A), λ_k are the relaxation parameters, and w_i^k are positive iteration dependent weights which must sum up (over i) to one, for every $k \geq 0$.

We employed this algorithm with unity relaxation, i.e., $\lambda_k = 1$, for all $k \geq 0$, with equal and constant weights, meaning that $w_i^k = 1/m$ for all i and all k, and using a uniform starting image x^0, for which for any given view (projection angle) v

$$\sum_{j=0}^n x_j^0 = \sum_{i \in I_v} \langle a^i, x^0 \rangle, \tag{12.7}$$

where I_v is a set of all projection lines from the view v.

For testing our binary steering method with Cimmino's reconstruction algorithm, under the above described circumstances, we used the three test phantoms (see Figs. 12.3, 12.4, and 12.5, top left images) of Fishburn et al. [9]. These same phantoms were also used by Vardi and Lee [8], by Salzberg, Rivera-Vega and Rodriguez [14], by Gritzmann et al. [10], and by Patch [15].

We demonstrate the performance of the binary steering method by showing along with each of the three phantoms its reconstructions using 2, 3, and 4 views. Two views are the two orthogonal views along the Cartesian axes in the plane, the three views include additionally a diagonal view at 45° (view of the direction $(1, 1)$ in [9]) and the four views include also another diagonally oriented view at 135°. The three view run is employing the same view directions as used by Fishburn et al. [9].

The only reconstruction parameter that is being changed in the tests presented here is the number of iterations, where an iteration is counted as a complete sweep through all equations. The number of iterations was chosen so as to minimize the data error e_p, i.e., to minimize the sum of the absolute values of the differences between the line sums in the phantom and the reconstructed image. Following are the observations based on our tests.

In the tests using two views the data error dropped quickly down to a certain value already after a small number of iterations. Top right images in Figs. 12.3, 12.4, and 12.5 show, by way of example, the reconstructions using 25, 25, and 200 iterations, respectively, having data errors 16, 28, and 34, respectively. The number of image errors e_i, i.e., the number of locations at which the reconstructed image disagrees with the phantom, is 34, 50, and 96, respectively. Further decrease of the data error was (for the given values of our reconstruction parameters: ϵ, and sequences λ_k, t_k, α_k, β_k) only very slow when increasing the number of iterations. For example, it took as much as 90,000 iterations to decrease the data errors to 8, 4, and 12, respectively. The image errors at the same time slightly increased to the values 48, 70, and 110, respectively.

In the tests using three views we needed 220 and 70 iterations to find a solution for the phantoms 1 and 2, respectively, (see bottom right images in Figs. 12.3 and 12.4; note that the solution we obtained for phantom 1 differs from the phantom by the switching chain of length six). Since phantom 3 is substantially more difficult to reconstruct, it needed more iterations. The data error for it stabilized at about 3,000 iterations (see Fig. 12.5, bottom right; $e_p = 6$, $e_i = 36$). To find a solution free of data errors it took as much as 500,000 iterations for our choice of parameters. For other reconstruction parameters the exact solution might be obtained earlier. This solution differs from the phantom at 58 locations, representing a set of switching chains. It is as good as any other solution based on the data alone. To be able to reconstruct the particular solution of the original phantom we would need to utilize some additional prior information on the reconstructed images (see, e.g., Chapter 8 by Matej, Vardi, Herman, and Vardi).

```
 1  ...................................00000      ..............................................
 2  ...................................oo         ..............................................
 3  ................11................o.o         ..................11..........................
 4  ...............1111...............o..o        .................1111.........................
 5  .....11........1111.............1..o...o       ....•11.........1111.............1.......
 6  ....1111.......1111.........111.....          ....1111........1111..........111....
 7  ...11111.......1111111.........11111....      ...•11111........111111-........1111-...
 8  ..1111111......1111111.........11111....      ...1111111.......1111111.........11111....
 9  ..11111111.....1111111..111....1111111..      ..•11111111.....1111111...---.....11111-...
10 ..111111111...11111111111111....11111111..    ..111111111•••1111111111111....111111-...
11 ..1111111111111111111111111111...11111111..   ..11111111111111111111111111•..11111111..
12 ..11111111111111111111111111111..11111111..   ..11111111111111111111111111••11111111..
13 ..111111111111111111111111111111111111111..   ..111111111111111111111111111111111111111..
14 ..111111111111111111111111111111111111111..   ..111111111111111111111111111111111111111..
15 ..111111111111111111111111111111111111111..   ..111111111111111111111111111111111111111..
16 ..111111111111111111111111111111111111111..   ..111111111111111111111111111111111111111..
17 ..111111111111111111111111111111111111111..   ..111111111111111111111111111111111111111..
18 ..111111111111111111111111111111111111111..   ..111111111111111111111111111111111111111..
19 ..111111111111111111111111111111111111111..   ..111111111111111111111111111111111111111..
20 ..111111111111111111111111111111111111111..   ..111111111111111111111111111111111111111..
21 ..111111111111111111111111111111111111111..   ..111111111111111111111111111111111111111..
22 ..111111111111111111111111111111111111111..   ..111111111111111111111111111111111111111..
23 ..111111111111111111111111111111111111111..   ..111111111111111111111111111111111111111..
24 ..111111111111111111111111111111111111111..   ..111111111111111111111111111111111111111..
25 ..1111111111111111111111111111111111111....   ..1111111111111111111111111111111111111••..
26 ..111111111111111111111........1111111....    ..111111111111---111111111•..•••.---11111•....
27 ..111...................................      ..---...............••.....
28 ..............................................  ..............................................
29 ..............................................  ..............................................
```

```
 1  ..............................................  ..............................................
 2  ..............................................  ..............................................
 3  ................11............................  ..................11..........................
 4  ...............1111...........................  .................1111.........................
 5  .....11........1111.............1......        ....-1.........11111•............1.......
 6  ....1111.......1111.........111....           ....1111........1111..........111....
 7  ...11111.......1111111.........11111....      ...•11111........111111-........1111....
 8  ..1111111......1111111.........11111....      ...1111111.......1111111.........11111....
 9  ..11111111.....1111111..111....1111111..      ..11111111.....1111111...111.....1111111..
10 ..111111111...11111111111111....11111111..    ..111111111...1111111111111111....11111111..
11 ..1111111111111111111111111111...11111111..   ..11111111111111111111111111...11111111..
12 ..11111111111111111111111111111..11111111..   ..11111111111111111111111111...11111111..
13 ..111111111111111111111111111111111111111..   ..111111111111111111111111111111111111111..
14 ..111111111111111111111111111111111111111..   ..111111111111111111111111111111111111111..
15 ..111111111111111111111111111111111111111..   ..111111111111111111111111111111111111111..
16 ..111111111111111111111111111111111111111..   ..111111111111111111111111111111111111111..
17 ..111111111111111111111111111111111111111..   ..111111111111111111111111111111111111111..
18 ..111111111111111111111111111111111111111..   ..111111111111111111111111111111111111111..
19 ..111111111111111111111111111111111111111..   ..111111111111111111111111111111111111111..
20 ..111111111111111111111111111111111111111..   ..111111111111111111111111111111111111111..
21 ..111111111111111111111111111111111111111..   ..111111111111111111111111111111111111111..
22 ..111111111111111111111111111111111111111..   ..111111111111111111111111111111111111111..
23 ..111111111111111111111111111111111111111..   ..111111111111111111111111111111111111111..
24 ..111111111111111111111111111111111111111..   ..111111111111111111111111111111111111111..
25 ..1111111111111111111111111111111111111....   ..1111111111111111111111111111111111111....
26 ..111111111111111111111........1111111....    ..111111111111111111111........1111111....
27 ..111...................................      ..1-1•..........................
28 ..............................................  ..............................................
29 ..............................................  ..............................................
```

FIGURE 12.3. Phantom 1 (top left) and its reconstructions using 2 views (top right; $K = 25$, $e_p = 16$ and $e_i = 34$, where K is the number of iterations, e_p is the data error and e_i represents the number of places at which the reconstructed image disagrees with the phantom), 3 views (bottom right; $K = 220$, $e_p = 0$ and $e_i = 6$) and 4 views (bottom left; $K = 22$, $e_p = 0$ and $e_i = 0$); "." and "1" represent the values zero and one, respectively, in the phantom and at the correct locations in the reconstructions; "-" and "*" represent incorrect values of zero and one, respectively, in the reconstructions; the "o"s in the phantom (top left) show directions of the line sums in the three views case.

```
 1      ....................................          ....................................
 2      ....................................          ....................................
 3      ......11..............1111111111........       .....11.............11111-1---...........
 4      ..111111..........111111111111.........        ..111111*...........111111111---......
 5      ..1111111.........111111111111111.......       ..1111111*........11111111111111--....*..
 6      ..1111111......11111111111111111.....          ..11111111**.....11111111111111--...**..
 7      ..111111111....11111111111111111...1..         ..11111111*...-11111111111111--...*1..
 8      ..11111111111111111111111111111111.11..        ..11111111111111111111111111111111*11..
 9      ..111111111111111111111111111111111111..       ..11111111111111111111111111111111111..
10      ..11111111111111111111111111111111111..        ..11111111111111111111111111111111111..
11      ..11111111111111111111111111111111111..        ..11111111111111111111111111111111111..
12      ..11111111111111111111111111111111111..        ..11111111111111111111111111111111111..
13      ..11111111111111111111111111111111111..        ..11111111111111111111111111111111111..
14      ..11111111111111111111111111111111111..        ..11111111111111111111111111111111111..
15      ..11111111111111111111111111111111111..        ..11111111111111111111111111111111111..
16      ..11111111111111111111111111111111111..        ..11111111111111111111111111111111111..
17      ..11111111111111111111111111111111111..        ..11111111111111111111111111111111111..
18      ..11111111111111111111111111111111111..        ..11111111111111111111111111111111111..
19      ..11111111111111111111111111111111111..        ..11111111111111111111111111111111111..
20      ..1111111111111111111111111111.....1111..       ..11111111111111111111111111****..--11..
21      ..1111111111111.111111111111......111..         ..11111111---.111111111111****...-11..
22      ...111111111......1111111.1........11..         ..*111111----.....1111111*1*.......--..
23      ...................1111..........11..           ..................1111..........--..
24      ...................1....................        ...................1..................
25      ....................................          ....................................
26      ....................................          ....................................


 1      ....................................          ....................................
 2      ....................................          ....................................
 3      ......11..............1111111111........       .....11.............1111111111.........
 4      ..111111..........111111111111.........        ..111111..........111111111111........
 5      ..1111111.........111111111111.......          ..1111111.........111111111111.......
 6      ..1111111......11111111111111111.....          ..1111111......1111111111111111.......
 7      ..111111111....11111111111111111...1..          ..111111111....11111111111111111...1..
 8      ..11111111111111111111111111111111.11..         ..11111111111111111111111111111111.11..
 9      ..111111111111111111111111111111111111..       ..11111111111111111111111111111111111..
10      ..11111111111111111111111111111111111..        ..11111111111111111111111111111111111..
11      ..11111111111111111111111111111111111..        ..11111111111111111111111111111111111..
12      ..11111111111111111111111111111111111..        ..11111111111111111111111111111111111..
13      ..11111111111111111111111111111111111..        ..11111111111111111111111111111111111..
14      ..11111111111111111111111111111111111..        ..11111111111111111111111111111111111..
15      ..11111111111111111111111111111111111..        ..11111111111111111111111111111111111..
16      ..11111111111111111111111111111111111..        ..11111111111111111111111111111111111..
17      ..11111111111111111111111111111111111..        ..11111111111111111111111111111111111..
18      ..11111111111111111111111111111111111..        ..11111111111111111111111111111111111..
19      ..11111111111111111111111111111111111..        ..11111111111111111111111111111111111..
20      ..1111111111111111111111111111.....1111..       ..1111111111111111111111111111......1111..
21      ..1111111111111.111111111111.......111..         ..11111111111.11111111.111........111..
22      ...111111111......1111111.1........11..          ...111111111......1111111.1.........11..
23      ...................1111..........11..            ..................1111..........11..
24      ...................1....................         ...................1..................
25      ....................................          ....................................
26      ....................................          ....................................
```

FIGURE 12.4. Phantom 2 (top left) and its reconstructions using 2 views (top right; $K = 25$, $e_p = 28$ and $e_i = 50$), 3 views (bottom right; $K = 70$, $e_p = 0$ and $e_i = 0$) and 4 views (bottom left; $K = 22$, $e_p = 0$ and $e_i = 0$); "." and "1" represent values zero and one, respectively, in the phantom and at the correct locations in the reconstructions; "-" and "*" represent incorrect values of zero and one, respectively, in the reconstructions.

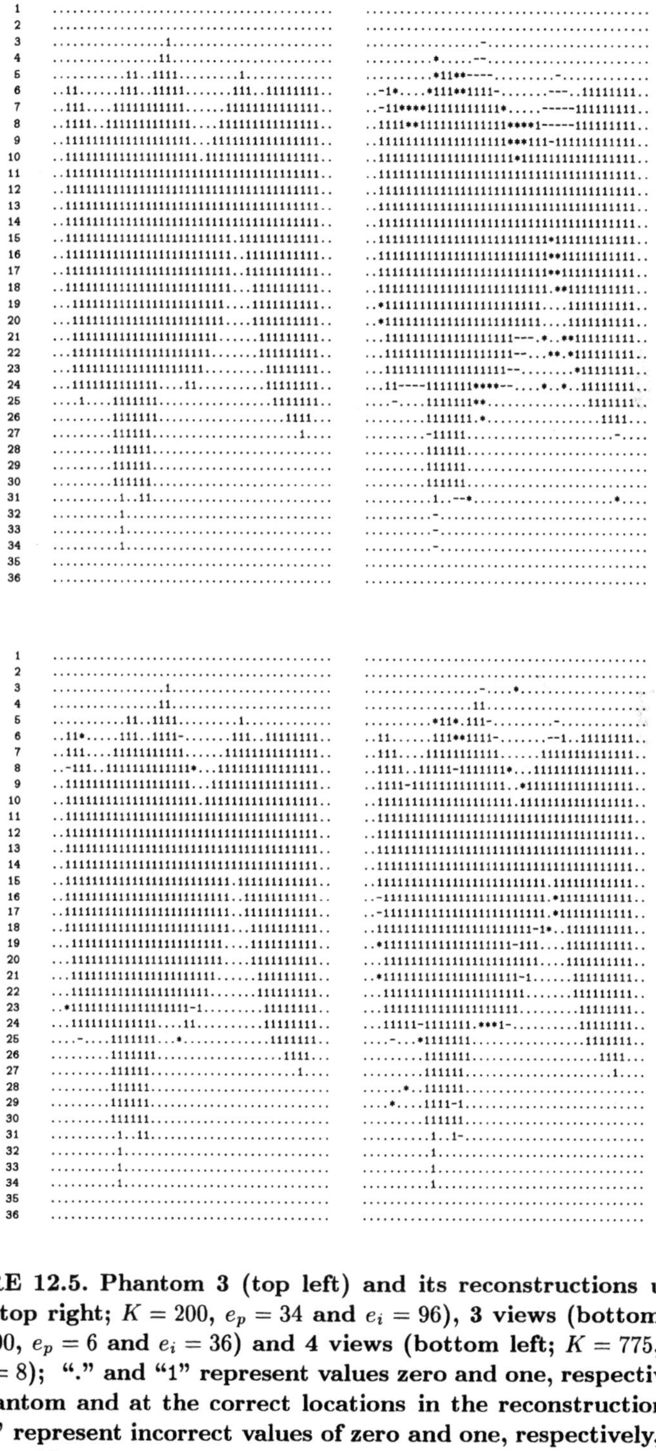

FIGURE 12.5. Phantom 3 (top left) and its reconstructions using 2 views (top right; $K = 200$, $e_p = 34$ and $e_i = 96$), 3 views (bottom right; $K = 3000$, $e_p = 6$ and $e_i = 36$) and 4 views (bottom left; $K = 775$, $e_p = 0$ and $e_i = 8$); "." and "1" represent values zero and one, respectively, in the phantom and at the correct locations in the reconstructions; "-" and "*" represent incorrect values of zero and one, respectively, in the reconstructions.

Finally, regarding the four views situation, we needed only 22, 22, and 775 iterations to find solutions (see bottom left images in Figs. 12.3, 12.4, and 12.5) for the given three phantoms, respectively. Note, that the solution for the third phantom differs from the phantom by a switching chain of length eight.

While adding more directions to the first two makes the discrete reconstruction problem "harder" from the computational complexity point of view, we experience in the computations better initial results. This is, of course, so because adding directions supplies the iterative algorithm with more information, thus enabling it to work "better."

Although the results of our preliminary computational experiments, presented in this section, are in no way exhausting, they clearly suggest that the underlying ideas of Herman [11], as refined and extended here, are a viable tool for binary steering of nonbinary iterative reconstruction algorithms.

12.4   Conclusions

The method proposed in this chapter is to reconstruct binary images by using nonbinary iterative reconstruction algorithms in conjunction with an additional mechanism to steer the nonbinary iterates toward an acceptable binary solution. The steering mechanism is independent of the particular choice of the nonbinary reconstruction algorithm and the overall process can be applied to three-dimensional binary image reconstruction once posed as a system of linear equations. The numerical results obtained by our preliminary computational experimentations encourage us to continue this line of research.

Efforts need to be invested in studying the effects of different sequences α_k, β_k, t_k and other parameters involved in the binarization and conflict settlement operations. Different nonbinary reconstruction algorithms need to be tried out within this methodology and full three-dimensional binary reconstruction problems must be solved with it to assess its efficiency. It should be possible to study the proposed scheme also from a mathematical point of view to determine bounds on the errors as functions of the parameters involved.

Acknowledgments

We thank Attila Kuba and Gabor Herman for many useful discussions and Stavros Zenios for help with the figures. We are grateful to Sven de Vries and Peter Gritzmann for their valuable comments on a draft of this paper. This work was supported by the National Institutes of Health Grants

HL-28438 and CA-54356 and by a research grant from the Israel Science Foundation, founded by the Israel Academy of Sciences and Humanities.

References

[1] G. T. Herman and A. Kuba (Eds.), "Special Issue on Discrete Tomography," *International Journal of Imaging Systems and Technology* **9**, No. 2/3, 1998.

[2] S.-K. Chang, "The reconstruction of binary patterns from their projections," *Communications of the ACM* **44**, 21-25 (1971).

[3] H. H. Bauschke and J. M. Borwein, "On projection algorithms for solving convex feasibility problems," *SIAM Review* **38**, 367-426 (1996).

[4] Y. Censor and S. A. Zenios, *Parallel Optimization: Theory, Algorithms, and Applications* (Oxford University Press, New York), 1997.

[5] C. L. Byrne, "Iterative algorithms for deblurring and deconvolution with constraints," *Technical Report, Department of Mathematical Sciences, University of Massachusetts at Lowell, Lowell, MA* (1997).

[6] C. L. Byrne, "Accelerating the EMML algorithm and related iterative algorithms by recalled block-iterative (RBI) methods," *IEEE Transactions on Image Processing* **IP-7**, 100-109 (1998).

[7] G. T. Herman, "Algebraic reconstruction techniques in medical imaging," In C. T. Leondes, *Medical Imaging Systems Techniques and Applications: Computational Techniques*, (Gordon and Breach, Overseas Publishers Association (OPA), Amsterdam), pp. 1-42, 1998.

[8] Y. Vardi and D. Lee, "Discrete Radon transform and its approximate inversion via the EM algorithm," *International Journal of Imaging Systems and Technology* **9**, 155-173 (1998).

[9] P. Fishburn, P. Schwander, L. Shepp, and R. Vanderbei, "The discrete Radon transform and its approximate inversion via linear programming," *Discrete Applied Mathematics* **75**, 39-61 (1997).

[10] P. Gritzmann, D. Prangenberg, S. de Vries, and M. Wiegelmann, "Success and failure of certain reconstruction and uniqueness algorithms in discrete tomography," *International Journal of Imaging Systems and Technology* **9**, 101-109 (1998).

[11] G. T. Herman, "Reconstruction of binary patterns from a few projections," In A. Günther, B. Levrat and H. Lipps, *International Computing Symposium 1973*, (North-Holland Publ. Co., Amsterdam), pp. 371-378, 1974.

[12] G. T. Herman, *Image Reconstruction from Projections: The Fundamentals of Computerized Tomography* (Academic Press, New York), 1980.

[13] N. Gastinel, *Linear Numerical Analysis* (Hermann, Paris), 1970.

[14] P. M. Salzberg, P. I. Rivera-Vega, and A. Rodriguez, "Network flow model for binary tomography on lattices," *International Journal of Imaging Systems and Technology* **9**, 147-154 (1998).

[15] S. K. Patch, "Iterative algorithms for discrete tomography," *International Journal of Imaging Systems and Technology* **9**, 132-134 (1998).

Chapter 13

Reconstruction of Binary Images via the EM Algorithm

Yehuda Vardi[1]
Cun-Hui Zhang[2]

ABSTRACT The problem of reconstructing a binary function x defined on a finite subset of a lattice $\mathbb{Z}$, from an arbitrary collection of its partial sums is considered. The approach is based on (a) relaxing the binary constraints $x(i) = 0$ or 1 to interval constraints $0 \leq x(i) \leq 1$, $i \in \mathbb{Z}$, and (b) applying a minimum distance method (using Kullback-Leibler's information divergence index as our distance function) to find such an x — say, $\hat{x}$ — for which the distance between the observed and the theoretical partial sums is as small as possible. (Turning this $\hat{x}$ into a binary function can be done as a separate postprocessing step: for instance, through thresholding, or through some additional Bayes modeling.) This minimum-distance solution is derived via a new EM algorithm that extends the often-studied EM/maximum likelihood (EM/ML) algorithm in emission tomography and certain linear-inverse problems to include lower- and upper-bound constraints on the function x. Properties of the algorithm including convergence and uniqueness conditions on the solution (or parts of it) are described.

13.1 Introduction

Let x be a binary function defined on a finite subset of a lattice, $x(i) = 0$ or 1, $i \in \mathbb{Z}$. Let $L_1, \ldots, L_m$ be a collection of subsets of the lattice $\mathbb{Z}$, and let

$$y_j = \sum_{i \in L_j} x(i), \qquad j = 1, \ldots, m, \tag{13.1}$$

and consider the problem of reconstructing the function f from the knowledge of the partial sums $y_1, \ldots, y_m$. This problem can be viewed as the discrete version of the Radon transform's inversion, and it is the key problem in "discrete tomography." (See the special issue on discrete tomography

---

[1]Rutgers University, Department of Statistics, Piscataway NJ 08854-8019, USA, E-mail: vardi@stat.rutgers.edu

[2]Rutgers University, Department of Statistics, Piscataway NJ 08854-8019, USA, E-mail: czhang@stat.rutgers.edu

of the *International Journal of Imaging Systems and Technology* (1998) for a collection of papers on the subject.) Recently, Vardi and Lee [1] proposed the following approach: (a) Replace the binary constraint $x(i) = 0$ or 1 with the interval constant $0 \leq x(i) \leq 1$. (b) Apply the EM algorithm to minimize the Kullback-Leibler information divergence criterion (or KL-"distance" for short) between the left and right side of (13.1), subject to the interval constraint in (a), after a suitable rescaling of the problem.

The rescaling converts the components of (13.1) to probability vectors, and is needed because the KL-"distance" is naturally defined on *probability* vectors. We note that the KL-"distance" between two probability vectors, say $p = (p_1, \ldots, p_m)$ and $q = (q_1, \ldots, q_m)$, is

$$KL(p,q) = \sum_{j=1}^{m} p_j \log p_j/q_j, \qquad (13.2)$$

and it is not a distance function in a purely mathematical sense, but it does possess some of its important properties (e.g., $KL(p,q) \geq 0$ with equality iff $p = q$, and $KL(p,q) \to 0$ if $p_j \to q_j > 0$, $j = 1, \ldots, m$). It is particularly useful in comparing probability measures.

For the rescaling, rewrite (13.1) as

$$y_j = \sum_{i=1}^{k} x_i A_{ij}, \qquad j = 1, \ldots, m, \qquad (13.3)$$

where $i = 1, \ldots, k$ is a labeling of the set $\mathbb{Z}$; $x_i = x(i)$, and $A_{ij} = 1_{L_j}(i)$ $(= 1$ if $i \in L_j$, and $= 0$ if $i \notin L_j)$. The interval constraints are then

$$0 \leq x_i \leq 1, \qquad i = 1, \ldots, k. \qquad (13.4)$$

Define now

$$\hat{g}_j = y_j / \sum_{j'=1}^{m} y_{j'},$$

$$h_{ij} = A_{ij} / \sum_{j'=1}^{m} A_{ij'},$$

$$f_i = x_i \left(\sum_{j'=1}^{m} A_{ij'} \right) \bigg/ \sum_{j'=1}^{m} y_{j'}. \qquad (13.5)$$

This results in

$$1 = \sum_{i=1}^{k} f_i = \sum_{j=1}^{m} \hat{g}_i = \sum_{j=1}^{m} h_{ij}, \qquad i = 1, \ldots, m, \qquad (13.6)$$

where, for the first equality, we assumed that (13.3) holds true, so that

$$\sum_{i=1}^{k} f_i = \sum_{j=1}^{m}\sum_{i=1}^{k} x_i A_{ij} \Big/ \sum_{j'=1}^{m} y_{j'} = \sum_{j=1}^{m} y_j \Big/ \sum_{j'=1}^{m} y_{j'} = 1. \qquad (13.7)$$

With this rescaling, the constraints (13.4) are replaced by

$$0 \le f_i \le \sum_{j=1}^{m} y_j \Big/ \sum_{j=1}^{m} A_{ij}, \qquad (13.8)$$

and so (13.3)-(13.4) becomes

$$\hat{g}_j = \sum_{i=1}^{k} f_i h_{ij}, \qquad j = 1, \ldots, m, \qquad (13.9)$$

subject to

$$0 \le f \le b, \qquad \sum_{i=1}^{k} f_i = 1, \qquad (13.10)$$

where $b = (b_1, \ldots, b_k)$ and, from (13.8),

$$b_i = \sum_{j=1}^{m} y_j \Big/ \sum_{j=1}^{m} A_{ij}, \qquad i = 1, \ldots, k. \qquad (13.11)$$

A minimum KL-"distance" solution for (13.9) and (13.10) seeks to

$$\text{minimize} \quad \left\{ -\ell(f) + \sum_{j=1}^{m} \hat{g}_j \log \hat{g}_j \right\}, \qquad (13.12)$$

with respect to f, subject to:

$$0 \le f \le b, \qquad \sum_{i=1}^{k} f_i = 1, \qquad (13.13)$$

where ℓ is defined as

$$\ell(f) = \sum_{j=1}^{m} \hat{g}_j \log \sum_{i=1}^{k} f_i h_{ij}. \qquad (13.14)$$

This is, of course, equivalent to

$$\text{maximize} \quad \ell(f)$$

$$\text{subject to}: 0 \le f \le b, \qquad \sum_{i=1}^{k} f_i = 1. \qquad (13.15)$$

This problem has a statistical interpretation as a constrained maximum likelihood estimation problem from incomplete data and hence an EM algorithm would be useful.

The "standard" EM algorithm of emission tomography, with the iteration step

$$f_i \leftarrow f_i \sum_{j=1}^{m} h_{ij} \frac{\hat{g}_j}{g_j(f)}, \quad i = 1, \ldots, k, \tag{13.16}$$

where we define

$$g_i(f) = \sum_{i=1}^{k} f_i h_{ij}, \quad j = 1, \ldots, m, \tag{13.17}$$

and initialize with a strictly positive f, is known to converge to the maximizer of (13.15), when $b = (b_1, \ldots, b_k) = (\infty, \ldots, \infty)$ (i.e., no upper bounds). (Because of the maximum likelihood interpretation of the problem, the algorithm is often referred to as the EM/ML algorithm.) Problem (13.15) with upper bounds has the same statistical interpretation of a maximum likelihood (ML) estimation problem from incomplete data, but now the parameter space is constrained and the maximization problem is more complicated.

The EM algorithm of (13.16) is not applicable to (13.15) with true upper bound, and neither is the "naive-modification" to (13.16), which would truncate f_i if $f_i > b_i$ after each iteration of (13.16). Vardi and Lee [1] developed an alternative algorithm, which does solve (13.15), and demonstrated its efficacy on several examples. Vardi and Zhang [2] extended this work to also include lower bounds on f, where (13.15) is replaced with

$$\text{maximize} \quad \ell(f) = \sum_{j=1}^{m} g_j \log \sum_{i=1}^{k} f_i h_{ij}$$

$$\text{subject to} : a \le f \le b, \quad \sum_{i=1}^{k} f_i = 1, \tag{13.18}$$

where a and b are prespecified vectors satisfying $0 \le a \le b$ (i.e., $0 \le a_i \le b_i$, $i = 1, \ldots k$). Since the cases $\sum a_i = 1$ and $\sum b_i = 1$ are trivial, we shall assume in the rest of the paper $\sum a_i < 1 < \sum b_i$. Vardi and Zhang [2] developed a new EM algorithm for this problem, which further generalizes that of Vardi and Lee [1]. They proved convergence of the algorithm and gave a characterization, which is helpful in determining uniqueness of the zero-one components of the solution. The current paper is based on results from both Vardi and Lee [1] and Vardi and Zhang [2]. For the details of some proofs, related methodologies, and further applications in fields outside tomography, the reader is referred to these papers.

Because of the interpretation of (13.18) as a maximum likelihood estimation problem in statistics, any solution to (13.18) is referred to heretofore as a maximum likelihood estimator (MLE). There always exists an MLE, but it need not be unique.

13.2   The EM/ML algorithm

We denote the set of all probability vectors of length k by $\mathcal{F}$:

$$\mathcal{F} = \left\{ f = (f_1, \ldots, f_k) : \sum_{i=1}^{k} f_i = 1, \ f_i \geq 0 \right\} \tag{13.19}$$

and the set of probability vectors satisfying the lower and upper bound constraints by $\mathcal{F}_0$:

$$\mathcal{F}_0 = \{ f \in \mathcal{F} : a_i \leq f_i \leq b_i, \ i = 1, \ldots, k \}. \tag{13.20}$$

For $f \in \mathcal{F}$, define the "standard" EM/ML mapping of (13.16) as $\widetilde{M}(f)$:

$$\widetilde{M}_i(f) = f_i \sum_{j=1}^{m} h_{ij} \frac{\hat{g}_j}{g_j(f)}, \quad i = 1, \ldots, k. \tag{13.21}$$

The EM/ML algorithm for (13.18) is then:
Initialization:

$$f^{(0)} = (f_1^{(0)}, \ldots, f_k^{(0)}), \quad \sum_{i=1}^{k} f_i^{(0)} = 1, \quad a_i \leq f_i^{(0)} \leq b, \quad i = 1, \ldots, k.$$
$$\tag{13.22}$$

Iteration: for $n \geq 0$, E-step:

$$f^{(n+1/2)} = \widetilde{M}(f^{(n)}), \tag{13.23}$$

and, with $f^{(n+1)} = (f_1^{(n+1)}, \ldots, f_k^{(n+1)})$, M-step:

$$f^{(n+1)} = \text{argmax}_{p \in \mathcal{F}_0} \sum_{i=1}^{k} f_i^{(n+1/2)} \log p_i = M(f^{(n)}) \tag{13.24}$$

where we define

$$M(f) = \text{argmax}_{p \in \mathcal{F}_0} \sum_{i=1}^{k} \widetilde{M}_i(f) \log p_i. \tag{13.25}$$

For $f \in \mathcal{F}$ define

$$\xi(r, f) = \sum_{rf_i < a_i} a_i + r \sum_{a_i \leq rf_i < b_i} f_i + \sum_{rf_i \geq b_i} b_i \tag{13.26}$$

and let

$$r(f) = \min\{r; \xi(r, f) = 1\}$$
$$(=\text{smallest } r \text{ for which } \xi(r, f) \text{ is equal to one}) \qquad (13.27)$$

with the convention that $\min \emptyset = \infty$. An alternative expression for (13.26) is:

$$\xi(r, f) = \sum_{i=1}^{k} \max(a_i, \min(b_i, r f_i)), \qquad (13.28)$$

which is obviously nondecreasing and continuous in the variable r. Thus, $r(f)$ of (13.27) is uniquely defined on $\mathcal{F}$. In (13.27), $r(f)$ is the unique solution of $\xi(r, f) = 1$ if and only if (iff) $r(f)$ is an interior point of $\bigcup_i [a_i/f_i, b_i/f_i]$ (not necessarily connected). If $f_i > 0$ on $\{i : b_i > 0\}$, then $\xi(\infty, f) = \sum_i b_i > 1$ implies $r(f) < \infty$.

Proposition 13.1.   *Given $f \in \mathcal{F}$, the function $\sum_{i=1}^{k} f_i \log p_i$ is uniquely maximized on $\mathcal{F}_0$ at $p^* = (p_1^*, \ldots, p_k^*)$ such that $p_i^* = \max(a_i, \min(b_i, r(f) f_i))$ with the $r(f)$ in (13.27).*

Let $M(f) = (M_1(f), \ldots, M_k(f))$ be as in (13.25). Since $\widetilde{M}(f) \in \mathcal{F}$ for $f \in \mathcal{F}_0$,

$$M_i(f) = \max\{a_i, \min\{b_i, r(\widetilde{M}(f))\widetilde{M}_i(f)\}\}. \qquad (13.29)$$

Thus, with $r_{n+1/2} = r(f^{(n+1/2)})$, the M-step of the EM algorithm (i.e., step (13.24) above) is

$$f_i^{(n+1)} = \begin{cases} a_i, & \text{if } f_i^{(n+1/2)} r_{n+1/2} < a_i \\ b_i, & \text{if } f_i^{(n+1/2)} r_{n+1/2} \geq b_i \\ f_i^{(n+1/2)} r_{n+1/2}, & \text{otherwise.} \end{cases} \qquad (13.30)$$

The value of $r(f)$ is relatively easy to find. See also Rothblum and Vardi [3], (5.2). Let $r_1 \leq \cdots \leq r_s$ be the ordered values of $\{a_i/f_i, b_i/f_i : f_i > 0, 1 \leq i \leq k\}$. If $\xi(r_s, f) \leq 1$, then $r(f) = \infty$. Suppose $\xi(r_s, f) > 1$. (In the EM algorithm this is always true: $\xi(r_s, f) = \xi(\infty, f) = \sum_i b_i > 1$ with $f = f^{(n+1/2)}$, since $f_i^{(0)} > 0$ implies $f_i^{(n+1/2)} > 0$ for $b_i > 0$.) Since $\xi(r_1, f) = \sum a_i < 1$, we may define $\tilde{r} = r_\ell$ with $\ell = \max\{i : \xi(r_i, f) < 1\}$. It follows from (13.26)-(13.28) that

$$r(f) = \left(1 - \sum_{\tilde{r} f_i < a_i} a_i - \sum_{\tilde{r} f_i \geq b_i} b_i\right) \bigg/ \sum_{a_i \leq \tilde{r} f_i < b_i} f_i, \qquad (13.31)$$

as $\xi(r_{\ell+1}, f) \geq 1 > \xi(r_\ell, f)$ implies $\{i : a_i \leq r_\ell f_i < b_i, f_i > 0\} \neq \emptyset$.

Proof: Since $\sum_{i=1}^{k} f_i \log p_i$ is concave, p^* is the maximizer iff

$$\frac{\partial}{\partial t} \sum_{i=1}^{k} f_i \log\{(1-t)p_i^* - t p_i\}\bigg|_{t=0} = \sum_i \frac{f_i}{p_i^*}(p_i - p_i^*) \leq 0 \qquad (13.32)$$

for all $p = (p_i, \ldots, p_k) \in \mathcal{F}_0$, with the convention $0/0 = 0$, iff there exists a constant $\tilde{c}$ such that $f_i/p_i^* = \tilde{c}$ ($\geq \tilde{c}$, or $\leq \tilde{c}$) for $a_i < p_i^* < b_i$ ($p_i^* = b_i > a_i$, or $p_i^* = a_i < b_i$). If such $\tilde{c}$ is unique for the given f, then $r(f) = 1/\tilde{c}$ is the unique solution of $\xi(r, f) = 1$. Otherwise, $\tilde{c}$ can be taken as the largest possible value and $f_i/b_i = \tilde{c}$ for some i, giving $r(f) = 1/\tilde{c}$. $\qquad\square$

For the case of no lower bound (i.e., $a_i = 0$, $i = 1, \ldots, k$), which occurs in discrete tomography applications, Vardi and Lee [1] proposed also a version of the EM/MC algorithm that replaces the sorting of the ratios b_i/f_i, $i = 1, \ldots, k$, as described above, with an iterative step (finite number of iterations) in each M-step, and is further described in Section 13.4 below.

Discussion of the EM algorithm and its applications can be found in Dempster, Laird, and Rubin [4], Herman [5], Shepp and Vardi [6], Vardi, Shepp, and Kaufman [7], and Vardi and Lee [8], among others.

13.3 Properties of the algorithm

The algorithm (13.22)–(13.24) converges monotonically in the sense that $\ell(f^{(n)}) \leq \ell(f^{(n+1)})$ and $f^{(n)} \to f^*$. We summarize the results below.

Theorem 13.1. *Suppose $\sum_{i=1}^k h_{ij} > 0$ for all j with $\hat{g}_j > 0$. Then, $\ell^* = \sup_{f \in \mathcal{F}_0} \ell(f)$ is finite, the set of MLEs $\mathcal{F}_0^* = \{f \in \mathcal{F}_0 : \ell(f) = \ell^*\}$ is nonempty, and the sequence $\{f^{(n)}, n \geq 1\}$ converges monotonically (in the sense of $\ell(f^{(n)}) \leq \ell(f^{(n+1)}), n = 0, 1, \ldots)$ to an MLE $f^* \in \mathcal{F}_0^*$,*

$$\lim_{n \to \infty} f^{(n)} = f^*, \qquad \lim_{n \to \infty} \ell(f^{(n)}) = \ell^*, \tag{13.33}$$

provided that $f_i^{(0)} > 0$ for all $1 \leq i \leq k$. Furthermore, $\hat{f}$ is an MLE ($\ell(\hat{f}) = \ell^*$) if and only if $g(\hat{f}) = g(f^*)$.

Remark. If $\sum_{i=1}^k h_{ij} = 0$ and $\hat{g} > 0$ for some j, then $\ell^* = -\infty$.

Theorem 13.1 extends the results of Cover [9], Csiszár and Tusnády [10], and Vardi, Shepp, and Kaufman [7] from $\mathcal{F}_0 = \mathcal{F}$ (i.e., $a_i = 0$ and $b_i = 1$) to general $\mathcal{F}_0$. Note that $M(\cdot) = \widetilde{M}(\cdot)$ when $\mathcal{F}_0 = \mathcal{F}$. The proof of Theorem 13.1 is given in Section 13.6.

The solution f^* obtained as a point of convergence of the algorithm may or may not be unique, depending on whether the problem (13.18) has a unique solution. In discrete tomography we are particularly interested in solutions that lie on the boundary of the constraint set. That is, solutions that satisfy $f_i = a_i$ or b_i (in discrete tomography $a_i = 0$). Theorem 13.2 below is helpful in partially identifying which coordinates of f_i^* are uniquely determined as boundary points for all solution points.

Let $\mathcal{F}^*$ denote the solution set of (13.18) as in Theorem 13.1:

$$\mathcal{F}_0^* = \{f \in \mathcal{F}_0 : \ell(f) = \ell^*\}, \tag{13.34}$$

and define

$$A = \{i : f_i = a_i, \forall f \in \mathcal{F}_0^*\} \text{ and } B = \{i : f_i = b_i, \forall f \in \mathcal{F}_0^*\}. \quad (13.35)$$

So A and B, respectively, are the coordinates on which all solutions, f^*, necessarily attain the lower and upper bounds, respectively. The following theorem does not quite characterize A and B, but gives nontrivial lower-bound-sets A' and B', such that $A' \subseteq A$ and $B' \subseteq B$. We do not know if it is possible to improve these lower-bound-sets but our experiments show that they are useful in the context of discrete tomography.

Theorem 13.2.   *Let f be an MLE (i.e., a solution of (13.18)). Define*

$$C_i(f) = \sum_{j=1}^{m} h_{ij} \frac{\hat{g}_j}{g_j(f)} \quad \left(= \frac{\widetilde{M}_i(f)}{f_i}, \text{ for } f_i > 0 \right), \quad i = 1, \ldots, k, \quad (13.36)$$

$$A' = \{i : C_i(f) < 1/r(\widetilde{M}(f))\} \text{ and } B' = \{i : C_i(f) > 1/r(\widetilde{M}(f))\}, \quad (13.37)$$

where r and $\widetilde{M}$ are given in (13.27) and (13.21), respectively. Then

$$A' \subseteq A \quad and \quad B' \subseteq B. \quad (13.38)$$

We propose to use $PDP = (|A'| + |B'|)/k$, the proportion of determined points to characterize the quality of the estimate f^*. Theorem 13.2 follows immediately from the corollary to Proposition 13.2 in Section 13.6.

13.4   Implementations and experiments

Vardi and Lee [1] suggested also an alternative M-step (see (13.24) and (13.30)) based on the following iterative procedure that terminates in a finite number of steps.

Begin:

$$p_i^{\text{old}} = f_i^{(n+1/2)}, \quad i = 1, \ldots, k \quad (13.39)$$

Iterate:

$$p_i^{\text{new}} = \begin{cases} \lambda^{-1} p_i^{\text{old}} & \text{if } p_i^{\text{old}} < b_i, \\ b_i & \text{if } p_i^{\text{old}} \geq b_i, \end{cases} \quad (13.40)$$

$i = 1, \ldots, k$, where λ is a scaling factor guaranteeing summability to 1 and is given by

$$\lambda = \frac{\sum_i p_i^{\text{old}} I[p_i^{\text{old}} < b_i]}{1 - \sum_i b_i I[p_i^{\text{old}} \geq b_i]}. \quad (13.41)$$

(The summation is for $i = 1, \ldots, k$.)

Stop: Terminate (with an optimal solution for (13.24)) as soon as $\mathbf{p}^{\text{new}} = \mathbf{p}^{\text{old}}$. When this occurs (always after a finite number of steps), set $\mathbf{f}^{(n+1)} = \mathbf{p}^{\text{new}}$. This results in the following implementation of the algorithm for discrete tomography applications:

Initialization: (13.22) $a_i = 0$, $i = 1, \ldots, k$

E-Step: (13.23)

M-Step: (13.39) and (13.40)

This algorithm was applied in Vardi and Lee [1] to the three examples of Fishburn *et al.* [11]. Each of the three examples is made up of a 0-1 array (these "phantoms" are displayed in Fig. 13.1 below, with a "." standing for 0), and the available data for each of these are the horizontal, vertical, and diagonal line sums: namely the row and column margins, and the diagonal margins [in direction (1,1)]. Almost all of phantom 1 is uniquely determined by these line sums, all of phantom 2 is uniquely determined by these line sums, while phantom 3 has considerable portions of nonuniqueness as discussed in Fishburn *et al.* [11].

The EM/ML reconstructions for the three phantoms are displayed in Fig. 13.2, below. In these figures a recovered value, x say, is displayed as "." if $x < 0.4$, as "1" if $x > 0.6$, and as the first decimal digit after roundoff if $0.4 \leq x \leq 0.6$. Details regarding computation time, experiments (including noisy data), related displays, and another shortcut-algorithm are given in Vardi and Lee [1].

When $f_{i_0}^* = x$ and x is an extreme value, 0 or 1, the natural question to ask is whether this is a uniquely determined value for all solutions f^* at coordinate i_0, or maybe there are other possible solutions of (13.18) (i.e., points of convergence of the EM/ML algorithm) for which the recovered value at coordinate i_0 is an interior value $0 < x < 1$. Theorem 13.2 gives a method for answering this question. The method is implemented here as a post-processing step as follows:

Determining sets of uniqueness of zero-one : Let $f^{(N)}$ denote the best solution generated by the EM/ML algorithm (after N iterations). Take this value as f^* and define

$$
\begin{array}{lll}
\text{(a)} & \bar{A} = \{i; f_i^* > 0\}, & \\[2mm]
\text{(b)} & \bar{B} = \{i; f_i^* < b_i\}, & \\[2mm]
\text{(c)} & C_i = \displaystyle\sum_{j=1}^{m} h_{ij} \frac{\hat{g}_j}{g_j(f^*)}, & \\[4mm]
\text{(d)} & C^+ = \displaystyle\max_{i \in \bar{A}}\{C_i\}, & (13.42) \\[3mm]
\text{(e)} & C^- = \displaystyle\min_{i \in \bar{B}}\{C_i\}, & \\[3mm]
\text{(f)} & A' = \{i; C_i < C^-\}, & \\[2mm]
\text{(g)} & B' = \{i; C_i > C^+\}. &
\end{array}
$$

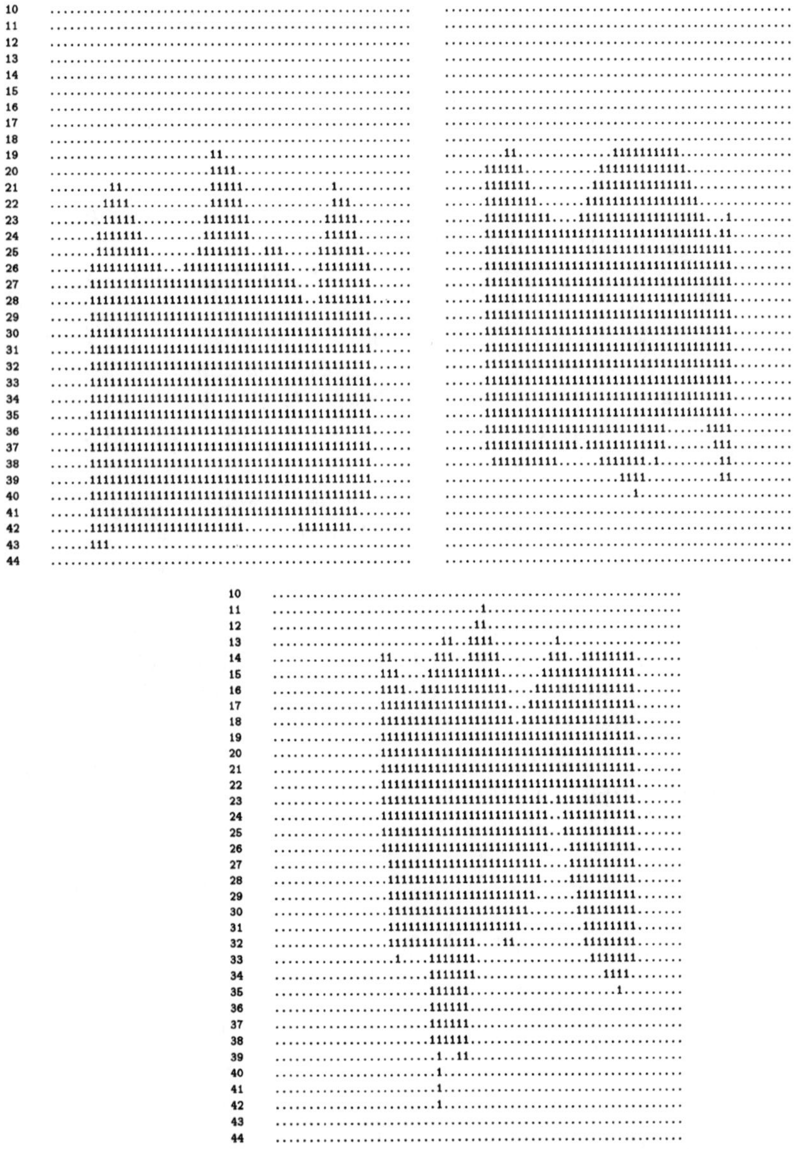

FIGURE 13.1. Three binary functions (phantoms) taken from [11]; '·' stands for 0.

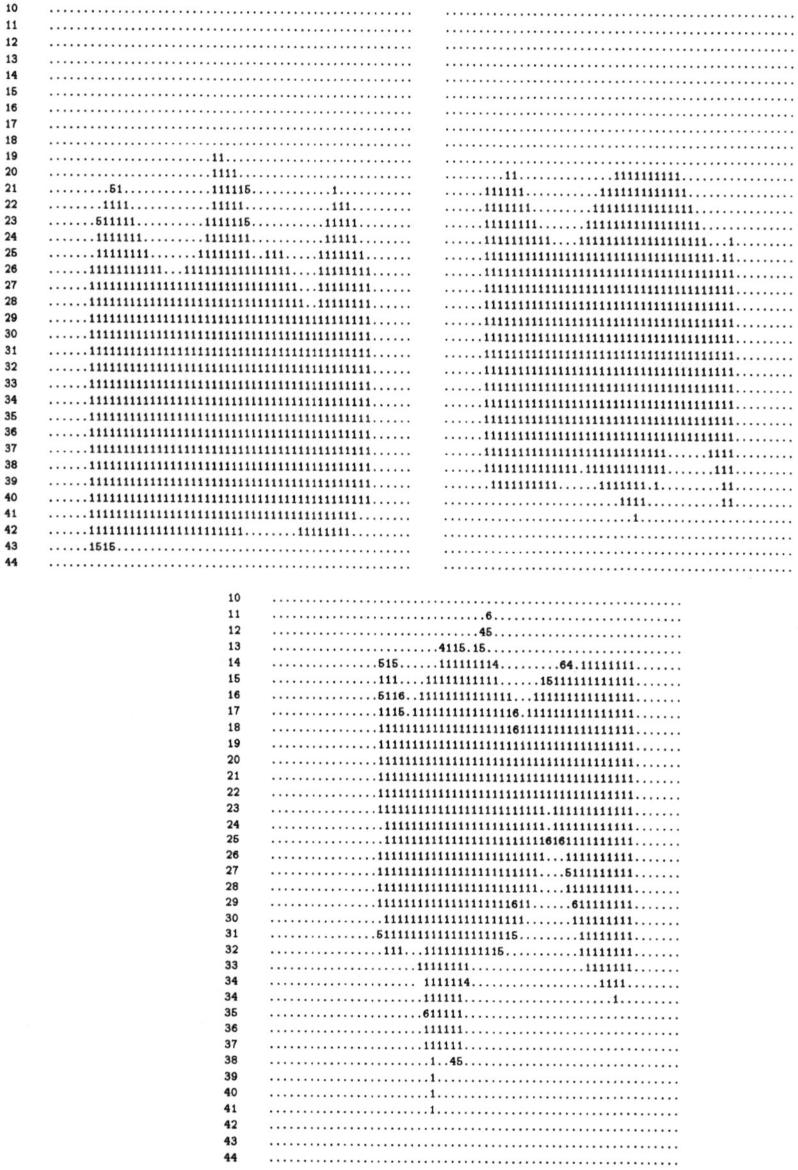

```
10 ..........................................          ..........................................
11 ..........................................          ..........................................
12 ..........................................          ..........................................
13 ..........................................          ..........................................
14 ..........................................          ..........................................
15 ..........................................          ..........................................
16 ..........................................          ..........................................
17 ..........................................          ..........................................
18 ..........................................          ..........................................
19 ..................11......                          ..........................................
20 ...............1111.....                   ..........11.............1111111111...........
21 ......51........111115...........1....     ....111111...........1111111111111....
22 ....1111........11111.........111....      ....111111............11111111111111....
23 ....511111.......1111115........11111......  ....11111111.........11111111111111111....
24 ....1111111........1111111.......11111......  ....111111111....111111111111111111111...1........
25 ....11111111.......11111111..111....1111111......  ....11111111111111111111111111111111111111.11........
26 ....1111111111...11111111111111....11111111.....  ....1111111111111111111111111111111111111111111....
27 ...1111111111111111111111111111111...11111111.....  ....11111111111111111111111111111111111111111111....
28 ...11111111111111111111111111111111..11111111.....  ....111111111111111111111111111111111111111111111....
29 ...111111111111111111111111111111111111111111111.....  ....1111111111111111111111111111111111111111111....
30 ....1111111111111111111111111111111111111111111.....  ....111111111111111111111111111111111111111111111....
31 ....1111111111111111111111111111111111111111111.....  ....111111111111111111111111111111111111111111111....
32 ....1111111111111111111111111111111111111111111.....  ....111111111111111111111111111111111111111111111....
33 ....1111111111111111111111111111111111111111111.....  ....111111111111111111111111111111111111111111111....
34 ....1111111111111111111111111111111111111111111.....  ....111111111111111111111111111111111111111111111....
35 ....1111111111111111111111111111111111111111111.....  ....1111111111111111111111111111111111111111111....
36 ....1111111111111111111111111111111111111111111.....  ....111111111111111111111111111111111111111111....
37 ....1111111111111111111111111111111111111111111.....  ....11111111111111111111111111111111.....1111....
38 ....1111111111111111111111111111111111111111111.....  ....1111111111111.1111111111111.......111....
39 ....1111111111111111111111111111111111111111111.....  ....1111111111......1111111.1........11....
40 ....1111111111111111111111111111111111111111111.....  ..........................1111..........11.......
41 ....11111111111111111111111111111111111111111.....  ............................1......................
42 ....1111111111111111111111111........11111111....
43 ....1515.........................
44 ........................................
```

```
10 ..........................................
11 ...............................6..........................
12 ...............................45.........................
13 ........................4115.15...........................
14 .................515......111111114........64.11111111.......
15 ...............111...11111111111......1511111111111.......
16 ...............5116..11111111111111...11111111111111.......
17 ...............1115.11111111111116.11111111111111.......
18 ...............1111111111111111116111111111111111.......
19 ...............11111111111111111111111111111111.......
20 ...............1111111111111111111111111111111.......
21 ...............1111111111111111111111111111111.......
22 ...............1111111111111111111111111111111.......
23 ...............1111111111111111111111.1111111111.......
24 ...............11111111111111111111.1111111111.......
25 ...............11111111111111111111111161611111111.......
26 ...............11111111111111111111...11111111.......
27 ...............111111111111111111111....51111111111.......
28 ...............11111111111111111111....1111111111.......
29 ...............111111111111111116611......61111111111.......
30 ...............111111111111111111111.......11111111.......
31 ...............51111111111111111116.......11111111.......
32 ...............111...1111111111115...........1111111.......
33 ...............11111111.................11111111.......
34 ...............1111114..................1111.......
35 ...............611111......
36 ...............111111.......
37 ...............111111.......
38 ...............1..45.......
39 ...............1.......
40 ...............1.......
41 ...............1.......
42 ..........................................
43 ..........................................
44 ..........................................
```

FIGURE 13.2. EM/ML reconstructions of phantoms in Fig. 13.1.
Numerical thresholding: $\hat{x} < 0.4 \Rightarrow x \leftarrow$ '.', $\hat{x} > 0.6 \Rightarrow x \leftarrow$ "1",
$0.4 \leq \hat{x} \leq 0.6 \Rightarrow x \leftarrow$ first decimal digit (i.e., 4, 5, or 6).

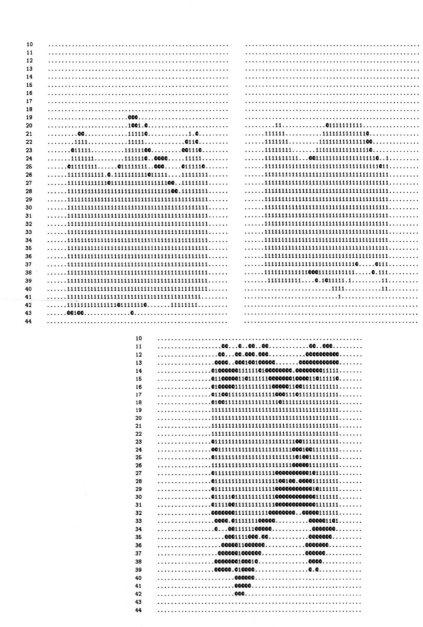

FIGURE 13.3. Determination of unique parts of the solution for all three phantoms of Fig. 13.1, using the method of Theorem 13.2 and (13.43): "1" stands for $i \in B'$, "." for $i \in A'$, and "@" for $i \neq A' \cup B'$.

In (13.42-f) and (13.42-g), one can replace C^- and C^+ with $(C^- - \epsilon)$ and $(C^+ + \epsilon)$, respectively, for numerical stability. Here ϵ is a small number, say 10^{-6}, within the tolerance of the convergence criterion of the EM/ML algorithm. From Theorem 13.2, we have:

$$i \in A' \Rightarrow f_i^* = 0 \text{ for all } f^*, \text{ which solve } (13.13),$$
$$i \in B' \Rightarrow f_i^* = 1 \text{ for all } f^*, \text{ which solve } (13.13). \qquad (13.43)$$

We believe that with increased attention to numerical accuracy the (already very good) results as displayed in Fig. 13.3 can be improved.

13.5 Further comments

On some related approaches: The EM/ML approach here is to minimize the KL-"distance" between the left and the right sides of (13.1), which (after rescaling) becomes (13.10). That is:

$$\text{minimize } KL\left(\hat{g}_j, \left\{\sum_i f_i h_{ij}\right\}\right) \quad \text{s.t. } 0 \leq f \leq 1. \qquad (13.44)$$

The KL-"distance" is not symmetric in its arguments, and so if we decide to switch the arguments and

$$\text{minimize } KL\left(\left\{\sum_i f_i h_{ij}\right\}, \hat{g}_j\right) \quad \text{s.t. } 0 \leq f \leq 1, \qquad (13.45)$$

the flavor of the approach (as a minimum distance method) remains very similar, but it would lead to different algorithm(s). In fact, the popular algebraic reconstruction technique ART (MART) of Gordon, Bender, and Herman [12] are algorithms for solving equation (13.45) without the box constraints. Both are special cases of the more general Bregman [13] algorithm for interval constraints (see algorithm 6.4.1 in Censor and Zenios [14]). Extensions to handle interval constraints are in Censor *et al.* [15] (see algorithm 6.9.2 in Censor and Zenios [14]). Byrne [18] surveyed some of these and the EM/ML algorithm, and proposed a cross-entropy measure of distance. He did not discuss the case of interval constraints. To the best of our knowledge, convergence properties of any of the ART-type algorithms which accommodate interval constraints are unknown in the inconsistent case. We note in this connection that Censor [16] presented a regularized version of MART and remarked that the behavior of MART in the inconsistent case is unknown; and Herman [17] noted that in the inconsistent case, MART may not maximize entropy. Section VI of Byrne [18] proposed a convergent algorithm, but still did not consider interval constraints.

More on the binary constraint: Following the approach in Fishburn *et al.* [11], we substitute the binary constraint $f(x) = 0$ or 1 with $0 \leq f(z) \leq 1$. Equivalently, in terms of the problem of reconstructing a set from its projections, this replaces the set constraint with a fuzzy-set constraint in the reconstruction. This is acceptable in algebraically consistent cases that have a unique solution. Also, for problems that are partially uniquely determined (see Aharoni, Herman, and Kuba [19] and Fishburn *et al.* [11] for sufficient conditions), our method identifies parts of the image that are uniquely determined (Theorem 13.2, and the implementation in (13.43)). However, for consistent and undetermined cases (with many solutions) or for inconsistent and overdetermined cases (no solution), the algorithm will produce an image $x(i)$ with $0 < x(i) < 1$ for some $i \in \mathbb{Z}$. We do not have a detailed proposal of how to redistribute these values to achieve a completely binary-valued function $x(i)$. An obvious (natural) approach is by thresholding. A more sophisticated approach could be to use the output image from our algorithm as an input image for a Bayesian image model as proposed, for instance, in Chan, Herman, and Levitan [20]. Clearly, this topic alone could be a basis for much further research, and for now we use thresholding in our experiments. Other approaches for the binary reconstruction problem are discussed — for example, in Herman [17] (and the references therein) — for ART-like methods and in Chang [21] for reconstructing 2D, 0-1 arrays from their margins.

13.6   Proofs

In this section, we prove the convergence of the iterative sequences in the EM algorithm. We shall first provide a characterization of local MLEs under the additional constraint that $f_i = 0$ on a set of i. This characterization and the continuity of certain functionals involved in the EM algorithm provide the convergence of the log-likelihood sequence $\ell(f^{(n)})$. The convergence of $f^{(n)}$ is proved based on that of $\ell(f^{(n)})$ and some inequalities about the KL-"distance" between $f^{(n)}$ and the set of MLEs (i.e., solution set of (13.18)). Some of the more technical details of the convergence proof are given in the Appendix and in Vardi and Zhang [2].

13.6.1   *Characterization of local MLEs*

Let $\mathcal{F}_0$ be as in (13.20). For $I \subseteq \{i : a_i = 0 < b_i\}$, define

$$\mathcal{F}_I = \{(f_1, \ldots, f_k) \in \mathcal{F}_0 : f_i = 0, \forall i \in I\},$$

$$\ell_I^* = \sup_{f \in \mathcal{F}_I} \ell(f), \quad \ell^* = \ell_\emptyset^* = \sup_{f \in \mathcal{F}_0} \ell(f),$$

and

$$\mathcal{F}_I^* = \{f \in \mathcal{F}_I : \ell(f) = \ell_I^*\}. \qquad (13.46)$$

Proposition 13.2 (ii) below provides a characterization of the MLE in the spaces $\mathcal{F}_I$. For the empty set $I = \emptyset$, $\mathcal{F}_\emptyset = \mathcal{F}_0$, so that $\mathcal{F}_\emptyset^* = \{f \in \mathcal{F}_0 : \ell(f) = \ell^*\}$ is the set of MLEs. Note that $\mathcal{F}_0$ and $\mathcal{F}_\emptyset^*$ become $\mathcal{F}_I$ and $\mathcal{F}_I^*$, respectively, if b_i are replaced by zero for all $i \in I$. Although the characterization is a consequence of the conditions of Kuhn and Tucker [22], a simple proof is provided here so that the paper is self-contained.

For $f = (f_1, \ldots, f_k) \in \mathcal{F}_0$ define $\ell'(f) = (\ell_1'(f), \ldots, \ell_k'(f))$ by

$$\ell_i'(f) = \frac{\partial \ell(f)}{\partial f_i} = \sum_{j=1}^m \hat{g}_j h_{ij}/g_j(f), \qquad (13.47)$$

with $\ell(f)$ in (13.14) and $g_j(f)$ in (13.17).

Proposition 13.2.   *Let I be a subset of $\{i : a_i = 0 < b_i\}$. Suppose $\mathcal{F}_I \neq \emptyset$ and $\ell_I^* > -\infty$. (i) The set $\mathcal{F}_I^*$ of local MLEs in (13.46) is nonempty and convex. (ii) For $f \in \mathcal{F}_I$, $f \in \mathcal{F}_I^*$ iff there exists a constant c (dependent on f) such that*

$$\ell_i'(f) \begin{cases} \leq c, & \text{if } f_i = a_i < b_i \\ = c, & \text{if } a_i < f_i < b_i \\ \geq c, & \text{if } f_i = b_i > a_i, \end{cases} \qquad (13.48)$$

for all $i \notin I$. (iii) Let $c(f)$ be the largest possible c satisfying (13.48). Then, $c(f) = 1/r(\tilde{M}(f))$ with $r(\cdot)$ and $\tilde{M}(\cdot)$ as in (13.27) and (13.21), respectively. (iv) On $\mathcal{F}_I^*$, $c(f)$ is a constant and $g(f)$ and $\ell'(f)$ are both constant vectors.

Proof: (i) Since $\ell(f)$ is concave and nonpositive and $\mathcal{F}_I$ is convex, $\mathcal{F}_I^*$ is nonempty and convex for finite ℓ_I^*.

(ii) Since the likelihood $\ell(f)$ is concave, $f \in \mathcal{F}_I^*$ iff

$$\left(\frac{\partial}{\partial t}\right)\ell\big((1-t)f + tp, f\big)\Big|_{t=0} = \sum_{i=1}^k \ell_i'(f)(p_i - f_i) \leq 0 \qquad (13.49)$$

for all $p = (p_1, \ldots, p_k) \in \mathcal{F}_I$. Checking this condition for those p such that $p_i \neq f_i$ only at two indices $i = i_1$ and $i = i_2$, we find that (13.48) holds for $f \in \mathcal{F}_I^*$. On the other hand, since $\sum_i p_i = 1$, (13.48) implies (13.49) via

$$\begin{aligned} \sum_{i=1}^k \ell_i'(f)(p_i - f_i) &= \sum_{i=1}^k \{\ell_i'(f) - c\}(p_i - f_i) \\ &= \sum_{f_i = a_i} \{\ell_i'(f) - c\}(p_i - a_i) \\ &\quad + \sum_{f_i = b_i} \{\ell_i'(f) - c\}(p_i - b_i) \leq 0. \qquad (13.50) \end{aligned}$$

(iii) We shall prove $c(f) = 1/r(\tilde{M}(f))$. For $f \in \mathcal{F}_0$ define

$$\Delta(f) = Q\big(M(f), f\big) - Q(f, f) \qquad (13.51)$$

with the $Q(p, f) = \sum_{i=1}^{k} \tilde{M}_i(f) \log p_i$ and $M(\cdot)$ is as in (13.25). Let $f \in \mathcal{F}_I^*$. Since $M(\cdot)$ is the EM mapping and $M(f) \in \mathcal{F}_I^*$, $0 \leq \Delta(f) \leq \ell(M(f)) - \ell(f) = 0$. Thus $M(f) = f$ on $\mathcal{F}_I^*$ by the uniqueness in 13.1, and by (13.21) and (13.47)

$$\ell_i'(f) = \tilde{M}_i(f)/f_i = \tilde{M}_i(f)/M_i(f). \qquad (13.52)$$

If $a_{i_0} < f_{i_0} < b_{i_0}$ for some i_0, then c is unique in (13.48), and by (13.29) and (13.52) $1 = r(\tilde{M}(f))\tilde{M}_{i_0}(f)/M_{i_0}(f) = r(\tilde{M}(f))c$ with $c = c(f)$. Otherwise, the maximal value of c in (13.48) is reached at the smallest $\ell_i'(f) = \tilde{M}_i(f)/M_i(f)$ over $\{i : f_i = b_i > a_i\}$, while $r(\tilde{M}(f))$ is the largest $b_i/\tilde{M}_i(f) = M_i(f)/\tilde{M}_i(f)$ over the same set as the solution set of $\xi(r, \tilde{M}(f)) = 1$ is the closed interval

$$\Big[\max_{f_i = b_i} b_i/\tilde{M}_i(f), \ \min_{f_i = a_i} a_i/\tilde{M}_i(f)\Big] \qquad (13.53)$$

in view of (13.26) and (13.27). Again, $c(f)r(\tilde{M}(f)) = 1$.

(iv) Since $\ell_I^* > -\infty$ and $\hat{g}_j > 0$, by (13.17) and (13.14) $g_j(f)$ is bounded away from 0 on $\mathcal{F}_I^*$ for all j. Let f and f' be two members of $\mathcal{F}_I^*$. By the convexity of $\mathcal{F}_I^*$, $(1-t)f + tf' \in \mathcal{F}_I^*$ for $0 \leq t \leq 1$ and

$$\Big(\frac{\partial}{\partial t}\Big)^2 \ell\big((1-t)f + tf'\big)\Big|_{t=0} = -\sum_{j=0}^{m} \hat{g}_j (g_j(f))^{-2}(g_j(f') - g_j(f))^2 = 0, \quad (13.54)$$

which implies $g(f) = g(f')$. Thus, by (13.47) $g(f)$ and $\ell'(f)$ are constant vectors on $\mathcal{F}_I^*$.

Let f' and f'' be two distinct members of $\mathcal{F}_I^*$. We shall prove $c(f') = c(f)$ for $f = (f' + f'')/2 \in \mathcal{F}_I^*$. Let $\tilde{I} = \{i : f_i' \neq f_i'' \text{ or } a_i < f_i < b_i\} \neq \emptyset$. For $i \in \tilde{I}$, $\ell_i'(f') = \ell_i'(f) = c(f)$ due to $a_i < f_i < b_i$. If $c(f') = \ell_i'(f')$ for some $i \in \tilde{I}$, then $c(f') = c(f)$. Assume $c(f') \neq \ell_i'(f')$ for all $i \in \tilde{I}$. By (ii) f_i' is either a_i or b_i and $f_{i_1}'' < f_{i_1}' = b_{i_1}$ for some $i_1 \in \tilde{I}$ due to $f' \neq f''$, so that $c(f) = \ell_{i_1}'(f) = \ell_{i_1}'(f') \geq c(f')$ by (ii). On the other hand, $f_{i_2}'' > f_{i_2}' = a_{i_2}$ for some $i_2 \in \tilde{I}$, so that $c(f) = \ell_{i_2}'(f) = \ell_{i_2}'(f') \leq c(f')$ by (ii). Hence, $c(f') = c(f)$.
□

Corollary 13.1. Let $A_I = \{i : f_i = a_i, \forall f \in \mathcal{F}_I^*\}$ and $B_I = \{i : f_i = b_i, \forall f \in \mathcal{F}_I^*\}$. Then, $\{i : \ell_i'(f) < c(f)\} \subseteq A_I$ and $\{i : \ell_i'(f) > c(f)\} \subseteq B_I$ for all $f \in \mathcal{F}_I^*$.

13.6.2 Convergence of the algorithm

If $\sum_{i=1}^{k} h_{ij} = 0$ and $\hat{g}_j > 0$ for some j, then $\ell^* = -\infty$. If $\hat{g}_j = 0$ for some j, the problem is equivalent to an identical one with smaller m via renormalization after removing the j-th cell. Thus, we assume without loss of generality in the sequel that $\hat{g}_j > 0$ and $\sum_{i=1}^{k} h_{ij} > 0$ for all $j = 1, \ldots, m$.

We need a number of lemmas for the proof of Theorem 13.1. Lemma 13.1 provides the continuity of mappings involved in the EM/ML algorithm. Lemma 13.2 ensures the existence of the MLE and the connectedness of the accumulation points of $\{f^{(n)}\}$.

Lemma 13.1. *Let $r(f)$, $\tilde{M}(f)$, $M(f)$ and $\Delta(f)$ be given by (13.27), (13.21), (13.25), and (13.51), respectively. Then, $r(f)$ is continuous on $\mathcal{F}$, and $\tilde{M}(f)$, $M(f)$ and $\Delta(f)$ are continuous on $\{f \in \mathcal{F}_0 : \ell(f) \geq \ell_0\}$ for all $\ell_0 > -\infty$.*

Remark. Since $\xi(r, f)$ in (13.26) is not strictly increasing in general, the use of infimum in the definition of $r(f)$ is crucial to ensure its continuity.

Lemma 13.2. *If $\ell(f^{(0)}) > -\infty$, then the set of accumulation points $\tilde{\mathcal{F}}$ of $\{f^{(n)}\}$ is a nonempty compact subset of $\mathcal{F}^* = \{f \in \mathcal{F}_0 : \Delta(f) = 0, \ell(f) > -\infty\}$, and $f^{(n+1)} - f^{(n)} \to 0$. Furthermore, $\mathcal{F}^*$ is the union of these $\mathcal{F}_I^*$ in (13.46) with $I \subseteq \{i : a_i = 0 < b_i\}$.*

Proof of Theorem 13.1. By (13.14), $-\infty < \ell(f^{(0)}) \leq \ell^* \leq 0$. The nonemptyness of $\mathcal{F}_\emptyset^*$ follows from Proposition 13.2 (i). First, we need to prove that the set of accumulation points $\tilde{\mathcal{F}}$ of $\{f^{(n)}\}$ is a subset of $\mathcal{F}_\emptyset^*$. Let $\tilde{f} \in \tilde{\mathcal{F}}$. By Lemma 13.2, $\tilde{f} \in \mathcal{F}_I^*$ for some I, so that by 13.2 (ii) and (iii) it suffices to prove $\ell_i'(\tilde{f}) \leq 1/r(\tilde{M}(\tilde{f})) = c(\tilde{f})$ for all i with $\tilde{f}_i = 0 < b_i$. Let $\tilde{f}_i = 0 < b_i$. Since $a_i = 0 < b_i$ and $f_i^{(0)} > 0$, $f_i^{(n)} > 0$ for all n. Since $f^{(n+1)} - f^{(n)} \to 0$ by Lemma 13.2 and $\tilde{f}$ is an accumulation point, there exists a subsequence $\{n'\}$ such that $0 = a_i < f_i^{(n'+1)} < f_i^{(n')} < b_i$ and $f^{(n')} \to \tilde{f}$. It follows from (13.29), (13.21), (13.47) and the continuity of $r(\tilde{M}(\cdot))$ and $\ell'(\cdot)$ that

$$1 > f_i^{(n'+1)}/f_i^{(n')} = r(\tilde{M}(f^{(n')}))\ell_i'(f^{(n')}) \to r(\tilde{M}(\tilde{f}))\ell_i'(\tilde{f}). \qquad (13.55)$$

Thus, $\ell_i'(\tilde{f}) \leq 1/r(\tilde{M}(\tilde{f})) = c(\tilde{f})$ for all i with $\tilde{f}_i = 0 < b_i$ and $\tilde{f} \in \mathcal{F}_\emptyset^*$.

The convergence of $f^{(n)}$ to an MLE f^*, in the sense of $\|f^{(n)} - f^*\| \to 0$, follows from several inequalities in Vardi and Zhang [2]. An alternative is to consider the problem via Csiszár and Tusnády [10]. See, for example, the treatment of Csiszár and Tusnády [10] in Vardi, Shepp, and Kaufman [7].

13.7 Appendix

Proof of Lemma 13.1. The continuity of $r(\cdot)$ is clear when the solution of $\xi(r, f) = 1$ is unique at f, as $\xi(r, f')$ is continuous in (r, f') at $(r(f), f)$ and $\xi(r, f)$ is strictly increasing in r at $r(f)$ when f is fixed. If the solution of $\xi(r, f) = 1$ is not unique, then the index set $\{1, \ldots, k\}$ can be partitioned into three disjoint subsets I, I' and I'' such that

$$\max_{i \in I'} b_i/f_i < \min_{i \in I''} a_i/f_i, \qquad \sum_{i \in I'} b_i + \sum_{i \in I'' \cup I} a_i = 1, \qquad (13.56)$$

$a_i < b_i$ for $i \in I' \cup I''$, and $I = \{i : a_i = b_i \text{ or } f_i = 0\}$. In this case, $r(f) = \max_{i \in I'} b_i/f_i$. Note that $I' \neq \emptyset$ due to $\sum_{i=1}^{k} a_i < 1$. Suppose (13.56) holds and let ϵ be a small positive number. For $f' \in \mathcal{F}$ close enough to f, (13.56) implies $\max_{i \in I'} b_i/f_i' < r(f) + \epsilon < \min_{i \in I''} a_i/f_i'$, so that

$$\xi\big(r(f) + \epsilon, f'\big) \geq \sum_{i \in I'} b_i + \sum_{i \in I'' \cup I} a_i = 1, \qquad (13.57)$$

which implies $r(f') \leq r(f) + \epsilon$. On the other hand, for $r < r(f)$, $\xi(r, f) < 1$ and

$$\xi(r, f') - 1 \leq r \sum_{i=1}^{k} |f_i' - f_i| + \xi(r, f) - 1 < 0 \qquad (13.58)$$

for $\sum_i |f_i' - f_i| < \{1 - \xi(r, f)\}/r$. This proves the continuity of $r(\cdot)$. Since $g_j(f)$ is bounded away from zero in $\{f \in \mathcal{F} : \ell(f) \geq \ell_0\}$, $\tilde{M}(f)$ is continuous by (13.21), so that $r(\tilde{M}(f))$ is continuous. The continuity of $M(\cdot)$ and $\Delta(\cdot)$ follows from (13.29), (13.51), (13.25) and the continuity of $r(\cdot)$ and $\tilde{M}(\cdot)$. This proves Lemma 13.1.

Proof of Lemma 13.2. Since $-\infty < \ell(f^{(0)}) \leq \ell^* \leq 0$ and $f^{(n)} \to f^{(n+1)} = M(f^{(n)})$ is an EM algorithm,

$$0 \leq \Delta(f^{(n)}) \leq \ell(f^{(n+1)}) - \ell(f^{(n)}) \to 0, \qquad (13.59)$$

so that the sequence $\{f^{(n)}\}$ visits the set $\{f : \Delta(f) > \epsilon\}$ only finitely many times for all $\epsilon > 0$. Thus, $\tilde{\mathcal{F}} \subseteq \mathcal{F}^*$, as $\Delta(f)$ is continuous on $\mathcal{F}(f^{(0)}) = \{f \in \mathcal{F}_0 : \ell(f) \geq \ell(f^{(0)})\}$ by Lemma 13.1. Since $\mathcal{F}(f^{(0)})$ is compact, $\mathcal{F}^*$ is compact.

Since $M(f)$ is uniquely defined, $M(f) = f$ on $\mathcal{F}^*$. Since $M(f)$ is continuous by Lemma 13.1, $f^{(n'+1)} - f^{(n')} \to M(\tilde{f}) - \tilde{f} = 0$ as $f^{(n')} \to \tilde{f} \in \mathcal{F}^*$ along any subsequences $\{n'\}$. Hence, $f^{(n+1)} - f^{(n)} \to 0$ by the compactness of $\mathcal{F}(f^{(0)})$.

Let $Q(p, f)$ be as in (13.51). By (13.21) and (13.47), $(\partial/\partial p_i)Q(p, f)|_{p=f} = \ell_i'(f)$ if $f_i > 0$ and $(\partial/\partial p_i)Q(p, f) = 0$ if $f_i = 0$. Set $I(f) = \{i : f_i = 0 < b_i\}$ for $f \in \mathcal{F}_0$. Since $Q(p, f)$ is concave in p, for fixed f it is maximized at $p = f$ (i.e., $M(f) = f$) iff

$$\left(\frac{\partial}{\partial t}\right) Q((1-t)f + tp, f)\Big|_{t=0} = \sum_{i=1}^{k} \ell_i'(f)(p_i - f_i) \leq 0 \qquad (13.60)$$

for all $p \in \mathcal{F}_{I(f)}$. By Proposition 13.2 (ii) and (13.49), (13.60) is also equivalent to $f \in \mathcal{F}^*_{I(f)}$. Thus $\mathcal{F}^*$ is the union of these $\mathcal{F}^*_I$. Note that $\mathcal{F}^*_{I(f)} = \mathcal{F}^*_I$ for $I(f) \supseteq I$ if $f_i' = 0$ for all $i \in I(f) \setminus I$ and some $f' \in \mathcal{F}^*_I$.

Acknowledgments

We thank David Lee for his generous technical help, and the NSF and NSA for supporting our research.

References

[1] Y. Vardi and D. Lee, "The discrete Radon transform and its approximate inversion via the EM algorithm," *International J. Imaging Systems and Techn.* **9**, 155-173 (1998).

[2] Y. Vardi and C.-H. Zhang, "Estimating mixing probabilities subject to lower and upper bound constraints with applications," *Technical Report #97-006, Department of Statistics, Rutgers University, Piscataway, NJ* (1997).

[3] U. Rothblum and Y. Vardi, "Maximum likelihood estimation of cell probabilities in constrained multinomial models," *J. Statist. Computation and Simulation,* **61**, 141-161 (1998).

[4] A. P. Dempster, N. M. Laird, and R. B. Rubin, "Maximum likelihood from incomplete data via the EM algorithm (with Discussion)," *J. R. Statist. Soc. B* **39**, 1-38 (1977).

[5] G. T. Herman, "Reconstruction of binary patterns from a few projections," In A. Günther, B. Levrat, and H. Lipps, *International Computing Symposium 1973*, (North-Holland Publ. Co., Amsterdam), pp. 371-378, 1974.

[6] L. A. Shepp, and Y. Vardi, "Maximum likelihood reconstruction for emission tomography," *IEEE Trans. Med. Imaging* **1**, 113-122 (1982).

[7] Y. Vardi, L. A. Shepp and L. Kaufman, "A statistical model for positron emission tomography (with Discussion)," *J. Amer. Statist. Assoc.* **80**, 8-37 (1985).

[8] Y. Vardi and D. Lee, "From image deblurring to optimal investments: Maximum likelihood solutions for positive linear inverse problems (with Discussion)," *J. R. Statist. Soc. B* **55**, 569-612 (1993).

[9] T. M. Cover, "An algorithm for maximizing expected log investment return," *IEEE Trans. Inform. Theory* **30**, 369-373 (1984).

[10] I. Csiszár and G. Tusnády, "Information geometry and alternating minimization procedures," *Statist. Decis.*, Suppl. 1, 205-237 (1984).

[11] P. Fishburn, P. Schwander, L. Shepp, and R. Vanderbei, "The discrete Radon transform and its approximate inversion via linear programming," *Discrete Applied Mathematics* **75**, 39-61 (1997).

[12] R. Gordon, R. Bender, and G. T. Herman, "Algebraic reconstruction techniques (ART) for three-dimensional electron microscopy and x-ray photography," *J. Theoret. Biol.* **29**, 471-481 (1970).

[13] L. M. Bregman, "The relaxation method of finding the common point of convex sets and its application to the solution of problems in convex programming," *U.S.S.R. Comput. Math. and Math. Phys.* **7**, 200-217 (1967).

[14] Y. Censor and S. A. Zenios, *Parallel Optimization: Theory, Algorithms, and Applications* (Oxford University Press, New York), 1997.

[15] Y. Censor, A. R. De Pierro, T. Elfving, G. T. Herman, and A. N. Iusem, "On iterative methods for linearly constrained entropy maximization," In A. Wakulicz, *Numerical Analysis and Mathematical Modeling*, (PWN - Polish Scientific Publishers, Warsaw), pp. 145-163, 1990.

[16] Y. Censor, "Finite series-expansion reconstruction methods," *Proc. IEEE* **71**, 409-419 (1983).

[17] G. T. Herman, "Applications to maximum entropy and Bayesian optimization methods to image reconstruction from projections," In C. P. Smith and W. T. Grandy, Jr., *Maximum-Entropy and Bayesian Methods in Inverse Problems*, (D. Reidel Publishing Company, Dordrecht, The Netherlands), pp. 319-338, 1985.

[18] C. L. Byrne, "Iterative image reconstruction algorithms based on cross-entropy minimization," *IEEE Trans. on Image Processing* **2**, 96-103 (1993).

[19] R. Aharoni, G. T. Herman, and A. Kuba, "Binary vectors partially determined by linear equation systems," *Discrete Math.* **171**, 1-16 (1997).

[20] M. T. Chan, G. T. Herman, and E. Levitan, "Bayesian image reconstruction using image-modeling Gibbs priors," *Int. J. Imaging Sys. Tech.* **9**, 85-98 (1997).

[21] S-K. Chang, "The reconstruction of binary patterns from their projections," *Comm. of the ACM* **14**, 21-25 (1971).

[22] H. W. Kuhn and A. W. Tucker, "Nonlinear programming." *Proc. Second Berkeley Symp. Math. Statist. Probab.* **1**, 481-492 (1951).

Chapter 14

Compact Object Reconstruction

Ali Mohammad-Djafari[1]
Charles Soussen[2]

ABSTRACT In this chapter we first present a review of the methods for the tomographic reconstruction of a compact homogeneous object that lies in a homogeneous background. Then we focus on contour estimation and polyhedral shape reconstructions. We give some sufficient conditions to obtain exact reconstructions from a complete set of projections in the 2D case and present some extensions to the 3D case. Finally, due to the inherent difficulties of the exact reconstruction methods and their inappropriateness for practical situations, we propose an approximate reconstruction method that can handle the situation of very limited-angle projections.

14.1   Introduction

We consider the reconstruction of a compact homogeneous object from its X-ray projections, assuming that the object lies in a homogeneous background. To show the originality and relationship of our method with other available ones, we first classify these methods into three categories:

1. Methods that discretize the object into voxels and use an appropriate model for their distribution to enforce the homogeneities of the background and of the interior of the object (see for example [1–4]). The main advantage of these methods is that the relation between the data and the unknown parameters can be assumed linear. However, there are two main drawbacks: the huge number of the parameters to estimate (equal to the number of voxels of the image) and the fact that the defined models do not constrain the object to be compact and to have a closed contour.

2. Methods that estimate the surface of the object by modeling it as a

---

[1]Laboratoire des Signaux et Systèmes (CNRS-ESE-UPS), Supélec, Plateau de Moulon, 91190 Gif-sur-Yvette, France, E-mail: djafari@lss.supelec.fr

[2]Laboratoire des Signaux et Systèmes (CNRS-ESE-UPS), Supélec, Plateau de Moulon, 91190 Gif-sur-Yvette, France, E-mail: soussen@lss.supelec.fr

level set of a continuous function (see for example [5]). The principle of this approach is to estimate directly the closed contour of the object. Consequently, these methods eliminate the last drawback of the discretization into voxels. However, to implement this method, the 3D function whose level set gives the surface of the object must be constructed. Therefore, the cost of its computation remains large.

3. Methods that directly estimate the geometrical shape of the object from the projections. The number of unknown parameters is drastically reduced compared to other methods, but the relation between the data and these parameters is no longer linear. Two subclasses of this approach can be derived: the methods using simple shapes with a very small number of parameters (see for example [6]), and those modeling the object shape by more general deformable templates.

In the following, we will focus especially on the case of polyhedral shapes. This modeling is actually a generalization of the polygonal modeling in 2D, which will be studied in a first step. We will summarize the sufficient conditions to obtain exact reconstructions of polygonal shapes and give some extensions to the 3D case.

We will see that these conditions are unfortunately too restrictive in practical situations. Consequently, we will abandon the exact reconstruction to the benefit of an approximate one. We will propose a regularization method to estimate directly the object shape (the vertices of the polygon in 2D and those of the polyhedron in 3D) from a few noisy projections. Some simulation results comparing the relative performances of these approaches will finally be presented.

14.2   Review of methods

For the purpose of this review, we consider the 2D case and the parallel projections model:

$$\mathcal{R}_{r,\phi}(f) = \iint_{\mathbb{R}^2} f(x,y)\, \delta(r - x\cos\phi - y\sin\phi)\, \mathrm{d}x\, \mathrm{d}y \qquad (14.1)$$

where f is the density function of the object named $\mathcal{P}$, $\mathcal{R}_{r,\phi}(f)$ is the X-ray transform of f, $\phi \in [0, \pi[$, $r \in \mathbb{R}$ and δ denotes the Dirac delta function. This relation leads to the following formulation of the direct problem:

$$p(r, \phi) = \mathcal{R}_{r,\phi}(f) + n(r, \phi) \qquad (14.2)$$

or more succinctly

$$p = \mathcal{R}(f) + n \qquad (14.3)$$

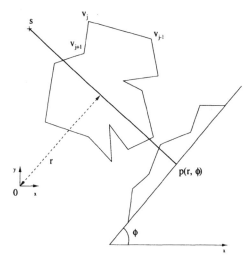

FIGURE 14.1. Geometric definition of the projection of a polygonal shape.

where p is the projection data and n represents the errors of modeling and measurement. (See Fig. 14.1 for a graphical definition of a projection in the case where the object is the interior of a polygonal shape.)

We consider hereafter the particular case where the density function can be defined by:

$$f(x,y) = \begin{cases} 1 & \text{if } (x,y) \in \mathcal{P}, \\ 0 & \text{otherwise} \end{cases} \qquad (14.4)$$

where $\mathcal{P}$ is assumed to be a compact region. The extension of the following description to other projection geometries and to the 3D case is straightforward.

14.2.1 Classical pixel representation approach

The first approach consists of discretizing equation (14.2) to obtain a linear relation:

$$p = Rf + n \qquad (14.5)$$

where:

- f and p are two vectors that contain, respectively, the discretized values of the object $f(x,y)$ (the pixel values of the image) and of the projection data $p(r,\phi)$;

- n is a vector that represents the errors of modeling, discretization, and measurement; and

- R is a matrix, whose (i,j)-th element is the length of the i-th ray through the j-th pixel.

Then, a solution can be defined as the minimizer of the compound criterion

$$J(f) = Q(p - Rf) + \lambda \Omega(f), \tag{14.6}$$

where λ is the regularization parameter and functions Q and Ω, respectively, reflect our prior knowledge of the noise and of the image. Q and Ω usually have the following form:

$$Q(g) = \sum_{j=1}^{n_p} q(g_j) \text{ and } \Omega(f) = \sum_{j=1}^{n_f} \omega_j(f) \tag{14.7}$$

where:

- q is a real function satisfying $q(x) = q(|x|)$ and is increasing on $[0, \infty)$;

- ω_j is also a real function (see Subsection 14.5.1 for some possible choices);

- n_f and n_p are the dimensions of vectors f and p, and g_j denote the elements of g.

This is the classical regularization approach to this image reconstruction problem.

One can also interpret $J(f)$ as the maximum a posteriori (MAP) criterion in the Bayesian estimation framework where $\exp[-Q(p - Rf)]$ represents the likelihood term and $\exp[-\lambda \Omega(f)]$ the prior probability law.

This approach has been successfully used in many applications (e.g., [1,2,7,8]) but the cost of its solution is huge due to the dimension of f, even though the matrix R is sparse. Much work has been done on choosing appropriate regularization functionals or equivalently appropriate prior probability laws for f to enforce some particular properties of the image such as smoothness, positivity or piecewise smoothness [9–12]. Among these, one can mainly mention the types of functions $\Omega(f)$ that enforce the binary assumption of the object (see Chapter 16 by J. Sachs and K. Sauer).

14.2.2   Level-set approach

The second approach consists in modeling directly the closed contour of the object as the zero-crossing (or any level set) of a smooth function $u(x, y)$:

$$\partial P = \{(x, y) : u(x, y) = 0\}. \tag{14.8}$$

Since the object P and the background are both assumed homogeneous, f satisfies:

$$f(x, y) = \begin{cases} 1 & \text{if } u(x, y) > 0, \\ 0 & \text{if } u(x, y) < 0. \end{cases} \tag{14.9}$$

The main idea is to define a time evolution for u, consequently also for the contour $\partial \mathcal{P}$ and for function f, such that:

$$\partial \mathcal{P}(t) = \{(x,y) : u(x,y,t) = 0\}. \tag{14.10}$$

This evolution must be such that as time goes to infinity, we obtain a function f, which is a solution to the inverse problem (14.3), in a least square (LS) sense. In other words, the evolution of u and consequently of the corresponding contour $\partial \mathcal{P}$ and of the object is such that the LS criterion

$$J(f) = \|p - \mathcal{R}(f)\|^2 \tag{14.11}$$

decreases during the evolution. In this approach, the function u describes a surface (of a heat wave) and the evolution of the contour $\partial \mathcal{P}(t)$ is restricted to be perpendicular to this surface. This means that the variation of the interior region $(\delta x, \delta y)$ is such that

$$(\delta x, \delta y) = \alpha(x,y,t) \frac{\nabla u}{|\nabla u|}. \tag{14.12}$$

The Level-Set approach has been originally developed by Osher and Sethian [13] for problems involving the motion of curves and surfaces and then has been adapted to computer vision and referred to as *snakes* or *active contour models* by many authors [5,14–17]. It has also been recently applied to inverse problems [18]. This approach needs a pixel representation of the image and its calculation cost becomes huge in 3D imaging systems. We are presently working on the extension of this approach to the minimization of a regularized criterion instead of the LS criterion (14.11) and on its implementation in 2D and 3D tomographic image reconstruction.

14.2.3   Shape reconstruction approach

The principle of this approach is to estimate directly the geometrical shape of the object from the projections. We consider two classes of shape modeling:

1. **Parametric shapes**:
   A very small number of parameters describe the shape and it is possible to relate analytically the projections to these parameters. For example, a superposition of elliptical homogeneous regions might be chosen:

   $$f(x,y) = \sum_{k=1}^{n_e} d_k \, f_k(x - x_k, y - y_k) \tag{14.13}$$

   where

   $$f_k(u,v) = \begin{cases} 1 & \text{if } \left(\frac{u}{a_k}\right)^2 + \left(\frac{v}{b_k}\right)^2 < 1, \\ 0 & \text{otherwise} \end{cases} \tag{14.14}$$

with obvious notation. Note $\boldsymbol{\theta} = \{d_k, x_k, y_k, a_k, b_k, \ k = 1, \ldots, n_e\}$ the vector of parameters defining the parametric model of the image (it contains the density values, the coordinates of the center and the values of the radii of each ellipse). The analytical calculation of the projections is straightforward, and the relation (14.2) between the data and the unknown parameters becomes:

$$p(r, \phi) = h(r, \phi; \boldsymbol{\theta}) + n(r, \phi) \qquad (14.15)$$

where $h(r, \phi; \boldsymbol{\theta})$ has an analytic expression in $\boldsymbol{\theta}$. If the noise is assumed to be zero mean, white and Gaussian, the LS and the maximum of likelihood estimate are equal and given by

$$\boldsymbol{\theta}_{LS} = \arg\min_{\boldsymbol{\theta}} \left\{ \|p(r, \phi) - h(r, \phi; \boldsymbol{\theta})\|^2 \right\}. \qquad (14.16)$$

This approach has also been used with success in image reconstruction [6]. But its range of applicability is limited to the cases where the parametric models are actually appropriate.

2. **Deformable templates**:
   The contour of the object can be modeled using deformable templates (see for example [19, 20]). In the case where the template is a spline function, the parameters are the control points of the spline. The polygonal shape can be considered a particular case of this category of methods, in which the control points are directly the vertices of the polygon. The reconstruction problem becomes equivalent to the estimation of these parameters as in the previous case, but there is no analytical relation between the data and these parameters.

14.3   Polygonal and polyhedral shape modeling

We consider in this section the modeling of the object by a polygonal or polyhedral region with a fixed number n_v of vertices. The aim of this shape reconstruction becomes the estimation of the coordinates of the vertices from the data. Note that in 2D as in 3D, a set of vertices define in a unique way a convex polygon (polyhedron) but may define many different non-convex ones. Hence, there are two subclasses of these methods:

1. those which assume that the shapes are convex, a case for which much work has been done [21–23];

2. those which do not assume the shape convexity but estimate an approximate solution. The proposed method belongs to this category.

In the 2D case, the work of Milanfar, Karl, and Willsky [24–26] is of interest. They propose a method for estimating the coordinates of the vertices of a polygon from the moments of its projections, whether it is convex or not, and study the conditions for an exact reconstruction. We first summarize the main results of this approach and propose new extensions in the 3D case.

14.3.1 Exact reconstruction of polygonal shapes in 2D

The object $\mathcal{P}$ is here the interior of a polygon. It is completely determined by the number of its vertices n_v and their sequence. We denote the complex coordinates of the vertices by $\{v_1, v_2, \ldots, v_{n_v}\}$ (see Fig. 14.1). Following the X-ray transform $\mathcal{R}_{r,\phi}(f)$ defined in (14.1) and the particular model for f in (14.4), it is easily shown that there is a relation between the geometric moments of the projections:

$$h_k(\phi) = \int_{\mathbb{R}} \mathcal{R}_{r,\phi}(f)\, r^k\, dr \tag{14.17}$$

and the geometric moments of the object:

$$\mu_{p,q} = \iint_{\mathcal{P}} f(x,y)\, x^p y^q\, dx\, dy. \tag{14.18}$$

For all integers k and all ϕ in $[0, \pi[$, this relation is

$$h_k(\phi) = \sum_{j=0}^{k} \binom{k}{j} \cos^{k-j}(\phi) \sin^j(\phi)\, \mu_{k-j,j}. \tag{14.19}$$

From the geometric moments of $\mathcal{P}$, it is possible to compute the harmonic moments c_k:

$$c_k = \iint_{\mathcal{P}} f(x,y)\, v^k\, dx\, dy, \quad \text{with } v = x + iy \tag{14.20}$$

by the relation:

$$c_k = \sum_{j=0}^{k} \binom{k}{j} i^j \mu_{k-j,j}. \tag{14.21}$$

The above formulations are valid for any shape. In the polygonal shape case, the harmonic moments are themselves related to the coordinates v_j by:

$$\tau_k = k(k-1)\, c_{k-2} = \sum_{j=1}^{n_v} a_j v_j^k \tag{14.22}$$

for all $k \geq 2$, where the coefficients a_j are independent of k. From the relation (14.22), it is possible to deduce a linear system independent of the coefficients a_j:

$$\mathcal{M}_{n_v}\, p^{(n_v)} = t^{(n_v)}, \tag{14.23}$$

where:

- $\mathcal{M}_{n_v}$ is an $n_v \times n_v$ invertible matrix whose coefficients only depend on $\{\tau_2, \ldots, \tau_{2n_v-2}\}$;

- $p^{(n_v)} = [p_{n_v}, \ldots, p_1]^T$ is such that the following equation is satisfied for all complex numbers v:

$$Q(v) = \prod_{j=1}^{n_v} (v - v_j) = v^{n_v} + p_1 v^{n_v - 1} + \cdots + p_{n_v - 1} v + p_{n_v}. \quad (14.24)$$

Note that $p^{(n_v)}$ uniquely determines the vertices v_j if the polygon is non-degenerate; and

- $t^{(n_v)} = [\tau_{n_v}, \ldots, \tau_{2n_v-1}]^T$.

Finally, there is also another relation between the coefficients a_j and v_j, which is derived from Green's theorem in the complex plane and the Cauchy-Riemann equations for analytic functions [27, 28]. This relation is:

$$a_j = \frac{i}{2} \left(\frac{\bar{v}_{j-1} - \bar{v}_j}{v_{j-1} - v_j} - \frac{\bar{v}_j - \bar{v}_{j+1}}{v_j - v_{j+1}} \right), \quad (14.25)$$

where the overline denotes the complex conjugate. Consequently, if at least $2n_v - 2$ distinct projections are available, one can consider a reconstruction procedure as follows:

1. Select $2n_v - 2$ distinct values of ϕ: $\{\phi_0, \ldots, \phi_{2n_v-3}\}$;

2. From projections $p(r, \phi_j)$, calculate $\{h_k(\phi_j), \ j = 0, \ldots, 2n_v - 3\}$ for all k in $\{0, \ldots, 2n_v - 3\}$ using (14.17);

3. For $k = 0$ to $2n_v - 3$, calculate $\{\mu_{k-j,j}, \ j = 0, \ldots, k\}$ using (14.19);

4. Calculate $\{c_k, \ k = 0, \ldots, 2n_v - 3\}$ using (14.21);

5. Calculate $\{v_j, \ j = 1, \ldots, n_v\}$ using (14.23) and (14.24);

6. If the polygon is assumed convex then stop – it is determined.
   If not – an ordering for $\{v_j, \ j = 1, \ldots, n_v\}$ has to be defined. This is done by the following procedure:

   (a) Calculate $\{a_j, \ j = 1, \ldots, n_v\}$ using (14.22), call this estimate a_0;

   (b) Calculate $\{a_j, \ j = 1, \ldots, n_v\}$ using (14.25) for all possible orderings $\{a_m\}$;

(c) Choose the ordering set of vertices v_j that gives the best fit between $\boldsymbol{a}_0$ and $\boldsymbol{a}_m$. A L_2 or a L_1 distance can be used to measure the fitness.

Note that direct relations are available for steps 2 and 4 whereas steps 3 and 5 require inversions. Milanfar *et al.* [24] derived these relations and gave sufficient conditions for the existence and uniqueness of these two inversions:

1. For any value of N, the geometric moments up to order N of an object $\{\mu_{k-j,j},\ j = 0, \ldots, k,\ k = 0, \ldots, N\}$ are uniquely determined from the $N + 1$ first moments of $N + 1$ distinct projections of this object $\{h_k(\phi_j),\ j, k = 0, \ldots, N\}$.

2. The vertices $\{v_j,\ j = 1, \ldots, n_v\}$ of any non-degenerate polygon are uniquely determined from all the moments τ_k, with $k \leq 2n_v - 1$.

Combining these results and the definition of τ_k in (14.22), the polygon $\{v_j,\ j = 1, \ldots, n_v\}$ is uniquely determined from the $2n_v - 2$ first moments of $2n_v - 2$ distinct projections $\{h_k(\phi_j),\ j, k = 0, \ldots, 2n_v - 3\}$.

14.3.2 Exact reconstruction of polyhedral shapes in 3D

The extension of this result to the 3D case is not obvious. Its first step relates the geometric moments of the object $\mathcal{P}$ to the moments of its projections and is summarized below. As in the 2D case, this relation is valid for any 3D binary object, even if it is not compact. For the second step, we could unfortunately not find an easy analytical relation between the geometric moments of a polyhedron and the coordinates of its vertices. Consequently, we decided to abandon this objective, and we propose estimation of an ellipsoid whose moments up to the second order match those of the real object. As will be seen in the following, at least three distinct projections are needed to uniquely determine such an ellipsoid. In practice, we will use this result as an initialization for an approximate method, which then iteratively estimates the vertices of the polyhedron directly from the projection data.

Reconstruction of the geometric moments from projections

For the sake of simplicity, we consider here parallel projections. The direction vector of a projection is named $\vec{u}$ and the corresponding detector plane $(\mathcal{T})$ is described by two vectors $\vec{v}$ and $\vec{w}$ which are orthogonal to $\vec{u}$. The origin of $(\mathcal{T})$ is the projection of the point of coordinates $(0, 0, 0)$ on $(\mathcal{T})$ along $\vec{u}$. With spherical coordinates notations (see Fig. 14.2), let

$$\vec{u} = [\sin\theta\cos\phi, \sin\theta\sin\phi, \cos\theta]^T \qquad (14.26)$$

with $\theta \in [0, \pi]$ and $\phi \in [0, 2\pi[$, and define $\vec{v}$ and $\vec{w}$ by

$$\vec{v} = [-\cos\theta\cos\phi, -\cos\theta\sin\phi, \sin\theta]^T \text{ and } \vec{w} = [\sin\phi, -\cos\phi, 0]^T. \quad (14.27)$$

With this notation, the line directed by $\vec{u}$ and cutting the plane $(\mathcal{T})$ in

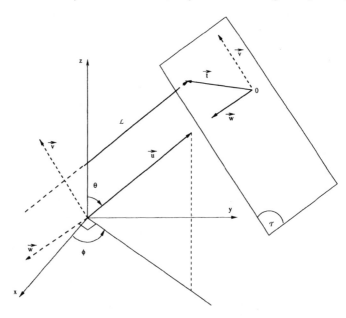

FIGURE 14.2. Geometric definition of a projection.

$\vec{t} = a\vec{v} + b\vec{w}$ has the following equations:

$$
\begin{aligned}
r_{\theta,\phi}(x,y,z) &= z\sin\theta - x\cos\theta\cos\phi - y\cos\theta\sin\phi &= a \\
s_{\theta,\phi}(x,y,z) &= x\sin\phi - y\cos\phi &= b
\end{aligned}
\quad (14.28)
$$

and the X-ray transform relating $f(x, y, z)$ and the projection $p(a, b, \vec{u})$ can be written as a function of $\vec{t}$, θ and ϕ by

$$
\begin{aligned}
p(\vec{t}, \theta, \phi) &= \iiint_{\mathbb{R}^3} f(x,y,z)\, \delta_2 \left[\begin{array}{c} r_{\theta,\phi}(x,y,z) - a \\ s_{\theta,\phi}(x,y,z) - b \end{array} \right] \mathrm{d}x\, \mathrm{d}y\, \mathrm{d}z \\
&= \iiint_{\mathcal{P}} \delta_2 \left[\left(\begin{array}{c} r_{\theta,\phi}(x,y,z) \\ s_{\theta,\phi}(x,y,z) \end{array} \right) - \vec{t} \right] \mathrm{d}x\, \mathrm{d}y\, \mathrm{d}z, \quad (14.29)
\end{aligned}
$$

where δ_2 is the 2D Dirac distribution. Then, every square integrable function $F\left(\vec{t}\right)$ satisfies the following property:

$$
\iint_{\mathbb{R}^2} p(\vec{t}, \theta, \phi)\, F\left(\vec{t}\right) \mathrm{d}\vec{t} = \iiint_{\mathcal{P}} F \left[\begin{array}{c} r_{\theta,\phi}(x,y,z) \\ s_{\theta,\phi}(x,y,z) \end{array} \right] \mathrm{d}x\, \mathrm{d}y\, \mathrm{d}z. \quad (14.30)
$$

Taking $F\left(\vec{t}\right) = F((a,b)^{T}) = a^{l}b^{m}$ for any integers l and m, we obtain an expression of the moments of the projection p. These moments are defined by

$$h_{l,m}(\theta, \phi) = \iint_{\mathbb{R}^{2}} a^{l} b^{m} p(\vec{t}, \theta, \phi) \, d\vec{t} \qquad (14.31)$$

and have the following expression:

$$h_{l,m}(\theta, \phi) = \iiint_{\mathcal{P}} (z \sin \theta - x \cos \theta \cos \phi - y \cos \theta \sin \phi)^{l} \cdot$$
$$(x \sin \phi - y \cos \phi)^{m} \, dx \, dy \, dz, \qquad (14.32)$$

that is, for $\theta \neq \frac{\pi}{2}$ and $\phi \neq \frac{\pi}{2} \, mod(\pi)$,

$$h_{l,m}(\theta, \phi) = \cos^{l}(\theta) \cos^{m}(\phi) \iiint_{\mathcal{P}} (z \tan \theta - x \cos \phi - y \sin \phi)^{l} \cdot$$
$$(x \tan \phi - y)^{m} \, dx \, dy \, dz. \qquad (14.33)$$

We can of course derive from (14.32) a general relation between $h_{l,m}(\theta, \phi)$ and the set $\{\mu_{i,j,k}, \ i+j+k=n\}$ where $n = l + m$ and $\mu_{i,j,k}$ denote the geometric moments of $\mathcal{P}$:

$$\mu_{i,j,k} = \iiint_{\mathcal{P}} x^{i} y^{j} z^{k} \, dx \, dy \, dz. \qquad (14.34)$$

Note that all the n-order moments of the projection depend only on the n-order geometric moments of $\mathcal{P}$ and that the relation corresponding to $l = 0$ is very similar to (14.19), obtained in the 2D case. For a fixed value of n, it is possible to derive the n-order geometric moments of the object $\{\mu_{i,j,k}, \ i+j+k=n\}$ from the n-order moments of at least $n+1$ projections $h_{l,m}(\theta_{j}, \phi_{j}), \ j \in \{0, \dots, m\}, \ l+m=n)$ in the following way:

1. $l = 0$.
   Derive $\{\mu_{j,n-j,0}, \ j = 0, \dots, n\}$ from $\{h_{0,n}(\theta_{j}, \phi_{j}), \ j \in \{0, \dots, n\}\}$.

2. For $l = 1$ to n
   Let $m = n - l$ and derive $\{\mu_{j,m-j,l}, \ j = 0, \dots, m\}$ from $\{h_{l,m}(\theta_{j}, \phi_{j}), \ j \in \{0, \dots, m\}\}$.

It is indeed possible to show that if at least m distinct projections (θ_{j}, ϕ_{j}) are available, the linear system linking $\{h_{l,m}(\theta_{j}, \phi_{j}), \ j \in \{0, \dots, m\}\}$ and $\{\mu_{j,m-j,l}, \ j = 0, \dots, m\}$ is invertible, with the coefficients $\{\mu_{i,j,k}, \ k < l\}$ considered as known [29].

Note that the previous calculations have to be done for each value of n. Consequently, if we want to compute the geometric moments of the object up to order N, at least $N + 1$ projections must be given.

Of course, in practice, it is strongly recommended to use more than $N + 1$ data and then to apply a least-square method for the resolution of the linear systems described above.

Elements of reconstruction of a polyhedron from geometric moments

The generalization of the 2D results to the 3D case is far from being obvious because of the complexity of the description of a polyhedron. Indeed, a polyhedron is defined by not only the sequence of its vertices but also by the description of all its facets $\{\mathcal{P}_l,\ l = 1, ..., f_p\}$. We denote in the following $\vec{n}_l = \left(n_x^l, n_y^l, n_z^l\right)^T$ the unit normal vector to facet $\mathcal{P}_l$, which is directed to the exterior of $\mathcal{P}$, and n_w^l the real number such that $n_x^l x + n_y^l y + n_z^l z + n_w^l = 0$ is an equation of the plane containing this face.

For a given polyhedron $\mathcal{P}$, one can establish a procedure that provides a direct and exact relation between the geometric moments $\mu_{i,j,k}$ and the coordinates of the vertices [30]. We do not give the explicit formulation of this relation, since it is very complex. However, we summarize hereafter the process that yields such a relation. For a fixed value of (i, j, k), the development of $\mu_{i,j,k}$ is obtained in several steps:

1. The use of the divergence theorem:

$$\iiint_{\mathcal{P}} \operatorname{div}\left(\vec{F}\right)(x, y, z)\ \mathrm{d}x\,\mathrm{d}y\,\mathrm{d}z = \iint_{\partial \mathcal{P}} \vec{F}(x, y, z) \cdot \vec{n}\ \mathrm{d}A, \quad (14.35)$$

where $\vec{n}$ is the normal vector to the surface on its border points $\partial \mathcal{P}$. This equation with a particular field, for instance

$$\vec{F}_{i,j,k}(x, y, z) = \left(\frac{x^{i+1} y^j z^k}{i+1}, 0, 0\right), \quad (14.36)$$

can be used to decompose $\mu_{i,j,k}$ in equation (14.34) into a surface integral on the border of $\mathcal{P}$, which is equal to a sum of surface integrals of a polynomial function $G_{i,j,k}(x, y, z)$ on each face $\mathcal{P}_l$ of $\mathcal{P}$.

2. For a fixed value of l in $\{1, ..., f_p\}$, the transformation of the surface integral

$$\iint_{\mathcal{P}_l} G_{i,j,k}(x, y, z)\ \mathrm{d}A \quad (14.37)$$

to another surface integral over one of the planes $(x = 0)$, $(y = 0)$ or $(z = 0)$. If for example, the face $\mathcal{P}_l$ is not perpendicular to the z-axis, then the following equation holds:

$$\iint_{\mathcal{P}_l} G_{i,j,k}(x, y, z)\ \mathrm{d}A =$$

$$\frac{1}{|n_z^l|} \cdot \iint_{\Pi(\mathcal{P}_l)} G_{i,j,k}\left(x, y, -\frac{1}{n_z^l}(n_x^l x + n_y^l y + n_w^l)\right)\ \mathrm{d}x\,\mathrm{d}y, \quad (14.38)$$

where $\Pi(\mathcal{P}_l)$ denotes the projection of $\mathcal{P}_l$ on the axis $(z = 0)$. The obtained integral is now a surface integral on the interior of the polygon defined by $\Pi\,(\mathcal{P}_l)$. Of course, one has to select for each face $\mathcal{P}_l$ one of the planes $(x = 0)$, $(y = 0)$ or $(z = 0)$, which are not perpendicular to $\mathcal{P}_l$. The one usually chosen corresponds to the greatest value of $|n_x^l|$, $|n_y^l|$ and $|n_z^l|$. Note that the choice of this plane is the source of great complexity in the expression of $\mu_{i,j,k}$ as an explicit function of the coordinates of $\mathcal{P}$.

3. For each l in $\{1,\ldots,f_p\}$, the latter obtained expression is a linear combination of two-dimensional moments of the projected polygon whose vertices depend only on those of the face $\mathcal{P}_l$. Each of these moments can consequently be written as a function of the vertices of the projected polygon, due to the results of Subsection 14.3.1, and then as a function of those of the original polyhedron.

Even if the number of vertices per face and the index of the vertices composing each face are assumed known, this formulation is not invertible since the latter expression depends on the coordinates of the normal vector to each face and these coordinates are not simply related to the vertex coordinates.

However, if we assume that the vertices of the polyhedron are located on an ellipsoid, then we can propose estimating its parameters from the data and then constructing the polyhedron from the ellipsoid. We actually have implemented this technique and used it for the initialization of the proposed approximate estimation method described in the next section.

We estimate this ellipsoid from:

- its center of mass (X_c, Y_c, Z_c);

- the directions of its principal axes $\vec{u}_i = \vec{u}(\theta_i, \phi_i)$ $(i \in \{1,\ldots,3\})$, where $\theta_i \in [0,\pi]$ and $\phi_i \in [0,2\pi[$. These directions are defined with spherical coordinates notations (see Fig. 14.2); and

- its radii $a_i, i \in \{1,\ldots,3\}$.

The center of mass of the ellipsoid is related to its moments of order 0 and 1 by:

$$X_c = \frac{\mu_{1,0,0}}{\mu_{0,0,0}} \quad Y_c = \frac{\mu_{0,1,0}}{\mu_{0,0,0}} \quad Z_c = \frac{\mu_{0,0,1}}{\mu_{0,0,0}} \tag{14.39}$$

and the other parameters can be deduced from $\{\mu_{i,j,k},\ i+j+k \leq 2\}$. Indeed, the matrix of inertia of the ellipsoid is

$$M_I = \begin{pmatrix} \mu_{0,2,0} + \mu_{0,0,2} & -\mu_{1,1,0} & -\mu_{1,0,1} \\ -\mu_{1,1,0} & \mu_{2,0,0} + \mu_{0,0,2} & -\mu_{0,1,1} \\ -\mu_{1,0,1} & -\mu_{0,1,1} & \mu_{2,0,0} + \mu_{0,2,0} \end{pmatrix}. \tag{14.40}$$

M_I is diagonalizable and its eigenvalues are $\frac{a_i^2}{5}\mu_{0,0,0}, i \in \{1,\ldots,3\}$. The corresponding normalized eigenvectors are the directions $\vec{u}_i$.

14.4   Description of the proposed method

As seen in the previous section, it is theoretically possible to estimate exactly a polygonal shape from the moments of its projections. However, the sufficient conditions on the exact reconstruction can not be fulfilled in many real applications, since at least $2n_v - 1$ projections are needed, where n_v is the number of vertices. They may not be available in practical situations, such as Non-Destructive Testing (NDT).

For this reason, and since an exact reconstruction is not possible in the 3D case, Mohammad-Djafari et al. [31, 32] recently proposed methods to compute approximate solutions to this problem, based on the regularization theory or its Bayesian estimation interpretation. In the following, we first summarize the 2D case and then give its extension to the 3D case:

1. *The 2D problem*

   The coordinates of the vertices of the polygonal region are estimated by minimizing the criterion

   $$J(v) = ||p - h(v)||^2 + \lambda\Omega(v), \qquad (14.41)$$

   where $v = \{v_j, \ j = 1,\ldots,n_v\}$ is the vector composed by the complex coordinates of the vertices, h represents the direct operator, which computes the projections for any given set v, and Ω is a function which reflects the regularity of the object contour. The following function is a possible choice for Ω:

   $$\Omega(v) = \sum_{j=1}^{n_v} |v_{j-1} - 2v_j + v_{j+1}|^2$$
   $$= 4 \sum_{j=1}^{n_v} \left| v_j - \frac{1}{2}(v_{j-1} + v_{j+1}) \right|^2, \qquad (14.42)$$

   where $v_{n_v+1} = v_1$. Note that $\left| v_j - \frac{1}{2}(v_{j-1} + v_{j+1}) \right|^2$ is the square of the Euclidean distance between the vertices v_j and the middle of the line segment joining its two neighbors. Therefore, this choice favors the shapes whose local radii of curvature are limited. There is also a probabilistic interpretation to this choice: v_j can be considered as complex random variables with the following Markovian laws:

   $$p(v_j|v) = p(v_j|v_{j-1}, v_{j+1})$$
   $$\propto \exp\left[-\frac{1}{2\sigma^2} |v_{j-1} - 2v_j + v_{j+1}|^2 \right]., \qquad (14.43)$$

   where σ is a parameter that fixes the scale of the shape curvature.

2. *The 3D problem*

   To simplify the problem of the estimation of the polyhedron, we assume that:

(a) the polyhedron is composed of only triangular facets.

(b) the neighborhood relations between the vertices themselves and between the vertices and the facets of the polyhedron are already defined.

Consequently, the polyhedron is represented by only its vertices. We denote n_v the number of vertices and $v_j = (x_j, y_j, z_j)$ their coordinates $(j = 1, \ldots, n_v)$. We also define the set of vertices by $v = \{v_j, j = 1, \ldots, n_v\}$. From the above assumptions, the coordinates of the vertices are estimated as in the 2D case by minimizing the criterion

$$J(v) = \|p - h(v)\|^2 + \lambda \Omega(v), \qquad (14.44)$$

with similar notation. The chosen regularizing function is

$$\Omega(v) = \sum_{j=1}^{n_v} \left\| v_j - \frac{1}{K_j} \sum_{i \in \mathcal{V}j} v_i \right\|^2, \qquad (14.45)$$

where $\mathcal{V}j$ stands for the neighborhood of v_j and K_j is the number of vertices that belong to this neighborhood. $\frac{1}{K_j} \sum_{i \in \mathcal{V}j} v_i$ represents the geometric center of all the neighbors of v_j. Hence, the defined function $\Omega(v)$ also favors the shapes whose local radii of curvature are limited.

In both cases, the criterion $J(v)$ is multimodal essentially because of the fact that h is a nonlinear function of v. Computing the optimal solution corresponding to its global minimum requires carefully designed algorithms. For this purpose, we propose the following strategies:

1. The use of a global optimization technique such as *simulated annealing* (SA), [33]. This technique is iterative and involves a parameter T_n called temperature, where n is the number of the corresponding iteration. The sequence of the temperatures (T_n) decreases, and converges to 0 as n goes to infinity. For a fixed value of n, the vertices v_j are sequentially visited. At the j-th step, only the vertex v_j is modified, according to a random procedure. v_j is generally sampled from a uniform, a Gaussian or using its prior probability distribution. Let v^j denote the vector v, in which v_j has been replaced by its new value. A decision rule indicating which of the configurations v and v^j has to be kept is the following:

   - if $J(v^j) < J(v)$ then accept the modification of v_j. The new object is $v := v^j$.
   - if $J(v) < J(v^j)$ then accept the configuration v^j with a probability proportional to

$$\exp\left(-\frac{J(v^j) - J(v)}{T_n} \right). \qquad (14.46)$$

There exist sufficient conditions on the sequence (T_n), which insure that this optimization algorithm converges to one of the global minima of J, whatever the initial configuration is. In practice, this technique gives satisfactory results (see the simulations in the next section), but requires a large number of iterations and some skill in choosing the first temperature T_0 and the cooling schedule. The overall computational cost is not very large, due to the fact that the calculation of the gradient of the criterion is not needed.

2. The use of a local optimization technique with an initial solution, if possible in the attractive region of the global optimum:

- the problem of the definition of an initial solution is then the most critical. In both 2D and 3D cases, we use the results of Section 14.3 to estimate the moments of the object up to the second order from the moments of its projections. In a second step, a polygon or a polyhedron is reconstructed such that its vertices are on an ellipse or an ellipsoid whose moments up to the second order match those calculated from the projections. This procedure is accurate enough to obtain a good initial solution.

- the local optimization technique is slightly different from the SA algorithm described above. The only difference with SA is that the new configuration after modification of v to v^j is accepted if and only if $J(v^j) < J(v)$. Such a technique in statistical image processing has been known as *Iterated Conditional Modes* (ICM) [33].

The next section will show some results describing the performances of these two methods as well as a comparison with some other classical methods.

14.5   Simulation results

14.5.1   2D reconstructions

To evaluate the performances of the proposed method and to keep the objective of using this method for NDT applications in which the number of projections is very small, we simulate a case where the real object is a polygon with $N = 40$ vertices (handmade) and calculate its projections for only 5 directions: $\phi = -45, -22.5, 0, 22.5$, and 45 degrees. We add a zero-mean, white, and Gaussian noise to simulate the measurement errors, with a S/N ratio equal to 20 dB.

Figure 14.3 represents the original object and the simulated projection data. From these data, we reconstruct the object by the proposed method, using both optimization techniques.

Projections

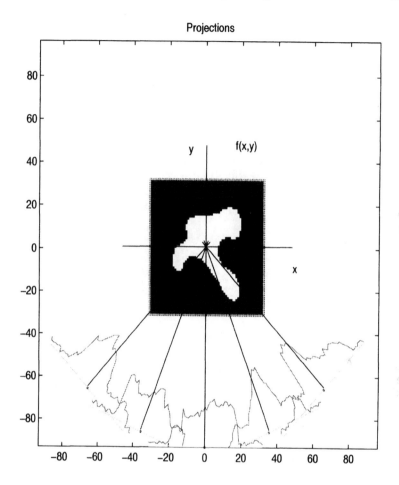

FIGURE 14.3. Original image and simulated projections data.

The original object, its initial reconstruction, some intermediate solutions and the final one, obtained after 200 iterations are represented on Fig. 14.4.

The final result and the ones obtained by some classical methods are compared on Fig. 14.5. We have considered the classical backprojection method, the level-set approach and pixel-based estimation approaches with different regularization functionals (see (14.7) for the definition of ω_j):

- the *Entropic laws* with

$$\omega_j(\boldsymbol{f}) = -f_j \log f_j. \tag{14.47}$$

The method is called *Maximum entropy regularized method;*

- the *Gaussian-Markovian laws* with the potential function:

$$\omega_j(\boldsymbol{f}) = \sum_{i \in \mathcal{V}j} |f_j - f_i|^2, \qquad (14.48)$$

where $\mathcal{V}j$ represents the pixels of the image that are adjacent to pixel j. The method is called *quadratic regularization method*; and

- the *Markovian laws* with non-convex potential functions, for example the truncated quadratic function:

$$\omega_j(\boldsymbol{f}) = \min_{i \in \mathcal{V}j} \left\{ |f_j - f_i|^2, 1 \right\}. \qquad (14.49)$$

The function q defined in (14.7) is chosen to be $q(x) = x^2$. In this last case, we use a Graduated Non Convexity (GNC) based optimization algorithm [12] to find the solution. For the sake of curiosity, we also show binary segmented images obtained by thresholding these last images. The threshold is chosen to be the mean of the maximum and minimum values of the reconstructed image.

The situation we simulated is close to a realistic non-destructive testing application. This is a very difficult situation, since the number of projections and their angles are very limited. It is evident from these simulations that the performance of the proposed method is significantly higher than that of the other techniques we have examined.

14.5.2 3D case

The following simulations correspond to the case of the estimation of a non-convex shape from 9 parallel projections on the same detector plane. As for the 2D simulations, a zero-mean Gaussian noise is added to the simulated projections. The S/N ratio is equal to 20 dB. Figure 14.6 represents the original object which is a polyhedron with 226 vertices and 448 facets, the chosen directions of the projections and the generated data.

The polyhedral reconstruction method is illustrated on Fig. 14.7. The initial reconstruction and an intermediate one are also represented. These reconstructions are obtained assuming that the object has 74 vertices and 144 facets. The chosen regularization parameter is $\lambda = 0.5$, and the plotted objects correspond to 0, 40 and 100 iterations. Their projections are also represented on this figure.

As in the 2D case, this situation is difficult since the number of projections is very limited and the projections have limited angles. The proposed method gives satisfaction, but we have not so far compared its performance with other techniques. In particular, a comparison with the one that involves a binary Markov modeling (see Chapter 16 by J. Sachs and K. Sauer in this book) would be of interest; we are presently working on this study.

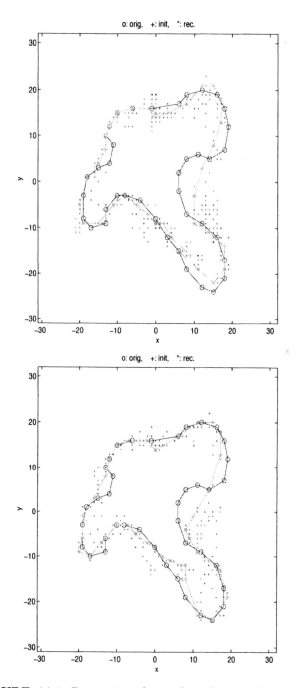

FIGURE 14.4. Reconstruction using simulated annealing and ICM algorithm. o) Original objects, +) Initializations, .) Evolution of the solutions during the iterations and ⋆) Final reconstructions.

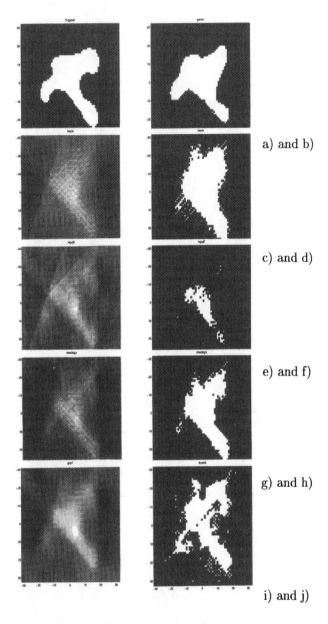

a) and b)

c) and d)

e) and f)

g) and h)

i) and j)

FIGURE 14.5. A comparison with backprojection and some other classical methods: a) Original object, b) Proposed method, c) Backprojection method, d) Binary threshold of c, e) Gaussian Markov modeling MAP reconstruction, f) Binary threshold of e, g) Maximum entropy regularized reconstruction, h) Binary threshold of g, i) Compound Markov modeling and GNC optimization algorithm using truncated quadratic potential function, j) Level-set approach.

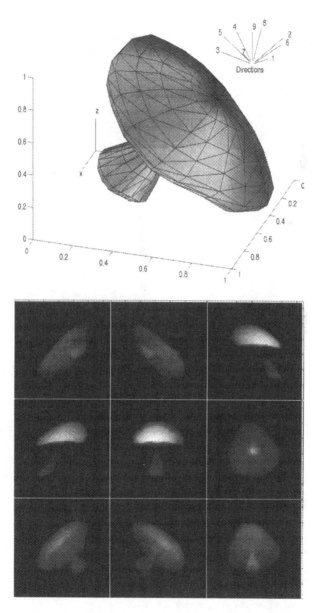

FIGURE 14.6. A 3D object, the directions of 9 parallel projections
and the corresponding projection data on the detector plane ($z=1.5$).
The images of the projections are ranked line by line. For example,
the first line corresponds to the three first projections.

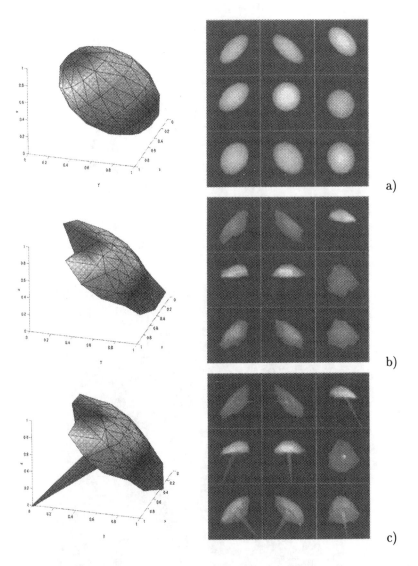

a)

b)

c)

FIGURE 14.7. Reconstructions of the object and their projections: a) initial reconstruction, b) reconstruction after 40 iterations, c) reconstruction after 100 iterations.

14.6 Conclusions

We first reviewed the reconstruction methods of a compact homogeneous object from its tomographic projection data. We then focused on the reconstruction of polygonal and polyhedral objects. We examined the conditions needed to obtain exact reconstructions in 2D and opened the question to the 3D case. Finally, since these conditions may not be fulfilled in practical applications, we proposed approximate solutions.

The proposed method is based on regularization or equivalently on the Bayesian MAP estimation framework, defining the solution as the optimizer of a compound criterion. To find the optimized solution, two algorithms have been examined:

- a global optimization method based on simulated annealing (SA) and

- a local descent-based method with a good initialization obtained using a moment-based method.

The final field of application of the proposed method is Non-Destructive Testing (NDT). X-rays are not the only type of data which are used. One may also use Ultrasound, Eddy currents, or even a combination of them.

We are presently working on the extension of this approach for these different imaging applications.

Acknowledgments

Both authors were visiting the University of Notre Dame, Notre Dame, Indiana, while working on this chapter. The authors would like to thank Ken Sauer for interesting discussions and for the proofreading of this chapter. This work has been partially supplied by a contract between DGA and CNRS: ERG 97-1055/A000/DSP/SREA/SC/PROSP.

References

[1] G. T. Herman, H. K. Tuy, K. J. Langenberg, and P. C. Sabatier, *Basic Methods of Tomography and Inverse Problems* (Adam Hilger, Bristol, UK), 1987.

[2] A. C. Kak and M. Slaney, *Principles of Computerized Tomographic Imaging* (IEEE Press, New York), 1987.

[3] K. D. Sauer and C. A. Bouman, "Bayesian estimation of transmission tomograms using segmentation based optimization," *IEEE Transactions on Nuclear Sciences* **39**, 1144-1152 (1992).

[4] K. D. Sauer and C. A. Bouman, "A local update strategy for iterative reconstruction from projections," *IEEE Transactions on Signal Processing* **SP-41**, 534-548 (1993).

[5] R. Malladi, J. A. Sethian, and B. C. Vemuri, "Shape modeling with front propagation: A level-set approach," *IEEE Transactions on Pattern Analysis and Machine Intelligence* **PAMI-17**, 158-175 (1995).

[6] D. J. Rossi and A. S. Willsky, "Reconstruction from projections based on detection and estimation of objects," *IEEE Transactions on Acoustics Speech and Signal Processing* **ASSP-32**, 886-906 (1984).

[7] G. Demoment, "Image reconstruction and restoration: Overview of common estimation structure and problems," *IEEE Transactions on Acoustics Speech and Signal Processing* **ASSP-37**, 2024-2036 (1989).

[8] S. Geman and D. McClure, "Statistical methods for tomographic image reconstruction," In *Proceedings of the 46th Session of the ISI, Bulletin of the ISI*, volume 52, pp. 5-21, 1987.

[9] L. Bedini, I. Gerace, and A. Tonazzini, "A deterministic algorithm for reconstructing images with interacting discontinuities," *Computer Vision and Graphics and Image Processing* **56**, 109-123 (1994).

[10] C. A. Bouman and K. D. Sauer, "A generalized Gaussian image model for edge-preserving MAP estimation," *IEEE Transactions on Image Processing* **IP-2**, 296-310 (1993).

[11] A. Mohammad-Djafari and J. Idier, "A scale invariant Bayesian method to solve linear inverse problems," In G. Heidbreder, *Maximum Entropy and Bayesian Methods* (Kluwer Academic Publishers, Dordrecht), pp. 121-134, 1996.

[12] M. Nikolova, J. Idier, and A. Mohammad-Djafari, "Inversion of large-support ill-posed linear operators using a piecewise Gaussian MRF," *IEEE Transactions on Image Processing* **7**, 571-585 (1998).

[13] S. Osher and J. A. Sethian, "Fronts propagating with curvature-dependent speed: Algorithms based on Hamilton-Jacobi formulations," *Journal of Computational Physics* **79**, 12-49 (1988).

[14] F. Catté, P. Lions, J. Morel, and T. Coll, "Image selective smoothing and edge detection by nonlinear diffusion," *SIAM Journal of Numerical Analysis* **29**, 182-193 (1992).

[15] R. T. Chin and K. F. Lai, "Deformable contours: Modeling and extraction," *IEEE Transactions on Pattern Analysis and Machine Intelligence* **PAMI-16**, 601-608 (1994).

[16] M. Kass, A. P. Witkin, and D. Terzopoulos, "Snakes: Active contour models," *International Journal of Computer Vision* **1**, 321-331 (1988).

[17] L. H. Staib and J. S. Duncan, "Parametrically deformable contour models," *Computer Vision and Pattern Recognition*, 98-103 (1989).

[18] F. Santosa, "A level-set approach for inverse problems involving obstacles," *Control, Optimisation and Calculus of Variations* **1**, 17-33 (1996).

[19] Y. Amit, U. Grenander, and M. Piccioni, "Structural image restoration through deformable templates," *Journal of Acoustical Society America* **86**, 376-387 (1991).

[20] K. M. Hanson, G. S. Cunningham, and R. J. McKee, "Uncertainty assessment for reconstructions based on deformable models," *International Journal of Imaging Systems and Technology* **8**, 506-512 (1997).

[21] D. Kölzow, A. Kuba, and A. Volcic, "An algorithm for reconstructing convex bodies from their projections," *Discrete and Computational Geometry* **4**, 205-237 (1989).

[22] J. L. Prince and A. S. Willsky, "Reconstructing convex sets from support line measurements," *IEEE Transactions on Pattern Analysis and Machine Intelligence* **12**, 377-389 (1990).

[23] J. L. Prince and A. S. Willsky, "Convex set reconstruction using prior shape information," *Computer Vision and Graphics and Image Processing* **53**, 413-427 (1991).

[24] P. Milanfar, W. C. Karl, and A. S. Willsky, "A moment-based variational approach to tomographic reconstruction," *IEEE Transactions on Image Processing* **25**, 772-781 (1994).

[25] P. Milanfar, W. C. Karl, and A. S. Willsky, "Reconstructing binary polygonal objects from projections: A statistical view," *Computer Vision and Graphics and Image Processing* **56**, 371-391 (1994).

[26] P. Milanfar, G. C. Verghese, W. C. Karl, and A. S. Willsky, "Reconstructing polygons from moments with connections to array processing," *IEEE Transactions on Signal Processing* **43**, 432-443 (1995).

[27] P. J. Davis, "Triangle formulas in the complex plane," *Mathematics of Computation* **18**, 569-577 (1964).

[28] P. J. Davis, "Plane regions determined by complex moments," *Journal of Approximation Theory* **19**, 148-153 (1977).

[29] C. Soussen and A. Mohammad-Djafari, "A 3D polyhedral shape reconstruction from tomographic projection data," *Technical Report, GPI-LSS, Gif-sur-Yvette, France* (1998).

[30] B. Mirtich, "Fast and accurate computation of polyhedral mass properties," *Journal of Graphic Tools* 1, 31-50 (1996).

[31] A. Mohammad-Djafari, "Shape reconstruction in X-ray tomography," In *Proc. of SPIE 97*, volume 3170, (SPIE, Bellingham, WA), pp. 240-251, 1997.

[32] A. Mohammad-Djafari, K. D. Sauer, Y. Khayi, and E. Cano, "Reconstruction of the shape of a compact object from a few number of projections," In *IEEE Int. Conf. on Image Processing (ICIP)*, volume 1, (IEEE, Piscataway, NJ), pp. 165-169, 1997.

[33] G. Winkler, *Image Analysis, Random Fields and Dynamic Monte Carlo Methods* (Springer Verlag, Berlin), 1995.

Part III

Applications

Chapter 15

CT-Assisted Engineering and Manufacturing

Jolyon A. Browne[1]
Mathew Koshy[2]

ABSTRACT
X-ray computed tomography (CT) is an important and powerful tool in industrial imaging for obtaining shape and dimensional information of industrial parts. It also serves to provide digital models of parts for inputs to new and emerging technologies in the manufacturing industry that have begun to embrace CT-assisted engineering and design. Since a large number of objects encountered in industrial CT are made either of a single homogenous material or a few homogenous materials, algorithms for discrete tomography should, in principle, yield CT images whose resolution and dimensional accuracy are superior to CT images obtained by conventional algorithms. This in turn should result in significant improvements in the accuracy of boundaries extracted from CT images for the creation of digital models of a large class of parts of interest in CT-assisted manufacturing. This chapter looks at some important applications in CT-assisted engineering and manufacturing that can benefit from the techniques of discrete tomography, and discuss some of the technical challenges faced in extracting boundaries with the degree of accuracy demanded for engineering and manufacturing applications.

15.1 Introduction

The tomographic reconstruction problem is concerned with the reconstruction of an object from a set of line integrals or line sums through the object. Mathematically, the object corresponds to a real-valued function defined over a subset of n-dimensional space, and the problem posed is to reconstruct the function from integrals or sums over subsets of its domain. The domain of the function is said to be continuous if it contains all points in a region in space; the range of the function is continuous if it can have any

---

[1] Advanced Research and Applications Corporation (ARACOR), 425 Lakeside Drive, Sunnyvale, CA 94086, USA, Email: browne@aracor.com

[2] Advanced Research and Applications Corporation (ARACOR), 425 Lakeside Drive, Sunnyvale, CA 94086, USA, Email: koshy@aracor.com

value in an interval of the real line. In general, the tomographic inversion problem may be continuous or discrete. In continuous tomography, both the domain and range of the function are continuous. In discrete tomography, the domain of the function may be either discrete or continuous, and the range of the function is a finite set of real, generally nonnegative, numbers. If the domain of the reconstructed function is continuous, the data used to reconstruct it consists of a set of line integrals of the function. If the domain is discrete, the data used to reconstruct the function is a set of line sums of the function. Most practical applications of tomography use reconstruction algorithms that solve the continuous tomography problem. These algorithms provide analytic solutions for obtaining the function from its line integrals; then the derived solution is discretized at the end for computer implementation [1, 2].

Over the years, reconstruction of a discrete-valued function from its line sums has been applied to diverse areas such as computer vision [3], electron microscopy [4], crystallography [5], and combinatorics [6]. Indeed, a large number of algorithms have been designed for the discrete tomography problem. In most of these algorithms, a merit function, expressed in terms of the measured data and the image to be reconstructed, is optimized. The optimization problem is typically solved using an iterative approach. In the context of medical and industrial tomography it is well-known that when the collected data are sparse and noisy, the iterative techniques based on the discrete tomography model are superior to those approaches based on the continuous model. However, their high computational complexity has made them unpopular in most applications of medical and industrial tomography. Nevertheless, the flexibility of the discrete-based algorithms in accommodating any tomographic geometry, and their ability to incorporate prior information of the object to be reconstructed, is unmatched by algorithms based on the continuous model.

In recent years, X-ray computed tomography (CT) [1, 2] has become an important and powerful tool in industrial imaging for obtaining shape and dimensional information of industrial parts [7]. Accurate dimensional measurements from CT images is a prerequisite in several new and emerging technologies in the manufacturing industry that has begun to embrace CT-assisted engineering and design. These technologies, such as rapid prototyping, rapid tooling, and reverse engineering, form the basis of agile manufacturing, a new manufacturing model that promises to revolutionize current manufacturing environments by reducing manufacturing complexity, increasing productivity, and reducing costs in many high-value manufacturing markets. As a starting point, these technologies require an accurate computer-aided design (CAD) model of the part of interest. The essence of CT-assisted engineering and manufacturing is to use X-ray CT to nondestructively provide a digital model of the object. In this case, one of the greatest technical challenges is to extract accurate boundaries from the CT image.

Images provided by industrial CT systems are reconstructed by algorithms derived from the continuous tomography model. However, a large fraction of the objects scanned in industrial CT systems are made of a single material, such as plastic, aluminum, or steel. Therefore the ideal reconstructed image should contain only two values: 0 for air, and a value associated with the material composing the object. In these environments, applying techniques of discrete tomography to utilize prior knowledge of the discrete set of values of the function to be reconstructed should yield CT images whose resolution and dimensional accuracy are superior to CT images obtained by conventional algorithms. This in turn should result in significant improvements in the accuracy of boundaries extracted from CT images for CAD models of a large class of parts of interest in CT-assisted engineering and design. If this promise is realized, then industrial Non-Destructive Evaluation (NDE) may very well be one of the truly exciting applications of discrete tomography in general, and binary tomography in particular.

This chapter will survey some important applications in NDE that may benefit from the renewed interest in discrete tomography. In particular, we will look at CT-assisted engineering and design in agile manufacturing, and see some of the critical technologies that can benefit from the techniques of discrete tomography. We will also see some of the technical challenges involved in making discrete tomography practical in CT-based engineering and manufacturing applications.

15.2 Agile manufacturing: A new manufacturing paradigm

Modern manufacturing environments typically embrace a combination of different technologies for reducing manufacturing complexity, achieving high levels of quality control, increasing productivity, and reducing cost. Coupled with this desire is a shift of manufacturing emphasis from traditional mass, undifferentiated production, and inventory management to small, custom production, reduced inventories, and just-in-time delivery that can more rapidly respond to market changes. Under this manufacturing approach, parts are designed, manufacturing process simulated, and product performance predicted with the aid of a computer. The goal is to be able to respond quickly to custom requests, even if the quantities are small. This manufacturing emphasis is sometimes called *agile manufacturing*, where agile means the ability to make any part at any time in any quantity for any customer, in short, *mass customization*. Agile manufacturing techniques do not preclude mass production methods; rather, by reducing the time and expense of development, agile manufacturing techniques make low-volume and/or custom production runs more feasible. This allows manufacturers

to produce small, custom lots cheaper and faster in niche markets that do
not support mass production.

A key aspect of agile manufacturing is obtaining accurate computer
models. This digital model is the gateway to three major activities that
are crucial to the agile manufacturing methodology: *reverse engineering*,
part metrology, and *computational modeling* (Fig. 15.1). Reverse engineering refers to the creation of a digital model, such as a computer-aided
design (CAD) model, from an existing part. Metrology is the process of
extracting geometric data from a component to compare with the original
design dimensions. Computational modeling is the process of using digital
models to predict performance of a part.

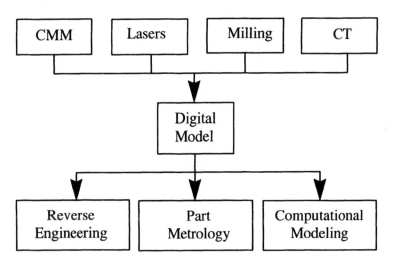

FIGURE 15.1. Facets of agile manuacturing.

Reverse engineering is required whenever a computer model, such as a
CAD description, of an existing part is needed. It provides a mechanism
for generating CAD models of parts that do not have such a description.
Examples of such scenarios are fairly common. For instance, an old part
may have been designed on paper before the use of computers, drawings
for old components may not exist, components lacking a CAD description
may be no longer in production, or the company that originally produced
a component may no longer be in business. A CAD model may be needed
for a part, such as an aircraft joystick or a computer mouse, which may
have been designed by sculpting and molding the model out of clay and so-
liciting feedback from end-users to achieve an ergonomic "feel" of the part.
Even new parts that were produced originally with a CAD model may need
to be reverse engineered. Such parts, for example, may have been modified during development to optimize performance or facilitate manufacture,
thereby making the original CAD files obsolete. Reverse engineering may

also be used on a first-article prototype at the end of the production line to compare the manufactured part with its CAD master to determine dimensional conformance, or to certify a particular manufacturing process.

Obtaining metrological information from a digital model is an important activity in many manufacturing operations. Geometrical information from the digital model of the manufactured part is used to compare part geometry with the original CAD geometry to verify that the part has been manufactured within design tolerances, to acquire statistics on geometrical variations from part to part, or to identify design changes that are needed to enhance manufacturability. In recent years computational modeling has become an invaluable tool in modern manufacturing. Geometrical information from the digital model of a part is used with material properties such as density to construct computer-aided engineering (CAE) models to analyze the performance of as-built parts against design requirements. Such CAE models may utilize finite-element [8] or other computational methods and may serve as the gateway to other sophisticated analyses such as fluid flow studies, solidification models, and fracture mechanics.

15.3 Obtaining the digital model

As shown in Fig. 15.1, four existing technologies offer the ability to create digital models of an object: coordinate measuring machines (CMMs), laser scanners, physical sectioning (i.e., milling) machines, and CT scanners. Traditionally, the first three of these technologies have been commonly used to obtain the digital model; however, all three suffer from serious limitations. CMM machines, which utilize a stylus to physically probe the surface of an object, often produce relatively sparse data sets containing ambiguites in data continuity and connectivity. Lasers are sensitive to surface finish and will not work well on objects with certain surfaces. Both CMMs and lasers require time-consuming setup procedures, require part-specific programming, have difficulty measuring internal passages or highly complex parts, and cannot provide information on structural defects. Milling machines are often used with other technologies, such as the CMM, to measure internal passages and structural defects, but they are slow, destroy the part, and are limited mainly to single-material objects. Moreover, physical sectioning provides information only about specific locations of the object; for example, the dimensions in selected planes or the porosity in specific regions. In addition, the very process of sectioning destroys any information about the cut-zones.

Computed tomography overcomes all of the shortcomings of the traditional methods. In particular, CT is indifferent to surface finish and can be used to inspect nondestructively the interior of an object of virtually any material composition. Thus, it can be used to provide complete dimensional and structural information for inaccessible regions of complex parts without the need for physical sectioning. Plus, the map of the X-ray linear attenuation coefficient obtained by CT can be used to extract density information about a part. Since this density information can be related to material properties, CT is an ideal method to develop an accurate finite element model of a component based on the as-manufactured material properties rather than on the as-designed properties.

The key image processing steps for converting a CT image of a part to its CAD representation have long been studied in image processing and computer vision [9–11]. These steps can be identified as five distinct operations as outlined in the following paragraphs.

The first step is *image segmentation*, whereby regions associated with the background and the different materials composing the object are unequivocally identified and separated. Candidate segmentation methods include threshold-based and gradient-based algorithms. The typical output of this step is an image approximating the original image but consisting of a small number of separate regions, each with an assigned identification number. If the object is made of a single material, for example, the resulting image would consist of only two types of pixels: those associated with the background, and those associated with the object. This image could be adequately represented with just two values: say, 1 for object pixels, and 0 for background pixels.

The second step is *image classification*, whereby segmented regions are decomposed into sets containing only connected pixels or voxels. In this step, the basic task is to determine the connectivity of regions with the same identification number. Image classification can be performed in several ways; one of the most basic approaches is to assume that pixels that share the same identification number with all nearest neighbor are connected. Connectivity is established either in plane (for a 2D image) or in space (for a 3D image). Each connected set identified corresponds to a different part of the object. The output of this step is a set of regions, each with a unique identification number, such that all pixels or voxels in a region are connected.

The third step is the extraction of the *image topology*. This is the process by which boundaries between regions are determined, and exterior and interior boundaries are established for each connected set. Each connected set has only one exterior border and any number of interior borders. The image topology accounts for the full hierarchy of sets and borders, and determines the relationship among the various components of the imaged object.

The fourth step is to *generate contours* (for a 2D image) or surfaces (for a 3D image) from the image topology. For a 2D image a contour is a closed set of points; for a 3D image a surface is a closed network of triangular or polygonal elements.

In the latter step, the boundaries of a contour or a surface are located to the nearest pixel or voxel. The fifth image processing step *refines the boundary values* to fractions of a pixel or a voxel. In other words, the coordinates of the boundaries are adjusted to provide sub-pixel or sub-voxel accuracy. One way of performing this refinement is to: (i) determine the normal at each point on the boundary from the local edge topology; (ii) extract the so-called edge response normal to the boundary from the original image data; and (iii) analyze the edge response based on a knowledge of the imaging process to determine a best estimate of the location of the edge.

If discrete tomography is used to reconstruct the object, the first step can be automatically eliminated, because the reconstructed image is already segmented. Furthermore, as we shall see in a later section, it is often possible to obtain a high resolution reconstruction using discrete tomography. In such a case, the fifth image processing step, which refines the boundaries using edge profiles can also be eliminated.

15.4   The role of computed tomography: Selected examples

Figure 15.2 shows the power of CT in creating digital models of components lacking an electronic description; then using the CT-derived models in a manufacturing process to create castings of the original part. (In manufacturing circles, *casting* refers to the creation of a component by cooling molten metal, plastic, or other materials in a mold.) At the top left of Fig. 15.2 is the photograph of a certified replica of the Liberty Bell. At top right is the digital 3D point cloud obtained from CT image data; here the points represent all surfaces of the object. The solid CAD model generated from the point cloud data is shown at bottom left in Fig. 15.2. This CAD model then served as input to a casting process to produce a copy, shown at bottom right, of the original replica.

The problem of generating digital models of highly complex parts is one that is easily addressed by means of CT. Figure 15.3 shows another type of digital model, a surface mesh, of an automobile transmission housing. As seen here, this part has a number of intricate passages which makes it difficult and time-consuming to render digitally by CMMs and lasers.

Figure 15.4 shows the application of CT to the problem of obtaining a CAD description of part where no such documentation exists. The specific example shown here is that of producing CAD drawings of a worn-out and undocumented control-rod mechanism of an aging nuclear power plant. The

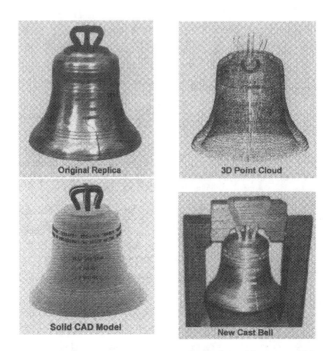

FIGURE 15.2. CT-assisted reverse engineering of parts with no electronic designs.

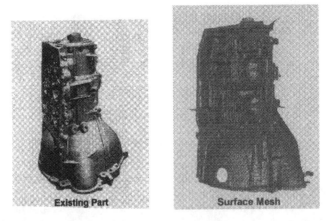

FIGURE 15.3. CT-assisted reverse engineering of a part too complex for CMMs, lasers, and milling machines.

control-rod, shown at top left of the figure, was scanned with an ARACOR CT system. A longitudinal section through the CT image, at bottom left, reveals the internal complexity of the part. Contours were extracted from the CT image, and loaded into a well-known CAD program; then a CAD engineer manipulated the data to produce the engineering drawings shown at the right.

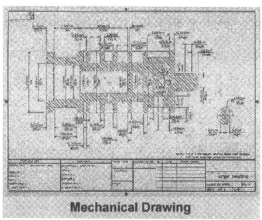

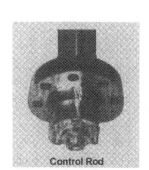
Control Rod

Mechanical Drawing

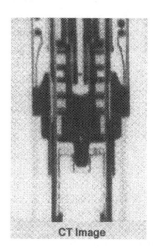
CT Image

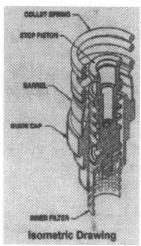
Isometric Drawing

FIGURE 15.4. CT-assisted reverse engineering of a part that has no documentation.

The use of CT-obtained digital models in part metrology is shown in Fig. 15.5. This illustrates an example of comparing digitally obtained part geometry with the original CAD model to analyze dimensional conformance. On the left of the figure is the original CAD model of a part. In the center is the point cloud derived from CT data obtained by scanning the part. The image on the right shows the variations between the CT-derived point cloud and original CAD model; this surface map illustrates the differences between the actual part and the CAD model.

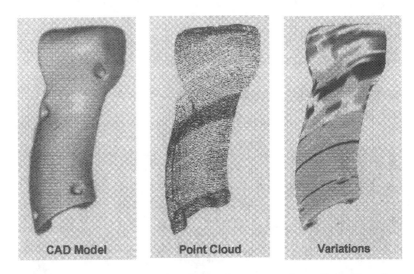

FIGURE 15.5. CT-assisted part metrology to analyze dimensional conformance.

Figure 15.6 illustrates the application of CT to creating digital models for computational modeling. Here we see an application to the study of solidification modeling to simulate the casting process on a computer. As mentioned earlier, the casting process requires the cooling of molten material in hollow molds called *tooling*. A tool is essentially two halves of a mating die with a center cavity corresponding to the shape of the desired component. Often complex cooling passages are added to the tooling to provide optimal conditions for cooling the molten material. In Fig. 15.6 the image at the top shows a CT-derived CAD model of the tool halves. At the bottom is a finite element-based solidification model used for simulating the casting process. Specifically, this model allows manufacturers to analyze how solidification will proceed, to determine where regions of shrink, porosity and stress will develop, and to obtain a multitude of critical parameters that can be used both for redesigning the tool or controlling the casting process.

The casting industry presents one of the most immediate applications for CT-assisted agile manufacturing. Figure 15.7 illustrates how activities of reverse engineering, part metrology, and computational modeling, all dictated by CT, combine with other technologies in the manufacturing industry to produce castings of components. The starting point for this process is a CAD model of the part of interest. If such a model is absent, CT is used to create one. Once a CAD description of the part is available, a CAD model of a casting tool is designed by modeling two mating halves of

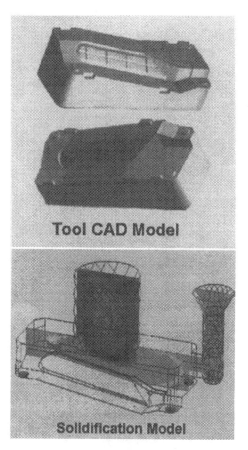

FIGURE 15.6. **CT-assisted computational modeling for solidification studies.**

a die block with a center cavity corresponding to the shape of the desired part.

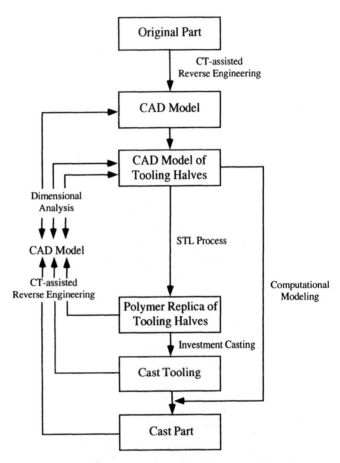

FIGURE 15.7. Integration of CT-assisted reverse engineering, metrology, and computational modeling to create castings of components.

The CAD model of the tooling halves is now used for two purposes. First it is used in computational modeling for solidification studies in the casting process. Second it serves as input to a process known as stereolithography (STL); this process uses lasers to build polymer replicas of the tooling halves from the CAD files. Before proceeding, the replicas are scanned via CT and a CAD description is obtained. The metrological information obtained from this CAD model is used to check for dimensional conformance with the original CAD model. Once the tooling replicas are deemed satisfactory, they are used in an investment casting process to cast the actual tooling out of a suitable alloy. The cast tools are scanned by CT to confirm dimensional accuracy with their CAD counterparts. The tools are now ready to be used to produce castings of the desired part. Here again, CT is used to check the cast part for dimensional conformance with the original CAD model.

Figure 15.8 illustrates the concept just described for the case of manufacturing replacements for an existing component. The upper left shows a photograph of an aerodynamically shaped plastic airfoil used in racing cars to keep wiper blades in close contact with the windshield. In this particular situation, no CAD model was available, so the part was reverse engineered using CT. The resulting CAD model is shown next to the photograph. The upper right shows the CAD model of the tooling halves that was created from the CAD model of the airfoil. The lower left shows a polymer replica of one of the tooling halves; this replica was obtained by the stereolithography process. Just above the replica, the corresponding investment cast tool half is shown. The cast tool halves were then used to mold the plastic replicas shown at the lower right.

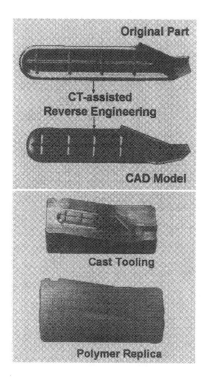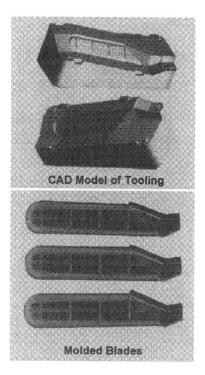

FIGURE 15.8. CT-assisted agile manufacturing in the casting of replacement parts.

15.5   The role of discrete tomography in improving the digital model

In the applications described in the previous section, the objects scanned by the CT system are made of either a single homogeneous material or, at most, a few homogeneous materials. Therefore, the X-ray linear attenuation coefficients (LACs) belong to a set of discrete numbers. This scenario is typical of a large number of objects encountered in industrial CT. As noted in Section 15.1, CT image reconstruction techniques typically solve the continuous tomography problem without using *a priori* information about the discrete nature of the X-ray linear attenuation coefficient (LAC) function to be reconstructed. Consequently, the reconstructed LAC function varies throughout the object, even in areas where it is known to be constant. Furthermore, at the boundary between the object and the background (air), the values gradually decrease to the neighborhood of zero (Fig. 15.9, top left).

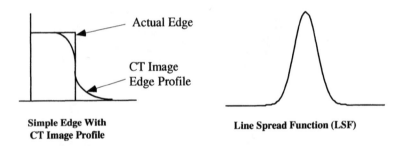

Simple Edge With CT Image Profile

Line Spread Function (LSF)

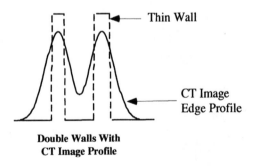

Double Walls With CT Image Profile

FIGURE 15.9. Edge profiles in CT.

The formation of this so-called *edge profile* can be modeled as the convolution of a square edge with a Line Spread Function (LSF) (Fig. 15.9, top). If the LSF is symmetric, then the edges of thick walls (Fig. 15.9, top left) can be calculated to sub-pixel accuracy, even without explicit knowledge of the LSF. However, in the case of thin walls, such a procedure is not possible (Fig. 15.9, bottom). If the LSF is known, an *image enhancement* or *deconvolution* step can improve the accuracy of the edge location. However, such a step is highly sensitive to noise in the image and to errors in the LSF. Therefore it is difficult to consistently estimate the positions of the edges.

One approach to improving accuracy is to impose constraints that reflect prior knowledge about the object. In particular, the discreteness of the LAC function can be applied as a constraint. It has been shown [12] that a binary object can be exactly reconstructed using only two orthogonal projections, provided that the object has no *switching components*. (A switching component is a special case of a switching set, defined in Chapter 8 by Matej, Vardi, Herman, and Vardi, whereby the set consists of binary elements; see also Chapter 3 by Kong and Herman.) This condition does not necessarily hold for many complex objects which are of interest in industrial tomography. However, in practice, several hundred projections are typically used, rather than just two. It has been shown that the use of additional views reduces, and sometimes eliminates, the ambiguity caused by the presence of switching components [13]; see also Chapter 12 by Censor and Matej, and Chapter 8 by Matej, Vardi, Herman, and Vardi. Results of this type offer the strong possibility that substantial improvements in resolution can be achieved by the application of the discreteness constraint in industrial tomography.

15.6   Technical challenges

As noted in the previous section, it is possible to obtain high-resolution discrete images when a large number of views are used. However, theoretical results that determine the maximum resolution that can be achieved using the discreteness constraint with a given number of views do not yet exist. Such results would help to fully determine the power of discrete tomography approach in CT-assisted engineering and manufacturing applications.

Most of the current methods for solving discrete tomography problems assume a small number of views. Research into efficient algorithms which can be applied to problems with many views would also be useful in determining its efficacy of applying the discreteness constrain in practical tomographic problems.

As with any imaging instrument, the CT scanner will produce a resolution-limited image. The best we can hope for is to use prior knowledge *and* a sufficient amount of data to minimize the extent to which the practical problems encountered in CT scanning tend to limit the ultimate resolution possible in reconstructed images. The techniques of discrete tomography applied to a large number of tomographic views offer the promise of pro-

ducing CT images whose resolution and dimensional accuracy are superior
to those obtained by conventional algorithms. This in turn should result in
significant improvements in the accuracy of boundaries extracted from CT
images for CAD models of a large class of parts of interest in CT-assisted
engineering and design. If this promise is realized, then CT-based industrial
NDE in general, and CT-assisted manufacturing in particular, will be an
important application of discrete tomography.

15.7   Conclusions

We have looked at some important applications in CT-based NDE that
may benefit from techniques of discrete tomography. In particular, we have
observed that discrete tomography has the potential to improve the accuracy of CT-derived digital models of a large class of industrial objects.
These digital models form the basis of new manufacturing technologies that
promise to revolutionize current manufacturing environments by reducing
manufacturing complexity, increasing productivity, and reducing costs.

Acknowledgments

Many of the figures presented in this paper have been derived from work
supported through the Ohio Edison Materials Technology Center (EMTEC)
from funds provided by the State of Ohio and the Defense Logistics Agency
(DLA). We would also like to thank Drs. James Stanley and Robert Yancey
for their contributions to an earlier version of this article.

References

[1] G. T. Herman, *Image Reconstruction from Projections: The Fundamentals of Computerized Tomography* (Academic Press, New York),
1980.

[2] A. C. Kak and M. Slaney, *Principles of Computerized Tomographic
Imaging* (IEEE Press, New York), 1988.

[3] J. L. C. Sanz, E. B. Hinkle, and A. K. Jain, *Radon and Projection
Transform-Based Computer Vision: Algorithms, A Pipeline Architecture, and Industrial Applications* (Springer Verlag, Berlin), 1988.

[4] M. C. San Martin, N. P. J. Stamford, N. Dammerova, N. Dixon, and
J. M. Carazo, "A structural model of the DnaB helicase from E. Coli
based on three-dimensional electron microscopy data," *J. Structural
Biology* **114**, 167-176 (1995).

[5] P. Schwander, C. Kisielowski, M. Seibt, F. H. Baumann, Y. Kim, and A. Ourmazd, "Mapping projected potential, interfacial roughness and chemical composition in general crystalline solids by quantitative transmission electron microscopy," *Phys. Rev. Lett.* **71**, 4150-4153 (1993).

[6] R. A. Brualdi and H. J. Ryser, *Combinatorial Matrix Theory* (Cambridge University Press, New York), 1991.

[7] N. J. Dusaussoy, Q. Cao, R. N. Yancey, and J. H. Stanley, "Image processing for CT-assisted reverse engineering and part characterization," *Proc. 1995 IEEE Intl. Conf. on Image Processing Vol. 3*, (IEEE Computer Society Press, California), pp. 33-36, 1995.

[8] R. N. Yancey, "Analysis of Stress Distributions in Metal-Matrix Composites with Variations in Fiber Spacing," *Ph.D. Dissertation, University of Dayton, Dayton, Ohio* (1997).

[9] A. Rosenfeld and A. C. Kak, *Digital Picture Processing*, Vol. 2 (Academic Press, New York), 1982.

[10] T. Y. Kong and A. Rosenfeld, "Digital topology: Introduction and survey," *Comp. Vis., Graphics, Image Process.* **48**, 357-393 (1989).

[11] J. K. Udupa, "Multidimensional digital boundaries," *CVGIP: Graphical Models Image Process.* **56**, 311-323 (1994).

[12] A. Kuba and A. Volčič, "Characterisation of measurable plane sets which are reconstructible from their two projections," *Inverse Problems* **4**, 513-527 (1988).

[13] A. Shilferstein and Y. T. Chen, "Switching components and the ambiguity problem in the reconstruction of pictures from their projections," *Pattern Recogn.* **10**, 327-340 (1978).

Chapter 16

3D Reconstruction from Sparse Radiographic Data

James Sachs, Jr.[1]
Ken Sauer[2]

ABSTRACT Nondestructive evaluation of materials through X-ray and γ-ray radiography has long been achieved by inferring three-dimensional structure from exposed films. Multiple views with varying positions of radioactive sources and the film have the potential for direct three-dimensional tomographic reconstruction for more detailed diagnosis of material flaws. The data are sufficiently sparse, however, to leave the reconstruction badly under-specified, requiring regularization and/or constraints to achieve meaningful results. In this chapter we discuss and illustrate the application of Bayesian binary 3D tomographic reconstruction to radiographs, including the several non-idealities frequently encountered in the field.

16.1 Introduction

Radiography is one of the most widely applied forms of data capture for nondestructive materials evaluation. Although most manufacturing processes to be monitored by X-ray will be outfitted with precise, calibrated systems offering a high degree of reproducibility, as discussed in Chapter 15 by Browne and Koshy, there remain a number of on-site inspection tasks that cannot be so tightly controlled. Evaluation of any objects too large or too remote for scanning by modern tomographic inspection systems, or permanently installed in a manner preventing free access may still be most practically "scanned" by radiographic film, using highly portable radioactive isotopes as sources, rather than accelerators or typical X-ray emitters [1,2]. The less precise control of data collection adds several types of uncertainty to our data not found in most tomographic work. In some such sparse-data applications, fusion of multiple data modalities [3] may allow improved diagnostics, but we will here restrict our consideration to

[1]Ford Motor Corporation, Product Development Center, PDC MD-331, 20901 Oakwook Blvd, P.O. Box 2053, Dearborn, MI 48121-2053, USA, E-mail: jsachs@ford.com

[2]University of Notre Dame, Department of Electrical Engineering, 275 Fitzpatrick Hall, Notre Dame, IN 46556, USA, E-mail: sauer@nd.edu

radiographic data.

The resulting films may be read by experts who usually must make a binary decision concerning the presence of a flaw in cast material or a weld. This sort of detection process may be adequately served by well-trained interpreters of radiographs. But if more complex decisions must be made concerning replacement or rejection of costly components, which can tolerate minor flaws, or those of certain positions and/or orientation, etc., three-dimensional rendering of the material and its flaws is invaluable. Given that each datum in the radiographs is approximately the integral projection of the material's attenuation along the line joining the radiograph pixel and the radioactive source, and given that the materials in which we are usually interested are homogeneous, the 3D reconstruction of few possible densities in the object's interior may be posed as a problem in discrete tomography in three dimensions.

The best method of estimating the 3D structure is not obvious. In addition to the data's resulting from this process being limited in quality due to the high attenuation typical of dense materials, the number of two-dimensional projections captured on film is typically quite small. Although backprojection-based techniques have been derived for the 3D tomographic problem [4–6], the paucity of projection data, badly violating the assumptions on which these algorithms are based, makes these techniques unsuitable for the problem. The reconstruction is highly under-specified also in the algebraic sense, since the number of voxels we wish to reconstruct is much larger than the number of measurements which are influenced by those voxels. Researchers have turned to statistical methods for this sort of case, relying on models of both the physical system of data collection, and the ensemble of possible objects [7–9]. In this framework, the pixel, or voxel values in the discretized domain of reconstruction are parameters in an estimation problem. Statistical methods can be applied with little or no modification to the "missing data" problem, which has been studied widely [7].

Our work in this domain centers primarily on maximum *a posteriori* probability (MAP) estimation of a random object, X, from observations, Y. The advantage of MAP over, for example, least mean-squared error estimation is that its solution is formulated as direct optimization problem which can be solved by iterative techniques, rather than potentially costly estimation of means. It also has the intuitive appeal of yielding the object "most likely," under the given models, to have caused the observed data.

The statistical model for the data is fixed by the physics of interactions between X-ray or γ-ray photons and matter, and the detection process on the receiving side. Simplification of the process is typically used, and results in a scatter-free model of photon travel, in which each photon either passes the entire distance from source to detector on a straight line, or is absorbed. This yields a relatively simple Poisson model for the data. The true interactions are more complicated, since for energies of interest,

Compton scattering is the principle phenomenon responsible for attenuation [2]. Many approaches to scatter compensation have been proposed, most based on deterministic models. We present a method for incorporating Compton scatter effects into a statistical estimation framework. This approach can include any stationary or nonstationary convolutional model for scatter distribution. Our experimental results include principally first order correction.

The Bayesian formulation requires a stochastic model for the object which is to be estimated from the radiographic data. This information is expressed by an *a priori* probability density function for X, often simply referred to as the prior density. This may also be viewed as simply a regularization process in which the logarithm of the density function for the random field is the regularizing functional. We take advantage of the restriction of our problems to homogeneous material containing voids, or flaws, of a second density to pose a binary estimation task. Restriction to a single void as, for example, in Chapter 14 by Mohammad-Djafari and Soussen, allows the reconstruction to be posed as estimation of the object's shape.

In the sections that follow, we first present the attributes of our problem that distinguish it from most of the others found in this book, that is, the numerous system non-idealities with which we must contend. We formulate the reconstruction problem statistically, taking into account the pervasive Compton scatter with pre-processing of radiographic data. With Monte Carlo simulations, we reproduce the principle scatter and Poisson counting noise effects and show the effectiveness of the pre-processing and nonlinear Bayesian reconstruction.

In some real data sets, gross non-idealities in the digitization process may dominate the nonlinear effects of scatter, in which case their compensation is the primary preprocessing step. A case study with real radiographs intended to mimic the problem of estimating relatively fine cracks in solids shows the distortion of poor digitization, compensation thereof, and relatively effective and accurate binary reconstruction for diagnostic interpretation.

16.2 Radiographic/tomographic data

16.2.1 Idealized photon counting model

We begin under the assumption that, though our radiographs may be corrupted by counting noise and other effects discussed below, the exposed film gives us information transformable into energy absorbed per pixel area on the film. Using standard theory for density of exposed, developed film, illuminated by light of intensity I_0, transmitted light intensity will be $I_t = I_0 e^{-D}$, where D is the photographic density at the given pixel [2].

Density is in turn proportional to the log of the total exposure. Exposure is approximately proportional to the number of photons arriving in the given pixel, which we will treat as a Poisson random variable, Y_i, whose realization is y_i. A simple inverse relationship therefore exists, ideally, between the Poisson photon counts and transmitted light in a digitizer of radiographs:

$$y_i \propto I_t^{-1}. \tag{16.1}$$

With a slight loss of generality and gain in simplicity, we assume that the average total photon counts directed along all rays are equal to y_T (generalization to varying dosage is relatively simple). The discretization of both the object and radiograph domains allows the forward projection operation to be described by the matrix A, whose i-th row we denote A_{i*}. A single forward projection from the 3D object x is then $p_i = A_{i*}x$. According to the simplest attenuation and photon counting models, Y_i is Poisson, with mean and variance $y_T e^{-p_i}$ [10].

For values of the Poisson mean typical of our applications, the log-likelihood function $\log \mathcal{P}(Y = y | X = x)$ can be approximated with negligible error as a quadratic function of the unknown object x [11]. Thus, whatever the Poisson model applied, our log-likelihood function, within a constant, will be of the form

$$\log \mathcal{P}(Y = y | X = x) \approx -1/2(p - Ax)^t D(p - Ax), \tag{16.2}$$

provided the quadratic approximation is made about the proper point. This yields a direct transformation from the digitization of film to a likelihood function for the object under study.

16.2.2 Compton scattering effects

Under the simplest scatter-free model, p and A are as described above, with D being a diagonal matrix with the photon counts, $\{y_i\}$ on its diagonal [11]. This model would be reasonably accurate if photons were simply absorbed by the materials, but the principle mechanism for attenuation in our problem is Compton scattering, whose angular distribution for these energies is decidedly forward [2]. Subsequent scatter events of the same photon have wider angular distribution, and the cumulative effect, especially given that in our application the majority of energy reaching the film have been scattered, is that direct utilization of photon counts is infeasible without some correction for scatter.

In order to realistically simulate radiographs including scatter effects, we employ Monte Carlo generation of photon counts in the data vector y. The source placement is illustrated in Fig. 16.1. The simulated radiographs are placed orthogonal to a line from the point source through the origin of the block, and are in contact with the side or edge of the block opposite the source. The rays are thus forced to penetrate along the greater path lengths in the material in this simulation. Each γ-ray photon is generated with a random orientation from the point source, and follows a pseudo-random path according the probability law for its path length before scattering [10]. This distribution depends on both the material and the photon energy. The change in path, and loss of energy at any scatter location are computed from the Klein-Nishina formula [12]. For simulations, we used an initial energy of 0.47 MeV, representative of ^{192}Ir. The resulting radiographs appear in Fig. 16.2, while the profile of the scattered placement of photons originally directed along a single ray appears in Fig. 16.3.

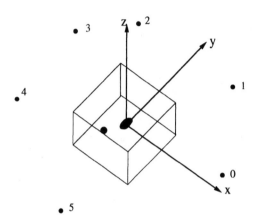

FIGURE 16.1. Geometry of Monte Carlo trials of inspection of 3×3×1.6 cm steel block irradiated by ^{192}Iridium. Sources are numbered from zero starting on the x-axis, and proceeding counter-clockwise, as viewed from above. The coordinates of the sources in (x, y, z), measured in cm, are: (5.0,0.5,0.0), (3.0,4.85,0.0), (-3.5,5.35,0.5), (-4.85,3.0,-0.5), (-4.85,-3.0,0.0), (0.5,-5.0,0.0). The block contains two voids, an ellipsoid at the origin, and smaller sphere at (-0.75,-0.75,0).

Various approaches have been suggested to compensate for the scattering problem, many of them designed for medical emission tomography. A common technique in transmission tomography is simple background scatter subtraction [13]. This method is based on the assumption that scattered photons are approximately uniform in intensity across the detecting area, and can therefore be considered an additive constant in y. Fahmi and Macovski [14] modeled the effects of scatter in X-ray images as being isotropic and stationary, and designed an iterative process to estimate a kernel representing the scatter. Other researchers have developed related techniques for scatter kernel estimation for both transmission and emission tomography [15]. But the strong forward orientation at the energies used to penetrate the dense materials in our applications may yield highly spatially varying scatter geometries if the object is not uniform in thickness.

The same sort of approximation, with accuracy similar to (16.2), is

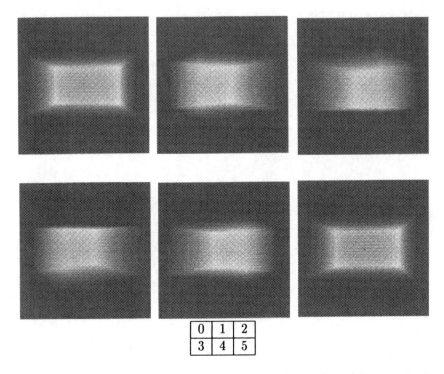

0	1	2
3	4	5

FIGURE 16.2. Monte Carlo generated radiographs with per-pixel dosage of $y_T = 5000$. Indices correspond to source numbers in the previous figure.

possible with linearized incorporation of scattered photons into the log-likelihood. This changes the definitions of p, A and D of (16.2), giving the operations represented by A and A^t much greater spatial support, and making any iterative reconstruction method far more costly. Fortunately, the gain in incorporating scatter into this case is primarily in a "first or-der" preprocessing step similar to a deconvolution operating only on the raw radiographic counts y, which can then be simply transformed into pro-jection data p [16]. As in, for instance, [14], we could estimate a "best" kernel for this convolution, but such cases as the geometry of Fig. 16.1 have scatter patterns which are much too varied. For radiograph 0 in the above Monte Carlo simulations, for example, we have used the scatter pat-tern estimated at the origin of the image to perform compensation for the entire film in Fig. 16.4(b). Reconstructions from data pre-processed in this manner are very poor. We have been unable to find any stationary method yielding reasonable quality for such an example. Using a kernel corrected by local means of scatter concentration from Monte Carlo trials using a defect-free version of the block under study [16], we achieve a compensated radiograph as shown in Fig. 16.4(c). The reconstructions from Monte Carlo

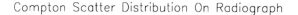

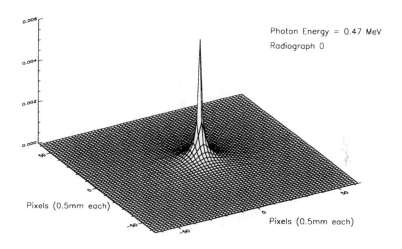

FIGURE 16.3. Spatial distribution of multiple Compton scatter for a single beam from the source to the origin of radiograph, with radiograph adjacent to material. The vast majority of effects are caused by those of fifth order scatter or lower.

data to follow all derive from data preprocessed in this manner.

As material thickness increases, scatter patterns become wider, unscattered photons become the minority and most of the radiographs' exposure results from these indirect arrivals. As we will see in Section 16.4, other non-idealities as well may corrupt real data.

16.3 3D maximum a posteriori reconstruction

16.3.1 Bayesian formulation

The approximate log-likelihood function of (16.2) may invite solution in terms of an x maximizing the log-likelihood for a maximum-likelihood (ML) estimate, but as is the case in most problems approached in the discrete tomography framework, the dimension of our x is typically much larger than that of y, the radiograph pixel values, and the solution is underspecified by the data. Constraining and/or penalizing the solution with *a priori* beliefs concerning X is perhaps most easily achieved by minimizing some simple objective function including the log-likelihood and a term penalizing high local variance. In the Bayesian estimation framework the common choice is the *a posteriori* probability (MAP) estimate, $\hat{x}_{MAP}$ of the object x from

Noiseless, Scatter–Free Projections

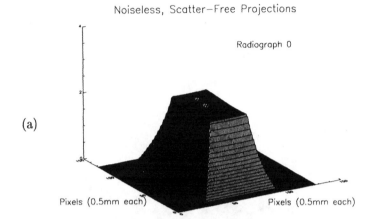

(a)

Scatter Correction by Stationary Linear Model

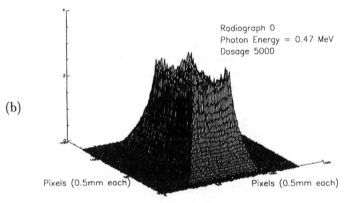

(b)

Scatter Correction by Nonstationary Linear Model

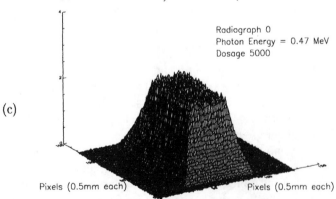

(c)

FIGURE 16.4. Linear (in photon counts) scatter correction by stationary and nonstationary convolution. Pixel values represent entries in the vector p.

the realization y of Y:

$$\hat{x}_{MAP} = \arg\max_x P(X = x | Y = y)$$
$$= \arg\max_x \{\log P(Y = y | X = x) + \log P(X = x)\}. \quad (16.3)$$

As an *a priori* model for the unknown x, the Markov random field (MRF) [17–19] provides a rich family of choices, with behavior described by the potential function penalizing various relationships among spatially adjacent voxels. The general form of the density function for the MRF is

$$P(X = x) = Z^{-1} \exp\{- \sum_{(i,j) \in C} a_{ij} \rho(x_i - x_j)\}. \quad (16.4)$$

The set C is the collection of all neighboring voxel pairs, and Z is a normalizing constant. In each of our prior models, the coefficients $\{a_{ij}\}$ are non-zero for the 26 neighboring voxels. Though our primary interest is in binary reconstructions using the Ising MRF [19], we show results with three important and common MRFs. All can, with inclusion of constraints, be described by the potential function

$$\rho(x_i - x_j) = \frac{|x_i - x_j|^q}{q\sigma^q}, \quad (16.5)$$

with q a parameter determining the degree of edge preservation, and σ a scaling factor related to the variance of voxel values. This type of MRF is known as the Generalized Gaussian MRF (GGMRF) [20], and includes the Gaussian for $q = 2$. For simplicity we here use $\gamma = (q\sigma^q)^{-1}$. Values of q near 2 represent models with higher probabilities of smooth transitions, while values near 1 represent those in which abrupt changes are equally as likely as gradual transitions. For many materials inspection problems, the value $q = 1$ is appealing, since sharp differences are commonly found at material interfaces.

The constraint to binary pixel values has been applied to tomographic estimation in several settings, particularly in very limited data cases [21–23]. For binary or m-ary reconstruction, we simply constrain pixel values to the given densities. In our applications, it is realistic to assume these densities known, but as is shown in Chapter 10 by Frese, Bouman, and Sauer, they could also be estimated during reconstruction. The value of γ may be estimated from data or from sample objects, but to this point we have not found such values generally satisfactory, and have instead either chosen values heuristically, or modified the MRF model to better accommodate the appearance of relatively rare exceptions to homogeneity with a more complex model [24].

Under most common models for data acquisition, rays are assumed parallel, or fan-beam with relatively dense and uniform exposure of all areas of the object. This is not the case with very sparse radiographic, cone beam

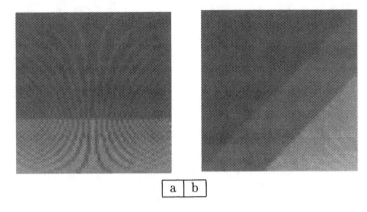

FIGURE 16.5. Nonuniform weighting of projection data across center slice with fan-beam geometry at (a) 0 degrees and (b) 45 degrees. Density is proportional to total weighting of entries in A for the given voxels.

data, especially when physical constraints require the radioactive sources to be placed relatively near the object and film. This makes the assumption of parallel beams at the object quite unrealistic, and slightly complicates the choice of weighting parameter, γ, for the prior model. In relatively homogeneous materials such as the metals we scan, γ is chosen with consideration of the relative weighting between entries in $A^t D A$ from (16.2) and γ. Unfortunately, the weighting of voxels in the log-likelihood function may vary widely as beams diverge. Figure 16.5 shows the examples of the central plane from the block in Fig. 16.1, with voxels and radiograph pixels having equal dimensions. The intensity in the figures is proportional to total weighting, at each voxel, of the likelihood term as expressed by $\sum_i A_{ij}$ for voxel j. If sources are limited to one side of an object, often the case [25], this effect may show widely varying degrees of influence of the prior density versus the likelihood, and degrees of regularization with wide spatial variation. Likelihood weighting may also vary spatially due to the greater influence of measurements of higher photon counts, due to the dependence of entries in D on y, or on scatter-corrected counts.

16.3.2   Reconstruction from simulated radiographs

In general, we hope to let the data dominate to the greatest extent possible, and one would prefer estimates which do not rely on prior beliefs or constraints, as would be the case if data were plentiful and of high SNR. But in sparse data problems, regularization by the log *a priori* probability density necessarily has a relatively strong influence on the MAP solution. Care must be taken, therefore, in choosing both the form of the model and its respective free parameters.

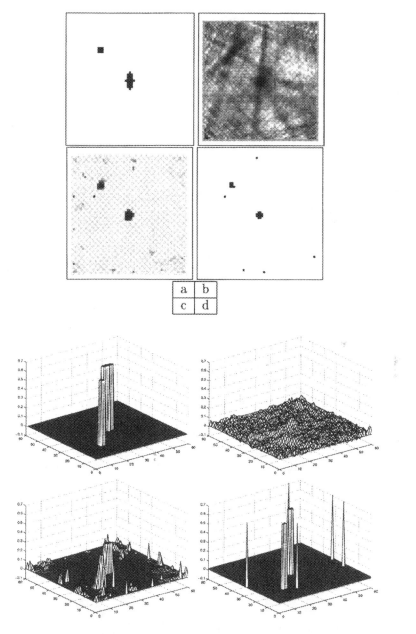

FIGURE 16.6. Center slice ($z = 0$) of block attenuation using various MRF *a priori* models. (a) Discretized original; (b) Gaussian prior;
(c) absolute-value penalty of local differences; (d) binary-valued MRF.
The expected dosage was 5000 photons per ray. Above: gray-scale representation. Below: plots, with values representing differences from
uniform material's attenuation.

The choice of model must also depend on the familiarity of the eventual expert observer with the attributes favored by each. An example of several reconstruction from the Monte Carlo generated data appears in Fig. 16.6. These slices are all from the central plane of the block in Fig. 16.1 of voxels measuring 0.5 mm on each side. These slices are taken from estimates under the MAP criterion, subject to the limitations of optimization discussed below.

Probably the least dramatic MRF choice is the Gaussian, discouraging abrupt changes while specifying an estimate that is a linear function of the projection observations. The relatively poor contrast reconstruction of Fig. 16.6(b) results from the severe quadratic penalization of local differences, but retains artifacts that are relatively easy to interpret. Modeling abrupt local differences as more probable while still penalizing them in terms of probability leads us to the MRF using the absolute value of local voxel differences as prior, illustrated in Fig. 16.6(c). This model tends to suppress overall contrast, but allows good definition of edges even in the presence of noise suppression. This reconstruction shows the dramatic improvement possible by using a "heavy-tailed" conditional distribution for local differences. Finally, in Fig. 16.6(d), we see the binary-constrained MAP reconstruction, in which the true, higher contrast between the homogeneous background and the voids can be maintained without sacrifice of noise suppression. It is this model that we apply most widely in nondestructive materials evaluation, where the assumption of few discrete levels of intensity or absorptivity fits physical reality to a great degree.

Because the likehood term, as explained above, exerts influence, which varies spatially, a single value for the parameter γ may cause smoothing to be nonhomogeneous. With the same simulation as in previous figures, the sequence of increasingly regularized reconstructions in Fig. 16.7 shows the much larger void at the center of the block being eliminated from the estimate before the smaller, which is located nearer the corner. This is due to the higher variance of the more attenuated measurements through the center, offsetting the larger signature of the center void on the radiographs.

16.3.3   Optimization considerations

The computational problem resulting for the MAP estimate has the form

$$\hat{x}_{MAP} = \arg\min_{x \in \Omega} \left\{ 1/2(\hat{p} - Ax)^T D(\hat{p} - Ax) + \gamma \sum_{(i,j) \in C} a_{ij} |x_i - x_j|^q \right\}.$$

$$(16.6)$$

The three models discussed above result in different forms of the convex optimization problem to be solved to find the MAP estimate. We employ an algorithm of greedy, sequential updates of voxel values, closely related to

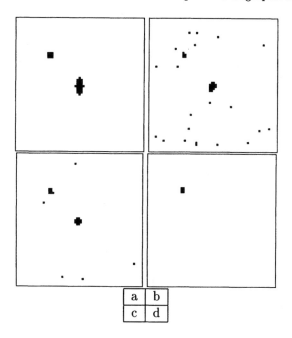

FIGURE 16.7. Original center slice ($z = 0$) of block (a) and reconstructions using binary *a priori* model with γ set to (b) 5.0; (c) 10.0,
(d) 15.0.

iterated conditional modes (ICM) [18], and known as iterative coordinate
descent (ICD). The application of such sequential estimation methods to
tomographic estimation is discussed in detail in [11]. The domain Ω may be
used to enforce constraints such as positivity, or restricted sets of density
values, as in our binary reconstruction, posing a discrete optimization problem. In spite of convexity, the binary constraint makes the optimization a
potentially more challenging numerical problem than the continuously valued reconstructions.

Although the computational burden of statistical methods such as those
proposed in this paper is much larger than most deterministic backprojection techniques, convergence of the MAP estimate under ICD is quite
rapid in iteration counts. All the plots in Fig. 16.8 show near convergence
of the *a posteriori* likelihood for the reconstructions above in a handful of
iterations, following initialization with an estimate corresponding to a solid
block. The Gaussian prior yields a relatively smooth quadratic cost profile,
which may require a dozen iterations to converge beyond any perceptible
change. The binary reconstruction typically has reached its final value in
5 to 7 complete iterations for this data set. But this may be only a local
minimum, and true maximization of the *a posteriori* probability remains
an important open problem in discrete tomography. Stochastic methods
such as simulated annealing sample a larger set of possible solutions, at

the expense of greatly increased computation. More heuristic techniques employing modified greedy descent from varied initial conditions offer a compromise between these extremes with potential improvement over ICD.

Convergence of Iterative Reconstructions

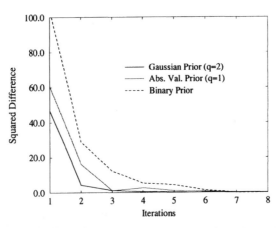

FIGURE 16.8. Convergence of ICD in terms of total squared difference between successive estimates of $60 \times 60 \times 32$-voxel reconstructions. Each case has $y_T = 5000$.

16.4   Physical radiographic experiments

On-site exposure of radiographs has traditionally been performed with limited concern for precision in recorded locations of films and sources, given that a human observer has variety of visual cues available for relative registration of objects in film. Application of tomographic reconstruction to these data presumes high precision in the known locations of both sources and pixels. Outside the laboratory, this may be impossible to achieve, leading to problems ranging from limited resolution of flaws or aberrations in materials to inconsistencies sufficient to preclude any useful tomographic inversion. Especially when sources are interior to an object whose walls are under study [25], control of placement may leave significant uncertainty. While our primary applications usually allow good precision in film placement, significant uncertainty is common in the coordinates of the radioactive sources, as well as in manually placed radiographic films.

The results of simulating error in assumed knowledge of source locations appear in Fig. 16.9. All sources in the simulation above were randomly displaced, independently and uniformly distributed within spheres centered

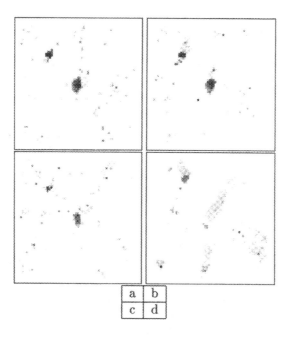

a	b
c	d

FIGURE 16.9. Reconstruction with increasing diameters of spherically uniformly distributed perturbation of source location. Reconstruction is from six radiographs, low dosage, using the absolute-value potential in the prior model. (a) Perfect placement of sources; (b) uncertainty radius = 0.3 cm; (c) 0.4 cm; (d) 0.5 cm.

on true locations. The resolution of the voids shown in the center slices deteriorates rapidly from little change in Fig. 16.9(b) at 0.3 cm radius to loss of both voids in Fig. 16.9(d). The relative sensitivity of reconstruction quality on the precision of source location compared to that of film location depends on the proximity of each to the irradiated object. In our simulation, the source is perhaps closer to the object than in typical applications. As a source retreats to infinite distance, an approximation necessary for parallel beam approximations frequently made for 3D cone-beam problems, uncertainty in film location dominates this type of system error.

Figure 16.10 illustrates a specimen used for tomographic reconstruction experiments under the auspices of Electricité de France, for the sake of evaluating reconstruction algorithms' performance in locating and sizing relatively fine fissures in thick steel structures. The block, 70 mm thick, has four cuts 0.25 mm in width and machined in the positions illustrated; depths vary from 5 mm to 30 mm. The seven [192]Iridium sources were placed, sequentially, one in the center and six on the perimeter of a circle with a diameter of 240 mm in a plane approx 390 mm above the block. The exposed film rested directly under the lower surface.

This experiment includes all the non-idealities discussed above, having

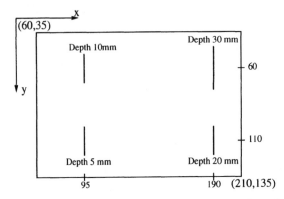

FIGURE 16.10. View from above of the center section, beginning at (60 mm, 35 mm), of steel block, 70 mm thick, with 0.25mm wide cuts with depths as indicated. Lengths are, clockwise from upper left, 20, 30, 20, and 20 mm.

an attenuation sufficient to yield a majority of the films' exposure from scattered radiation. Minor uncertainty in the placement of both sources and film occurs at the exposure stage, and again in the digitization. For this set of data, positions of radiographs are deduced from lead "markers" attached to the test block, whose shadows in digitized imagery, estimated from segmented masks of the letters, register locations of segments of the film containing information of interest. While it may appear less than impartial to pre-select the regions of reconstruction, it is exactly this sort of focused reconstruction that is envisioned in application. Complete reconstruction of entire objects of this size, still far smaller than systems to be inspected, is unnecessary and very costly computationally in current technology. Selective reconstruction of regions of interest is likely to remain the norm, since experts can still cover vast amounts of radiographic "territory" far faster than reconstructions can be done. Automatic detection of these regions of interest, either in the two-dimensional radiographic domain, or in three dimensions, is an open research problem.

The panels of data in Fig. 16.11 are segments taken from seven different films, with all capturing a single region of interest corresponding to the upper left cut of Fig. 16.10. They are captured after a form of corruption additional to those already discussed. The digitizer suffers from highly non-uniform illumination, varying widely within even one of these frames of less than 50 × 50 mm. This factor dominates the error of these data, necessitating systematic correction. Though in the future, more accurately calibrated digitizations may allow a direct transformation from data to photon counts as in (16.1), it is not practical in this case. We transform the recorded light transmission values into approximate projection measurements by fitting the images to the projections of a solid object. Let $r(m,n)$ be the digitized values of the radiograph, and $\tilde{p}(m,n)$ the projections of

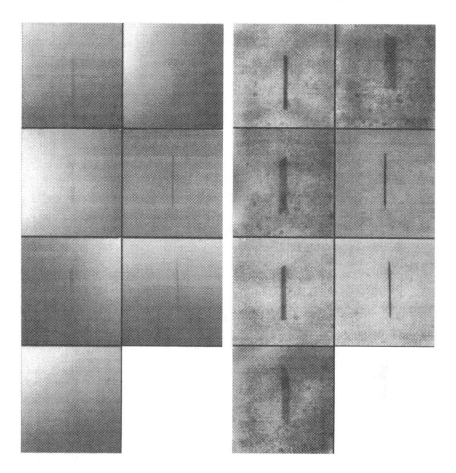

**FIGURE 16.11. Left: real radiographs with non-uniform illumination
in digitization. Right: radiographs after correction by least-squares fit
of fourth order.**

the solid block. The data $r(m,n)$ are approximated by the least-squares fit
of a two-dimensional polynomial surface (typically fourth order), $\tilde{r}(m,n)$.
The working approximations of the integral projections are then

$$p(m,n) = \frac{r(m,n)\tilde{p}(m,n)}{\tilde{r}(m,n)}. \qquad (16.7)$$

The corrected and enhanced radiograph segments are shown on the right
in Fig. 16.11. Following approximation of average dosage y_T, the weighting
matrix in the quadratic approximation of (16.2) can be computed from
$p(m,n)$, creating the same approximate likelihood as in Subsection 16.2.1.
For the sake of the MAP estimate, accurate determination of y_T is not
essential, since the solution will finally be determined by only the balance
between the values of y_T and γ.

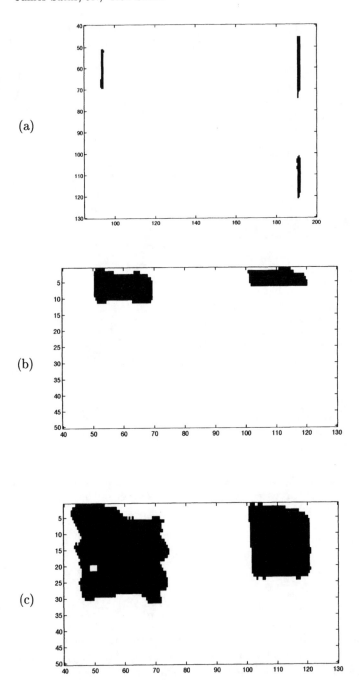

FIGURE 16.12. Slices of reconstructed block; (a) horizontal slice at $z = 10$ mm; (b) vertical slice at $x = 95$mm; (c) vertical slice at $x = 190$mm.

MAP reconstructions of the center portion of the block, while not precise, are accurate in determining location and depth of the voids. The correct extents are found in both the y and z directions, excepting failures primarily around edges of voids, especially near the plane $z = 0$. The horizontal slice of Fig. 16.12(a) also shows slices rendered as two to three pixels wide at this level, while their known width is only 0.25 mm, or one-half pixel width. We attribute this lack of resolution in part to imprecision in source placements and radiograph segment locations, with the effects illustrated in Fig. 16.9.

The reconstructions above, under realistic experimentation with radiographic film on-site nondestructive evaluation, offer an encouraging demonstration of the viability of three-dimensional tomography for this problem. While the quality of these results under the given radiographic signal-to-noise ratio may not be adequate for real diagnostics at present, improved precision in measurement and, particularly, in digitization are expected to allow substantially better resolution in the future. Further algorithmic refinements are certainly possible as well. The problem of source and radiographic placement error could be ameliorated by allowing perturbation of their coordinates alternating with reconstruction steps. This would risk loss of accuracy in absolute location of flaws in materials, but the exchange of this accuracy for greater precision in the shape and size of voids may well be a diagnostically worthwhile exchange. Given the difficulty of guaranteeing true maximization of *a posteriori* probability under the binary constraint, numerical improvements as well will be welcomed.

16.5   Conclusion

Tomographic reconstruction from radiographs has been shown viable and numerically feasible over the past decade. While this is a relatively specialized tomographic application, facilitating its expanded usage offers potentially improved visualization for diagnostics in many settings important to public safety and economy for infrastructure maintenance. It is the inherently discrete nature of the materials we wish to study which makes possible the quality of estimates thus far, and hope for future improvements. Several important problems remain to be addressed, which are unique to this arena, but further fundamental and algorithmic advances, as offered in the other chapters of this book, promise to enrich and advance the world of radiographic nondestructive evaluation more fully into three dimensions.

Acknowledgment

This research was funded in part by Electricité de France under Grants P21L03/2K3208/EP542, /EP602 and /02/EP648.

References

[1] R. Halmshaw, *Industrial Radiography: Theory and Practice* (Applied Science Publishers, London), 1982.

[2] L. E. Bryant, P. McIntire, and R. C. McMaster (Eds.), *Nondestructive Testing Handbook*, Second Edition (American Society for Nondestructive Testing, Columbus, Ohio), 1985, Volume 3.

[3] S. Gautier, J. Idier, A. Mohammad-Djafari, and B. Lavayssière, "X-ray and ultrasound data fusion," In *Proc. IEEE Int'l Conf. Image Proc.*, (IEEE, Piscataway, NJ), pp. (III)366-(III)369, 1998.

[4] A. C. Kak, "Computerized tomography with X-ray, emission, and ultrasound sources," *Proc. IEEE* **67**, 1245-1272 (1979).

[5] L. A. Feldkamp, L. C. Davis, and J. W. Kress, "Practical cone-beam algorithm," *J. Opt. Soc. Amer. A* **6**, 612-619 (1984).

[6] P. Grangeat, "Mathematical framework of cone beam 3D reconstruction via the first derivative of the Radon transform," In G. T. Herman, A. K. Louis and F. Natterer, *Mathematical Methods in Tomography*, (Springer-Verlag, Berlin), pp. 66-97, 1991.

[7] R. M. Ranggayyan, A. T. Dhawan, and R. Gordon, "Algorithms for limited-view computed tomography: An annotated bibliography and a challenge," *Applied Optics* **24**, 4000-4012 (1985).

[8] G. T. Herman, H. Hurwitz, A. Lent, and H-P. Lung, "On the Bayesian approach to image reconstruction," *Info. and Cont.* **42**, 60-71 (1979).

[9] K. M. Hanson and G. W. Wecksung, "Bayesian approach to limited-angle reconstruction in computed tomography," *J. Opt. Soc. Am.* **73**, 1501-1509 (1983).

[10] G. T. Herman, *Image Reconstruction from Projections: The Fundamentals of Computerized Tomography* (Academic Press, New York), 1980.

[11] C. Bouman and K. Sauer, "A unified approach to statistical tomography using coordinate descent optimization," *IEEE Trans. Image Proc.* **5**, 480-492 (1996).

[12] E. Segre, *Nuclei and Particles* (W. A. Benjamin, Reading, MA), 1977.

[13] G. H. Glover, "Compton scatter effects in CT reconstructions," *Med. Phys.* **9**, 860-867 (1982).

[14] H. Fahmi and A. Macovski, "Reducing the effects of scattered photons in X-ray projection imaging," *IEEE Trans. Med. Imaging* **8**, 56-63 (1989).

[15] J. Nuyts, H. Bosmans, and P. Suetens, "An analytical model for Compton scatter in a homogeneously attenuating medium," *IEEE Trans. Med. Imaging* **12**, 421-429 (1993).

[16] K. Sauer, J. Sachs, Jr., and C. Klifa, "Bayesian estimation of 3-D objects from few radiographs," *IEEE Trans. Nucl. Sci.* **41**, 1780-1790 (1994).

[17] S. Geman and D. Geman, "Stochastic relaxation, Gibbs distributions, and the Bayesian restoration of images," *IEEE Trans. Pattern Anal. and Mach. Intell.* **PAMI-6**, 721-741 (1984).

[18] J. Besag, "On the statistical analysis of dirty pictures," *J. Roy. Statist. Soc. B* **48**, 259-302 (1986).

[19] J. Marroquin, S. Mitter, and T. Poggio, "Probabilistic solution of ill-posed problems in computational vision," *J. Am. Stat. Assoc.* **82**, 76-89 (1987).

[20] C. Bouman and K. Sauer, "A generalized Gaussian image model for edge-preserving MAP estimation," *IEEE Trans. Image Proc.* **2**, 296-310 (1993).

[21] M. Soumekh, "Binary image reconstruction from four projections," In *Proc. IEEE Int'l Conf. Acoust., Speech and Sig. Proc.*, (IEEE, New York), pp. 1280-1283, 1988.

[22] J. M. Dinten, "Tomographie à partir d'un nombre très limité de projections, regularisation par des champs markoviens," *Doctoral Thesis, University of Paris XI* (1990).

[23] C. Klifa and B. Lavayssière, "3D reconstruction using a limited number of projections," In *Proc. SPIE Conf. Vis. Comm. and Im. Proc.*, (SPIE, Bellingham, WA), pp. 443-454, 1990.

[24] J. L. Sachs, Jr. and K. Sauer, "Object-oriented methods in Bayesian 3-D tomographic reconstruction from radiographs," In *Proc. 36th Midwest Symp. Circ. and Sys.*, (IEEE, Piscataway, NJ), pp. 241-244, 1993.

[25] C. Klifa, "Reconstruction tridimensionelle d'objets à partir d'un nombre très limité de projections: Application à la radiographie industrielle," *Ph.D. Thesis, Telecom Paris* (1991).

Chapter 17

Heart Chamber Reconstruction from Biplane Angiography

Dietrich G.W. Onnasch[1]
Guido P.M. Prause[2]

ABSTRACT In this chapter we describe an application of the binary tomography technique to routinely acquired biplane cardiac angiograms. The described model-based reconstruction approach aims to recover the 3D shape of the left or right heart chamber from the density profiles of orthogonal biplane ventriculograms. Several geometric and densitometric imaging errors need to be corrected in the clinical data before the moving heart chamber may be reconstructed slice-by-slice and frame-by-frame. The ventricular reconstructions allow for 3D visualization, volume determination, and regional wall motion analysis independently of the gantry setting used for image acquisition. The method has been applied to clinical angiograms and tested in left and right ventricular phantoms yielding a well shape conformity even with few model information. The results indicate that volumes of binary reconstructed ventricles are less projection-dependent compared to volume data derived by purely contour-based methods.

17.1   Introduction

In the clinical routine, the information content of digital biplane angiograms is often utilized to only a small extent. Biplane ventriculograms are mostly judged qualitatively by the cardiologists. Quantitative results such as diameters and volume data or contraction pattern analysis are based on silhouettes in the projection images without having knowledge of the actual 3D structure of the examined ventricle. One major goal of the work presented in this chapter was to exploit the potential of quantitative biplane angiography more completely by combining the geometric and densitometric information of the two views.

The described reconstruction approach aims to recover the 3D shape

---

[1]University of Kiel, Department for Pediatric Cardiology and Biomedical Engineering, Schwanenweg 20, D-24105 Kiel, Germany, E-mail: onnasch@pedcard.uni-kiel.de

[2]University of Bremen, MeVis – Center for Medical Diagnostic Systems and Visualization, Universitätsallee 29, D-28359 Bremen, Germany, E-mail: prause@mevis.de

of the left or right heart chamber from the density profiles of orthogonal biplane ventriculograms. After reconstruction, 3D visualization in different orientations is possible, new projection images and cross sections can be calculated, and the ventricular volume may be computed independently of the biplane view used for image acquisition. For a fully reconstructed cardiac cycle, the regional 3D wall motion can be analyzed, which may be helpful for an early detection of myocardial ischemia and infarction.

When applying binary tomography to images obtained from routine biplane angiography, an important problem is the deviation of the real input data from ideal projection data. As a result, this chapter deals not only with the pure algorithmic aspects of the reconstruction but also with the techniques of image acquisition and restoration as well as a proper preparation of the input data. Finally, results are presented from clinical ventriculograms.

17.2   Cardiac X-ray angiography

17.2.1   Image recording and processing

Cardiac X-ray angiography is a well-established method for examining congenital and acquired heart diseases. During the last two decades the technical equipment of the heart catheterization laboratory has been fundamentally improved — among other things — by the introduction of flexible multiaxial gantries and real time digital storage of the angiographic image series [1]. For the representation of the beating left or right ventricle a short bolus of contrast medium is injected through a catheter by a power injector while X-ray images are recorded with 12.5 to 60 images per second. The image chain consists of the X-ray tube, an anti-scatter grid, an electronic image intensifier, a television camera, an analog/digital converter and an image acquisition computer. The acquired image series, so-called cardiac angiograms, ventriculograms, or arteriograms, can be taken simultaneously in two planes with alternating pulsed radiation to reduce cross-scatter between the two image chains. For the techniques described here, we assume that the two X-ray projections are adjusted perpendicular to each other, the rotational angles as well as the distances between X-ray tube and image screen being recorded together with the angiogram. Typically, the images are stored at a resolution of $512 \times 512 \times 8$ bit.

Several techniques of image enhancement and restoration are available at the acquisition computer platform. As we are evaluating the projections of the opacified ventricle one important step is to remove all other structures from the images. This is done by subtracting an image before contrast injection from the images after contrast injection. Ideally, the gray values are now linearly related to the mass of the dye within the ventricle, and — assuming a homogeneous dye concentration — the relation is also linear with the penetrated volume.

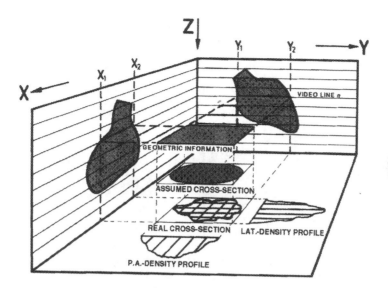

FIGURE 17.1. Shadow and densitometric information obtainable from orthogonal projections of a left ventricle for every video-line of a biplane X-ray angiogram. In the scheme parallel projection is assumed.

17.2.2 Quantitative biplane angiography

At the medical workstation, quantitative evaluations of angiograms are accessible to the cardiologist. These include quantification of coronary stenotic lesions and volume determination of the cardiac chambers and the myocardial mass. In addition, when the gray level information of ventriculograms is quantified in end-diastolic and end-systolic images the regurgitation of insufficient cardiac valves can be assessed by relating the regurgitating blood volume to the forward stroke volume. These methods are mostly applied to monoplane angiograms.

Less common are combined evaluations of biplane angiograms. Based on the geometric image information alone, quantitative biplane angiography (QBA) allows for the calculation of length and direction of the main axes of the heart in the thorax, the three-dimensional reconstruction of the coronary artery tree, and an improved calculation of the ventricular volume. For cross sections obtained from left ventricular casts [2], Fig. 17.2 presents some correction factors, which have to be applied when the cross-sectional area of the ventricle is calculated from the ventricular silhouette. In cardiology, often the so-called multiple-slices method is used for ventricular volume determination, whereby the sum over elliptical cross sections are multiplied by an averaged correction factor [3,4].

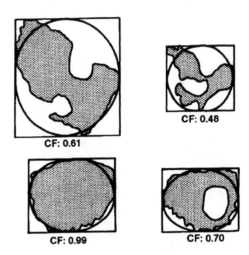

FIGURE 17.2. Typical end-systolic and end-diastolic left ventricular cross sections. The papillary muscles may lead to wholes or semicircular notches. The correction factors (CF) give the relation between the actual areas and the areas of the inscribed ellipses.

If the image intensity is utilized as an additional source of information, spatial assessment of the myocardial perfusion is possible, as well as the subject of this chapter: the reconstruction of the ventricular shape by use of binary tomography. In order to apply this technique to biplane ventricular angiograms, the following assumptions are made:

1. The biplane angiograms of the examined heart chamber are taken simultaneous and orthogonal to each other.

2. The contrast agent is evenly and completely distributed within each reconstructed ventricular cross section.

3. The heart chamber is not overlapped by other opacified structures, e.g., the aorta, the pulmonary artery, or the myocardium.

The ventricular contours are detected and the 3D shape of the heart chamber is reconstructed as a stack of binary slices from the biplane density profiles (Fig. 17.1).

However, clinical angiograms differ considerably from ideal projection data. The geometric and densitometric information of the images is degraded by several sources of error. The greater part of these errors — e.g., geometric distortion, scatter, and noise — is based on radiation physics and technical imperfections of the imaging system [1]. Others are caused by shortcomings of the angiographic visualization procedure such as incomplete dye filling and subtraction artifacts. To enable a binary reconstruction from routinely acquired angiograms, it is necessary to find robust and effective solutions to these inaccuracies.

17.3 Binary tomography

17.3.1 The problem

The problem of reconstructing a binary matrix from its column and row projections has attracted the attention of researchers for many years. Fundamental work on this topic was done in the late 1950s by the combinatorial mathematician Ryser [5]. The employment of the binary tomography approach for the 3D shape recovery of the heart chambers from two orthogonal angiograms was first proposed by Chang and Chow in 1973 [6]. To date, in the field of cardiology, a variety of algorithms have been published aiming at the reconstruction of either ventricular or coronary cross sections [6] — [16].

Consider two corresponding density profiles from a pair of orthogonal biplane angiograms, given by the column and row sums a_j and b_k. From the mathematical point of view, reconstructing the related real cross section is that of finding an assignment for $m \times n$ binary variables $x_{kj} \in \{0, 1\}$ solving a system of $m + n$ linear equations

$$\sum_{k=1}^{m} x_{kj} = a_j \, , \qquad \sum_{j=1}^{n} x_{kj} = b_k, \qquad (17.1)$$

where $j = 1, \ldots, n$ and $k = 1, \ldots, m$ under the restriction

$$\sum_{j=1}^{n} a_j = \sum_{k=1}^{m} b_k \, . \qquad (17.2)$$

Obviously, the problem is underestimated and ill-posed, i.e., Hadamard's conditions (existence, uniqueness, and continuity of the solution) are not fulfilled. As discussed extensively in the early chapters of this book, you may find exactly one, more than one, or no binary matrix satisfying a given pair of projection vectors (a, b). Ryser [5] introduced the most elementary projection-preserving operation on a binary matrix, the so-called *interchange* or *switching operation*, which allows to generate new solutions of a binary tomography problem from a given one. Generally, a binary 3D object is not uniquely determined by a pair of orthogonal 2D projection images. Especially for roughly symmetrically objects, there are different orientations producing nearly the same projection images. To overcome this problem of ambiguity, it is necessary to provide additional information about the heart chamber's shape and orientation. The algorithms mentioned above do this by introducing either geometric restrictions [6, 10, 11, 13] or by incorporating a priori knowledge [7–9, 12, 14]. Since real ventricular cross sections (Fig. 17.2) do not follow the required geometric constraints (symmetry, convexity, regularity etc.) algorithms of the second category should be preferred. The reconstruction program described in this work employs the model-based approach of Onnasch and Heintzen [8].

17.3.2 Probability-driven reconstruction

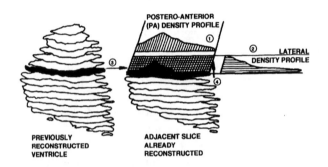

FIGURE 17.3. Information used in reconstructing the ventricle slice by slice. At the beginning of the reconstruction process, the earlier reconstructed slices are replaced by slices of a suitable ventricular model.

Contextual information may be incorporated into to the reconstruction approach if we consider not only isolated slices but also slices being adjacent in space or in time. This idea is illustrated in Fig. 17.3 for a right ventricle. As a first step of reconstruction problem we calculate for each element in rectangular array defined by the two density profiles the probability of belonging to the cross section. This probability is derived from the two profiles, from the beneath slice already reconstructed, and from the slice at the same location of the ventricle in the previously reconstructed state of contraction or relaxation. Based on the overall probability, the binary array is filled in a second step heeding that the row and column sums do not exceed the width of the respective profile.

As illustrated by the flow chart in Fig. 17.4, the binary reconstruction of the i-th ventricular cross section $B_{t,i}$ at phase t is based on the product $W_{t,i}$ of three probability arrays. The first one, the fundamental probability array $F_{t,i}$, is the outer product of the density profiles $a_{t,i}$ and $b_{t,i}$ being weighted by a 2D ramp filter to counteract the tendency of hiding holes inside the reconstructed cross sections. The other two probability arrays $T_{t,i}$ and $S_{t,i}$ strengthen the similarity of the slice to be reconstructed to the temporally and spatially adjacent binary slices $B_{t-1,i}$ and $B_{t,i-1}$. Nonexistent adjacent

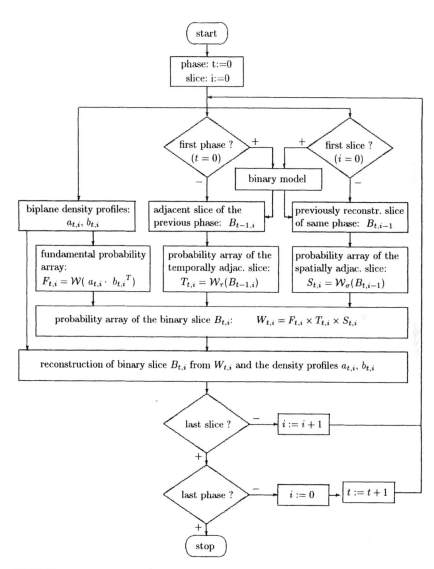

FIGURE 17.4. Flow chart of the model-based algorithm. The ventricular model is used only for the first cardiac phase ($t = 0$). For all following phases, the binary reconstruction of the preceding phase serves as a model. The ventricle is reconstructed slice by slice ($i := i + 1$) by setting the most probable elements provided the row and column sums do not exceed $a_{t,i}$ and $b_{t,i}$.

slices are substituted by the ventricular 3D model, which is previously rotated according to the gantry setting used for image acquisition.

The influence of the neighboring slices on the currently reconstructed slice $B_{t,i}$ is controlled by two weighting parameters τ and σ, respectively. The probability arrays $T_{t,i} = W_\tau(B_{t-1,i})$ and $S_{t,i} = W_\sigma(B_{t,i-1})$ are calculated from the temporally and spatially adjacent slices $B_{t-1,i}$ and $B_{t,i-1}$ as follows. The elements of the Gaussian-shaped 5×5 mask

$$M = \begin{pmatrix} .99 & .96 & .93 & .96 & .99 \\ .96 & .82 & .70 & .82 & .96 \\ .93 & .70 & .52 & .70 & .93 \\ .96 & .82 & .70 & .82 & .96 \\ .99 & .96 & .93 & .96 & .99 \end{pmatrix} \qquad (17.3)$$

are raised to the power of τ or σ, respectively, with $\tau, \sigma \geq 0$. In the binary arrays $B_{t-1,i}$ and $B_{t,i-1}$, each entry of value one is then successively multiplied with the masks M^τ and M^σ, respectively. Finally, the elements of the resulting matrices are multiplied with a factor of 10 and raised to the power of -1. The resulting probability arrays $T_{t,i}$ and $S_{t,i}$ are blurred versions of the adjacent slices $B_{t-1,i}$ and $B_{t,i-1}$. Setting the weighting parameters τ and σ to zero results into matrices $T_{t,i}$ and $S_{t,i}$ of ones and the combined probability array $W_{t,i}$ equals the fundamental probability array $F_{t,i}$. For values of τ and σ greater than zero, the impact of the neighboring slices on the slice under reconstruction increases exponentially.

Controlled by the total probability array $W_{t,i} = F_{t,i} \times T_{t,i} \times S_{t,i}$, the binary slice $B_{t,i}$ is filled up in two passes from the center to the periphery. In the first pass, the most probable elements are set from the centre to the peripheral alternatively for rows and columns. In the second pass, the borderline pixels are also filled; they must be connected to first-pass pixels to reduce the roughness of the slice contour. At each single step, the zero pixel of highest probability is switched to one only if the column and row projections do not exceed the density profiles $a_{t,i}$ and $b_{t,i}$. With the filling algorithm used, connected binary slices are favored but holes and small islands are reconstructed as well [8, 15, 16].

17.4   Input data restoration

A proper matching of corresponding density profiles in biplane X-ray projections requires an accurate correction of geometric image distortions both within and between both views. A correction method that is usable in the clinical routine must not disturb the work of the cathlab team. Thus, approaches based on periodically recorded calibration phantoms were not considered. Furthermore, the method should be fully automatic, robust, and capable of handling distortions that are changing with the gantry setting.

The main source for geometric distortions in the imaging chain is the image intensifier [17]. Depending on the manufacturer, the installation, and the selected field of view of the image intensifier, image intensifiers show different types of distortion [18] such as displacement, radial stretching caused by the curvature of the input phosphor (pincushion distortion) as well as twisting and S-shaped distortion due to geomagnetism and superimposed local magnetic fields. The amount of the last type of distortion depends on the orientation of the image intensifier relative to the magnetic field vector. A moving C-arm with a cm-grid attached to its image intensifier input screen shows a systematically rotating and shifting X-ray image [19].

The application of the binary tomography technique to biplane angiograms requires the determination of the ventricular contours and the calculation of corresponding density profiles in the two views. Both tasks are complicated due to the divergent X-ray geometry, image rotation, and inaccuracies of the gantry system. Therefore, an image pairing procedure was developed that offers a standardized biplane display of paired angiograms in order to simplify combined evaluations [15, 16, 19, 20].

First, the magnification of the geometrically corrected images is equalized utilizing the source-image intensifier-distances (SIDs) and effective pixel sizes of both imaging planes, and assuming the ventricle to be located at the isocentre. An absolute cm-scale related to the isocentre allows measurements of calibrated distances.

Next, the image rotation caused by angulations of the biplane gantry system is analyzed and compensated. A projection $A = (\alpha, \beta)$ is uniquely determined by the angle of rotation $\alpha \in (-180°, 180°)$ and the angle of angulation (or skew) $\beta \in (-90°, 90°)$. A biplane projection is determined by $A = (\alpha, \beta)$ and $B = (\gamma, \delta)$. For non-angulated biplane projections $A = (\alpha, 0°)$ / $B = (\gamma, 0°)$, e.g., frontal/lateral ($\alpha = 0°$ and $\gamma = 90°$) or right anterior oblique (RAO) / left anterior oblique (LAO) ($\alpha = -30°$ and $\gamma = 60°$), the central scan lines of both image coordinate systems lie within the so-called *isocentre plane* [20] or *meridional plane* [21] spanned by the two projection axes. In this case, the isocentre plane defines the patient's transversal plane (yz-plane) and corresponds to the central row of the two digitized image matrices.

For angulated biplane projections ($\beta \neq 0$ or $\delta \neq 0$), however, the isocentre plane is rotated out of the central matrix row in at least one view [19]. This image rotation is misleading for a human observer and a source of errors in identification and matching of corresponding structures in biplane angiograms. Therefore, the images of angulated biplane views are always rotated back and displayed in a non-rotated way with the isocentre plane at the central row of each image matrix (see upper panel of Fig. 17.6). The rotation angles ρ_A, ρ_B of both views are calculated directly from the angles of rotation and angulation $\alpha, \beta, \gamma, \delta$ depending on the equipment types of the two C-arm units [16, 19].

The three steps of image pairing — correction of geometric distortions, adjustment of magnification, and rotation — are performed simultaneously and fully automatically in a single bilinear transform. This reduces the number of spatial resamplings and gray value interpolations needed for each image to one, which increases both the speed and the accuracy of the calculation. The next step, the determination of corresponding density profiles in both planes (*epipolar lines*), however, requires user interaction, since small inaccuracies of the isocentric gantry system cause several unpredictable errors concerning the alignment of biplane images [19, 22]. The reasons for these inaccuracies are variations of the imaging parameters (SIDs, projection angles) around the measured values and deviations of the projection axes from the theoretically claimed isocentre (skew) [22]. Owing the relatively large size of the imaged object, ventricular angiograms are mainly affected by the skew, which results in a noticeable displacement of the biplane images. In order to compensate for this displacement error, the user must define a fixed vertical offset between the epipolar lines of both planes to make the lines coincide at clearly discernible reference points, e.g., the apex of the ventricle or the tip of the catheter [16].

17.5   Implemented algorithm

Before the gray values of routinely acquired biplane angiograms may be used as input for a binary tomography algorithm, the raw image data have to pass several phases of image correction and processing. The developed reconstruction program consists of three major parts: image pre-processing, binary ventricular reconstruction, and post-processing of the 3D ventricle. The following description provides an overview of the entire reconstruction process.

17.5.1   Pre-processing

Images digitized with a linear or *white compression* look-up table have to be logarithmically converted after acquisition, to obtain a linear relationship between gray values and X-ray absorption. For systems with a nonlinear density transfer function, an additional correction of the gray scale is necessary [1].

After selecting a cardiac cycle for 3D reconstruction, suitable pre-injection images for mask mode subtraction are determined. The images are reduced in spatial and gray-level resolution to reduce random noise. In case of poor contrast mixing, the weighted average of up to three consecutive pre- and post-injection angiograms may be taken to improve the dye homogeneity within the ventricle. The subtracted images are paired as discussed in the previous section. Each image pair of the cardiac cycle is loaded into the graphical interface for determination of the ventricular contours [15, 16].

Pixel values outside the ventricular contours are set to zero. The displacement of the images is compensated by a matrix shift. Now, the centers of gravity of the paired images should be located on epipolar lines representing the same reconstruction plane. In the geometrically corrected images, the density profiles are sampled along the epipolar lines using bilinear interpolation. The sampled values form the rows of the so-called *profile matrices*.

The profile matrices are densitometrically adjusted in two steps. This is necessary since different tube voltages, X-ray and light scatter as well as subtraction artifacts cause deviations of the integral values of the biplane density profiles (see eq. 17.2). After being globally adjusted to the same total value using linear regression, each pair of profiles is locally equalized to its average row sum [15].

The final pre-processing step is the scaling of the noncalibrated gray values to the spatial resolution (number of voxels) of the binary tomography cube. Since the concentration of dye in actual ventriculograms is generally not known and varies between apical and valvular cross sections, a slice-oriented scaling method was developed. This method assumes a homogeneous dye concentration not for the whole cavity but only within each reconstructed cross section. From the density profiles a_i, b_i and the ventricular model, a scaling factor s_i is calculated for each slice of the reconstruction cube

$$s_i = \min\left(\frac{l_{b_i}\, f_{b_i}}{\max(a_i)}, \frac{l_{a_i}\, f_{a_i}}{\max(b_i)}\right) , \qquad (17.4)$$

where $\max(a_i), \max(b_i)$ denote the maximum values of the density profiles and l_{a_i}, l_{b_i} their width in voxel. The factors $f_{a_i}, f_{b_i} \in (0, 1]$ represent the ratios between maximum value and width in the respective binary model slice. Equation (17.4) assures that $s_i \max(a_i) \leq l_{b_i}\, f_{b_i}$ and $s_i \max(b_i) \leq l_{a_i}\, f_{a_i}$ with equality in one of both relations.

17.5.2 Ventricular reconstruction

The algorithm of Onnasch and Heintzen [8], used for binary tomography in our program, largely reduces the ambiguity of the problem by incorporating a priori knowledge of the ventricle. In addition to the orthogonal density profiles, the similarity of cross sections adjacent in time or space is exploited. For the reconstruction of the first cardiac phase and the first slice of each phase, one of four ventricular 3D models is used. These binary models of size $64 \times 64 \times 64$ represent the averaged casts of 21 left and 22 right human ventricles in end-systole and end-diastole [2]. The resulting object was scaled to fill an isotropic cube of $128 \times 128 \times 128$ voxels, a spatial resolution that turned out to be a good compromise between a reduction of dye inhomogeneities and random noise and an adequate spatial accuracy.

17.5.3 Post-processing

The voxels of the binary data cube representing the reconstructed ventricle are resampled back to the epipolar lines. The surface of the binary ventricle is smoothed by applying a 3D morphological operation (an *opening* followed by a *closing*) with an isotropic ball structuring element of size $3 \times 3 \times 3$ [15]. For detection of isolated regions, the connected components of the reconstruction are calculated.

Finally, the result is analyzed and rendered as wire-frame or shaded surface object, allowing a free choice of the viewing point. If the reconstruction was carried out over a full cardiac cycle, the 3D contraction pattern of the ventricle can be displayed and studied in real time [23].

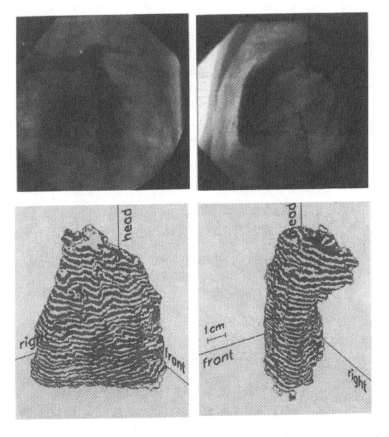

FIGURE 17.5. Posterior and lateral views of an end-diastolic right ventricle. Upper panels: the recorded angiographic projections, lower panels: the result of reconstruction in a wire frame representation.

17.6   Results

17.6.1   Patient data

The method was applied to several biplane angiograms that were recorded for diagnostic or interventional reasons in the clinical routine. The results for a right (RV) and a left ventricle (LV) are presented as examples.

The aim of the RV examination was to ensure the diagnosis of a suspected ventricular septum defect in a pediatric patient (10.9 kg). The images were recorded in the cranial/lateral-projection with 90 cm (A)/100 cm (B) SID, 17 cm field of view and 68 kVp (A)/78 kVp (B) the tube voltage. 18 ml contrast agent (Iopamidol 370) with a flow of 14 ml/s was injected into the RV via a balloon catheter. Figure 17.5 (upper panels) shows the end-diastolic biplane images used for reconstruction.

The LV image data were taken from a pediatric patient (9.2 kg), who was examined to check the result of a balloon dilatation applied to an aortic re-stenosis. For image acquisition, the gantry system was brought in the orthogonal angulated views $A = (-16°, 19°)$, $B = (70°, -29°)$ with SID of 88 cm (plane A) and 98 cm (plane B). The field of views of the image intensifiers were 14 cm. Using a pigtail catheter, 15 ml contrast agent with a flow of 12 ml/s was injected into the LV. The end-systolic images used for reconstruction are displayed in Fig. 17.6 after the first steps of pre-processing.

Both ventricles were binary reconstructed over a full cardiac cycle consisting of twelve (RV) and eleven (LV) biplane images with a temporal resolution of 40 ms. All images were first pre-processed as mentioned above and then interpolated to 128×128 matrices. For the reconstruction of the first cardiac phase (end-systole), the ventricular models were used. For the following phases, the previously reconstructed binary ventricles served as a model. During the whole reconstruction process, the weighting parameters were fixed to $\tau = 0.8$ and $\sigma = 1.0$. Results of reconstruction are given in the Figs. 17.5 and 17.6 in wire frame and shaded surface representations.

Absolute volume data were derived by multiplying the voxel volume of the reconstructed ventricle with the third power of the isocenter-related voxel size (0.71 mm for LV, 0.82 mm for RV). In Table 17.1, the LV and RV volume data determined with the binary reconstruction approach (BR) are compared with the results of the multiple-slices (MS) and area length method (AL). The listed values are: end-systolic volume (ESV), end-diastolic volume (EDV), stroke volume ($SV = EDV - ESV$) and ejection fraction ($EF = SV/EDV$). Whereas no further scaling was used for BR, phase dependent correction factors < 1 were applied to the volumes MS and AL determined from the size of the ventricular silhouette alone.

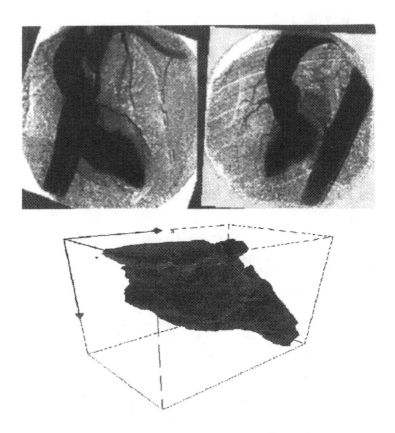

FIGURE 17.6. For an end-systolic left ventricle, the upper panel presents the orthogonal angiographic projections after mask mode subtraction, equalizing of magnification and compensation of image rotation. In the lower panel the result of binary reconstruction is given in a shaded surface representation.

Volume	LV			RV		
Data	BR	MS	AL	BR	MS	AL
ESV[ml]	7.6	(.55) 5.9	(.60) 5.5	13.7	(.50) 9.3	(.54) 9.8
EDV[ml]	21.3	(.72) 17.4	(.80) 16.9	34.0	(.58) 23.1	(.62) 24.7
SV[ml]	13.7	11.5	11.4	20.3	13.8	14.9
EF	0.64	0.66	0.67	0.60	0.60	0.60

TABLE 17.1. Left (LV) and right ventricular (RV) volume data derived with the binary reconstruction approach (BR), the multiple-slices (MS), and the area length method (AL). The correction factors used for MS and AL are based on the cast studies of [3, 4] and listed in parentheses.

17.6.2   Ventricular phantoms

The complete approach was tested in different phantom studies using regular-shaped test objects as well as left and right ventricular phantoms of known volume. To quantify the results *shape conformity* and *volume conformity* were calculated, which are the absolute differences of voxels or volumes, respectively, related to the average volume, minus 100% [15, 16].

The ventricular phantoms were projected in four orientations and the results of reconstruction were compared mutually. Without a model, the reconstructions of the left ventricular phantom showed a shape conformity of $87.2 \pm 1.9\%$ and a volume conformity of $98 \pm 1.4\%$ on the average. Using a model, there was only little improvement. The right ventricular phantom was reconstructed with a mean shape conformity of only $58.5 \pm 10.9\%$ and a volume conformity of $93.7 \pm 3.9\%$ when no model was used. Using a poor model, the two conformity values increased to $77.9 \pm 4.8\%$ and $96 \pm 3.2\%$, respectively.

Compared to the water displacement volume (71 ml), the reconstructed LV volume data (68 to 70.9 ml) was nearly the same (69 ± 1.3 ml). However, for the RV phantom the reconstructed volume data were between 78 and 89.3 ml with an overestimation of 17% on the average.

17.7   Discussion

We have demonstrated that it is possible to reconstruct the 3D shape of cardiovascular structures from high-quality, biplane X-ray angiograms. Slump and Gerbrands [9] and Pellot *et al.* [14] also developed algorithms for binary reconstruction of vascular structures that consider both a priori information and the resemblance between adjacent slices. An important difference to our approach is their assumption of an evenly distributed contrast density within the entire segment under study. This may be true for certain peripheral structures but based on our experience not for the heart chambers or vessels close to the heart. In addition, the reconstruction algorithm proposed by Pellot *et al.* is based on simulated annealing, which needs several iterations leading to execution times of several seconds per slice. Our algorithm is so fast, that — in the interest of saving storage space — the pre-processed densitometric profiles may be stored instead of the reconstructed binary arrays.

For the application of the presented approach in cardiology two conditions must be fulfilled: a binary data base of typical ventricular cross sections and an analysis of the density transfer function of the X-ray equipment. The data base is utilized in a twofold way: first during pre-processing for the assessment of the relative amount of contrast medium in each slice (17.4), which is necessary to scale the binary arrays slice by slice, and second during the process of probability-driven reconstruction to reduce the ambiguity in setting the elements of the binary array (Fig. 17.4). From our experiments with test objects we draw the conclusion that as a rule a rather coarse prototype is sufficient. However, without such a model, the shape conformity may be reduced significantly.

Since the homogeneity of the test objects was close to the optimum, the obtained shape and volume conformities should be taken as upper limits for clinical images. Nevertheless, the application of the method to human in vivo angiograms results into realistic shape reconstructions of single ventricular phases that show a consistent and coherent wall motion in the video animation.

The standard deviations between results of different views indicate that binary reconstructed volumes — especially of right ventricles — are less projection-dependent compared to volume data estimated with the multiple-slices or area length method without correction factors. The absolute volume of the left ventricular phantom was assessed correctly whereas the right ventricular phantom was overestimated by 17% on the average.

For the patients the real values of the ventricular volumes are not known. Compared to the values assessed geometrically from two orthogonal silhouettes in clinical angiograms and corrected by the appropriate correction factors (Table 17.1), the volumes determined by binary tomography seem to overestimate the ventricular size, too. However, the geometric methods AL and MS are affected by a standard deviation of about 10%.

The main reason for an overestimation could be the limited knowledge of the actual distribution of contrast agent inside the cavity. The applied scaling method tries to assess the contrast density slice-by-slice by claiming equality between the maximum density value and the ventricular diameter. As seen from the RV phantom experiments, this strategy may fail particularly for elongated cross sections oriented diagonally to the reconstruction matrix.

With respect to image acquisition, not all requirements are always fulfilled in the clinical setting. The deviation caused by a non-parallel projection can normally be neglected [15]. The limitation arising from an unevenly or incomplete contrast mixing within the reconstructed cross sections is more severe. Although not applied to the images used in this work, the dye-homogeneity of poor quality angiograms may be improved by averaging two or three consecutive frames. However, frame averaging introduces motion blur and tends to underestimate end-diastolic and overestimate end-systolic volumes.

Another prerequisite is that the heart chamber must not be superimposed by other opacified structures. That means, that the biplane orthogonal projection must be selected carefully and that no mitral or tricuspidal regurgitation is present. As a rule, cranially or caudally skewed projections must be used for an optimal angiographic visualization.

Despite of these limitations, the probability-driven reconstruction program allows the recovery of the dynamic 3D shape of the left or right heart chamber from routine biplane angiograms. Independent of the gantry setting used for image acquisition, the reconstructed ventricle may be analyzed in space and time. This is a big advantage compared to the conventional methods of 2D ventricular volume determination or contraction pattern analysis.

The information about the heart chamber's 3D morphology and function is obtained without additional burden to the patient and without recourse to modern volume image modalities such as ECG-gated magnetic resonance imaging, electron beam computed tomography or 3D echocardiography.

Acknowledgment

This work was partly supported by the Deutsche Forschungsgemeinschaft (DFG) under the grant On 8/1.

References

[1] K.-F. Kamm and D. G. W. Onnasch, "X-ray radiography," In P. Lanzer and M. Lipton, *Vascular Diseases: Principles and Technology*, (Springer-Verlag, Berlin), pp. 63-98, 1997.

[2] P. E. Lange, D. G. W. Onnasch, F. L. Farr, V. Malerczyk, and P. H. Heintzen, "Analysis of left and right ventricular size and shape, as determined from human casts. Description of the method and its validation," *Europ. J. Card.* **8**, 431-448 (1978).

[3] P. E. Lange, D. G. W. Onnasch, F. L. Farr, and P. H. Heintzen, "Angiocardiographic left ventricular volume determination. Accuracy, as determined from human casts, and clinical application," *Europ. J. Card.* **8**, 449-476 (1978).

[4] P. E. Lange, D. G. W. Onnasch, F. L. Farr, and P. H. Heintzen, "Angiocardiographic right ventricular volume determination. Accuracy, as determined from human casts, and clinical application," *Europ. J. Card.* **8**, 477-501 (1978).

[5] H. J. Ryser, "The combinatorial properties of matrices of zeros and ones," *Canad. J. Math.* **9**, 371-377 (1957).

[6] S.-K. Chang and C. K. Chow, "The reconstruction of three-dimensional objects from two orthogonal projections and its application to cardiac cineangiography," *IEEE Trans. Comp.* **C-22**, 18-28 (1973).

[7] G. T. Herman, "Reconstruction of binary patterns from a few projections," In A. Günther, B. Levrat, and H. Lipps, *International Computing Symposium 1973*, (North-Holland Publ. Co., Amsterdam), pp. 371-378, 1974.

[8] D. G. W. Onnasch and P. H. Heintzen, "A new approach for the reconstruction of the right or left ventricular form from biplane angiocardiographic recordings," In *Conf. Comp. Card. 1976*, (IEEE Comp. Soc. Press, Washington), pp. 67-73, 1976.

[9] C. H. Slump and J. J. Gerbrands, "A network flow approach to reconstruction of the left ventricle from two projections," *Comp. Graph. Im. Proc.* **18**, 18-36 (1982).

[10] A. Kuba, "The reconstruction of two-directionally connected binary patterns from their two orthogonal projections," *Comp. Vis. Graph. Im. Proc.* **27**, 249-265 (1984).

[11] R. O. Kenet, E. M. Herrold, J. P. Hill, J. Waltman, A. Diamond, P. Fenster, J. Barba, M. Suardiaz, and J. S. Borer, "Reconstruction of coronary cross-sections from two orthogonal digital angiograms," *Conf. Comp. Card. 1986*, (IEEE Comp. Soc. Press, Washington), pp. 273-276, 1987.

[12] Y. Bao, "A pyramidal approach to three-dimensional reconstruction of a vascular system from two projections," *Conf. Comp. Ass. Rad. CAR'89 Berlin*, Springer-Verlag, Berlin, pp. 317-321 (1989).

[13] Z. D. Bai, P. R. Krishnaiah, C. R. Rao, P. S. Reddy, Y. N. Sun, and L. C. Zhao, "Reconstruction of the left ventricle from two orthogonal projections," *Comp. Vis. Graph. Im. Proc.* **47**, 165-188 (1989).

[14] C. Pellot, A. Herment, M. Sigelle, P. Horain, H. Maître, and P. Peronneau, "A 3D reconstruction of vascular structures from two X-ray angiograms using an adapted simulated annealing algorithm," *IEEE Trans. Med. Imag.* **13**, 48-60 (1994).

[15] G. P. M. Prause, "Binäre Rekonstruktion der dreidimensionalen dynamischen Ventrikelgeometrie aus biplanen angiokardiographischen Bildserien," *Fortschritt-Bericht 121, Reihe 17 (Biotechnik)*, (VDI-Verlag, Düsseldorf), 1995.

[16] G. P. M. Prause and D. G. W. Onnasch, "Binary reconstruction of the heart chambers from biplane angiographic image sequences," *IEEE Trans. Med. Imag.* **15**, 532-46 (1997).

[17] J. M. Boone, J. A. Seibert, W. A. Barrett, and E. A. Blood, "Analysis and correction of imperfections in the image intensifier-TV-digitizer imaging chain," *Med. Phys.* **8**, 236-242 (1991).

[18] S. Rudin, D. R. Bednarek, and R. Wong, "Accurate characterization of image intensifier distortion," *Med. Phys.* **18**, 1145-1151 (1991).

[19] D. G. W. Onnasch and G. P. M. Prause, "Geometric image correction and iso-center calibration at oblique biplane angiographic views," In *Conf. Comp. Card. 1992*, (IEEE Comp. Soc. Press, Los Alamitos), pp. 647-650, 1992.

[20] G. P. M. Prause and D. G. W. Onnasch, "Biplane angiocardiography: General solution for pairing images taken from oblique views," In *Comp. Ass. Rad. CAR'93*, (Springer-Verlag, Berlin), pp. 547-552, 1993.

[21] H. P. Trivedi, "A semi-analytic method of determining stereo camera geometry from matched points in a pair of images: Coincident meridional planes, exact or noisy data," *Comp. Vis. Graph. Im. Proc.* **51**, 299-312 (1990).

[22] A. Wahle, E. Wellnhofer, I. Mugaragu, H.U. Sauer, H. Oswald, and E. Fleck, "Assessment of diffuse coronary artery disease by quantitative analysis of coronary morphology based upon 3-D reconstruction from biplane angiograms," *IEEE Trans. Med. Imag.* **14**, 230-241 (1995).

[23] O. Stützer and D. G. W. Onnasch, "Visualisierung der linken Herzkammer nach ihrer Binärrekonstruktion aus biplanen angiographischen Bildserien zur räumlichen Analyse des Kontraktionsablaufs," *Biomedizinische Technik* **41**, suppl. 1, 634-635 (1996).

Chapter 18

Discrete Tomography in Electron Microscopy

J. M. Carazo[1]
C. O. Sorzano[2]
E. Rietzel[3]
R. Schröder[4]
R. Marabini[5]

ABSTRACT *Structural biology is a very fast evolving field that provides key information to understand how biological processes happen in the cell. In essence, its aim is to obtain the three-dimensional structure of biological macromolecules, and then help to establish a link between structure and function. Among the different techniques that provide this three-dimensional information, in this chapter we will concentrate on the one normally referred to as* Three-dimensional Electron Microscopy *(3D EM), which provides information in the resolution range of between 0.5 to about 4 nanometers of protein and of complexes of proteins and nucleic acids by a process of three-dimensional reconstruction from projections. We seek to obtain information at the highest possible resolution level, and to this end we work toward incorporating into the reconstruction process as much experimental as well as* a priori *information as possible. This work is an assessment of the physical considerations that lead us to believe that discrete tomography has a role to play in this field, identifying the main problems to be addressed and the range of possible applications.*

[1]Centro Nacional de Biotecnología Campus Universidad Autónoma de Madrid, 28049 Madrid, Spain, E-mail: carazo@cnb.uam.es

[2]Centro Nacional de Biotecnología Campus Universidad Autónoma de Madrid, 28049 Madrid, Spain, E-mail: coss@cnb.uam.es

[3]MPI für med. Forschung, Jahnstr. 29, 69120 Heidelberg, Germany, E-mail: erietzel@mpimf-heidelberg.mpg.de

[4]MPI für med. Forschung, Jahnstr. 29, 69120 Heidelberg, Germany, E-mail: rasmus.schroeder@mpimf-heidelberg.mpg.de

[5]University of Pennsylvania, Department of Radiology, Medical Image Processing Group, Blockley Hall, Fourth Floor, 423 Guardian Drive, Philadelphia, PA 19104-6021, USA, E-mail: roberto@mipg.upenn.edu

18.1   Introduction

It is our quest as human beings to explore the environment, finding out *how things function*. In fact, one of the great challenges is to know how *we function ourselves*, as well as to understand the processes that regulate life in all its forms. Going to the level of detail, indeed all processes are governed by interatomic interactions, and our quest could then be regarded as ultimately find how these interactions happen and, eventually, how we can interfere with them. Structural biology is a specialty that studies the way biological specimens are built, always aiming at their description at the highest possible resolution, atomic resolution being the final goal.

Traditionally, the bulk of information in structural biology comes from X-ray diffraction studies, exploiting the low wavelength of X-ray photons to explore the biological matter. Some fifteen years ago a new technique started with the advent of two-dimensional (2D) *Nuclear Magnetic Resonance* (NMR). In essence, the two techniques can provide atomic information, although X-rays require three-dimensional (3D) crystals of the specimen under study, and NMR is only suitable for relatively small molecules [1, 2].

A radically different way to approach structural biology studies starts being recognized now, it is the so-called *three-dimensional electron microscopy* (3D EM). The principles are simple: transfer the biological specimen under study into the column of a transmission electron microscope (TEM) while preserving its structural integrity, obtain images of the specimen at different angles and, finally, apply a *reconstruction from projections* approach to obtain an estimation of the original volume of the macromolecule. This last step exploits the fact that — within certain approximations — the TEM images of thin biological samples are 2D projection images of the 3D structure of the specimen.

Even if the principles just described are simple, the control of all the parameters that govern these procedures has been a very difficult task that has attracted much experimental research over the last thirty years [3]. Today the situation is such that the barrier of the 1 nanometer resolution has been already passed in a number of key biological applications, and that in some cases even molecular quasi atomic resolution has been reached [4, 5]. It can then be stated that 3D EM is reaching maturity, and starts providing key 3D structural information in domains unreachable by either X-ray diffraction (due to the lack of 3D crystals) or NMR (due to the relatively large size of the specimens being studied).

However, and in contrast with the way other structural techniques approach the 3D reconstruction problem, 3D EM procedures make very little usage of any *a priori* knowledge about the specimen. In particular, no usage is made of the known biochemical and biophysical differences between the main components that form biological matter, even if they result in distinct differences in the value of the electron density in different areas of the macromolecule. Following this lead, and in the context of discrete tomography, we will assess in this chapter the possibility to use this *a priori* knowledge in the process of 3D reconstruction. It will be our final conclusion that the possibility exists, at least for some key application areas, provided that a number of problems are circumvented. The result of this usage of *a priori* knowledge should be an increase in resolution in the 3D reconstructions that would take us closer to provide definite answers to the way *we — and all biological matter around us — function.*

18.2 3D electron microscopy

The physics behind three-dimensional electron microscopy is conceptually simple. Consider a biological macromolecule in an aqueous environment. In order to visualize this complex under the high vacuum conditions of the transmission electron microscope, it is necessary either to cover the sample with some form of *mask* that stabilizes the sample in the microscope (a common technique is the one known as *negative staining*), or to bring the water environment into a special solid phase, known as *amorphous ice*, a technique usually referred to as *cryo electron microscopy* of vitrified samples. While the usage of masks normally reduces the achievable resolution, cryo electron microscopy has been proved to create a matrix in which the macromolecules are well preserved up to atomic resolution. (Other preparative conditions are also possible, although they are not as widespread as the ones just mentioned.)

Once the sample is in the microscope, a flux of electrons traveling along the optical axis of the microscope goes through the specimen. Under the assumption that the interaction of the electrons with the sample is *weak* (the so-called weak phase object — WPO — approximation), the image that is finally obtained can be regarded as a filtered *projection image*. The image forming model in the microscope then follows the simple equation:

$$G = Filter \otimes (H \cdot F + N), \qquad (18.1)$$

where G refers to the experimental image, F to the *true* specimen structure, H to the projection operator, N to a recording noise (assumed to be Gaussian), *Filter* is a filter function and $\otimes$ means convolution. This function describes the information transfer properties of the microscope largely dependent of the optical parameters of the instrument and the defocus of the image.

There are several possible strategies for data collection as well as 3D reconstruction algorithms that are used in 3D EM (for a review see [6,7]). In very broad terms, we can differentiate between two types of approaches. In the first case the specimen being imaged is considered *unique*, and then the different projection images have to be obtained by tilting the grid inside the microscope with the help of a goniometer. The second case starts from the hypothesis that the specimen under study has not a unique structure, but that — in fact — we have many (typically thousands) of equivalent specimens simultaneously under study. The schema is then to combine images from equivalent specimens as if they were indeed coming from one single specimen, and reconstruct in this way an average structure. In general, the work with *unique* specimens naturally happens when studying large and complex samples like, for instance, whole cellular organelles. On the other hand, when studying macromolecules the hypothesis that they all have the same 3D structure is usually correct.

A consideration that is always present in 3D EM is that the radiation level that the specimen receives should be kept low enough so as not to cause its structural degradation. When we work with large sets of equivalent specimens trying to obtain their average 3D structure, then the electron dose can be very low. Essentially, in this case we only need to obtain one image per specimen, and then thousands of images of equivalent specimens can be combined. Considering this argument in the context of the process of 3D reconstruction, it follows that working with *unique* specimens the number of images cannot be very large (since it is one single specimen that is receiving the cumulative electron dose), while there are no intrinsic limits to the number of images when working with collections of equivalent specimens. Typically we may be dealing with dozens of images in the first case, and with several thousands in the second case.

As far as reconstruction algorithms are concerned, historically the method most used is filtered backprojection with a specially tailored filter function [8], although iterative methods such as forms of SIRT [9] and ART [10] start being used. Also, some forms of maximum entropy algorithms have been used on a few occasions [11]. For the special case of specimen ordered either on 2D crystals or on helices, Fourier-based methods are normally used [3,12]. With respect to incorporating *a priori* information, there has been some exploratory work on the incorporation of constrains on spatial support limits, maximum energy, density intervals, as well as noise-related constrains using Projections Onto Convex Sets [13,14]. However the constraint of spatial support has been used effectively only in a few cases in practice [15], and no practical use of other signal-related constraints has been made so far.

We cannot finish this section without referring to the filter function that affects TEM images. This is a circularly symmetric function, which comes from intrinsic aberrations of the objective lenses, and it is usually referred to in the field as the *Contrast Transfer Function (CTF)*. It has the following approximate form in Fourier space if we assume that the electron beam is monochromatic and coherent [16–26].

$$\chi(\rho) = \sin\left(\pi\lambda\left(\Delta f\,\rho^2 - \frac{1}{2}C_s\,\rho^4\,\lambda^2\right)\right), \qquad (18.2)$$

where ρ is the distance from the origin in Fourier space (referred to in Fig. 18.1 as the frequency), C_s is the microscope spherical aberration coefficient, Δf is the defocus and λ is the electron wavelength. Plots of this function for two different values of Δf are presented in Fig. 18.1.

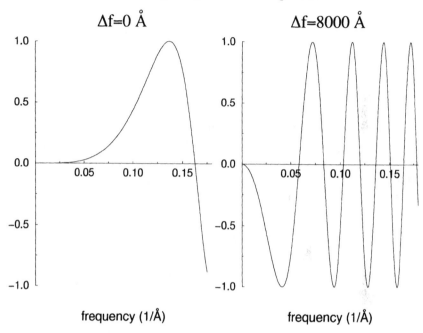

FIGURE 18.1. Contrast transfer function for two defocus values $\Delta f = 0$ Å and $\Delta f = 8000$ Å $C_s = 5.6$ mm. and $\lambda = 0.037$ Å.

In essence, the CTF has an oscillating behavior, and its only free parameters are the defocus Δf and the electron wavelength λ at which the microscope is operated (C_s is set for a given microscope). The way the CTF affects the image signal content is first a destruction of the information at certain frequencies (at the zeros of the CTF) and then a change of the amplitude and sign of the signal image in between alternate zeros. For more general cases in which the WPO approximation is no longer valid, the filter function (especially at low frequencies), becomes extremely difficult to understand, and only a rough approximate parametric model is available [7].

In the rest of this chapter we concentrate our attention to the case of working with ensembles of equivalent specimens under cryo electron microscopy conditions, trying to reach subnanometer resolution. It is our claim that discrete tomography has the capability to make a significant impact on this field, a potential that has not yet been exploited in practice. We review in the next section the main concepts that substantiate this claim, following with an exposition of some of the practical problems that will have to be overcome to solve experimental cases. Finally, we end up with a practical example and the main conclusions.

18.3   Discrete tomography in electron microscopy

When talking about discrete tomography in EM, a key consideration is the biochemical *a priori* knowledge of the specimen, or, in other words, the sample composition. Most biological macromolecules are such that they contain essentially two (protein and ice) or three (protein, ice, and nucleic acid) components. Each of these components has known and distinct biochemical and biophysical properties, including the electron density, which is the physical magnitude that is being measured in TEM images. The path to a discrete tomography application in this area is then to study in detail these differences in electron density between the different components of the macromolecule and the embedding aqueous media, and then use this knowledge to restrict the values in the final 3D reconstruction to those corresponding to these components.

The first step we have performed in this assessment of discrete tomography in 3D EM has been to design a proof-of-concept test aimed at measuring how the biochemical and biophysical differences between ice, protein and nucleic acids are reflected in the voxel values of a volume at a given resolution. To this end we have generated 3D volumes made of ice only, protein only and nucleic acid only. Once these volumes have been generated at atomic resolution, we calculate histograms sampling the volume at different resolutions.

Our tests suggest (Fig. 18.2) that the situation is as follows: at 0.25 nm, ice and protein histograms are slightly separated, while protein and nucleic acid histograms overlap extensively (although their average densities are different). The situation changes at lower resolution and at 0.75 nm ice, protein and nucleic acids histograms present a negligible overlapping.

The net result of the proof-of-concept test discussed in this section is that the range of possible voxel values corresponding to a biological macromolecule that appear when the biochemical and biophysical *a priori* information regarding their constituents is taken into account is indeed limited. The potential to use discrete tomography approaches is therefore a venue to be further explored in experimental cases.

18.4   Considering experimental applications: The problems

We have identified two basic problems to be addressed when considering concrete discrete tomography applications in 3D EM: one comes from the

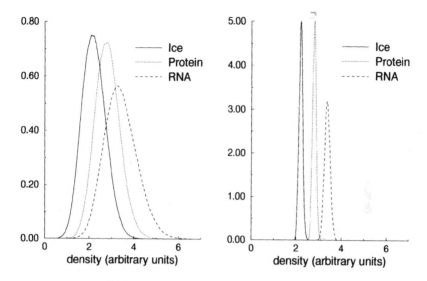

FIGURE 18.2. Histograms of the voxel values corresponding to volumes sampled using voxels of edge length equal to 0.25 nm (left) and 0.75 nm (right) obtained from volumes composed of either only ice or only protein or only RNA.

effect of the CTF on the images, and the other one from the discretization of the electron density values.

18.4.1   The Contrast Transfer Function (CTF)

The first problem, the effect of the CTF, has a key influence on the final reconstruction. This is so because the filter function will affect in a very pronounced way not only the "details" of the reconstruction provided by the high frequencies, but also the average values over large areas of the images that are determined by the low frequencies. Since it is clear that in the absence of a proper correction of the CTF the absolute value of each element of the volume is not directly related to the electron density value, it follows that some form of CTF restoration is a must for quantitative 3D electron microscopy and, obviously, for further considerations in a discrete tomography framework.

However, to perform a restoration process it is first very advisable to have an accurate model for the initial degradation process. In this latter respect, while there exits quite good parametric models for the CTF at medium and high frequencies, this is not the case for the low frequency region. This is so because the physical events dominating the behavior at these frequencies are a mixture of elastic and inelastic scattering events that do not lend themselves to be explained as a simple filter function. Indeed, the emerging solution to this low frequency modeling problem is to *exclude* totally the inelastic scattering events from the process of image formation, in such a way that the new imaging conditions allow the derivation of an approximate parametric model as the one proposed by Angert *et al.* [7]. To make this *exclusion* of inelastically scattered electrons possible, a special *energy filter* has to be implemented in the microscope in such a way that it selects only those electrons that have not lost energy while traversing the specimen. This process is usually referred to as *zero loss filtering*, and there are a number of technological alternatives implemented by the different microscope suppliers.

Starting from zero-loss filtered images, it is now possible to consider that the recorded images have been blurred by the effect of a filter function of the form described by Angert *et al.* [7] and then apply image restoration techniques. However, the very low signal to noise ratio — below 1 — of many electron microscopy images, specially those obtained by cryo microscopy (Fig. 18.3), coupled with the complex form of the filter function, makes this process difficult. For this reason, typically either several images at the same defocus are averaged before applying any restoration, or different images of the same specimen at different defocus are combined, or the CTF is directly incorporated into the reconstruction process [11, 26, 27].

FIGURE 18.3. Typical TEM image of the ribosome imaged in amorphous ice.

18.4.2   Discretization of the electron density of specimens

Considering that matter is composed of atoms, to think in terms of *discretizing* a magnitude — the electron density in this case — in similar terms as we think of discretizing (sampling) a continuous signal, is always a controversial topic. So far we have avoided a direct consideration of the atomic composition of matter by always working with voxel values, which are effectively *averaged electron densities* over regions containing many atoms.

However, when different constituents coexist in a given specimen, as it is always the experimental case, then the calculation of these averaged electron densities at the border between these constituents will necessarily mix different types of atoms. This effect leads to the appearance of many more voxel values than those corresponding to any of the constituents alone. Therefore, we will indeed have discrimination errors along the interaction surface between different components.

18.5   A practical application

Since the term *discrete tomography* is as yet totally alien to the structural electron microscopy community, we consider this chapter as a preliminary discussion of its potential. We complete this discussion with a demonstration of how the algorithms described in Chapter 9 by Chan, Herman, and Levitan can be used to restore electron microscopy reconstructions. (We use the term restoration for those techniques which are able to use *a priori* information to enhance the reconstruction quality.)

To try the effectiveness of the algorithm we have performed computer experiments with a phantom (see Fig. 18.4) as well as real data (see Fig. 18.5). A binary image resembling one slice of a true 3D protein (Fig. 18.4, left) was corrupted with zero-mean Gaussian noise (variance=0.9) (Fig. 18.4, middle) and then restored using the MAP method as described by Chan, Herman and Levitan (see the section "Recovering images corrupted by additive noise"). The result is shown in Fig. 18.4, right. Fig. 18.5, left shows a slice of a 3D reconstruction of a real specimen and the restoration is in Fig. 18.5, right. The results are promising (specially if we take into account that the priors and noise model used have been the ones proposed by Chan, Herman and Levitan and have not been optimized for this application, in particular the partial volume effect has not been modeled), suggesting that the electron microscopy images can be considerably improved using this image modeling method.

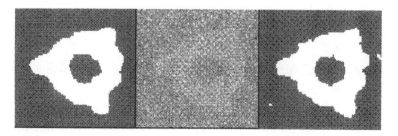

FIGURE 18.4. Original, noise contaminated, and restored images for one slice of phantom resembling a protein.

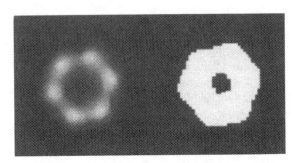

FIGURE 18.5. Slice of a previously reconstructed volume (namely the protein DnaB helicase of *E. Coli* (unpublished results), which does not contain nucleic acids) and MAP restored image of this slice.

18.6   Conclusions

For the growing field of 3D structural determination by EM at medium and high resolution, it is indeed the case that the specimen can be considered to be composed of discrete and basically homogeneous regions. In order for this biochemical and biophysical fact to became useful for improving the quality of the experimental images, zero-loss filtering, and CTF correction approaches have to be considered. Within the limits just set, the applicability of discrete tomography to this field seems to be justified.

Acknowledgments

This work has been funded, in part, by grants from Comisión Interministerial de Ciencia y Tecnología (Plan Nacional de Biotecnología) number BIO98-0761 and NATO number CRG 960070. Dr. Marabini holds a NATO postdoctoral fellowship.

References

[1] D. Sherwood, *Crystals, X-rays and Proteins* (Wiley, New York), 1976.

[2] G. Wagner, S. G. Hyberts, and T. F. Havel, "NMR structure determination in solution: A critique and comparison with X-ray crystallography," *Annu. Rev. Biophys. Biomol. Struct.* **21**, 167-198 (1992).

[3] D. J. De Rosier and A. Klug, "Reconstruction of three dimensional structures from electron micrographs," *Nature* **217**, 130-134 (1968).

[4] W. Kühlbrandt, D. N. Wang, and Y. Fujiyoshi, "Atomic model of plant light-harvesting complex by electron crystallography," *Nature*

367, 614-621 (1994).

[5] E. Nogales, S. G. Wolf, and K. H. Downing, "Structure of the alpha beta tubulin dimer by electron crystallography," *Nature* **391**, 199-203 (1998).

[6] R. Marabini, C. San Martín, and J. M. Carazo, "Electron tomography of biological specimens," In C. Roux and J. L. Coatrieux, *Contemporary Perspectives in Three-Dimensional Biomedical Imaging Studies in Health Technology and Informatics,* (IOS Press, Amsterdam), pp. 53-78, 1997.

[7] I. Angert, W. Jahn, K. C. Holmes, and R. R. Schröder, "A modified theory of image formation in a EFTEM," In H. A. Calderón and M. J. Yacamán, *Electron Microscopy 1998*, (Institute of Physics Publishing, Philadelphia), pp. 683-684, 1998, Volume 1.

[8] M. Radermacher, "The three-dimensional reconstruction of single particles from random and non random tilt series," *J. Electron Microsc. Tech.* **9**, 359-394 (1988).

[9] P. Penczek, M. Radermacher, and J. Frank, "3-Dimensional reconstruction of single particles embedded in ice," *Ultramicroscopy* **1**, 33-53 (1992).

[10] R. Marabini, G. T. Herman, and J. M. Carazo, "3D reconstruction in electron microscopy using ART with smooth spherically symmetric volume elements (blobs)," *Ultramicroscopy* **72**, 53-65 (1998).

[11] U. Skoglund, L. G. Öfverstedt, R. M. Burnett, and G. Bricogne, "Maximum-entropy three-dimensional reconstruction with deconvolution of the contrast transfer function: A test application with adenovirus," *J. Struct. Biol.* **117**, 173-188 (1996).

[12] R. Henderson and P. N. T. Unwin, "Three-dimensional model of purple membrane obtained by electron microscopy," *Nature* **257**, 28-32 (1975).

[13] J. M. Carazo and J. L. Carrascosa, "Restoration of direct Fourier three-dimensional reconstructions of crystalline specimens by the method of convex projections," *J. Microsc.* **145**, 159-177 (1987).

[14] J. M. Carazo and J. L. Carrascosa, "Information recovery in missing angular data cases: An approach by the convex projections method in three-dimensions," *J. Microsc.* **145**, 23-43 (1987).

[15] C. W. Akey and M. Radermacher, "Architecture of the Xenopus Nuclear-pore complex revealed by 3-dimensional cryoelectron microscopy," *J. Cell. Biol.* **122**, 1-19 (1993).

[16] H. P. Erickson and A. Klug, "Measurement and compensation of defocusing and aberrations by Fourier processing of electron micrographs," *Phil. Trans. Roy. Soc. Lond.* **261**, 105-118 (1971).

[17] F. A. Lenz, "Transfer of image information in the electron microscope," In U. Valdrè, *Electron Microscopy in Material Sciences*, (Academic Press, New York) pp. 540-569, 1971.

[18] F. Thon, "Phase contrast electron microscopy," In U. Valdrè, *Electron Microscopy in Material Sciences*, (Academic Press, New York) pp. 572-625, 1971.

[19] J. Frank, "The envelope of electron microscopic transfer functions for partially coherent illumination," *Optik* **38**, 519-536 (1973).

[20] R. H. Wade and J. Frank, "Electron microscope transfer functions for partially coherent axial illumination and chromatic defocus spread," *Optik* **49**, 81-92 (1977).

[21] Z. H. Zhou and W. Chiu, "Prospects for using an IVEM with a FEG for imaging macromolecules toward atomic resolution," *Ultramicroscopy* **49**, 407-416 (1993).

[22] K. H. Downing and D. A. Grano, "Analysis of photographic emulsions for electron microscopy of two-dimensional crystalline specimens," *Ultramicroscopy* **7**, 381-404 (1982).

[23] J. P. Langmore and M. F. Smith, "Quantitative energy-filtered electron microscopy of biological molecules in ice," *Ultramicroscopy* **46**, 349-373 (1992).

[24] R. H. Wade, "A brief look at imaging and contrast transfer," *Ultramicroscopy* **46**, 145-156 (1992).

[25] J. Frank, *Three Dimensional Electron Microscopy of Macromolecular Assemblies* (Academic Press, New York), 1996.

[26] J. Zhu, P. A. Penczek, R. Schröder, and J. Frank, "Three-dimensional reconstruction with contrast transfer function correction from energy-filtered cryoelectron micrographs: Procedure and application to the 70S escherichia coli ribosome," *J. Struct. Biol.* **118**, 197-219 (1997).

[27] L. D. Marks, "Wiener-filter enhancement of noisy HREM images," *Ultramicroscopy* **62**, 43-52 (1996).

Chapter 19

Tomography on the 3D-Torus and Crystals

Pablo M. Salzberg[1]
Raul Figueroa[2]

ABSTRACT We exhibit a fast Radon transform on an ambient space over a finite field which furnishes spatial limited-angle models for electron and X-ray tomography. These algorithms have applications in crystallography.

19.1   Introduction

Some discrete planar models were extensively studied in the earlier days of X-ray tomography (cf. [1–5], and references therein). In general, the tomographic problem involved in these models can be described in terms of a triple $(\Omega, \mathcal{L}, w)$; Ω being a square grid (or matrix) of points in the Euclidean plane, whereas each ray in $\mathcal{L}$ consists of a subset of points belonging to a straight strip in some direction. As part of the problem, we assume that unknown weights(or densities) $w_1 = w(P_1), w_2 = w(P_2), \ldots$, are assigned to the points of Ω. In order to know the value of these densities, we are allowed to "irradiate" along the rays in $\mathcal{L}$. Therefore, the problem can be stated as: *how can these values w_i be obtained from the line sums (or line weights) $w(L) = \sum_{P \in L} w(P)$ along each ray $L \in \mathcal{L}$?*

Thus, the solution of the tomographic problem leads to the inversion of a large matrix which in general, besides the amount of computation required, is an ill-conditioned problem. One of the simplest techniques used in computerized tomography that avoids inverting large matrices is the backprojection technique (BPT) introduced by Kuhl and Edwards [6].

In this contribution we exhibit a technique close to filtered BPT, which is based on combinatorial properties of lines in an affine geometry $\mathcal{G}$ on Ω. The reader is referred to [7] for an extensive and detailed coverage on this

[1]University of Puerto Rico, Department of Mathematics and Computer Sciences, P.O.Box 23355, Rio Piedras Campus, Puerto Rico 00931, E-mail: psalzber@goliath.cnnet.clu.edu
[2]University of Puerto Rico, Department of Mathematics and Computer Sciences, P.O.Box 23355, Rio Piedras Campus, Puerto Rico 00931, E-mail: rfiguero@goliath.cnnet.clu.edu

area.

There are several advantages in dealing with the discrete model we are proposing. A significant one is that the model gives us a simple solution also in the case of 3D tomography. This is not the case for the analytical models currently in use [8,9]. Moreover, it is a limited angle model, i.e., the beam of rays need only to sweep an angle less than 90° angle (a quadrant) for the planar case and less than an octant in the spatial model.

In Section 19.2 we exhibit a fast Radon transform on an ambient space $\mathcal{G}$ over a finite field which permits us to retrieve *any* (not necessarily binary) density distribution by means of a corrected average of the weights of the set (web) of lines passing through each point. Since this transform acts on each point individually, it allows us to reconstruct the density by means of parallel computations.

This transform furnishes the heuristic for a continuous model on the 3D-torus T^3 obtained by overlapping the lines of $\mathcal{G}$ with real (Euclidean) lines. This matter is discussed in Section 19.3.

In Section 19.4 we derive an heuristic for reconstructing from a few projections in the case of a binary tomography on lattices. These algorithms have applications in crystallography. We exhibit reconstructions of several phantoms proposed by P. Schwander.

19.2   A fast inverse transform

The tomographic problem that we consider in this section is of a more general nature than the binary problem.

To explain the main ideas underlying our model, let us assume that Ω is a cubic grid of points of prime order, say p, in the space. A geometry of *discrete* lines $\mathcal{L}$ on Ω can be introduced in a natural way by coordinating the points in Ω, i.e., by considering a coordinate system as shown in Fig. 19.1.

A line in $\mathcal{L}$ passing through $P \in \Omega$ and with direction m can be defined as the set

$$L_{P,m} = \{P + tm \mid t \in Z_p\}, \tag{19.1}$$

where Z_p is the field of integers (mod p), and P, $m \in Z_p^3$ (as shown in Fig. 19.2 for a planar case; in that figure m refers to the second coordinate of the slope vector $(1, m)$).

Let us denote by $\mathcal{G} = AG(Z_p, 3)$, the set of lines in a 3D-affine space. Lines in any affine geometry have the following four properties:

(i) Given two different points P and Q, there is one and only one line containing (or incident to) P and Q.

(ii) Given two different points P and Q, there is at least one line passing through P and not containing Q.

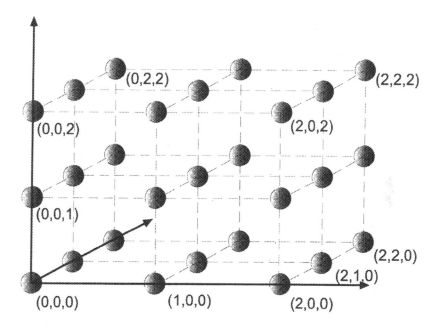

FIGURE 19.1. Coordinating $\Omega \subset Z^3$ canonically.

(iii) Two different lines are disjoint (parallel) or intersect at one point.

(iv) Every line has the same number of points.

These four properties imply that given any point $P \in \Omega$, the *web of lines* $\mathcal{L}_P = \{L_1, ..., L_k\}$ *through* P satisfies the following equalities, as can be noticed from Fig. 19.3:

(I) $L_i \cap L_j = \{P\}$, for any $i \neq j$, and

(II) $\bigcup_{i=1}^{k} L_i = \Omega$.

Properties (I) and (II) can be rephrased as follows: *any point* $Q \in \Omega - \{P\}$ *belongs to one and only one line of the web* $\mathcal{L}_P$ *through* P. Obviously P belongs to all lines in the web.

Now, let us denote by $w(L) = \sum_{Q \in L} w(Q)$ the weight of each line $L \in \mathcal{L}$. Thus, $\{w(L) \mid L \in \mathcal{L}\}$ constitutes the input data set of our tomography problem. To find the unknown density $w(P)$ associated with any point $P \in \Omega$, notice that (I) and (II) above imply $\sum_{L \in \mathcal{L}_P} w(L) = w(\Omega) + (k - 1)w(P)$ from which we can obtain the $w(P)$. This procedure is illustrated in Fig. 19.4 below.

Remark 19.1. *Properties (i)-(iv) are not exclusive for affine geometries. Indeed,* $\mathcal{L} = \{(P, Q) \mid P, Q \in \Omega\}$, *where* Ω *is any finite set, satisfies (i)-(iv).*

420   Pablo M. Salzberg, Raul Figueroa

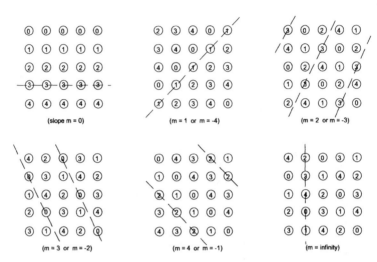

FIGURE 19.2. Sets of parallel lines in the planar $AG(Z_5, 2)$ in each of the six possible directions. Points in different lines are assigned different labels.

Remark 19.2.   *From properties (I) and (II) it can be easily seen that there are $k = (p^3 - 1)/(p - 1)$ lines in the web of lines through any point $P \in \Omega$. In fact, each line has p points, $|\Omega| = p^3$, and $k = |\mathcal{L}_P|$ satisfies $kp - (k - 1) = p^3$, where $|\cdot|$ denotes cardinality.*

When dealing with the tomographic problem given by the triple $(\Omega, \mathcal{L}, w)$, the preceding discussion suggests that some appropriate structure must be imposed on the set $\mathcal{L}$ in order to retrieve the individual weights in a convenient way. This ideas can be presented in a more general setting as follows, which in turn show the kind of conditions to be imposed on $\mathcal{L}$.

We call $\mathcal{A} \subset 2^\Omega$ an *algebra* in Ω if $\mathcal{A}$ is closed under the set operations of union and complementation, and $\Omega \in \mathcal{A}$. Within this framework, a real-valued function (or functional) $w : \mathcal{A} \to \Re$ is *additive* if it satisfies $w(A_1 \cup A_2) = w(A_1) + w(A_2)$, whenever A_1, $A_2 \in \mathcal{A}$ are disjoint. As a consequence of these definitions, an additive functional w defined on $\mathcal{A}$ satisfies the following two properties:

a) $w(A_1 \cup A_2) = w(A_1) + w(A_2) - w(A_1 \cap A_2)$, for any pair A_1, $A_2 \in \mathcal{A}$, and

b) $w(A_1 - A_2) = w(A_1) - w(A_2)$, for any pair A_1, $A_2 \in \mathcal{A}$ such that $A_2 \subset A_1$.

Theorem 19.1.   *Let $\mathcal{S} = (\Omega, \mathcal{A}, w)$, where w denotes an additive functional over an algebra $\mathcal{A}$ in Ω. Let $\{L_1, \ldots, L_k\} \subset \mathcal{A}$ denote a web in Ω; i.e., a subset of $\mathcal{A}$ satisfying the following three conditions:*

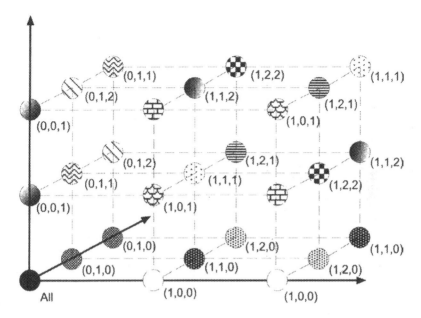

FIGURE 19.3. Web of lines in $AG(Z_3, 3)$ through the origin. Lines in different directions are represented with different patterns.

1. $k \geq 2$,

2. $w(L_i \cap L_j) = w(\cap_{i=1}^k L_i)$, for $1 \leq i \neq j \leq k$, and

3. $w(\Omega) = w(\cup_{i=1}^k L_i)$.

Then,

$$w(\cap_{i=1}^k L_i) = \frac{1}{k-1} \left(\sum_{i=1}^k w(L_i) - w(\Omega) \right).$$ (19.2)

Proof: From properties a) and b) in the roster preceding the statement, it follows that $w[(L_i - \cap_{s=1}^k L_s) \cap (L_j - \cap_{s=1}^k L_s)] = 0$, for $1 \leq i \neq j \leq k$. Therefore, $w(\Omega) = w(\cup_{i=1}^k L_i) = w[\cup_{i=1}^k (L_i - \cap_{s=1}^k L_s) \cup \cap_{s=1}^k L_s] = \sum_{i=1}^k w(L_i) - (k-1)w(\cap_{i=1}^k L_i)$. $\square$

Returning to the above question, Theorem 19.1 shows that a sufficient set of requirements to be satisfied by $\mathcal{L}$ is the following, where we define $\mathcal{L}_P = \{L \in \mathcal{L} \mid P \in L\}$:

1. $|\mathcal{L}_P| \geq 2$, for every $P \in \Omega$, where $|\cdot|$ denotes cardinality,

2. $L \cap L' = \{P\}$, for any $P \in \Omega$ and L, $L' \in \mathcal{L}_P$ such that $L \neq L'$, and

3. $\bigcup \mathcal{L}_P = \Omega$, for every $P \in \Omega$.

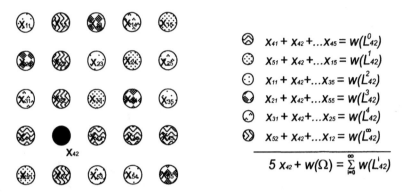

$$X_{41} + X_{42} + ... X_{45} = w(L_{42}^0)$$
$$X_{51} + X_{42} + ... X_{15} = w(L_{42}^1)$$
$$X_{11} + X_{42} + ... X_{35} = w(L_{42}^2)$$
$$X_{21} + X_{42} + ... X_{55} = w(L_{42}^3)$$
$$X_{31} + X_{42} + ... X_{25} = w(L_{42}^4)$$
$$X_{52} + X_{42} + ... X_{12} = w(L_{42}^\infty)$$

$$5 X_{42} + w(\Omega) = \sum_{i=0}^{\infty} w(L_{42}^i)$$

FIGURE 19.4. This figure shows how to retrieve the density of the displayed entry.

The next result follows as a consequence of Theorem 19.1 and the fact that the set $\mathcal{L}$ of lines of any affine space satisfies the three conditions in the above roster.

Corollary 19.1.   *Let $\mathcal{G} = AG(F_q, d)$ be a d-dimensional affine geometry over the finite field F_q (where $d \geq 2$, $q = p^n$ for some prime p and $n \in N$). Let Ω and $\mathcal{L}$ denote the sets of points and lines in $\mathcal{G}$, and let $w : \Omega \to \Re$ be a real-valued function, extended additively to any subset in $\mathcal{P}(\Omega)$. If $\mathcal{L}_P \subset \mathcal{L}$ denote the web of lines passing through any given point $P \in \Omega$ then, for any given $P \in \Omega$,*

$$w(P) = \frac{1}{|\mathcal{L}_P| - 1}\left(\sum_{L \in \mathcal{L}_P} w(L) - w(\Omega) \right). \qquad (19.3)$$

This transform is essentially a corrected average of the weights of the lines in the web radiating from the point to be reconstructed. It is clear that the reconstruction can be performed simultaneously on each point, allowing us to program the computational work in a highly parallel fashion.

The reader is referred to [10–12] (and references therein), for others Radon transforms on ambient spaces over finite fields.

19.3   The continuous case

Notice that the inversion transform given by equation (19.3) is based on discrete lines. However, in practical applications such as in the case of X-ray tomography, or in transmission electron microscopy, rays represent the continuous path of atomic particles. This leads us to explore the possibility of overlapping the lines of the finite geometry $\mathcal{G}$ with real (Euclidean) lines. This is feasible only when $q = p$, i.e., when q is a prime number. In order to tackle this approach, let $G = \{0, 1, ..., p-1\}^3$ be a cubic lattice (of prime order p) imbedded in Z^3. As we mentioned in the preceding section, we can endow G with a structure of affine space $\mathcal{G} = AG(Z_p, 3)$ in a canonical form: the $p^2(p^2 + p + 1)$ lines in $\mathcal{L}$ are given by the sets

$$\widetilde{L}_{b,m} = \{b + tm \quad (\text{mod } p) \mid t \in \Re\}, \tag{19.4}$$

where $b, m \in Z_p^3$, and $\Re$ denotes the real numbers.

Thus, (19.4) is obtained from (19.1) by allowing t to vary continuously. These sets can be regarded as lines immersed in a 3D-torus $T_p^3 = \Re^3/(Z_p)^3$.

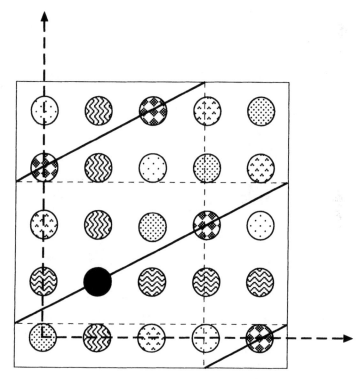

FIGURE 19.5. A line on the torus overlapping a discrete line of the affine geometry.

The next step is to "irradiate" along the p^2 parallel lines in each of the $p^2 + p + 1$ directions given by $\{(m_1, m_2, 1), (m_1, 1, 0), (1, 0, 0)\}$, where $m_1, m_2 \in Z_p$. To reconstruct the density at a given point we just consider the line sums along the web of lines passing through that point.

At this point it is worthwhile to mention that the directions of the toroidal lines need not necessarily be those described in terms of $m = (m_1, m_2, m_3)$ in (19.4). Furthermore, different directions can lead to the same discrete lines in the affine geometry, as it is shown in the following result where, as described above, we assume that G is any cubic lattice of order p imbedded in Z^3 and T_p^3 is the 3D-torus overlapping G.

Theorem 19.2.   *Any toroidal line $\widetilde{L}$ in T_p^3 containing two points of the lattice G must contain exactly p points of G. Moreover, the intersection $L = \widetilde{L} \cap G$ between the toroidal line and the lattice coincides with a line of the affine geometry $\mathcal{G}$, i.e., $L \subset \mathcal{L}$ (see Fig. 19.6).*

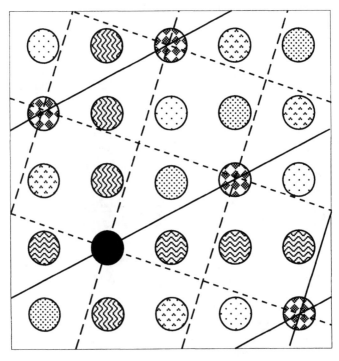

FIGURE 19.6. Any line on the torus with rational direction cosines and passing through a lattice point must contain exactly one discrete line of the affine geometry induced on the lattice.

Proof: We can assume, without any lost of generality, that one of the intersection points is the origin. Let $(r_1, r_2, r_3) \in \Re^3$ be the direction cosines of the line. By hypothesis,

$$t(r_1, r_2, r_3) = (m_1, m_2, m_3) \in Z^3 - \{(0,0,0)\}, \qquad (19.5)$$

for some $t \in \Re$. Therefore, $\gcd(p, m_1, m_2, m_3) = 1$ which implies $\gcd(m_i, p) = 1$ for at least one $i = 1, 2, 3$, where gcd denotes the greatest common divisor. Assume, for instance, that $\gcd(m_2, p) = 1$. Therefore, $t(r_1, r_2, r_3)$ can be rewritten as $\tau(m_1/m_2, 1, m_3/m_2)$ for some $\tau \in \Re$. In order for $\tau(m_1/m_2, 1, m_3/m_2) \in Z^3$, τ must take on values in the ideal (m_2). On the other hand, since $\gcd(m_2, p) = 1$, then $\{0, m_2, 2m_2, ..., (p-1)m_2\}$ constitutes a complete residue system modulo p, and therefore the toroidal line passes through exactly k points of the lattice. This line coincides with the line $L_{0,m}$ of the affine geometry, m being the slope vector $m = (m_1, m_2, m_3)$ (mod p). Finally, notice that if

$$m_1' \equiv m_1 \pmod{p}, \quad m_2' \equiv m_2 \pmod{p} \quad and \quad m_3' \equiv m_3 \pmod{p}, \quad (19.6)$$

then both toroidal lines $\widetilde{L}_{b,m}$ and $\widetilde{L}_{b,m'}$ not necessarily coincides but must 'generate' the same line in the affine geometry $\mathcal{G}$.

□

Remark 19.3.   *Theorem 19.2 is particularly important in electron transmission microscopy where there are severe limitations on the tilt angle of the specimen. It asserts, for instance, that we can use toroidal lines with arbitrarily small direction cosines with respect to any zone axes to generate all the lines in the affine geometry. However, since each toroidal line is formed by a flat bundle of parallel segments, the tilt angle will be admissible only when the distance between two consecutive segments of the toroidal line are greater than the resolution power of the instrument.*

19.4   Binary tomography on lattices

19.4.1   Binary tomography and crystals

In general, binary tomography problems deal with the reconstruction of black and white images from the knowledge of all parallel projections of that image along a set of directions. This problem has been considered for over twenty years, with motivation coming mainly from (biplane) angiography [8, 13] and from industrial imaging (e.g., of radioactive materials).

Recently, an important application of binary tomography was proposed by Peter Schwander *et al.* in connection with the study of the atomic structure of crystal lattices [14, 15]. Using transmission electron microscopy, Schwander developed a technique (QUANTITEM) that measures the variation of the sample potential from general lattice images of structurally perfect crystalline materials, requiring no knowledge of the image conditions. This technique, which can be applied to a wide range of materials — including semi-conducting metallic elements and alloys — can be used to count approximately the number of atoms in each atomic column of a crystal, in case that the atoms reside on coherent lattices, with no compositional inhomogeneities in the beam direction. Since the crystal can be tilted along different zone axes, all column sums can be known along a small set of directions. The goal is to reconstruct the atomic configuration of the crystal from the knowledge of the approximate number of atoms in each atomic column along a small set of directions (see Fig. 19.7).

As indicated in [14, 15], this knowledge may be used to measure the chemical transition between two regions of known composition in crystalline materials. In general, this research opens the way for the study of a

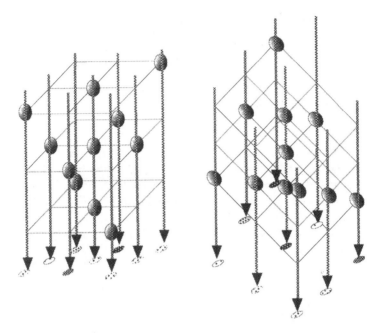

FIGURE 19.7. Using transmission electron microscopy, Schwander _et al._ developed a technique to count approximately the number of atoms in each atomic column of a crystal, in the case there is only one type of atom [14, 15].

variety of important inter-facial reactions at the atomic level such as surface roughening during oxidation, which are important for the development of the silicon technology necessary for electronic devices.

The application of known algorithms poses a problem because the tilt range of the crystal is normally restricted for several reasons. The most important problem being the obstruction to the electron path produced by the case supporting the specimen (at high angles), which in commercial instruments limits the tilt angle to around $\pm 60°$ angle. Indeed, the maximum tilt angle influences the resolution of the reconstruction by limiting the amount of Fourier space sampled [8, 9]. In addition, a large number of projections recorded with high precision (taken at increments of at most $\pm 0.1°$) are required, condition that can not be fulfilled in Schwander's procedures in which it is possible to measure projections only within a cone of about $15°$.

19.4.2 _Stating the binary tomography problem_

The previous theory shows how to reconstruct any density function defined on a p^d-lattice ($d \geq 2$, and p prime) from all p^{d-1} parallel line sums along $(p^d - 1)/(p - 1)$ directions, i.e., along all the lines in $\mathcal{L}$. In what follows we tackle the *binary tomography problem*, which can be modeled by considering the ordinary integer lattice Z^d, where $d \geq 2$. A binary function with *finite* support $w : Z^d \to \{0, 1\}$ is known only by its line sums (projections) along any parallel line in each of k given directions. The problem is to reconstruct the actual function w from these projection data. Recalling our previous notation, we assume that the line sums are known along all lines in a subset $\mathcal{B} \subset \mathcal{L}$, closed under parallelism, i.e., for any line $L \in \mathcal{B}$, this set contains all lines parallel to L.

Figure 19.8 shows that we can not expect, in general, a unique solution. It is still an open problem to determine the minimum number of directions necessary to guarantee uniqueness. Obviously, in the 3D affine geometry $p^2 + p + 1$ directions are sufficient for uniqueness. This remark suggest the following definition. We say that a reconstruction w_R is *feasible* if w and w_R have the same projections along any parallel line in each of the given k directions.

Within the framework described above, a pioneer work on binary tomography that considers all parallel projections along a small set of directions was written by Fishburn *et al.* [16]. They show that some specific configurations, called additive sets, can be reconstructed from the knowledge of the line sums along any parallel line in only two directions. In general, however, when a reduced number of directions is considered there is not uniqueness, which poses a threat to any effort of finding a good feasible solution, i.e., a reconstruction close enough to the unknown configuration. Some significant contributions on this problem are due to Aharoni *et al.* [17] and Kuba [18].

On the other hand, from a computational point of view, the problem of finding feasible solutions is NP-complete for $k \geq 3$, for most classes of sets appearing in applications. Nevertheless, there are some algorithms available to find solutions in polynomial time under certain circumstances; we now give a summary of them.

An interesting methodology was recently developed by Fishburn *et al.* [19]. Here, the binary function w to be reconstructed from its projections is relaxed to be a "fuzzy set", i.e., it is replaced by a function taking values in the interval $[0, 1]$. Under this relaxation, the problem of finding a feasible solution can be treated as a linear programming problem, for which there are well-known efficient algorithms. However, if $w^{-1}(1)$ is not additive then the solution produced by the linear programming algorithms is, in general, fuzzy (i.e., not binary). Another interesting approach using this relaxation technique in conjunction with the EM algorithm was presented in [20]. Working in a different direction, the first author and collaborators presented in [21] a network-flow approach to the reconstruction of binary functions on planar or spatial latices, as well as an outline of an approximation theory.

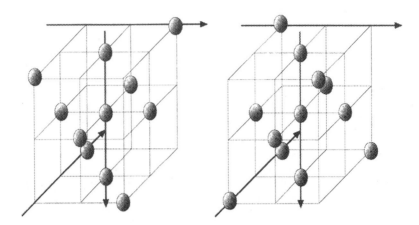

FIGURE 19.8. The solution may be not unique, as can be easily seen by counting the line sums in both cases.

19.5   The reconstruction algorithm

In what follows we exhibit a highly parallelizable algorithm based on a *maximum likelihood principle*, but first we need to introduce some notation.

Let $\mathcal{B}$ denote a subset of $\mathcal{L}$ that includes all parallel lines in the given directions. As it can be noticed from Fig. 19.5 (or Fig. 19.6), each $L \in \mathcal{B}$ is a bundle of 'parallel' subsets. We denote these subsets by $\{L_1, ..., L_{k_L}\}$. Clearly, the set of raw data (i.e., the information obtained from the scanner) consists of the $w(L_i)$'s for each $L \in \mathcal{B}$.

Next we introduce a measure of the *discrepancy* between w and w_R on $L_i \subset L \in \mathcal{B}$ in terms of $d(L_i) = w(L_i) - w_R(L_i)$, where w_R denote the reconstructed binary function. In turn, this discrepancy is extended additively to $\mathcal{B}$ as $d(L) = \sum_{L_i \subset L} d(L_i)$. Once the discrepancy d is defined on every line of $\mathcal{B}$, we introduce the function $s : \Omega \to \Re$, defined by $s(P) = \sum_{L \in \mathcal{B}_P} d(L)$, which plays a key role in our algorithm. Notice that d, and therefore s, are defined in terms of known data. A global measure of discrepancy, which we refer to as the *total absolute discrepancy* is given by $|d| = \sum_{L_i \subset L \in \mathcal{B}} |d(L_i)|$. Finally, let D denote the set of slopes associated with those directions included in $\mathcal{B}$.

Initially, the heuristic involved in this algorithm consists in interpreting the values $s(P) = \sum_{L \in \mathcal{B}_P} w(L)$ (since $w_R = 0$) as the *likelihood* that either $w(P) = 1$ or $w(P) = 0$. In fact, recall from (19.3) that if $\mathcal{B}_P = \mathcal{L}_P$, i.e., if $\mathcal{B}_P$ contains all the directions in the affine geometry, then $w(P)$ can be obtained from $s(P)$ by a very simple *increasing* affine transformation, namely, $w(P) = (|\mathcal{B}_P| - 1)^{-1}(s(P) - w(G))$. In applications, $|\mathcal{B}_P|$ is significantly less than $|\mathcal{L}_P|$ and we can not expect that our inverse transformation yields an exact reconstruction at P. Therefore, we interpret $s(P)$ as the likelihood for the occurrence of 0 or 1 at P in the following manner: the higher the value of $s(P)$ as compared with the value at other points in G, the greater the likelihood that $w(P) = 1$; the lower the value, the greater the likelihood that $w(P) = 0$.

The algorithm proceeds as follows:

Step 0. Initialize $w_R = 0$.

Step 1. At each point $P \in G$ compute $s(P) = \sum_{L \in \mathcal{B}_P} d(L)$. Let S denote the matrix whose entries are these values.

In the following step we introduce a reconstruction function w_{R_m}, for each direction $m \in D$. Here, $s(P) = \sum_{L \in \mathcal{B}_P} d(L)$ is interpreted as the *likelihood for changing* the value of w_R at P. In other words, if $s(P)$ is a large or small percentile in the distribution of values of S along $L_i \subset L$, then we consider as high the likelihood that the current value $w_R(P)$ is incorrect.

Step 2. For each direction $m \in D$ (initialize $w_{R_m} = w_R$), and for each line $L \in \mathcal{B}$ in this direction let us consider each L_i as described above. Evaluate $d(L_i)$. A positive value means that w_R, as obtained in previous steps, turned 'off' more points than necessary in L_i. Then, sort the values of the array $\{s(P) \mid P \in L_i\}$ and turn 'on' the points associated with the $d(L_i)$ largest values in this array, i.e., assign them the value $w_{R_m}(P) = 1$. Analogously, if $d(L_i) < 0$, turn 'off' the $|d(L_i)|$ points $P \in L_i$ with the smallest value $s(P)$.

Step 3. Let w'_R be the average of all w_{R_m} for each direction $m \in D$. Thus, $w'_R(P) = (|D|)^{-1} \sum_{m \in D} w_{R_m}(P)$, for each $P \in G$, where $|D|$ denotes the number of directions we are considering. Then define w_R by splitting the values of w'_R in two, i.e., by assigning 1 to those points whose associated values w'_R are in the upper 50 percentile. Borderline points to both classes could be assigned either $w_R(P) = 1$ or $w_R(P) = 0$, whatever is better to decrease the total discrepancy $|d|$.

Step 4. Repeat Steps 1-3 until the total absolute discrepancy $|d|$ does not decreases.

19.6   Final remarks and examples

Notice that Step 1 of the algorithm does not involve all the available information. Indeed, the particular values $\{w(L_i)\}$ are not considered in this step; we use only the grouped values $w(L) = w(L_1) + ... + w(L_{k_L})$. For this reason, a reconstruction obtained at this stage by splitting in two the values in S, i.e., by assigning value 1 to those above or equal to the 50

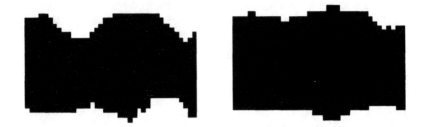

FIGURE 19.9. Left) Schwander's Phantom 1. Right) Its reconstruction after Step 1 of the algorithm. $D = \{-1, 0, 1, \infty\}$.

percentile of the distribution of values, and 0 otherwise, would look like in Fig. 19.9, where the phantom was kindly provided by P. Schwander.

When Steps 1-3 are applied to the same phantom considered in Fig. 19.9, they furnish the reconstruction shown in Fig. 19.10.

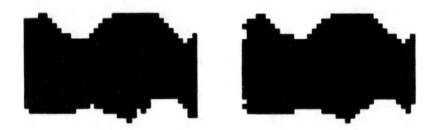

FIGURE 19.10. Left) Schwander's Phantom 1. Right) Its reconstruction after Steps 1-3 of the algorithm. $D = \{-1, 0, 1, \infty\}$.

Figure 19.11 shows the final reconstruction attained with this algorithm.

To measure the quality of a reconstruction, Herman [1] introduced the *relative mean error (rme)*. For the reconstruction in Fig. 19.10 (a single iteration) $rme = 0.026$. For the reconstruction in Fig. 19.11 (after two additional iterations) $rme = 0.009$. Moreover, for matrices of this size (61×61), each iteration takes about 0.34 seconds with a 200Mhz PC, computed sequentially, and with a program not specifically designed to optimize speed.

Remark 19.4.   *Another meaningful measure related to the rme can be obtained from $|d|$, with the advantage that it can be computed from the available data. A simple transformation of $|d|$, namely $(|D| \times |w^{-1}(1)|)^{-1}|d|$, yields the average number of errors per direction relative to the total number of 1's. This index seems to be highly correlated to the rme. In fact, when it is used as a factor for predicting the value of rme by means of linear regression (based on hundreds of reconstructions), the coefficient of multiple determination R^2 is about .95.*

FIGURE 19.11. Left) Schwander's Phantom 1. Right) Reconstruction of the phantom given in the preceding figures with the complete algorithm.

Figures 19.12 and 19.13 show (right side) additional reconstruction of phantoms kindly provided by P. Schwander, of size 61×61 (left side), which are believed to be representative of real crystals [19]. For the first reconstruction $D = \{-1, 0, 1, \infty\}$, while for the second D contains two additional directions with slopes 2 and -2, respectively.

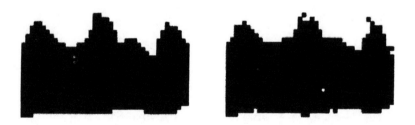

FIGURE 19.12. Left) Phantom provided by P. Schwander. Right) Reconstruction using $D = \{-1, 0, 1, \infty\}$. Here, $rme = 0.044$ after two iterations of the algorithm.

An extension of the preceding theory toward a spatial limited-angle model for computerized tomography of continuous objects is outlined in [22–24]. This extension is based on the inversion transform given in Corollary 19.1. The reader is referred to [25, 26] for a discussion of the behavior of webs of lines on the torus.

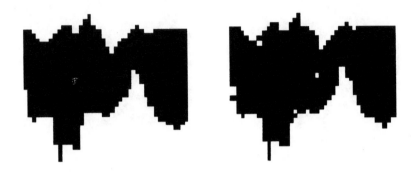

FIGURE 19.13. Left) Phantom provided by P. Schwander. Right) Reconstruction for $D = \{-2, -1, 0, 1, 2, \infty\}$**. In this case,** $rme = 0.020$ **after eight iterations of the algorithm.**

Acknowledgments

The authors are indebted to Prof. Larry A. Shepp for his comments on an earlier version of this algorithm, which resulted in a substantial improvement of the same. They are also thankful to the Editors for their multiple suggestions and corrections to the original manuscript. The first author is partially supported by NIH, MBRS Program, under grant 5S-06GM08102.

References

[1] G. T. Herman, "Two direct methods for reconstructing pictures from their projections: A comparative study," *Computer Graphics and Image Processing* **1**, 123-144 (1972).

[2] R. A. Gordon, "A tutorial on ART (Algebraic Reconstruction Techniques)," *IEEE Trans. Nuclear Science* **21**, 78-93 (1974).

[3] R. A. Brooks and G. Di Chiro, "Theory of image reconstruction in computed tomography," *Radiology* **117**, 561-572 (1975).

[4] R. A. Brooks and G. Di Chiro, "Principles of computer assisted tomography (CAT) in radiographic and radioisotopic imaging," *Physics in Medicine and Biology* **21**, 689-732 (1976).

[5] G. T. Herman and R. M. Lewitt, "Overview of image reconstruction from projections," In G. T. Herman, *Image Reconstruction from Projections: Implementation and Applications* (Springer-Verlag, Berlin), pp. 1-7, 1979.

[6] D. E. Kuhl and R. Q. Edwards, "Reorganizing data from transverse section scans of the brain using digital processing," *Radiology* **91**, 975-983 (1968).

[7] M. Hall, Jr., *Combinatorial Theory*, Second Edition, (John Wiley and Sons, New York), 1986.

[8] S. K. Chang and C. K. Chow, "The reconstruction of a three-dimensional object from two orthogonal projections and its applications to cardiac cineangiography," *IEEE Trans. Comput.* **22**, 18-28 (1973).

[9] A. Klug and R. A. Crowther, "Three-dimensional image reconstruction from the viewpoint of information theory," *Nature* **238**, 435-440 (1972).

[10] E. D. Bolker, "The finite Radon transform," In R. L. Bryant, V. Guillemin, S. Helgason, and R. O. Wells, Jr., *Integral Geometry*, (American Mathematical Society, Providence, RI), pp. 27-50, 1987.

[11] E. L. Grinberg, "The admissibility theorem for the hyperplane transform over a finite field," *J. Combinatorial Th., Series A* **53**, 316-320 (1990).

[12] J. P. S. Kung, "Reconstructing finite Radon transforms," *Nuclear Physics B (Proc. Suppl.)* **5A**, 44-49 (1988).

[13] G. T. Herman, "Reconstruction of binary patterns from a few projections," In A. Günther, B. Levrat and H. Lipps, *International Computing Symposium 1973*, (North-Holland Publ. Co., Amsterdam), pp. 371-378, 1974.

[14] C. Kisielowski, P. Schwander, F. H. Baumann, M. Seibt, Y. Kim, and A. Ourmazd, "An approach to quantitative high-resolution transmission electron microscopy of crystalline materials," *Ultramicroscopy* **58**, 131-155 (1995).

[15] P. Schwander, C. Kisielowski, M. Seibt, F. H. Baumann, Y. Kim, and A. Ourmazd, "Mapping projected potential, interfacial roughness, and composition in general crystalline solids by quantitative transmission electron microscopy," *Phys. Rev. Let.* **71**, 4150-4153 (1993).

[16] P. C. Fishburn, J. C. Lagarias, J. A. Reeds, and L. A. Shepp, "Sets uniquely determined by projections on axes. II. Discrete case," *Disc. Math.* **91**, 149-159, 1991.

[17] R. Aharoni, G. T. Herman, and A. Kuba, "Binary vectors partially determined by linear equation systems," *Disc. Math.* **171**, 1-16, 1997.

[18] A. Kuba, "Reconstruction of unique binary matrices with prescribed elements," *Acta Cybern.* **12**, 57-70 (1995).

[19] P. Fishburn, P. Schwander, L. Shepp, and R. J. Vanderbei, "A discrete Radon transform and its approximate inversion via linear programming," *Disc. Appl. Math.* **75**, 39-61 (1997).

[20] Y. Vardi and D. Lee, "The discrete Radon transform and its approximate inversion via the EM algorithm," *Int. J. Imaging Syst. and Technol.* **9**, 155-173 (1998).

[21] P. M. Salzberg, P. E. Rivera-Vega, and A. Rodriguez, "Network flow models for binary tomography on lattices," *Int. J. Imaging Syst. and Technol.* **9**, 147-154 (1998).

[22] P. M. Salzberg, "Tomography in projective spaces: a heuristic for limited-angle reconstructive models," *SIAM J. Matrix Anal. Appl.* **9**, 393-398 (1988).

[23] P. M. Salzberg, "An application of finite field theory to computerized tomography: A spatial limited-angle model," In G. L. Mullen and P. Shiue *Finite fields, Coding Theory, and Advances in Communications and Computing*, (Marcel Dekker, New York), pp. 395-402, 1992.

[24] P. M. Salzberg, A. Correa, and R. Cruz, "On a spatial limited-angle model for X-ray computerized tomography," In *Tomography, Impedance Imaging and Integral Geometry*, (Amer. Math. Soc., Providence, RI), pp. 25-33, 1994.

[25] R. Figueroa and P. M. Salzberg, "Pencil of lines on the 2-D torus," *Ars Combinatoria* **37**, 235-240 (1994).

[26] P. M. Salzberg and R. Figueroa, "Incidence pattern of a pencil of lines in the n-dimensional torus," *Congressus Numeratium* **97**, 197-204 (1993).

Chapter 20

A Recursive Algorithm for Diffuse Planar Tomography

Sarah K. Patch[1]

ABSTRACT Diffuse tomography generalizes the standard discrete tomography problem, permitting anisotropic scattering. The diffuse problem involves more unknowns, and also more data. Markov transition probabilities are recovered from measurements taken at all pairs of input/output ports on the boundary. A recursive algorithm is used to solve the problem on a general $n \times n$ lattice in the plane.

20.1 Introduction

Diffuse tomography models photon transport on a discrete lattice as a Markov process and lends itself to recursive inversion. There are two major differences between discrete and diffuse tomography: scatter and the physical meaning of both data and unknowns. Physically, discrete tomographic data represents the object's density integrated along the path between source and detector. Diffuse tomographic data represents the probability with which a particle travels between the same source and detector; see Fig. 20.1. Scatter of near-infrared radiation used for optical imaging motivated the diffuse tomographic model [1] which considers *all* paths through the imaging object, not just straight paths. In diffuse tomography, we assume that data is collected all around the imaging object, whereas in discrete tomography measurements are taken only corresponding to straight lines from source to detector; see Fig. 20.1. Because the diffuse tomographic model is more complicated, we must measure more data in order to have any hope of solving the inverse imaging problem. Scatter-free diffuse tomographic data can be converted to discrete tomographic data just as raw CT data is preprocessed, by taking $-ln(I_{meas}/I_0)$, where I_{meas} = measured intensity of radiation passing through the imaging object and I_0 = intensity of radiation incident upon the object [2].

The author's work in diffuse tomography began with a study of consis-

---

[1]General Electric Company Corporate Research and Development, Industrial Electronics Laboratory, KW B405, PO Box 8, Schenectady, NY 12301-0008, USA, E-mail: patch@crd.ge.com

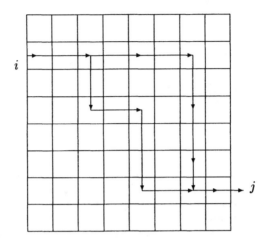

FIGURE 20.1. Two (out of infinitely many) possible paths taken by a diffuse tomograhic particle through an 8×8 system from the source at port i to the detector at port j. Notice that in discrete tomography, the data corresponding to ports i and j is considered *only* if a view along the direction vector between i and j is measured.

tency conditions upon diffuse tomographic data [3]. These conditions result from the Markovian nature of diffuse tomographic systems and are trivially fulfilled in the specific discrete tomographic setup. Therefore, range conditions are mentioned only in passing.

Subsection 20.2.1 describes the diffuse tomographic model in the plane and contrasts it to the discrete tomographic model. Diffuse tomography's forward model is governed by a nonlinear matrix equation:

$$Q = Pio + Pih \, (I - Phh)^{-1} \, Pho, \qquad (20.1)$$

where Q is the input/output matrix and the one step Markov transition matrices Pio, Pih, Phh, and Pho pertain to Markov transitions between incoming, hidden, and outgoing states. Computing Q from the one step transition matrices constitutes the forward problem. The imaging problem is the inverse problem: given Q, recover Pio, Pih, Phh, and Pho. The inverse problem is *underdetermined* [3] and therefore has *families* of solutions. The general discrete tomography problem does not take scatter into account. However, when imaging structured objects, like crystals, discrete tomography permits an *unique* solution from data corresponding to only *two* views [4].

Diffuse tomographic image reconstruction is done by recursively splitting the imaging object. See Fig. 20.2. At each recursive level a $n \times n$ system is broken into four $\frac{n}{2} \times \frac{n}{2}$ subsystems and their data sets are written in terms of the parent $n \times n$ system's data *plus* $8n$ parameters. Families of solutions

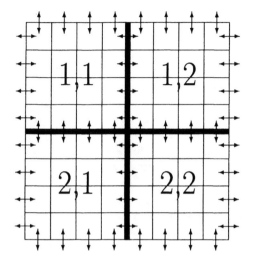

FIGURE 20.2. Decomposition of an 8 × 8 system into four 4 × 4 subsystems. The thick lines separate the subsystems. Only states that are considered when solving for the subsystems' data are denoted with arrows.

for the subsystems' data sets are easily found. These data sets, however, do not obey range conditions for diffuse tomographic systems and depend upon $4n^2 \geq 8n$ parameters. Range conditions upon the data imply that the data sets should depend upon only $8n$ parameters, where

$$8n = \# \text{ measured data} - \# \text{ independent consistency conditions.} \quad (20.2)$$

Enforcing range conditions not only restores self consistency to the model, but also eliminates all superfluous parameters. In fact, the bulk the algorithm's work is devoted to enforcing range conditions.

The overarching concept behind the inversion algorithm is recursion. The recursive inversion algorithm depends upon matrix manipulations to simplify solutions and eliminate parameters (Section 20.4). This chapter generalizes the work of the author for the 4 × 4 problem [5]. New techniques for eliminating extra parameters from the solutions for $n \times n$ systems are presented.

20.2 Diffuse tomography model

The fundamental differences between diffuse and "discrete" tomography are scatter and their physical interpretations. Diffuse tomographic data is the sum over all possible paths between source and detector of the probabilities with which a particle traverses that path. If we were to presuppose that the probabilities over all non-straight (i.e., scattered) paths are identically zero, the resulting data set has the same information content as discrete tomographic data. Let Σ equal the sum of densities along path L. Σ is the discrete tomographic data corresponding to path L and $e^{-\Sigma}$ is the corresponding diffuse tomographic data. The discrete data pertains to the *density* of the imaging object along path L, whereas the diffuse tomographic data pertains to the *probability* with which particles travel along path L. The relationship between the data sets is clear, but their physical meanings lend themselves to different reconstruction techniques. We exploit the probabilistic (in fact, Markovian) nature of diffuse tomography by recursively splitting the system into smaller and smaller subsystems.

In diffuse tomographic systems particles travel between pixels in the plane. Consider an $n \times n$ array of pixels in the plane. On each outer face there are two devices. One device shoots photons across the outside edge into the neighboring pixel; the other device detects photons which leave the system, but does *not* register their exit times. For each of the $4n$ outside edges we shoot photons into the system and measure outgoing radiation at each of the $4n$ ports. These data are stored as a $4n \times 4n$ transition matrix, Q. Within the system, photons travel either horizontally or vertically, do not interact with each other, and may be absorbed within a pixel; see Fig. 20.1. Photons move according to a Markov process. The probabilities with which a photon moves to a neighboring pixel depend upon its previous, as well as present, location. In this two step formulation the state space consists of locations. We redefine the state space so that photons move according to a one step Markov process. In the new state space a single state consists of the photon's location and direction of travel.

There are three different types of these Markov states: incoming, hidden, and outgoing. (Outgoing states are absorbing.) Particles incident to the same pixel from *different* directions need not behave alike. For each pixel and incident direction the sum of the absorption probability and the four possible transition probabilities must be identically one. Therefore, we neglect the absorption probability. Each pixel corresponds to

4 incident directions $\times$ 4 active trans. probs. = 16 trans. probs.

These probabilities are the nonzero entries of the Markov transition matrix M. M is sparse and may be written as a block matrix with four nontrivial subblocks:

$$M = \begin{bmatrix} \Theta & Pih & Pio \\ \Theta & Phh & Pho \\ \Theta & \Theta & I \end{bmatrix} \tag{20.3}$$

See Fig. 20.1 for the sizes of these subblocks. Their physical meaning is described in the following sections. A 2×2 system is shown in Fig. 20.3.

matrix	relevant transitions	size original	size modified
Pio	inc-out	$4n \times 4n$	$4n \times 4n$
Pih	inc-hid	$4n \times (16n^2 - 4n)$	$4n \times 4n$
Phh	hid-hid	$(16n^2-4n) \times (16n^2-4n)$	$4n \times 4n$
Pho	hid-out	$(16n^2 - 4n) \times 4n$	$4n \times 4n$

TABLE 20.1. The nontrivial subblocks of the one-step transition matrix M for both the original formulation and also the "modified" problem.

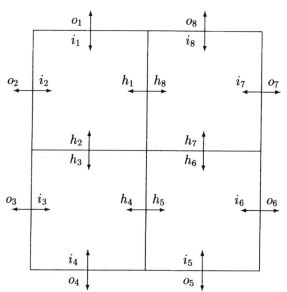

FIGURE 20.3. Incoming, hidden, and outgoing states are labeled with i's, h's, and o's, respectively. Also, the 4×4 submatrices representing travel *across* the system are generically of rank 2.

20.2.1 Forward problem

The upper right block of M contains one-step transition probabilities from incoming to outgoing states. The measured data, Q, is the upper right corner of $\lim_{k \to \infty} M^k$. Therefore, the forward map can be written as the matrix equation

$$Q = Pio + Pih\ Pho + Pih\ Phh\ Pho + Pih\ Phh^2\ Pho + \cdots$$

$$= Pio + Pih \sum_{n=0}^{\infty} Phh^n\ Pho$$

$$= Pio + Pih\ (I - Phh)^{-1}\ Pho \qquad (20.4)$$

The forward map takes $16n^2$ transition probabilities to the $4n \times 4n$ data matrix Q. The domain of the forward map lies in the unit cube in $\mathbb{R}^{16n^2}$. Furthermore, none of these transition probabilities is permitted to be zero. Q_i^j represents the probability that a photon which enters the system at source i eventually exits the system at detector j. Q provides no time-of-flight information, which would give the pathlength traveled by the particle. Because Q is a transition matrix acceptable solutions lie in the unit cube in $\mathbb{R}^{16n^2}$ and satisfy

$$0 \le \sum_{\lambda=1}^{4n} Q_i^{\lambda} \le 1, \qquad i = 1, 2, \ldots, 4n \qquad (20.5)$$

20.2.2 Consistency conditions

Although $Q : \mathbb{R}^{16n^2} \to \mathbb{R}^{16n^2}$, the range of the forward map is not of dimension $16n^2$. Range conditions appear as rank deficient submatrices of Q. Each of these rank deficient submatrices represents travel from one "side" of the system to the other "side." Let b be a virtual barrier separating the two sides of the system composed of $\#b$ hidden states. The Markovian nature of the system can be used to show that the corresponding submatrix is generically of rank $\#b$. A $n \times n$ system is subject to $8n(n-1)$ independent conditions [3, 6].

Notation: Let $Q_{\mathbf{r}}^{\mathbf{c}}$ denote the submatrix of Q taken from rows $\mathbf{r}$ and columns $\mathbf{c}$. Let $dQ_{\mathbf{r}}^{\mathbf{c}}$ denote the determinant of this submatrix. Furthermore, let $a : b$ denote $a, a+1, \ldots, b$ where $a, b \in \mathbb{N}$ and $a < b$.

For example, the data matrix for a 2×2 system has many rank deficient submatrices of rank two. The submatrix representing travel from left to right, $Q_{1:4}^{5:8}$, is generically rank two, as is $Q_{5:8}^{1:4}$. See Fig. 20.3. Similarly, the submatrices $Q_{3:6}^{1:2,7:8}$ and $Q_{1:2,7:8}^{3:6}$ are generically of rank two as well.

$$
\begin{bmatrix}
o & x & & & & & & \\
x & o & & & & & & \\
& & o & x & & & & \\
& & x & o & & & & \\
& & & & o & x & & \\
& & & & x & o & & \\
& & & & & & o & x \\
& & & & & & x & o
\end{bmatrix}
\qquad
\begin{bmatrix}
x & & & & & & o & \\
& o & & & & & & x \\
& & o & & x & & & \\
& & x & & o & & & \\
& & & & & o & & x \\
& & & & & x & & o \\
x & & & & & & o & \\
o & & & & & & x &
\end{bmatrix}
$$

FIGURE 20.4. The array on the left represents the block structure of and *Pho* **(and of course** A**) for a modified** $n \times n$ **problem where** $n = 2^k$, $k \in \mathbb{N}$. **The array on the right gives the off diagonal block structure for modified transition matrices** *Pih*. **Each** x **and** o **represents a nontrivial** $\frac{n}{2} \times \frac{n}{2}$ **block in diffuse tomography; in discrete tomography the blocks corresponding to** o **are identically zero.** *Phh* **and** *Pio* **share the block structures of** *Pih* **and** *Pho* **in diffuse tomography.**

20.3 Recursive solution

Although the final goal is to recover the microscopic transition probabilities for each pixel from boundary value data, the purpose of this section is more modest. The original $n \times n$ system is broken into four $\frac{n}{2} \times \frac{n}{2}$ subsystems; $4n^2$ parameter families of the subsystems' data sets are computed from the data set for the $n \times n$ array. (Here $n = 2^k$, $k \in \mathbb{N}$.)

A "trick" is used to solve the inverse problem for a 2×2 system; the recursive scheme presented here takes advantage of the same "trick" many times over [7]. The "trick" requires invertibility of *Pho*, a non-square matrix for $n > 2$. By considering only the $4n$ hidden states dividing an $n \times n$ system into four $\frac{n}{2} \times \frac{n}{2}$ subsystems, the "modified" transition matrices are square. In fact, they have the same *block structure* as their 2×2 counterparts. See Fig.s 20.2 and 20.4. The only difference is that each entry of a 2×2 transition matrix is now a $\frac{n}{2} \times \frac{n}{2}$ *block* of the modified transition matrices for the $n \times n$ system. Note that the entries of these modified transition matrices are the data for the $\frac{n}{2} \times \frac{n}{2}$ subsystems. For example, if $Q11$, $Q12$, $Q21$, and $Q22$ and the data matrices for each of the four subsystems shown in Fig. 20.2, then

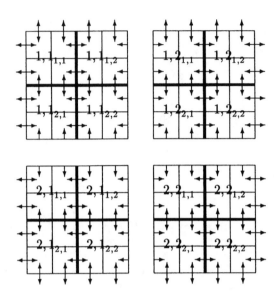

FIGURE 20.5. Decomposition of a 8×8 system into four 4×4 subsystems which are subsequently decomposed into 2×2 sub-subsystems. The thick lines separate the 2×2 subsystems.

$$Pho = \begin{bmatrix} Q11^{1-6,15,16}_{7-14} & & & \\ & Q21^{3-10}_{1,2,11-16} & & \\ & & Q22^{7-14}_{1-6,15,16} & \\ & & & Q12^{1,2,11-16}_{3-10} \end{bmatrix}. \tag{20.6}$$

Equation (20.4) expresses the data generated by the $n \times n$ system in terms the $\frac{n}{2} \times \frac{n}{2}$ subsystems' data. Note that the only "bad" term in (20.4) is $(I - Phh)^{-1}$ and define $A \equiv Pho^{-1}$. The governing equations may be written as a matrix equation of degree three in A, Pio, Phh, and Pih:

$$(Q - Pio) A (I - Phh) - Pih = 0. \tag{20.7}$$

The following notation is useful in manipulating (20.7), a matrix equation whose summands are functions of sparse block matrices.

Notation: $[M : N]$ denotes the concatenation of matrices M and N (where M and N have the same number of rows). *left*, *right*, *top*, and *bot* denote any choice of one half of the states on the left, right, top, and bottom of the system. There are $\binom{n}{n/2}$ possibilities for each. Finally, let $\mathbf{i} = \frac{(i-1)n}{2} + 1, \ldots, \frac{in}{2}$ for $i = 1, \ldots, 8$, see Fig. 20.6.

It is possible to solve for each of the nontrivial subblocks of Pio, Pih,

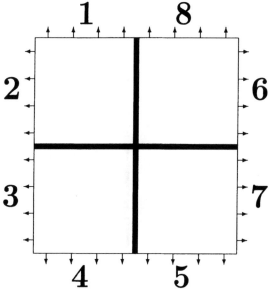

FIGURE 20.6. Groups of states are labeled 1, 2, ..., 8. For the 8×8 system shown above each group consists of four states.

Phh, and Pho as functions of A and Q [5]. The following blocks will be used later to eliminate some of the parameters A_i^j from the solutions:

$$Phh_{12}^3 = Pho_{12}^{12} \, (Q_{right}^{12})^{-1} \, Q_{right}^{34} \, A_{34}^3 \tag{20.8}$$

$$Pio_{12}^{12} = Q_{12}^{12} - [Q_{12}^{78}(Q_{bot}^{78})^{-1}Q_{bot}^{12}A_{12}^1 : Q_{12}^{34}(Q_{right}^{34})^{-1}Q_{right}^{12}A_{12}^2] \, Pho_{12}^{12} \tag{20.9}$$

$$Pih_{12}^3 = [Q_{12}^{34} - (Q_{12}^{12} - Pio_{12}^{12}) \, (Q_{right}^{12})^{-1} \, Q_{right}^{34}] \, A_{34}^3 \tag{20.10}$$

Expressions for other nontrivial blocks of Phh, Pio, and Pih take the same forms as the solutions in (20.8) through (20.10). The next sections parallel work done in [8] and are included here for completeness and the understanding of the reader.

20.4   Elimination of parameters

The data for each of the $\frac{n}{2} \times \frac{n}{2}$ subsystems is written in terms of Q and the $16n^2$ nonzero entries of A, as done above in expressions (20.8), (20.9), and (20.10). These data, however, do not conform to the range conditions described in Subsection 20.2.2; see Fig. 20.7. Enforcing these range conditions amounts to requiring that various $(\frac{n}{2} + 1) \times (\frac{n}{2} + 1)$ minors of each subsystem's newly found data sets be identically zero and results in polynomials in the $4n^2$ nonzero A_i^js. Fortunately, these polynomials factor into

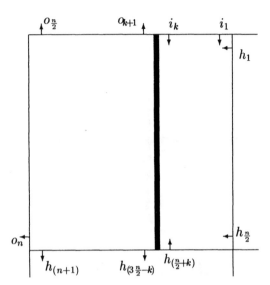

FIGURE 20.7. The 1,1 subsystem and the states corresponding to $Q11^k_{rl}$, the kth right-left rank deficient submatrix of $Q11$, a $(\frac{n}{2} + 2k) \times (3\frac{n}{2} - 2k)$ matrix of rank $\frac{n}{2}$.

a product of terms such that the zero-valued term is linear. Although there are many such conditions, only $4(n^2 - 2n)$ of them are independent. $8n$ of the parameters A^j_is in the solutions for Pho, Phh, Pih, and Pio cannot be eliminated by virtue of these range conditions.

The simplest range conditions force submatrices of the modified transition matrix Pho to be identically zero. Since $A = Pho^{-1}$, entries of A furthest from the diagonal are identically zero.

Theorem 20.1. *A has band width $(n + 1)$.*

Proof: Recall that $A = Pho^{-1}$ is block diagonal with four $n \times n$ blocks along the diagonal. For $k = 1, \ldots, (\frac{n}{2} - 1)$, let $Q11^k_{rl}$ be the matrix representing travel across $Q11$ from the rightmost $(\frac{n}{2} + 2k)$ incoming ports to the remaining $(3\frac{n}{2} - 2k)$ ports on the left. rank $Q11^k_{rl} = \frac{n}{2}$ which implies rank $Pho^{(k+1):n}_{1:\frac{n}{2}+k} = \frac{n}{2}$. For $(\frac{n}{2} + k) < j \leq n$,

$$\text{rank } Pho^{(k+1):n}_{1:(j-1),(j+1):n} \leq (n - k - 1) \qquad \text{so,}$$
$$\text{rank } Pho^{1:(k-1),(k+1):n}_{1:(j-1),(j+1):n} \leq (n - 2) \qquad (20.11)$$

However, $A^j_k = (-1)^{j+k} dPho^{1:(k-1),(k+1):n}_{1:(j-1),(j+1):n} / dPho^{1:n}_{1:n} = 0.$

The same argument holds upon the hidden-outgoing blocks within the other "hidden-outgoing" submatrices to prove the claim.   □

These identities account for one quarter of the conditions upon the parameters A_i^js. See Fig. 20.8 for the block structure of A. Another quarter of the conditions are listed below.

$$0 = \left[I_k : \Theta_k^{(n-k)} \right] (Q_{right}^{12})^{-1} Q_{right}^{34} A_{34}^{(\frac{3}{2}n-k)}$$

$$0 = \left[\Theta_k^{(n-k)} : I_k \right] (Q_{bot}^{12})^{-1} Q_{bot}^{78} A_{78}^{(7\frac{n}{2}+k+1)}$$

$$0 = \left[I_k : \Theta_k^{(n-k)} \right] (Q_{bot}^{78})^{-1} Q_{bot}^{12} A_{12}^{(\frac{n}{2}-k)}$$

$$0 = \left[\Theta_k^{(n-k)} : I_k \right] (Q_{left}^{78})^{-1} Q_{left}^{56} A_{56}^{(5\frac{n}{2}+k+1)}$$

$$0 = \left[\Theta_k^{(n-k)} : I_k \right] (Q_{right}^{34})^{-1} Q_{right}^{12} A_{12}^{(\frac{n}{2}+k+1)} \qquad (20.12)$$

$$0 = \left[I_k : \Theta_k^{(n-k)} \right] (Q_{top}^{34})^{-1} Q_{top}^{56} A_{56}^{(5\frac{n}{2}-k)}$$

$$0 = \left[\Theta_k^{(n-k)} : I_k \right] (Q_{top}^{56})^{-1} Q_{top}^{34} A_{34}^{(3\frac{n}{2}+k+1)}$$

$$0 = \left[I_k : \Theta_k^{(n-k)} \right] (Q_{left}^{56})^{-1} Q_{left}^{78} A_{78}^{(7\frac{n}{2}-k)}$$

These conditions can be used to eliminate $8 \sum\limits_{k=1}^{(\frac{n}{2}-1)} k = n(n-2)$ of the A_i^js from the solutions for Pio, Pih, Phh, and Pho in terms of Q and A. The first identity in (20.12) is derived below, using the following notation:

Notation: Define Θ_r^c to be the $r \times c$ zero matrix and I_k to be the $k \times k$ identity matrix.

Theorem 20.2. $\Theta_k^1 = \left[I_k : \Theta_k^{(n-k)} \right] (Q_{right}^{12})^{-1} Q_{right}^{34} A_{34}^{(\frac{3}{2}n-k)}$ where $k < \frac{n}{2}$.

Proof: Notice from Fig. 20.7 that

$$\text{rank} \left[Pho_{1:(\frac{n}{2}+k)}^{(k+1):n} \qquad Phh_{1:(\frac{n}{2}+k)}^{(n+1):(3\frac{n}{2}-k)} \right] = \frac{n}{2} \qquad (20.13)$$

Recall the solution formula for Phh (20.8) and write

$$Phh_{1:(\frac{n}{2}+k)}^{(n+1):(3\frac{n}{2}-k)} = Pho_{1:(\frac{n}{2}+k)}^{12} v^{1:(\frac{n}{2}-k)} \qquad (20.14)$$

where $\mathbf{v}$ is defined as

$$\mathbf{v} = (Q_{right}^{12})^{-1} Q_{right}^{34} A_{34}^{34} \qquad (20.15)$$

$$\begin{bmatrix} A_1^1 & A_1^2 & A_1^3 & \\ A_2^1 & A_2^2 & A_2^3 & A_2^4 \\ A_3^1 & A_3^2 & A_3^3 & A_3^4 \\ & A_4^2 & A_4^3 & A_4^4 \end{bmatrix}$$

$$\begin{bmatrix} A_1^1 & A_1^2 & A_1^3 & A_1^4 & A_1^5 & & & \\ A_2^1 & A_2^2 & A_2^3 & A_2^4 & A_2^5 & A_2^6 & & \\ A_3^1 & A_3^2 & A_3^3 & A_3^4 & A_3^5 & A_3^6 & A_3^7 & \\ A_4^1 & A_4^2 & A_4^3 & A_4^4 & A_4^5 & A_4^6 & A_4^7 & A_4^8 \\ A_5^1 & A_5^2 & A_5^3 & A_5^4 & A_5^5 & A_5^6 & A_5^7 & A_5^8 \\ & A_6^2 & A_6^3 & A_6^4 & A_6^5 & A_6^6 & A_6^7 & A_6^8 \\ & & A_7^3 & A_7^4 & A_7^5 & A_7^6 & A_7^7 & A_7^8 \\ & & & A_8^4 & A_8^5 & A_8^6 & A_8^7 & A_8^8 \end{bmatrix}$$

FIGURE 20.8. Zero structures of blocks along the diagonals of A for 4×4 and 8×8 systems, respectively.

Combining (20.13) through (20.15) implies rank $\left[Pho_{1:(\frac{n}{2}+k)}^{(k+1)n} \quad Pho_{1:(\frac{n}{2}+k)}^{12} v^{1:(\frac{n}{2}-k)} \right] = \frac{n}{2}$

where $k \le (\frac{n}{2}-1)$. Since rank $Pho_{1:(\frac{n}{2}+k)}^{(k+1):n} = \frac{n}{2}$, it is sufficient to force for each $k < \frac{n}{2}$, and $\alpha = 1, \dots, k,$

$$0 = \left| \, Pho_{1:\frac{n}{2},(\frac{n}{2}+\alpha)}^{(\frac{n}{2}+1):n} \quad Pho_{1:\frac{n}{2},(\frac{n}{2}+\alpha)}^{1:k} v_{1:k}^{(\frac{n}{2}-k)} \, \right|$$

$$= \sum_{\eta=1}^{k} v_\eta^{(\frac{n}{2}-k)} \left| \, Pho_{1:\frac{n}{2},(\frac{n}{2}+\alpha)}^{(\frac{n}{2}+1):n} \quad Pho_{1:\frac{n}{2},(\frac{n}{2}+\alpha)}^{\eta} \, \right| \qquad (20.16)$$

$$= \sum_{\eta=1}^{\alpha} v_\eta^{(\frac{n}{2}-k)} \, dPho_{1:\frac{n}{2},(\frac{n}{2}+\alpha)}^{\eta,(\frac{n}{2}+1):n} \qquad (20.17)$$

Equation (20.17) follows from (20.16) because for $\eta > \alpha$, $dPho_{1:\frac{n}{2},(\frac{n}{2}+\alpha)}^{\eta,(\frac{n}{2}+1):n} \equiv 0$. Since (20.17) holds for k different values of α, it is a homogeneous system of k equations for $\{v_\eta^{(\frac{n}{2}-k)}\}_{\eta=1,2,\dots,k}$. The Jacobian for this system is lower triangular and has a generically nonzero determinant, $\prod_{\eta=1}^{k} dPho_{1:\frac{n}{2},(\frac{n}{2}+\eta)}^{\eta,(\frac{n}{2}+1):n}$. Therefore, $0 = v_\alpha^{(\frac{n}{2}-k)}$, which proves the claim. $\square$

The identities in Theorems 20.1 and 20.2 give $2n(n-2)$ independent conditions upon the A_i^js. In Section 20.7 the following $2n(n-2)$ linear conditions upon the remaining A_i^js are derived by enforcing the rest of the consistency conditions upon the subsystems' data. These conditions are listed below:

$$0 = \left(dQ^{j,(2n+1):(7\frac{n}{2}-k)}_{\beta,(7\frac{n}{2}+k+1):4n,34} \right)^{j=1,\ldots,n}_{\beta=(\frac{7n}{2}-k+1),\ldots,(\frac{7n}{2}+k)} \cdot A^{(k+1)}_{12}$$

$$0 = \left(dQ^{j,(3\frac{n}{2}+k+1):3n}_{\beta,(n+1):(3\frac{n}{2}-k),78} \right)^{j=1,\ldots,n}_{\beta=(\frac{3n}{2}-k+1),\ldots,(\frac{3n}{2}+k)} \cdot A^{(n-k)}_{12}$$

$$0 = \left(dQ^{j,1:(\frac{n}{2}-k),78}_{\beta,(\frac{n}{2}+k+1):n,56} \right)^{j=(n+1),\ldots,2n}_{\beta=(\frac{n}{2}-k+1),\ldots,(\frac{n}{2}+k)} \cdot A^{(n+k+1)}_{34}$$

$$0 = \left(dQ^{j,(5\frac{n}{2}+k+1):4n}_{\beta,(2n+1):(5\frac{n}{2}-k),12} \right)^{j=(n+1),\ldots,2n}_{\beta=(\frac{5n}{2}-k+1),\ldots,(\frac{5n}{2}+k)} \cdot A^{(2n-k)}_{34}$$

$$0 = \left(dQ^{j,1:(3\frac{n}{2}-k)}_{\beta,(3\frac{n}{2}+k+1):2n,78} \right)^{j=(2n+1),\ldots,3n}_{\beta=(\frac{3n}{2}-k+1),\ldots,(\frac{3n}{2}+k)} \cdot A^{(2n+k+1)}_{56} \qquad (20.18)$$

$$0 = \left(dQ^{j,(7\frac{n}{2}+k+1):4n,12}_{\beta,(3n+1):(7\frac{n}{2}-k),34} \right)^{j=(2n+1),\ldots,3n}_{\beta=(\frac{7n}{2}-k+1),\ldots,(\frac{7n}{2}+k)} \cdot A^{(3n-k)}_{56}$$

$$0 = \left(dQ^{j,(n+1):(5\frac{n}{2}-k)}_{\beta,(5\frac{n}{2}+k+1):3n,12} \right)^{j=(3n+1),\ldots,4n}_{\beta=(\frac{5n}{2}-k+1),\ldots,(\frac{5n}{2}+k)} \cdot A^{(3n+k+1)}_{78}$$

$$0 = \left(dQ^{j,(\frac{n}{2}+k+1):2n}_{\beta,1:(\frac{n}{2}-k),56} \right)^{j=(3n+1),\ldots,4n}_{\beta=(\frac{n}{2}-k+1),\ldots,(\frac{n}{2}+k)} \cdot A^{(4n-k)}_{78}$$

These identities are derived by simplifying solutions for the unknown transition probabilities (equations (20.8), (20.9), and (20.10)), and using matrix identities from Section 20.6.

20.5 Conclusion

Equations (20.8), (20.9), and (20.10) give a $4n^2$ parameter family of data sets for $\frac{n}{2} \times \frac{n}{2}$ subsystems in terms of the $n \times n$ parent system's data. The most difficult step in the derivation is reducing the number of parameters from $4n^2$ to $8n$ and is done by enforcing range conditions upon the subsystems' data. These conditions are expressed most succinctly in Theorems 20.1, 20.2, and equation (20.18).

In order to recover the microscopic transition probabilities the recursion must continue until the 2×2 base case is solved. If $n = 2^k$ then k recursions are required. Denote the recursive levels by $r = 0, 1, \ldots, (k-1)$. At the rth recursion 4^r systems of size $(\frac{n}{2^r}) \times (\frac{n}{2^r})$ are subdivided and $8(\frac{n}{2^r})$ parameters are introduced per system. After all k recursions the transition probabilities are functions of

$$\sum_{r=0}^{(k-1)} 4^r \, 8(\frac{n^r}{2}) = 8n \sum_{r=0}^{(k-1)} 2^r = 8n(2^k - 1) = 8n(n-1) \qquad (20.19)$$

parameters. This number is optimal, (or rather minimal), because there are $8n(n-1)$ independent consistency conditions amongst the data [3]. Only by measuring additional data can the inverse problem be uniquely solved. Time-of-flight data, for example, may serve to close the system.

Clearly, the limiting case of isotropic scattering will be unstable because isotropic *Pho* matrices at the 2×2 level are singular. The continuum limit of the isotropic discrete model is a diffusion equation, well-suited to forward and ill-suited to inverse problems. The other extreme is discrete tomography.

Comparing "diffuse" and "discrete" tomography, scatter can be thought of as an added wrinkle that enriches the "diffuse" model of particle transport. Because of scatter, the diffuse tomographic model requires relatively more unknowns and unique solution to the inverse problem requires relatively more measured data.

20.6   Appendix I — Matrix identities

Solutions for subblocks of the one step Markov matrix, M, are matrix expressions in subblocks of A and Q. Furthermore, the constraints (20.12) upon the parameters in A are matrix identities. In order to derive the remaining constraints, more involved matrix identities are required. We begin with a few elementary identities, then incorporate range conditions (described in Section 20.2.2) and Graßmann-Plücker identities to construct more elaborate identities amongst minors of Q.

20.6.1   Elementary identities

For any matrix, Q, cofactor expansions of submatrices multiplied by other submatrices can be computed analytically. Let $\alpha, \beta, \gamma, \eta, \kappa \in \mathbb{N}^k$.

$$(Q_\alpha^\gamma)^{-1} Q_\alpha^\eta = \left(\frac{dQ_\alpha^{\gamma_1, \gamma_2, \ldots, \gamma_{i-1}, \eta_j, \gamma_{i+1}, \ldots, \gamma_n}}{dQ_\alpha^\gamma} \right)_{i,j} \qquad (20.20)$$

$$Q_\kappa^\gamma (Q_\alpha^\gamma)^{-1} Q_\alpha^\eta = Q_\kappa^\eta - (1/dQ_\alpha^\gamma)(dQ_{\kappa_i,\alpha}^{\eta_j,\gamma})_{i,j} \qquad (20.21)$$

Furthermore, for our block diagonal matrix A,

$$I = A_{(2\alpha-1):2\alpha}^{(2\alpha-1):2\alpha} Pho_{(2\alpha-1):2\alpha}^{(2\alpha-1):2\alpha}$$

$$= A_{(2\alpha-1):2\alpha}^{(2\alpha-1)} Pho_{(2\alpha-1)}^{(2\alpha-1):2\alpha} + A_{(2\alpha-1):2\alpha}^{2\alpha} Pho_{2\alpha}^{(2\alpha-1):2\alpha} \qquad (20.22)$$

where $\alpha = 1,2,3,4$.

20.6.2 Graßmann identities

The identities which embed Graßmannians $G(k,n)$ in $\mathbf{P}^{\binom{n}{k}-1}$ are used in the following section to simplify the remaining "incoming-hidden" constraints. These algebraic conditions upon minors of a matrix prove useful in the next section.

A cursory explanation of the embedding can be found in [7]. For a more thorough exposition see [9,10].

Let $\mathbf{\Lambda}$ be a matrix with k rows and n columns where $k < (n-1)$,
$$I = (i_1, i_2, i_3, \ldots, i_{(k-1)}) \text{ index } (k-1) \text{ distinct columns of } \mathbf{\Lambda}, \text{ and}$$
$$J = (j_1, j_2, j_3, \ldots, j_{(k+1)}) \text{ index } (k+1) \text{ distinct columns of } \mathbf{\Lambda}.$$
Then, the Graßmann relations are

$$\sum_{\lambda=1}^{k+1} d\mathbf{\Lambda}^{(i_1, i_2, \ldots, i_{k-1}, j_\lambda)} \, d\mathbf{\Lambda}^{(j_1, j_2, \ldots, j_{\lambda-1}, j_{\lambda+1}, \ldots, j_{k+1})} = 0 \qquad (20.23)$$

Combining identity (20.20) with Graßmann-Plücker relations results in

$$
\begin{aligned}
& (dQ_{\kappa_i,\alpha}^{\gamma_k,\beta})_{i,k} \, (Q_\alpha^\gamma)^{-1} Q_\alpha^\eta \\
&= (dQ_{\kappa_i,\alpha}^{\gamma_k,\beta})_{i,k} \left(\frac{dQ_\alpha^{\gamma_1,\gamma_2,\ldots,\gamma_{k-1},\eta_j,\gamma_{k+1},\ldots,\gamma_n}}{dQ_\alpha^\gamma} \right)_{k,j} \\
&= \frac{-1}{dQ_\alpha^\gamma} \sum_{k=1}^n (-1)^k \left(dQ_{\kappa_i,\alpha}^{\gamma_k,\beta} \, dQ_\alpha^{\eta_j,\gamma_1,\gamma_2,\ldots,\gamma_{k-1},\gamma_{k+1},\ldots,\gamma_n} \right)_{i,j} \\
&= \left(dQ_{\kappa_i,\alpha}^{\eta_j,\beta} - \frac{dQ_\alpha^\beta}{dQ_\alpha^\gamma} dQ_{\kappa_i,\alpha}^{\eta_j,\gamma} \right)_{i,j}
\end{aligned}
\qquad (20.24)
$$

Finally, the Laplace expansion and Graßmann-Plücker relations can be used to simplify the minor

$$\left| dQ_{\beta_i,\alpha}^{\kappa_j,\gamma} \right|_{i,j=1,\ldots,m} = dQ_{\beta,\alpha}^{\kappa,\gamma} (dQ_\alpha^\gamma)^{m-1} \quad \text{where } \beta, \kappa \in \mathbf{R}^m \text{ and } \alpha, \gamma \in \mathbf{R}^n \qquad (20.25)$$

20.6.3 Range conditions

In the following section, Graßmann-Plücker relations and the Laplace expansion of a determinant are often used in conjunction with range conditions. For example, range conditions upon Q imply

$$dQ_{\delta;34}^{j,78} \equiv 0 \quad \text{for each } j = (2n+1), \ldots, 3n, \quad \delta = 1, \ldots, n \qquad (20.26)$$

Furthermore, for $\gamma = (3n+1), \ldots, (7\frac{n}{2} - k)$, and $\alpha = (\frac{n}{2} - k + 1), \ldots, (\frac{n}{2} + k)$

$$Q_{1:(\frac{n}{2}-k),\alpha,(7\frac{n}{2}-k+1):4n}^{(\frac{n}{2}+k+1):2n} \text{is a } (n+1) \times (3\frac{n}{2} - k) \text{ matrix of rank } n \text{ and}$$

$$Q_{1:(\frac{n}{2}-k),\alpha,(7\frac{n}{2}-k+1):4n}^{\gamma,(\frac{n}{2}+k+1):2n} \text{is a } (n+1) \times (3\frac{n}{2} - k + 1) \text{ rank } n \text{ matrix.}$$

Adding a few more rows to these rank deficient rectangular matrices results in rank deficient square matrices. Therefore,

$$dQ_{1:(\frac{n}{2}-k),\alpha,(3n+1):\gamma-1,\gamma+1:4n}^{(\frac{n}{2}+k+1):2n} = 0 = dQ_{1:(\frac{n}{2}-k),\alpha,\mathbf{78}}^{\gamma,(\frac{n}{2}+k+1):2n} \tag{20.27}$$

These identities are used to derive another $2n(n-2)$ conditions upon the remaining A_i^js in the following section.

20.7 Appendix II — Enforcing range conditions

In this appendix the remaining range conditions upon the subsystems' data are enforced. The submatrices of $Q11$, $Q12$, $Q21$, and $Q22$ which should be rank deficient and (primarily) represent travel from incoming states to hidden states are used. Consider now the "incoming-hidden" submatrix

$$Q11_{tb}^k = \begin{bmatrix} Pio_{1:(\frac{n}{2}+k)}^{(\frac{n}{2}+k+1):n} & Pih_{1:(\frac{n}{2}+k)}^{3,(7\frac{n}{2}+1):(4n-k)} \\ Pho_{1:k}^{(\frac{n}{2}+k+1):n} & Phh_{1:k}^{3,(7\frac{n}{2}+1):(4n-k)} \end{bmatrix} \tag{20.28}$$

$Q11_{tb}^k$ should be of rank $\frac{n}{2}$. Only for $k = (\frac{n}{2} - 1)$ can $Q11_{tb}^k$ be factored to derive linear conditions upon the A_i^js. Rather than forcing all of $Q11_{tb}^k$ to be rank $\frac{n}{2}$ we undertake a less ambitious endeavor, forcing

$$\text{rank} \begin{bmatrix} Pio_{1:(\frac{n}{2}+k)}^{(\frac{n}{2}+k+1):n} & Pih_{1:(\frac{n}{2}+k)}^3 \\ Pho_{1:k}^{(\frac{n}{2}+k+1):n} & Phh_{1:k}^3 \end{bmatrix} = \frac{n}{2} \tag{20.29}$$

The ramifications of this requirement are clarified in two steps. In claim 20.1 the conditions in (20.29) are shown to be *linear* in the A_i^js. The unfortunately complicated coefficients in these conditions are simplified in claim 20.2.

Thanks to identities (20.21) and (20.22) the solution for Pio_{12}^{12} can be written quite succinctly

$$Pio_{12}^{12} = M^1 + \left(\frac{dQ_{i,right}^{j,\mathbf{34}}}{dQ_{right}^{\mathbf{34}}} \right)_{i,j} \tag{20.30}$$

$$\text{where} \quad M^1 \equiv \left(\frac{dQ_{i,bot}^{j,\mathbf{78}}}{dQ_{bot}^{\mathbf{78}}} - \frac{dQ_{i,right}^{j,\mathbf{34}}}{dQ_{right}^{\mathbf{34}}} \right)_{i,j} A_{12}^1 \, Pho_1^{12} \tag{20.31}$$

All of the nonzero blocks of Pio can be written in such simple form. These simpler solutions for Pio can be used to simplify solutions for subblocks of Pih. For instance, substituting (20.30) and several matrix identities of the forms shown in (20.21) and (20.24) into equation (20.10) yields

$$Pih_{12}^3 = M^1 \left(Q_{right}^{12} \right)^{-1} Q_{right}^{\mathbf{34}} A_{\mathbf{34}}^3 \tag{20.32}$$

See [11] for details.

Lemma 20.1. *Forcing $Q11_{tb}^k$ to be rank $\frac{n}{2}$ for each k implies*

$$(l)_{1:(\frac{n}{2}+k)}^{(k+1)} \in \text{colspan}\left(dQ_{i,right}^{j,34}\right)_{i=1,2,\ldots,(\frac{n}{2}+k)}^{j=(\frac{n}{2}+1+k),\ldots,n} \qquad (20.33)$$

Proof: The matrix in (20.29) may be rewritten using the following definitions

$$l \equiv \left(\frac{dQ_{i,bot}^{j,78}}{dQ_{bot}^{78}} - \frac{dQ_{i,right}^{j,34}}{dQ_{right}^{34}}\right)_{i=1,\ldots,n}^{j=1,\ldots,n} A_{12}^1$$

$$D \equiv \left(\frac{dQ_{i,right}^{j,34}}{dQ_{right}^{34}}\right)_{i=1,\ldots,n}^{j=1,\ldots,n}$$

$$S_1 \equiv \begin{bmatrix} \Theta_{(\frac{n}{2}+k)}^{(\frac{n}{2}-k)} \\ I_{(\frac{n}{2}-k)} \end{bmatrix} \qquad (20.34)$$

$$S_2 \equiv \left(Q_{right}^{12}\right)^{-1} Q_{right}^{34} A_{34}^3$$

and recall the definition of M^1. The blocks of (20.29) can be written as follows:

$$Pio_{1:(\frac{n}{2}+k)}^{(\frac{n}{2}+k+1):n} = l_{1:(\frac{n}{2}+k)} Pho_1^{(\frac{n}{2}+k+1):n} + D_{1:(\frac{n}{2}+k)}^{(\frac{n}{2}+k+1):n}$$

$$Pih_{1:(\frac{n}{2}+k)}^3 = l_{1:(\frac{n}{2}+k)} Pho_1^{12} S_2 \qquad (20.35)$$

$$Phh_{1:k}^3 = Pho_{1:k}^{12} S_2$$

Then matrix (20.29) equals

$$\begin{bmatrix} l_{1:(\frac{n}{2}+k)} Pho_1^{(\frac{n}{2}+k+1):n} + D_{1:(\frac{n}{2}+k)}^{(\frac{n}{2}+k+1):n} & Pih_{1:(\frac{n}{2}+k)}^3 \\ \hline Pho_{1:k}^{(\frac{n}{2}+k+1):n} & Phh_{1:k}^3 \end{bmatrix} \qquad (20.36)$$

$$= \begin{bmatrix} D_{1:(\frac{n}{2}+k)}^{(\frac{n}{2}+k+1):n} & \Theta \\ \hline \Theta & \Theta \end{bmatrix} + \begin{bmatrix} l_{1:(\frac{n}{2}+k)} Pho_1^{(\frac{n}{2}+k+1):n} & l_{1:(\frac{n}{2}+k)} Pho_1^{12} S_2 \\ \hline Pho_{1:k}^{(\frac{n}{2}+k+1):n} & Pho_{1:k}^{12} S_2 \end{bmatrix}$$

$$= \begin{bmatrix} D_{1:(\frac{n}{2}+k)}^{(\frac{n}{2}+k+1):n} & \Theta \\ \hline \Theta & \Theta \end{bmatrix} + \begin{bmatrix} l_{1:(\frac{n}{2}+k)} \\ I_k \quad \Theta_k^{n-k} \end{bmatrix} Pho_1^{12} \begin{bmatrix} S_1 & S_2 \end{bmatrix}$$

Since $Pih_{1:(\frac{n}{2}+k)}^3$ is generically of rank $\frac{n}{2}$ and Pho_1^{12} has only $\frac{n}{2}$ rows,

$$\text{rank} \begin{bmatrix} l_{1:(\frac{n}{2}+k)} \\ I_k \quad \Theta_k^{(\frac{n}{2}-k)} \end{bmatrix} Pho_1^{12} [S_1 : S_2] = \frac{n}{2} \qquad (20.37)$$

Therefore, colspan $\begin{bmatrix} l_{1:(\frac{n}{2}+k)} \\ I_k \quad \theta_k^{(\frac{n}{2}-k)} \end{bmatrix}$ has dimension $\frac{n}{2}$. In order to enforce condition (20.29) we require that

$$\text{colspan} \begin{bmatrix} D_{1:(\frac{n}{2}+k)}^{(\frac{n}{2}+k+1):n} \\ \Theta \end{bmatrix} \in \text{colspan} \begin{bmatrix} l_{1:(\frac{n}{2}+k)} \\ I_k \quad \theta_k^{n-k} \end{bmatrix} \tag{20.38}$$

equivalently, colspan $D_{1:(\frac{n}{2}+k)}^{(\frac{n}{2}+k+1):n} \in$ colspan $l_{1:(\frac{n}{2}+k)}^{(k+1):\frac{n}{2}}$. However, identity (20.25) allows one to check that rank $D_{1:(\frac{n}{2}+k)}^{(\frac{n}{2}+k+1):n} = (\frac{n}{2}-k)$. Therefore, the requirement (20.38) might as well be written

$$\text{colspan } D_{1:(\frac{n}{2}+k)}^{(\frac{n}{2}+k+1):n} = \text{colspan } l_{1:(\frac{n}{2}+k)}^{(k+1):\frac{n}{2}}, \tag{20.39}$$

which proves the claim. □

Claim 20.1 implies *linear* conditions upon the A_i^js:

$$0 = \left| \left(dQ_{i,right}^{j,\mathbf{34}} \right)_{i=1,\ldots,(\frac{n}{2}-k),\alpha}^{j=(\frac{n}{2}+k+1),\ldots,n} \quad : \quad l_{1:(\frac{n}{2}-k),\alpha}^{(k+1)} \right| \tag{20.40}$$

for each $k = (\frac{n}{2}-1), (\frac{n}{2}-2), \ldots, 1$ and $\alpha = (\frac{n}{2}-k+1), \ldots, (\frac{n}{2}+k)$. Recall the definition of l (20.34).

Repeated use of Graßmann-Plücker relations, range conditions, and the Laplace expansion are used in [11] to simplify these conditions. The result is given in the following

Lemma 20.2. *The conditions in (20.40) are equivalent to*

$$\Theta_{2k}^1 = \left(dQ_{\beta,(7\frac{n}{2}+k+1):4n,\mathbf{34}}^{j,(2n+1):(7\frac{n}{2}-k)} \right)_{\beta=(\frac{7n}{2}-k+1),\ldots,(\frac{7n}{2}+k)}^{j=1,\ldots,n} \cdot A_{12}^{(k+1)} \tag{20.41}$$

Furthermore, for all k from 1 to $(\frac{n}{2}-1)$ equation (20.41) forms a system of $\frac{n}{2}(\frac{n}{2}-1)$ independent conditions upon $\{A_i^{(k+1)}\}$.

Proof: To see this, fix k and compute the determinant of the first $2k$ columns of the Jacobian:

$$\left| dQ_{\beta,(7\frac{n}{2}+k+1):4n,\mathbf{34}}^{j,(2n+1):(7\frac{n}{2}-k)} \right|_{\beta=(7\frac{n}{2}-k+1),\ldots,(7\frac{n}{2}+k)}^{j=1,\ldots,2k} \tag{20.42}$$

$$= dQ_{(7\frac{n}{2}-k+1):4n,\mathbf{34}}^{1:2k,(2n+1):(7\frac{n}{2}-k)} \left(dQ_{(7\frac{n}{2}+k+1):4n,\mathbf{34}}^{(2n+1):(7\frac{n}{2}-k)} \right)^{2k-1} \neq 0 \tag{20.43}$$

The Jacobian in (20.42) is simplified by the identity (20.25) in line (20.43), which is generically nonzero. Therefore, the conditions in (20.41) are independent. Similar arguments apply to other "incoming-hidden" rank deficient submatrices and yield the identities (20.18), which can be used to eliminate another $2n(n-2)$ of the A_i^js from the solutions for $Q11$, $Q12$, $Q21$, and $Q22$. The end result is $8n$ parameter families of solutions for the $\frac{n}{2} \times \frac{n}{2}$ subsystems' data. $\qquad\square$

Acknowledgment

This work was done during a NSF post-doctoral fellowship at the Institute for Mathematics and its Applications in Minneapolis, MN.

References

[1] J. Singer, F. A. Grünbaum, P. Kohn, and J. Zubelli, "Image reconstruction of the interior of bodies that diffuse radiation," *Science* **248**, 990-993 (1990).

[2] G. T. Herman, *Image Reconstruction from Projections: The Fundamentals of Computerized Tomography*, (Academic Press, New York), 1980.

[3] S. K. Patch, "Consistency conditions in diffuse tomography," *Inverse Problems* **10**, 199-212 (1994).

[4] S. K. Patch, "Iterative algorithm for discrete tomography," *International Journal of Imaging Systems and Technology* **9**, 132-134 (1998).

[5] S. K. Patch, "Recursive recovery of a family of Markov transition probabilities from boundary value data," *Journal of Mathematical Physics* **36**, 3395-3412 (1995).

[6] F. A. Grünbaum and S. K. Patch, "How many parameters can one solve for in Diffuse Tomography," In G. Papanicolaou, A. Friedman, and R. Gulliver *I.M.A. Workshop on Inverse Problems in Waves and Scattering*, (Springer-Verlag, New York), pp. 219-236, 1995.

[7] F. A. Grünbaum and S. K. Patch, "The use of Graßmann identities for inversion of a general model in diffuse tomography," In *Proceedings of the Lapland Conference on Inverse Problems*, (Saariselkä, Finland), 1992.

[8] S. K. Patch, "Diffuse tomography modulo Graßmann and Laplace," *Journal of Mathematical Physics* **37**, 3283-3305 (1996).

[9] W. V. D. Hodge and D. Pedoe, *Methods of Algebraic Geometry*, (Cambridge University Press, Cambridge, UK) 1968.

[10] P. Griffiths and J. Harris, *Principles of Algebraic Geometry*, (Wiley and Sons, New York) 1978.

[11] S. K. Patch, "Sufficiency and simplicity of range conditions for diffuse tomgraphic systems," *Technical Report #97-07, Scientific Computing and Computational Mathematics, Stanford University, Stanford, CA* (1997).

Chapter 21

From Orthogonal Projections to Symbolic Projections

Shi-Kuo Chang[1]

ABSTRACT Symbolic projections are applicable to pictorial information retrieval and spatial reasoning problems where the relative spatial locations of objects are of interest. In this chapter the elements of the Theory of Symbolic Projection are introduced. 2D string representations of symbolic pictures are described. A survey of various applications is provided.

21.1 Introduction

The orthogonal projections of a binary picture give a concise characterization of the original picture [1]. A natural generalization is to introduce orthogonal projections for gray-level pictures where the pixel value can be a number between 0 and L-1 (L being the number of gray-levels), and the column sums and row sums are obtained by summing the gray-level values. Such orthogonal projections have been extensively studied and used in pattern recognition and other applications, most notably computerized tomography.

Another natural generalization is to introduce orthogonal projections for symbolic pictures where each pixel value can be the label of an object or a set of labels. This generalization leads to the concept of symbolic projections.

What are symbolic projections? How can symbolic projections be applied to pictorial information retrieval and spatial reasoning? A simple example will first be presented to illustrate the concept.

Figure 21.1(a) shows a picture with a house, a car and a tree. This picture is called a *symbolic picture*, as opposed to an actual image, because it contains objects that have symbolic names: house, tree, car, etc. Suppose the objective is to find out whether there is a tree to the southeast of the house. The x-projection of the above symbolic picture can be constructed as follows:

The names of objects in each column of the symbolic picture are pro-

---

[1] Department of Computer Science, University of Pittsburgh, Pittsburgh, PA 15260, USA, E-mail: chang@cs.pitt.edu.

jected onto the x-axis. The $<$ symbol is inserted to distinguish the objects belonging to different columns. Thus the x-projection is:

x-projection: house car $<$ tree

Similarly, the y-projection [2] is:

y-projection: house $<$ tree $<$ car

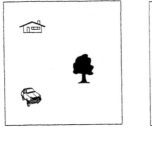 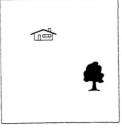

(a)   (b)

FIGURE 21.1. A symbolic picture (a) and its subpicture (b).

Unlike the projections of a mathematical function, the projections of a symbolic picture are strings. A pair of two symbolic projections is called a *2D string* [2].

The statement "there is a tree to the southeast of a house" corresponds to the symbolic picture shown in Fig. 21.1(b). This picture has the following symbolic projections:

x-projection: house $<$ tree

y-projection: house $<$ tree

We immediately notice "house $<$ tree" is a subsequence of "house car $<$ tree" and "house $<$ tree" is a subsequence of "house $<$ tree $<$ car." In this case, the two symbolic pictures can be perfectly reconstructed from the two corresponding pairs of symbolic projections. Therefore, the above statement can be verified to be true, just by checking the subsequence property of the 2D strings involved.

---

[2]The definition of y-projection in this chapter differs from the definition previously used by the author and other researchers, so that it can be consistent with the other chapters.

The Theory of Symbolic Projection was first developed by Chang and co-workers [2] based upon the above described intuitive concept. It forms the basis of a wide range of image information retrieval algorithms. It also supports pictorial-query-by-picture, so that the user of an image information system can simply draw a picture and use the picture as a query.

Many researchers have since extended this original concept, so that there is now a rich body of theory as well as empirical results. The extended Theory of Symbolic Projection can deal with not only point-like objects, but also objects of any shape and size [3,4]. Moreover, the Theory can deal with not only one symbolic picture, but also multiple symbolic pictures, three-dimensional pictures, a time sequence of pictures, etc. [5].

The purpose of this chapter is to introduce the elements of Symbolic Projection Theory as a complement of the Theory of Discrete Computed Tomography. 2D string representations of symbolic pictures are described in Section 21.2 . The matching of pictures using 2D strings is described in Section 21.3. The remaining five sections review the various applications of symbolic projections.

21.2   2D string representations of symbolic pictures

Let Σ be a set of symbols, or the vocabulary. Each symbol could represent a pictorial object, a pixel, etc.

Let A be the set { '=' , '<', ':' }, where '=', '<' and ':' are three special symbols not in Σ. These symbols will be used to specify spatial relationships between pictorial objects.

A *1D string* over Σ is any string $x_1 \, x_2 \ldots x_n$, $n \geq 0$, where the x_i's are in Σ.

A *2D string* over Σ, written as (u,v), is defined to be

$$(x_1 \, y_1 \, x_2 \, y_2 \ldots y_{n-1} \, x_n, \, x_{p(1)} \, z_1 \, x_{p(2)} \, z_2 \ldots z_{n-1} \, x_{p(n)})$$

where

$x_1 \ldots x_n$ is a 1D string over Σ;

p: $\{1, \ldots, n\} \to \{1, \ldots, n\}$ is a permutation over $\{1, \ldots, n\}$;

$y_1, \ldots, y_{n-1}$ is a 1D string over A.

$z_1, \ldots, z_{n-1}$ is a 1D string over A;

We can use 2D strings to represent pictures in a natural way. As an example, consider the picture shown in Fig. 21.2.

The vocabulary is $\Sigma = \{a, b, c, d\}$. The 2D string representing the above picture f is,

$(a = d < a = b < c , a = a < b = c < d)$

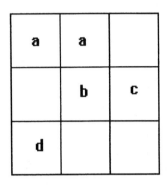

FIGURE 21.2. A picture f.

$$= (x_1\ y_1\ x_2\ y_2\ x_3\ y_3\ x_4\ y_4\ x_5,\ x_{p(1)}\ z_1\ x_{p(2)}\ z_2\ x_{p(3)}\ z_3\ x_{p(4)}\ z_4\ x_{p(5)})$$

where

$x_1\ x_2\ x_3\ x_4\ x_5$ is $adabc$;

$p(1)=1,\ p(2)=3,\ p(3)=4,\ p(4)=5,\ p(5)=2$;

$x_{p(1)}\ x_{p(2)}\ x_{p(3)}\ x_{p(4)}\ x_{p(5)}$ is $aabcd$;

$y_1\ y_2\ y_3\ y_4$ is $=\ <\ =\ <$;

$z_1\ z_2\ z_3\ z_4$ is $=\ <\ =\ <$.

In the above, the symbol '$<$' denotes the left-right spatial relation in string u, and the below-above spatial relation in string v. The symbol '$=$' denotes the spatial relation "approximately at the same spatial location as." The symbol '$:$' denotes the relation "in the same set as." Therefore, the 2D string representation can be seen to be the *symbolic projection* of picture f along the x- and y- directions.

In the 2D string representation, the operators '$=$' can be omitted. Therefore in the above example, the 2D string can be rewritten as ($ad < ab < c$, $aa < bc < d$).

If we are only interested in the *relative spatial relationships* between objects, we can rewrite '$<<$' to '$<$' to obtain the *reduced 2D string*. For example, the reduced 2D string of ($a << b,ab$) is ($a < b,ab$). Other types of 2D strings can be found in [2].

A *symbolic picture f* is a mapping M x $M \to W$, where $M = \{1, 2, \ldots, m\}$, and W is the power set of Σ (the set of all subsets of V). The empty set ϕ then denotes a null object. In Fig. 21.2, the "blank slots" can be filled by empty set symbols, or null objects. The above picture is,

$f(1,1) = \{a\}\ f(1,2) = \phi\ f(1,3) = \{d\}$;

$f(2,1) = \{a\}\ f(2,2) = \{b\}\ f(2,3) = \phi$;

$f(3,1) = \phi\ f(3,2) = \{c\}\ f(3,3) = \phi$.

It is easy to see that from f, we can construct the 2D string (u,v). The above example already illustrates the algorithm. Conversely, from the 2D string (u,v), we can reconstruct f. As an example, suppose the 2D string is $(x_1\ x_2 < x_3{:}x_4 < x_5,\ x_2\ x_3{:}x_4 < x_1\ x_5)$, where the notation $x_3{:}x_4$ indicates x_3 and x_4 are in the same set. We first construct the picture shown in Fig. 21.3, based upon 1D string u, by placing objects having the same spatial location (i.e., objects related by the '=' operator) in the same "slot."

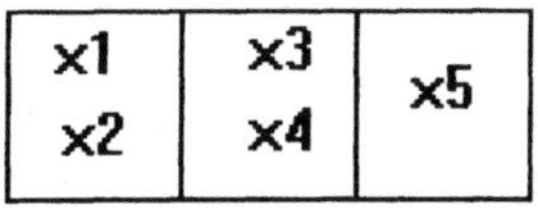

FIGURE 21.3. Reconstruction based upon 1D string u.

Next, we utilize 1D string v to construct the final picture, as shown in Fig. 21.4.

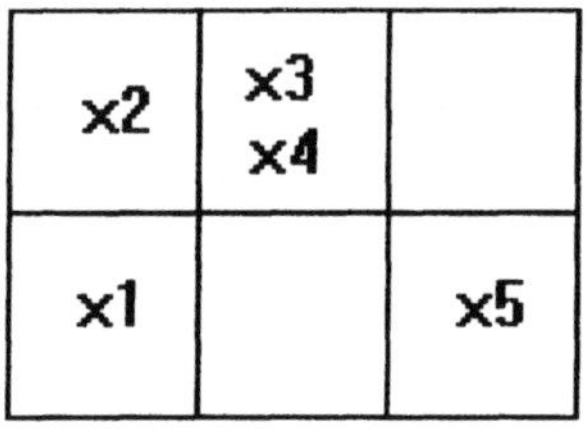

FIGURE 21.4. Reconstruction based upon 1D string v.

If all the symbols in a 2D string are distinct, the reconstructed picture is unique. If, however, there are identical symbols in the 2D string, then in general there may be several different reconstructed pictures. For example, the 2D string $(a < a, a < a)$ may represent a picture with a in both the upper-left and lower-right slots, or a picture with a in both the upper-right and lower-left slots. How to characterize such ambiguous pictures for different types of 2D strings is discussed in [2].

21.3   Picture matching

The 2D string representation provides a simple approach to perform sub-picture matching on 2D strings. The *rank* of each symbol in a string u, which is defined to be one plus the number of '<' preceding this symbol in u, plays an important role in 2D string matching. We denote the rank of symbol b by $r(b)$. For example, symbols in the string "$ad < b < c$" have ranks 1, 1, 2, 3, respectively, and symbols in the string "$a < c$" have ranks 1, 2, respectively.

A substring where all symbols have the same rank is called a *local substring*.

A string α is *s-contained* in a string β, if α is a subsequence of a permutation string of β.

A string α is a *type-k 1D subsequence* of string β, if (a) α is s-contained in β, and (b) if $a_1 w_1 b_1$ is a substring of α, a_1 matches a_2 in v and b_1 matches b_2 in β, then

(type-0) $r(b_2)-r(a_2) \geq r(b_1)-r(a_1)$ or $r(b_1)-r(a_1)=0$;
(type-1) $r(b_2)-r(a_2) \geq r(b_1)-r(a_1)>0$ or $r(b_2)-r(a_2)=r(b_1)-r(a_1)=0$;
(type-2) $r(b_2)-r(a_2)=r(b_1)-r(a_1)$.

Now we can define the notion of type-k (k=0, 1, 2) 2D subsequence as follows. Let (u,v) and (u',v') be the 2D string representation of f and f', respectively. (u',v') is a *type-k 2D subsequence* of (u,v) if (a) u' is type-k 1D subsequence of u, and (b) v' is type-k 1D subsequence of v. If the above is true, we say f' is a *type-k sub-picture* of f.

In Fig. 21.5, $f1$, $f2$ and $f3$ are all type-0 sub-pictures of f; $f1$ and $f2$ are type-1 sub-pictures of f; only $f1$ is type-2 sub-picture of f. The 2D string representations are:

f $(ad < b < c, a < bc < d)$;
$f1$ $(a < b, a < b)$;
$f2$ $(a < c, a < c)$;
$f3$ $(ab < c, a < bc)$.

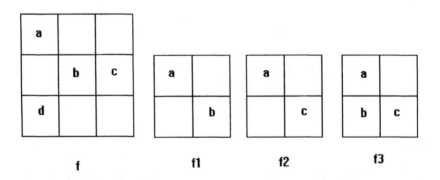

FIGURE 21.5. Picture matching examples, where $f1$ is a type-2 subpicture of f, $f2$ is a type-1 subpicture of f, and $f3$ is a type-0 subpicture of f.

Therefore, to determine whether a picture f' is a type-k sub-picture of f, we need only determine whether (u',v') is a type-k 2D subsequence of (u,v). The picture matching problem thus becomes a 2D string matching problem.

In type-1 subsequence matching, each local substring in u should be matched against a local substring in v. For example, in Fig. 21.5 substring "a" in $a < c$ of $f2$ is a subsequence of "ad" in $ad < b < c$ of f, and substring "c" in $a < c$ is a subsequence of "c" in $ad < b < c$. Notice the skipping of a rank is allowed in type-1 subsequence matching. Therefore, the type-1 subsequence matching problem can be considered as a two-level subsequence matching problem, with level-1 subsequence matching for the local substrings, and level-2 subsequence matching for the "super-string" where each local substring is considered as a super-symbol, and super-symbol u_1 matches super-symbol v_1 if u_1 is a subsequence of v_1.

Type-2 subsequence matching is actually simpler, because the rank cannot be skipped. That is to say, if local substring u_1 of u matches local substring v_1 of v, then substring u_i of u must match substring v_i of v for any i greater than 1. In the example shown in Fig. 21.5, $v =$ "$a < c$" of $f2$ is not a type-2 subsequence of "$ad < b < c$" of f.

21.4   Computer-aided design database

The 2D string representation is an efficient way to represent symbolic pictures, allowing an effective means for queries on image databases, spatial reasoning, visualization and browsing. At the same time, we note that the performance of the 2D string iconic indexing depends on the abstraction from segmented images to symbolic pictures [6]. Many researchers have been looking for good abstraction techniques from iconic images to symbolic representation [7–11]. The iconic indexing approach should be combined with pattern recognition so that iconic indices can be automatically created.

In the following we describe some typical applications of the Theory of Symbolic Projection to image information retrieval. These are based upon papers by researchers from many different countries and are indicative of the diversity of potential applications.

A CAD database for ships supports queries to retrieve ships with "2 cranes on the hull with a superstructure behind them and a mast, radar and funnel on the superstructure." To process such queries Hildebrandt and Tang applied the symbolic projection technique in 3D to symbolic voxel models [12].

CAD data is usually stored in one of two forms: the boundary representation or the constructive solid geometry form. In the boundary representation an object is segmented into non-overlapping faces. Each face is modeled by bounding edges and edges by end vertices. So the object is modeled by a tree of depth three. In constructive solid geometry there are primitives such as cylinders, boxes, and cones combined and modified by operations such as union, intersection, difference, rotation, and scale. The database catalog of the CAD database is assumed to contain a simple voxel model generated from the CAD data for queries.

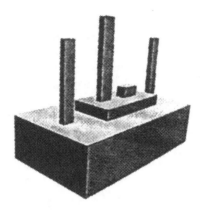

FIGURE 21.6. Voxel ship model.

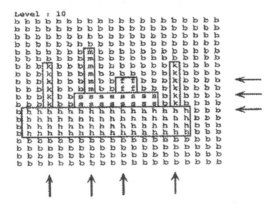

FIGURE 21.7. Slice of voxel model: h=hull, s=superstructure, k=kingpost, m=mast, and f=funnel. The arrows indicate a single type-1 match returned for the query pattern of Fig. 21.8.

GIS databases typically store a collection of co-registered two dimensional images of certain properties such as brightness, spot height and slope, together with vector data such as roads, rivers, and contours. Layers of raster data can be interpreted directly as images and grouped together to give voxel data. Vector data would have to be first converted into low resolution raster data and then used as image or voxel data. The simplified 2D representation could then be used on each band in the GIS to index spatial information, and it may be possible to use the three dimensional form to index spatial relations between all bands.

The simple voxel model encodes a three-dimensional object into slices. An example is illustrated in Fig. 21.6, which shows a 20 by 20 by 20 voxel model. Such models could be used to index a collection of CAD models and would allow 3D spatial queries. A slice through this model is shown in Fig. 21.7, where the letters 'h', 's', 'k', 'm', and 'f' denote "hull," "super-structure," "kingpost," "mast," and "funnel," respectively.

```
pattern:
Level : 0        Level : 1
k m f k          k m f k
k s s k          k s s k
h h h h          h h h h
```

FIGURE 21.8. A query pattern.

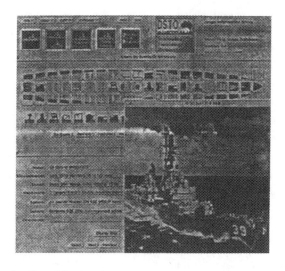

FIGURE 21.9. Graphical user interface combining textual and symbolic query with image retrieval.

In Fig. 21.8, a 3 by 4 by 2 pattern for a type-1 query is shown. A single type-1 match returned is indicated by the arrows in Fig. 21.7. This search pattern would be used with query "Find ship with 2 kingposts above hull with superstructure in between them and mast followed by funnel above superstructure."

A graphical user interface was constructed for a prototype ship database application (Fig. 21.9). For textual information associated with a ship, typical database forms were employed. To enter and display the spatial relations in the database, a graphical interface was employed where icons representing objects could be placed on the grided outline of a hull, viewed from above (top of Fig. 21.9). From this input, the required spatial relations could be determined and placed in a relational table to perform the database query. In addition to type-k queries, the system also supports pairwise relations matching so that similar patterns can be found more efficiently.

21.5   Geographical information systems

The application of Theory of Symbolic Projection to Geographical Information Systems was studied by Yuguo Sun [13].

Sun generalized the 2D G-string [5] to the 2D T-string. The 2D T-string is able to represent three different types of qualitative spatial relations, i.e., topological relations, ordering relations, and auxiliary relations. The topological relations describe local spatial relations, such as equal, disjoint, meet, edge, contain, and partial overlap. The ordering relations are the two basic global spatial relations < and | (edge-to-edge concatenation). The auxiliary relations include surround, partially surround, and quasi-partially surround. The cutting mechanism basically follows the cutting mechanism for the G-string, but refined by additional rules so that only the necessary cutting lines important to one of the above types of relations will be drawn. Techniques for constructing the 2D T-string from the symbolic picture, and for spatial reasonings, have been developed. Since they are similar to the techniques described in [14], the details will not be presented here.

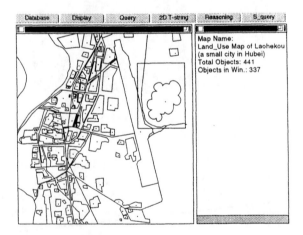

FIGURE 21.10. Land use map.

An experimental Spatial Relations Retrieval System based upon the 2D T-String was implemented for geographical information retrieval. The sys-

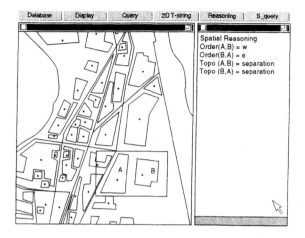

FIGURE 21.11. Example of spatial reasoning.

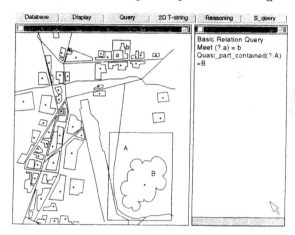

FIGURE 21.12. Basic spatial relation query.

tem supports spatial reasoning, basic spatial relation query, complex spatial relation query and similarity query. The geographical data are shown in the land use map of the Laohekou City in Hubei Province of China; see Fig. 21.10. The map contains 441 objects, and 337 of them are displayed in the window area. Fig. 21.11 is an example of spatial reasoning. The user selects a rectangular area of interest. The ordering relations ("A is to the west of B," and "B is to the east of A") and topological relations ("A and B are separated spatially") can be derived from the 2D T-string and displayed in the window area on the right.

Figure 21.12 illustrates basic spatial relation query. The system can find out that object B meets object A, and object B is quasi-part-contained in A.

Figure 21.13 illustrated complex spatial relation query. The system can

466   Shi-Kuo Chang

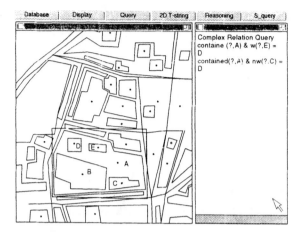

FIGURE 21.13. Complex spatial relation query.

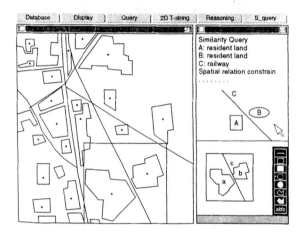

FIGURE 21.14. Similarity query.

find out that object D is contained in A and to the west of E, and object D is contained in A and to the northwest of C.

Figure 21.14 illustrates similarity query. The query is shown in the upper right window, where A and B are resident land, and C is the railway, and their approximate spatial relations are as shown. The result is displayed in the lower right window.

For similarity retrieval, time-consuming graph matching is required. However, in practical applications, the targets are restricted to a prespecified small window area, and the constraints include not only spatial constraints, but also constraints on the objects' attribute values such as shape, color, etc. Therefore, similarity retrieval can be computed in a reasonable time.

21.6   Retrieval of similar Chinese characters

Although many methods have been proposed to solve the problem of Chinese character retrieval, the problem of retrieval spatially similar Chinese characters still remains. There are several motivations to consider the retrieval of similar Chinese characters. First, it can be useful in learning Chinese characters. The structurally similar Chinese characters can be retrieved and presented to the student, so that the student can remember the components of the characters and their meanings. Second, similarity retrieval is also useful for Chinese character recognition because it is capable of clustering similar characters.

Chang and Lin applied the Symbolic Projection Theory to Chinese character retrieval [15], by regarding the Chinese character as a symbolic picture. As illustrated in Fig. 21.15(a), the original image corresponds to a Chinese character. Pattern recognition algorithm can be applied to segment the image into four major components A, B, C, and D, as illustrated in Fig. 21.15(b).

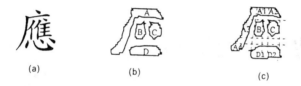

(a)   (b)   (c)

FIGURE 21.15. The original Chinese character (a), the symbolic picture (b), and the segmented symbolic picture (c).

The technique of orthogonal relations [16] can then be applied to discover the important orthogonal relations and convert the symbolic picture into the 2D string. As illustrated in Fig. 21.15(c), the following orthogonal relations are discovered:

$Ortho - relation(B,A) = \{A1, A3\}$
$Ortho - relation(C,A) = \{A2, A3\}$
$Ortho - relation(B,D) = \{D1\}$
$Ortho - relation(C,D) = \{D2\}$

Therefore, A is segmented into four pieces, and D is segmented into two pieces. The 2D string is (A4 < A3 < A1 B D1 < A2 C D2, A4 D1 D2 < A3 B C < A1 A2). Given a Chinese character, it can be transformed into the 2D string and then matched against the 2D strings of other Chinese characters. By using type-0, type-1 or type-2 matching and a cost algorithm, Chang and Lin can find weakly similar, partially similar or strongly similar Chinese characters.

In a related application, 2D strings have been applied to the retrieval and recognition of handwritten signatures [17].

21.7   Three-dimensional image database querying

An extension of 2D strings to deal with three dimensional imaged scenes was proposed in [18]. The approach relies on the consideration that two-dimensional iconic queries and 2D string-based representations are effective for the retrieval of images representing 2D objects or very thin 3D objects, but they might not allow an exact definition of spatial relationships for images representing scenes with 3D objects. In fact in this case, an incorrect representation of the spatial relationships between objects may result due to two distinct causes. First, 2D icons cannot reproduce scene depth. The 2D icon overlapping can be used only to a limited extent since it impacts on the understandability of the query. Second, as demonstrated by research in experimental and cognitive psychology, the mental processes of human beings simulate the physical world processes. Computer-generated line drawings representing 3D objects are regarded by human beings as 3D structures and not as image features, and they imagine spatial transformations directly in 3D space.

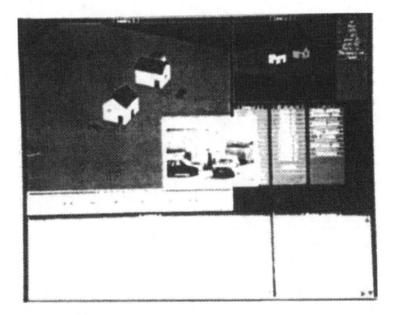

FIGURE 21.16. Querying a three-dimensional scene using pairwise 3D relations.

Therefore, an unambiguous correspondence is established between the iconic query and image contents, if the spatial relationships referred to are those between the objects in the scene represented in the image, rather than those between the objects in the image. The dimensionality of data structures associated with icons must follow the dimensionality of the objects in the scene represented in the image. A 3D structure should be employed for each icon to describe a 3D scene. An example is illustrated in Fig. 21.16.

Representations of images are derived considering 3D symbolic projections of objects in the 3D imaged scene. Thirteen distinct operators, corresponding to the interval logic operators, distinguish all the possible relationships between the intervals corresponding to the object projects on each axis.

Retrieval systems employing this ternary representation of symbolic projections have been expounded in [18] and [19]. In these approaches, the user reproduces a three-dimensional scene by placing 3D icons in a virtual space and sets the position of the camera in order to reproduce both the scene and the vantage point from which the camera was taken. A spatial parser translates the visual specification into the representation language and retrieval again is reduced to a matching between symbolic strings.

21.8   Medical image database system

The 2D string has been used in recognizing fungi in medical research [20]. This section describes the incorporation of 2D strings in a medical image database system.

Radiological examinations are extremely important in health care. X-ray film is the medium conventionally used for medical image archival purposes. A PACS (Picture Archiving and Communication System) is a computer system that supports digital image handling in a hospital environment. Facilities typically provided by a PACS include image entry, archiving, communication, presentation, etc. A PACS is connected by high-speed network with the HIS (Hospital Information System), in order to handle textual patient data together with images.

Such new environment opens a whole new world of possibilities for the utilization of medical images in the clinical environment, including computer assisted diagnosis, radiotherapy planning, surgery planning, medical training, etc. Medical image indexing and retrieval by content, in particular, play a special role in this net setting.

I^2C is an image database system that has been developed as a platform for the design, implementation, and evaluation of medical image indexing and retrieval by content schemes [21]. This system allows the user to define regions of interest (ROI) on the query image, and adjust the relative importance of different regions as well as their characteristics. The user can draw a sketch and adjust the search parameters, to direct the image retrieval process. The main concept in the design of I^2C are image classes and image description types. An image class encapsulates algorithms for the organization, processing and indexing of the images in it. When a request for retrieval is placed with I^2C, it is directed to the appropriate class. The concept of the image description type encapsulates all the details of an indexing and retrieval by content scheme, including the use of 2D strings.

References

[1] S. K. Chang, "The reconstruction of binary patterns from their projections," *Communications of the ACM* **14**, 21-25 (1971).

[2] S. K. Chang, Q. Y. Shi, and C. W. Yan, "Iconic indexing by 2D strings," *IEEE Transactions on Pattern Analysis and Machine Intelligence* **PAMI-9**, 413-428 (1987).

[3] S. K. Chang, E. Jungert, and Y. Li, "Representation and retrieval of symbolic pictures using generalized 2D strings," In *Proc. of SPIE Visual Communications and Image Processing Conference*, pp. 1360-1372, 1989.

[4] E. Jungert, "Extended symbolic projections as a knowledge structure for spatial reasoning and planning," In J. Kittler, *Pattern Recognition* (Springer-Verlag, Berlin), pp. 343-351, 1988.

[5] S. K. Chang and E. Jungert, *Symbolic projection for image information retrieval and spatial reasoning* (Academic Press, London), 1996.

[6] S. K. Chang, C. W. Yan, T. Arndt, and D. Dimitroff, "An intelligent image database system," *IEEE Trans. on Software Engineering* **SE-14** 681-688 (1988).

[7] S. K. Chang and S. H. Liu, "Indexing and abstraction techniques for pictorial databases," *IEEE Transactions on Pattern Analysis and Machine Intelligence* **PAMI-6**, 475-484 (1984).

[8] S. L. Tanimoto, "An iconic/symbolic data structuring scheme," *Pattern recognition and artificial intelligence* (Academic Press, New York), pp. 452-471, 1976.

[9] L. G. Shapiro and R. M. Haralick, "A spatial data structure", *Technical Report CS 79005-R, Dept. Comput. Sci., Virginia Polytech. Inst. and State University*, 1979.

[10] M. Sties, B. Sanyal, and K. Leist, "Organization of object data for an image information system," In *Proceedings 3rd Int. Joint Conference on Pattern Recognition*, pp. 863-869, 1976.

[11] A. Klinger, M. L. Rhode and V. T. To, "Accessing image data," *Int. J. Policy Analysis Information Syst.* **1**, 171-189 (1978).

[12] J. W. Hildebrandt and K. Tang, "Symbolic two and three dimensional picture retrieval," In *Workshop on Two and Three Dimensional Spatial Data: Representation and Standards* (Australian Pattern Recognition Society, Perth, WA), 1992.

[13] Y. G. Sun, "Description of Topological Spatial Relations and Representation of Spatial Relations using 2D T-String," *Ph.D. Thesis, Wuhan Surveying Technology University, Wuhan, China*, 1993.

[14] S. Y. Lee and F. J. Hsu, "Spatial reasoning and similarity retrieval of images using 2D C-string knowledge representation," *Pattern Recognition* **25**, 305-318 (1992).

[15] C. C. Chang and D. C. Lin, "Utilizing the concept of longest common subsequence to retrieve similar chinese characters," *Computer Processing of Chinese and Oriental Languages* **8**, pp. 177-191 (1994).

[16] S. K. Chang and E. Jungert, "A Spatial Knowledge Structure for Visual Information Systems," In T. Ichiakawa, R. Korfhage and E. Jungert, *Visual Languages and Applications* (Plenum Publishing Co, New York), pp. 277-304, 1990.

[17] I. K. Sethi and K. Han, "Use of local structural association for retrieval and recognition of signature images," In W. Niblack and R. C. Jain, *SPIE Proceedings of Storage and Retrieval for Image and Video Databases III* (SPIE, Bellingham, WA) **2420**, pp. 125-134, 1995.

[18] A. Del Bimbo, M. Campanai, and P. Nesi, "A three-dimensional iconic environment for image database querying," *IEEE Transactions on Software Engineering* **SE-19**, 997-1011 (1993).

[19] A. Del Bimbo, E. Vicario, and D. Zingoni, "A spatial logic for symbolic description of image contents," *Journal of Visual Languages and Computing* **3**, pp. 267-286 (1994).

[20] M. L. Dorf, A. F. Mahler, and P. F. Lehmann, "Incorporating semantics into 2D strings," In D. Cizmar, *Proceedings of 22nd Annual ACM Computer Science Conference* (ACM, New York), pp. 110-115, 1994.

[21] S. Kostomanolakis, M. Lourakis, C. Chronaki, Y. Kavaklis, and S. C. Orphanoudakis, "Indexing and retrieval by pictorial content in the i^2C image database system," *Technical report, Institute of Computer Science, Foundation for Research and Technology-HELLAS, Heraklion, Crete, Greece*, 1993.

Index